Guide to Physical Therapist Practice

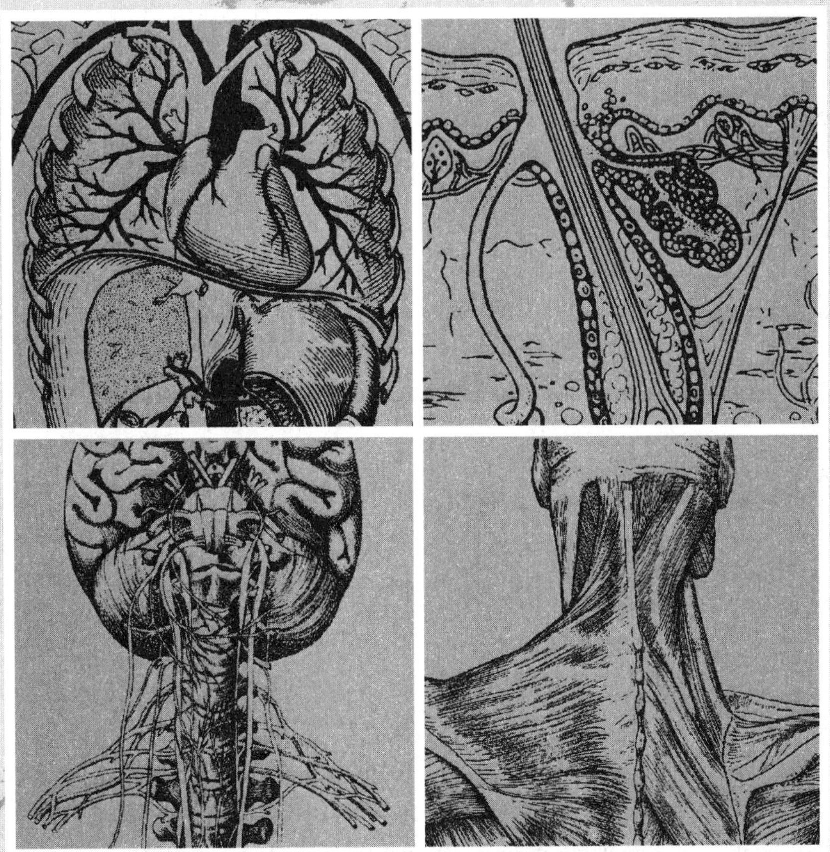

Second Edition

Revised June 2003
Originally published as: Guide to Physical Therapist Practice. 2nd ed. *Phys Ther*. 2001;81:9-744.

American Physical Therapy Association
Alexandria, Virginia

Guide to Physical Therapist Practice

Project Editors, *Guide to Physical Therapist Practice, Second Edition* and Interactive Guide CD-ROM (1999-2002)

Joanell Bohmert, PT, MS
Marilyn Moffat, PT, PhD, FAPTA
Cynthia Zadai, PT, MS, CCS, FAPTA

Task Force on Development of Catalog of Tests and Measures, Interactive Guide CD-ROM (1998-2001)

Laurence Benz, PT, MPT, ECS, OCS
Katherine Biggs, PT
Joanell Bohmert, PT, MS
David Boyce, PT, MS, ECS, OCS
Lori Thein Brody, PT, MS, SCS
Michael Fillyaw, PT, MS
Lisa Giallonardo, PT, PhD, OCS
Sandra Kaplan, PT, PhD
Kathleen Kline Mangione, PT, PhD, GCS
Marilyn Moffat, PT, PhD, FAPTA
Lisa Saladin, PT, BMR, MSc
Steven Tepper, PT, PhD
R Scott Ward, PT, PhD
Cynthia Zadai, PT, MS, CCS, FAPTA

Editorial Review Group, Catalog of Tests and Measures, Interactive Guide CD-ROM (2001)

Ross Anthony Arena, PT
Charles Ciccone, PT, PhD
Rebecca Craik, PT, PhD, FAPTA
Anthony Delitto, PT, PhD, FAPTA
Senobia Crawford, PT, PhD
Michael Fillyaw, PT, MS
G Kelley Fitzgerald, PT, PhD
Arlene Greenspan, PT, PhD
Jan Gwyer, PT, PhD
Karen Hayes, PT, PhD
Chris Hughes, PT, PhD
Jay Irrgang, PT, PhD
Diane Jette, PT, DSc
Gregory Karst, PT, PhD
Kathleen Kline Mangione, PT, PhD, GCS
Philip McClure, PT, PhD
Irene McEwen, PT, PhD
Michael Mueller, PT, PhD
Claire Peel, PT, PhD
Stella Prevost, PT, MS, CCS
Daniel Riddle, PT, PhD

APTA Staff

Practice and Research Division
Andrew Guccione, PT, PhD, FAPTA, Senior Vice President; Sarah Miller, Assistant to the Senior Vice President
Department of Practice: Donna Bernhardt Bainbridge, PT, PhD, ATC, Director; Lisa Culver, PT, MBA, and Nancy Goode, PT, MA, Associate Directors; Bobbie Jo Ellis and Michele Katsouros, Senior Administrative Assistants
Information Services Department: Tracy Temanson, Director; Nicole Orton, Senior Administrative Assistant
Research Services Department: Marc Goldstein, EdD, Director; Andrea Mink, Senior Administrative Assistant

Communications Division
Nancy Perkin Beaumont, CAE, Senior Vice President
Publications Department: Lois Douthitt, Director; Jan Reynolds, Associate Director; Evynn Blaher, Assistant Managing Editor

---

Second edition © 2001, 2003 by the American Physical Therapy Association (APTA). Second edition was published in the January 2001 issue of *Physical Therapy* [Guide to Physical Therapist Practice. 2nd ed. *Phys Ther.* 2001;81:9–744] and was revised June 2003.
ISBN 1-887759-85-9

Preferred Physical Therapist Practice Patterns℠ is a service mark of the American Physical Therapy Association (APTA).

Interactive Guide to Physical Therapist Practice With Catalog of Tests and Measures, Version 1.1 © 2002, 2003 by the American Physical Therapy Association (APTA). Available on CD-ROM only. ISBN 1-887759-87-5

First edition © 1997, 1999 by the American Physical Therapy Association (APTA). First edition was published in the November 1997 issue of *Physical Therapy* [Guide to Physical Therapist Practice. *Phys Ther.* 1997;77:1163-1650] and was revised April and July 1999.

Art adapted with permission from: *Dorland's Illustrated Medical Dictionary*. 28th ed. Philadelphia, Pa: WB Saunders Co; 1994:131, Plate 2; 1535, Figure. Williams PL, Warwick R, eds. *Gray's Anatomy*. 37th ed. New York, NY: Churchill Livingstone Inc; 1989: 868, Figure 7-12. Clemente CD, ed. *Gray's Anatomy*. 30th ed. Philadelphia, Pa: Lea & Febiger; 1985:514, Figure 6-42.

Guide to Physical Therapist Practice, First Edition

APTA Board of Directors Oversight Committee (1995-1997)

Marilyn Moffat, PT, PhD, FAPTA, APTA President (1991-1997)
Andrew Guccione, PT, PhD, FAPTA
Jayne Snyder, PT, MA

Project Advisory Group (1995-1997)

Joanell Bohmert, PT, MS
Jan Gwyer, PT, PhD
Laurita Hack, PT, PhD
Roger Nelson, PT, PhD, FAPTA
Jules Rothstein, PT, PhD, FAPTA (1995-1996)
Cynthia Zadai, PT, MS, CCS, FAPTA

Panels (1995-1997)

Musculoskeletal
Lisa Giallonardo, PT, MS, OCS, Chair
Lori Thein Brody, PT, MS, SCS
John Gose, PT, MS, OCS
Terry Holley, PT, MHS, GCS
Lindsay McNulty, PT, MPH, GCS
Erin Patterson, PT, MS, OCS
Julie Pauls, PT, MS, ICCE

Neuromuscular
Donna Cech, PT, MS, PCS, Chair
Richard Bohannon, PT, EdD, NCS
Nancy Byl, PT, PhD, MPH
Kathleen Fincher, PT, MS, PCS
Diane Nicholson, PT, PhD, NCS
Kirsten Potter, PT, MS, NCS
Gerry Stone, PT, MEd, GCS

Cardiopulmonary
Ellen Hillegass, PT, EdD, CCS, Chair
Gary Brooks, PT, MS, CCS
Lawrence Cahalin, PT, MA, CCS
Dianne Carrio, PT, MEd, GCS
Nancy Ciesla, PT

Integumentary
Debra Metzger-Donovan, PT, MS, Chair
Katherine Biggs, PT
Carrie Sussman, PT
Pamela Unger, PT
R Scott Ward, PT, PhD

Task Force to Review Practice Parameters and Taxonomy Documents (1994-1995)

Marilyn Moffat, PT, PhD, FAPTA
Andrew Guccione, PT, PhD, FAPTA
Roger Nelson, PT, PhD, FAPTA
Jayne Snyder, PT, MA

Practice Parameters Project Core Group (1993-1994)

Roger Nelson, PT, PhD, FAPTA, Chair and Board Liaison
John Barbis, PT, MA, OCS
Eileen Hamby, PT, DBA
Catherine Page, PT, PhD (1993)
Robert Post, PT, PhD
Gretchen Swanson, PT, MPH
Marilyn Moffat, PT, PhD, FAPTA *(ex officio)*

APTA Staff

Volume I: A Description of Patient Management

Department of Practice
Robert Mansell, PT, MS (1991-1996), Director

Part Two: Preferred Practice Patterns

Health Policy Division
Jerome Connolly, PT, Senior Vice President
Department of Practice: Jack Front, PT, MBA, Director;
Lisa Culver, PT, MBA, Maureen Lynch, PT, MA,
Allen Wicken, PT, MS, Associate Directors; Debbie Greene,
Senior Administrative Assistant

The Guide also is available as an interactive CD-ROM. *Interactive Guide to Physical Therapist Practice With Catalog of Tests and Measures* contains the *Guide to Physical Therapist Practice, Second Edition*; lists of approximately 500 specific tests, with annotations on reliability and validity of measurements; and more than 1,500 references for articles on reliability and validity, hyperlinked to article abstracts on PubMed, the online version of MEDLINE. All text is searchable using keywords, multiple terms, and ICD-9-CM codes. For more information, visit APTA's Web site, www.apta.org.

Preface to the First Edition November 1997

All health care professions are accountable to the various publics that they serve. The American Physical Therapy Association (APTA) has developed *Guide to Physical Therapist Practice* ("the Guide") to help physical therapists analyze their patient/client management and describe the scope of their practice. The Guide is necessary not only to daily practice but to preparation of students. It was used as a primary resource by the Commission on Accreditation in Physical Therapy Education (CAPTE) during its revision of evaluative criteria for physical therapist professional education programs and is an essential companion document to *The Normative Model of Physical Therapist Professional Education, Version 97*.

Specifically, the Guide is designed to help physical therapists (1) enhance quality of care, (2) improve patient/client satisfaction, (3) promote appropriate utilization of health care services, (4) increase efficiency and reduce unwarranted variation in the provision of services, and (5) promote cost reduction through prevention and wellness initiatives. The Guide also provides a framework for physical therapist clinicians and researchers as they refine outcomes data collection and analysis and develop questions for clinical research.

Groups other than physical therapists are important users of the Guide. Health care policymakers and administrators can use the Guide in making informed decisions about health care service delivery. Third-party payers and managed care providers can use the Guide in making informed decisions about reasonableness of care and appropriate reimbursement. Health care and other professionals can use the Guide to coordinate care with physical therapist colleagues more efficiently.

As the Guide is disseminated throughout the profession and to other groups, the process of revision and refinement will begin. We thank our colleagues who helped us make the Guide a reality.

Marilyn Moffat, PT, PhD, FAPTA
(APTA President, 1991-1997)
Andrew Guccione, PT, PhD
Jayne Snyder, PT, MA
APTA Board Oversight Committee

Foreword to the Second Edition
January 2001

The *Guide to Physical Therapist Practice* ("the Guide"), Parts One and Two, has represented a living document, with a life that has already spanned more than 8 years. The first edition of the Guide was the result of the expertise contributed by almost 1,000 physical therapist members of the American Physical Therapy Association. Each individual shared not only his or her knowledge and skills, but also time, energy, and commitment to a document that has dramatically affected the practice environment. The Guide has been used in ways and by people we never had imagined—becoming an invaluable resource to clinicians, educators, administrators, legislators, and payers throughout the health care community.

This second edition is a testament to its evolutionary nature. In reviewing the pages of this edition, you will know that its strengths have been shaped by its users—all of whose comments and questions received serious consideration. Hundreds of members have worked to respond to those suggestions and to the demands of a changing practice environment, thereby ensuring that the Guide encompasses the full scope of current physical therapist practice. To all of them, I extend the deep appreciation of our profession and its Association.

The Guide will continue to grow and be revised based on research evidence and on changes in examination and intervention strategies within practice. I invite you to be a part of its life by bringing to the Association your questions, comments, and suggestions. Our united participation in this evolutionary process will keep the Guide at the forefront of the profession.

Ben F Massey, Jr, PT
President
American Physical Therapy Association

Table of Contents

Introduction: Concepts, Development, and Content Overview

Part One: A Description of Patient/Client Management

Chapter 1 Who Are Physical Therapists, and What Do They Do?

Chapter 2 What Types of Tests and Measures Do Physical Therapists Use?

Chapter 3 What Types of Interventions Do Physical Therapists Provide?

Part Two: Preferred Physical Therapist Practice Patterns[SM]

Chapter 4 Musculoskeletal

Chapter 5 Neuromuscular

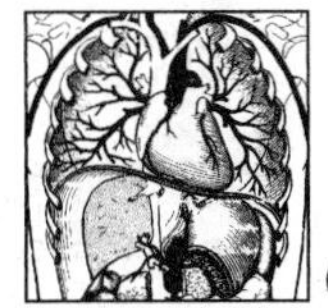

Chapter 6 Cardiovascular/Pulmonary

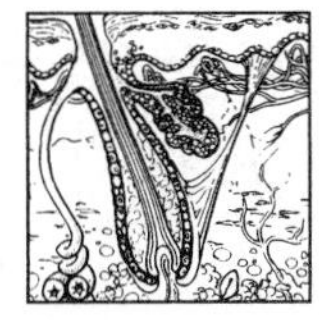

Chapter 7 Integumentary

Appendixes

Indexes

INTRODUCTION:

Concepts, Development, and Content Overview

- What Is Physical Therapy?
- How and Why Was the Guide Developed?
- On What Concepts Is the Guide Based?
- What Does the Guide Contain?

Content in this Introduction corresponds to "About the Guide" and "Understanding Physical Therapist Practice" in the Interactive Guide CD-ROM

What Is Physical Therapy?

Corresponds to "Who Are Physical Therapists" in the Interactive Guide CD-ROM

Physical therapy is a dynamic profession with an established theoretical and scientific base and widespread clinical applications in the restoration, maintenance, and promotion of optimal physical function. For more than 750,000 people every day in the United States, physical therapists:

- Diagnose and manage movement dysfunction and enhance physical and functional abilities.

- Restore, maintain, and promote not only optimal physical function but optimal wellness and fitness and optimal quality of life as it relates to movement and health.

- Prevent the onset, symptoms, and progression of impairments, functional limitations, and disabilities that may result from diseases, disorders, conditions, or injuries.

The terms "physical therapy" and "physiotherapy," and the terms "physical therapist" and "physiotherapist," are synonymous.

As essential participants in the health care delivery system, physical therapists assume leadership roles in rehabilitation; in prevention, health maintenance, and programs that promote health, wellness, and fitness; and in professional and community organizations. Physical therapists also play important roles both in developing standards for physical therapist practice and in developing health care policy to ensure availability, accessibility, and optimal delivery of physical therapy services. Physical therapy is covered by federal, state, and private insurance plans. The positive impact of physical therapists' services on health-related quality of life is well accepted.

As clinicians, physical therapists engage in an examination process that includes taking the patient/client history, conducting a systems review, and performing tests and measures to identify potential and existing problems. To establish diagnoses, prognoses, and plans of care, physical therapists perform evaluations, synthesizing the examination data and determining whether the problems to be addressed are within the scope of physical therapist practice. Based on their judgments about diagnoses and prognoses and based on patient/client goals, physical therapists provide interventions (the interactions and procedures used in managing and instructing patients/clients), conduct reexaminations, modify interventions as necessary to achieve anticipated goals and expected outcomes, and develop and implement discharge plans.

The American Physical Therapy Association (APTA), the national membership organization representing and promoting the profession of physical therapy, believes it is critically important for those outside the profession to understand the role of physical therapists in the health care delivery system and the unique services that physical therapists provide. APTA is committed to informing consumers, other health care professionals, federal and state governments, and third-party payers about the benefits of physical therapy—and, more specifically, about the relationship between health status and the services that are provided by physical therapists. APTA actively supports outcomes research and strongly endorses all efforts to develop appropriate systems to measure the results of patient/client management that is provided by physical therapists.

The patient/client management elements of examination, evaluation, diagnosis, and prognosis should be represented and reimbursed as physical therapy *only when they are performed by a physical therapist*. The patient/client management element of intervention should be represented and reimbursed as physical therapy only when performed by a physical therapist or by a physical therapist assistant performing selected interventions under the direction and supervision of a physical therapist in accordance with APTA positions, policies, standards, codes, and guidelines.

Physical therapists are the only professionals who provide physical therapy interventions. Physical therapist assistants are the only individuals who provide selected physical therapy interventions under the direction and supervision of the physical therapist. APTA recommends that federal and state government agencies and other third-party payers require physical therapy to be provided *only by physical therapists or under the direction and supervision of physical therapists*.

How and Why Was the *Guide* Developed?

Corresponds to "About the Guide" in the Interactive Guide CD-ROM

During the early 1990s, state legislative bodies began to request that health care professionals develop practice parameters. In February 1992, at the request of one of the American Physical Therapy Association's (APTA) state components, APTA's Board of Directors embarked on a process to determine whether practice parameters could be delineated for the profession of physical therapy. The Board initiated development of a document that would describe physical therapist practice—content and processes—both for members of the physical therapy profession and for health care policy makers and third-party payers (see Time Line, next page).

The initial foundation for the document was laid by the Board-appointed Task Force on Practice Parameters, whose work led to the appointment of the Task Force to Review Practice Parameters and Taxonomy. The deliberations of these task forces and the materials that they produced resulted in the Board's development of *A Guide to Physical Therapist Practice, Volume I: A Description of Patient Management* ("Volume I").[1] This document was approved in March 1995 by the Board. In June 1995, APTA's House of Delegates approved the conceptual framework on which Volume I was based and endorsed the Board's plan to develop Volume II using a process of expert consensus. Volume I was published in the August 1995 issue of *Physical Therapy*. Volume II was to be "composed of descriptions of preferred physical therapist practice for patient groupings defined by common physical therapist management." [Report to the 1997 House of Delegates, Processes to Describe Physical Therapy Care for Specific Patient Conditions, RC 32-95]

A Board-appointed Project Advisory Group and a Board Oversight Committee were charged to lead the Volume II project. The members of the Project Advisory Group were chosen on the basis of the following criteria:

- Broad knowledge of physical therapy
- Understanding of clinical policy development
- Familiarity with research in physical therapy
- Recognized decision-making abilities

In June 1995, the Project Advisory Group and the Board Oversight Committee met to refine the project design. That September, the Committee selected 24 physical therapists to serve on one of four panels: cardiopulmonary, integumentary, musculoskeletal, and neuromuscular. Each Project Advisory Group member was assigned as a liaison to one of the panels. Criteria for selection of panel members included the following:

- Experience in the subject area
- Knowledge of physical therapy literature
- Understanding of research and the use of data
- Expertise in documentation
- Experience in peer review
- Knowledge of broad areas of physical therapy
- Recognized ability to work with groups and reach a consensus
- Openness to a variety of treatment philosophies
- Willingness to commit to the entire project

Consideration also was given to creating panels whose collective clinical experience would represent a wide range of patient/client age groups and practice settings.

Between October 1995 and September 1996, the panels developed preferred practice patterns that were subsequently reviewed by more than 200 select reviewers. In addition, each pattern was reviewed by APTA's Risk Management Committee, by physical therapists with reimbursement expertise, by APTA's Reimbursement Department, and by APTA's legal counsel. In December 1996, revised drafts of the patterns were sent for broad-based review to more than 600 reviewers, to APTA chapter and section presidents, to APTA members with risk management and reimbursement expertise, and to other select reviewers. Input from the general membership was obtained during open forums at APTA Annual Conferences and APTA Combined Sections Meetings throughout 1996 and 1997.

In early 1997, Volume I and Volume II became Part One and Part Two of a single document ("the Guide"). Revisions were made to Part One to reflect Part Two. In March 1997, the Board of Directors approved the draft of Part Two; in June 1997, the House of Delegates approved the conceptual framework on which Part Two is based. The first edition of the Guide was published in the November 1997 issue of *Physical Therapy*.[2]

In 1998 and 1999, revisions were made to the Guide based on (1) input from both the general membership and the leadership of APTA and (2) changes in House of Delegates policies. These revisions were published in *Physical Therapy*.[3,4] During this period, the Association began developing forms (Appendix 6) to be used in clinical practice (both inpatient and outpatient settings) for documenting the five elements of patient/client management that are described in the Guide: examination, evaluation, diagnosis, prognosis (including plan of care), and interventions. In addition, a patient/client satisfaction assessment was developed for inclusion in the Guide (Appendix 7).[5]

In 1998, APTA began development of Part Three of the Guide to catalog the armamentarium of tests and measures that are used by physical therapists in the examination of patients/clients and in the documentation of patient/client management outcomes. (This part of the Guide, intended as a reference work, is available on CD-ROM only.) One task force was charged by APTA's Board to examine the available literature pertaining to tests and measures that are used in the assessment of the cardiovascular/pulmonary, integumentary, musculoskeletal, and neuromuscular systems. Another task force was charged to retrieve and review the available literature on tests and measures of health status, health-related quality of life, and patient/client satisfaction.

The two task forces met throughout 1999 and 2000 to search the peer-reviewed literature and develop a comprehensive list of tests and measures that are used in physical therapist practice. Field reviews were conducted, using APTA's Board, all APTA components (sections and state chapters), a sample of clinical specialists certified by the American Board of Physical Therapy Specialties (ABPTS), and APTA's general membership. Presentations of the work-in-progress were made at APTA Annual Conferences and APTA Combined Sections Meetings throughout 1999 and 2000.

To complete their charge to catalog the armamentarium of tests and measures that are used in physical therapist practice, the two task forces refined the template for documenting the history and systems review components of examination and for documenting intervention, based on the essential data elements of patient/client management described in the Guide. The documentation template (Appendix 6) was reviewed by all APTA components (sections and state chapters), a sample of clinical specialists certified by ABPTS, and APTA's general membership.

Throughout 1999 and 2000, Board-appointed Project Editors revised Part One and Part Two of the Guide to reflect input from the general membership, the Task Force on Development of Part Three of the *Guide to Physical*

Time Line for Development of the *Guide to Physical Therapist Practice*

1992	**APTA Board of Directors initiates development of document to describe physical therapist practice, appointing the Task Force on Practice Parameters and, later, the Task Force to Review Practice Parameters and Taxonomy.**
1995	***A Guide to Physical Therapist Practice, Volume I: A Description of Patient Management* is published in *Physical Therapy*. In fall 1995, panels begin developing preferred practice patterns for Volume II.**
1996	**Preferred practice patterns are reviewed by more than 600 field reviewers and are shared in open forums with the general membership at APTA Annual Conferences and Combined Sections Meetings.**
1997	**Volume I and Volume II become Part One and Part Two of the Guide. APTA Board and House of Delegates approve the draft and conceptual framework of Part Two, which is published, with Part One, in *Physical Therapy*.**
1998	**The Guide is released on CD-ROM. APTA develops Guide-based documentation forms for use in clinical practice; work begins on an instrument to measure patient/client satisfaction.**

Therapist Practice (Second Edition), and the leadership of APTA and to refine and clarify terminology and definitions used in the Guide.

In 2001, the Guide Project Editors further refined the catalog of tests and measures, and an Editorial Review Group reviewed the citations of articles on reliability and validity of measurements obtained using the tests and measures. The catalog of tests and measures is available only on the CD-ROM version of the Guide (*Interactive Guide to Physical Therapist Practice With Catalog of Tests and Measures*).

In 2002, APTA launched the "Hooked on Evidence" Web site (www.apta.org/Research), a grass-roots effort to develop a database of current research evidence on physical therapy interventions and foster evidence-based practice. Using Guide terminology and framework, "Hooked on Evidence" eventually will contain a catalog of interventions that is analogous to the Guide's catalog of tests and measures. "Hooked on Evidence" has the following objectives:

- Allow members to search a database of article critiques relevant to the field of physical therapy to build support for evidence-based practice
- Allow members to perform online reviews of the available literature in physical therapy
- Provide article critiques by experts in the field that will assist in rating the quality of a research study
- Serve as a Web portal for learning about evidence-based practice
- List useful web resources and other information consistent with evidence-based practice
- Disseminate position papers on topics of interest

Purposes of the Guide

APTA developed the *Guide to Physical Therapist Practice* as a resource not only for physical therapist clinicians, educators, researchers, and students, but for health care policy makers, administrators, managed care providers, third-party payers, and other professionals.

The Guide serves the following purposes:

1. To describe physical therapist practice in general, using the disablement model as the basis.
2. To describe the roles of physical therapists in primary, secondary, and tertiary care; in prevention; and in the promotion of health, wellness, and fitness.
3. To describe the settings in which physical therapists practice.
4. To standardize terminology used in and related to physical therapist practice.
5. To delineate the tests and measures and the interventions that are used in physical therapist practice.
6. To delineate preferred practice patterns (Preferred Physical Therapist Practice Patterns[SM]) that will help physical therapists (a) improve quality of care, (b) enhance the positive outcomes of physical therapy services, (c) enhance patient/client satisfaction, (d) promote appropriate utilization of health care services, (e) increase efficiency and reduce unwarranted variation in the provision of services, and (f) diminish the economic burden of disablement through prevention and the promotion of health, wellness, and fitness initiatives.

The Guide does not provide specific protocols for treatments, nor are the practice patterns contained in the Guide intended to serve as clinical guidelines. Clinical guidelines usually are based on a comprehensive search and systematic evaluation of peer-reviewed literature. The Institute of Medicine has defined clinical guidelines as "sys-

1999	**Guide revisions based on changes in House of Delegates policy are published. Task forces are formed to develop Part Three to standardize the armamentarium of tests and measures used in physical therapist practice.**
2000	**Part One and Part Two of the Guide are revised by Project Editors in preparation for publication of the Guide's second edition. Part Three undergoes field review. Development of the CD-ROM version of the Guide, to include Part Three, begins.**
2001	**The second edition of the Guide (Part One and Part Two) is published in *Physical Therapy* in January.**
2002	**The CD-ROM, *Interactive Guide to Physical Therapist Practice With Catalog of Tests and Measures,* Version 1.0—which contains Part Three—is released in April 2002.**
2003	**The second edition of *Guide to Physical Therapist Practice* is revised to be consistent with content in Version 1.1 of the *Interactive Guide;* both are released in June.**

tematically developed statements to assist practitioner and patient decisions about appropriate health care for *specific clinical circumstances* [emphasis added]."[6,7] The Guide was developed using expert consensus to identify common features of patient/client management for selected patient/client diagnostic groups. The Guide is a first step toward the development of clinical guidelines in that it provides patient/client diagnostic classifications and identifies the array of current options for care.

The preferred practice patterns identify the breadth of physical therapist practice. They are the boundaries within which the physical therapist may select and implement any of a number of clinical alternatives based on consideration of a wide variety of factors, including individual patient/client needs; the profession's code of ethics and standards of practice; and patient/client age, culture, gender roles, race, sex, sexual orientation, and socioeconomic status. *The Guide is not intended to set forth the standard of care for which a physical therapist may be legally responsible in any specific case.*

Future Development of the Guide

The *Guide to Physical Therapist Practice* is an evolving document that will be systematically revised as the physical therapy profession's knowledge base, scientific literature, and outcomes research develop and as examination and intervention strategies change. The Guide is the structure on which scientific evidence will be fastened, and, in turn, the evidence will reshape the structure.

Notification of revisions will be published annually in *Physical Therapy* and will be posted on APTA's Web site (www.apta.org).

References

1 A Guide to Physical Therapist Practice, Volume I: A Description of Patient Management. *Phys Ther.* 1995;75:707-764.

2 Guide to Physical Therapist Practice. *Phys Ther.* 1997;77:1163-1650.

3 Guide to Physical Therapist Practice. Revisions. *Phys Ther.* 1999;623-629.

4 Guide to Physical Therapist Practice. Revisions. *Phys Ther.* 1999;1078-1081.

5 Goldstein MS, Elliott SD, Guccione AA. The development of an instrument to measure satisfaction with physical therapy. *Phys Ther.* 2000;80:853-863.

6 Field M, Lohr K, eds. *Clinical Practice Guidelines: Directions for a New Program.* Washington, DC: Institute of Medicine, National Academy Press; 1990.

7 Field M, Lohr K, eds. *Guidelines for Clinical Practice: From Development to Use.* Washington, DC: Institute of Medicine, National Academy Press; 1992.

On What Concepts Is the Guide Based?

Corresponds to "Understanding Physical Therapist Practice" in the Interactive Guide CD-ROM

Three key concepts serve as the building blocks of the Guide and as the foundation of physical therapist practice:

- The disablement model typifies physical therapist practice and is the model for understanding and organizing practice.

- Physical therapist practice addresses the needs of both patients and clients through a continuum of service across all delivery settings—in critical and intensive care units, outpatient clinics, long-term care facilities, school systems, and the workplace—by identifying health improvement opportunities, providing interventions for existing and emerging problems, preventing or reducing the risk of additional complications, and promoting wellness and fitness to enhance human performance as it relates to movement and health. *Patients* are recipients of physical therapist examination, evaluation, diagnosis, prognosis, and intervention and have a disease, disorder, condition, impairment, functional limitation, or disability; *clients* engage the services of a physical therapist and can benefit from the physical therapist's consultation, interventions, professional advice, prevention services, or services promoting health, wellness, and fitness.

- Physical therapist practice includes the five essential elements of patient/client management (examination; evaluation; diagnosis; prognosis, including the plan of care; and intervention), which incorporate the principles of the disablement model.

The Disablement Model

The concept of *disablement* refers to the "various impact(s) of chronic and acute conditions on the functioning of specific body systems, on basic human performance, and on people's functioning in necessary, usual, expected, and personally desired roles in society."[1,2] Thus, the disablement model is used to delineate the consequences of disease and injury both at the level of the person and at the level of society. The disablement model provides the conceptual basis for all elements of patient/client management that are provided by physical therapists. The Guide uses an expanded disablement model[3,4] that provides both the theoretical framework for understanding physical therapist practice and the classification scheme by which physical therapists make diagnoses.

A number of disablement models have emerged during the past 3 decades; three models are shown in Figure 1. All of the disablement models attempt to better delineate the interrelationships among disease, impairments, functional limitations, disabilities, handicaps, and the "effects of the interaction of the person with the environment,"[5] though the effects themselves may be defined differently from model to model.

Nagi, a sociologist, was among the first to begin to challenge the appropriateness of the traditional medical classification of disease for understanding the genesis of disability. He put forth a theoretical formulation based on the concepts of disease or active pathology, impairment, functional limitation, and disability.[6-8] Based on Nagi's model, *active pathology* is the interruption of or interference with normal processes and the simultaneous efforts of the organism to restore itself to a normal state by mobilizing the body's defense and coping mechanisms; *impairment* is any loss or abnormality of anatomical, physiological, mental, or psychological structure or function; *functional limitation* is the restriction of the ability to perform a physical action, task, or activity

Figure 1. Three Disablement Models[a]

Nagi Scheme

Active Pathology	Impairment	Functional Limitation	Disability
Interruption or interference with normal processes, and efforts of the organism to regain normal state	Anatomical, physiological, mental, or emotional abnormalities or loss	Limitation in performance at the level of the whole organism or person	Limitation in performance of socially defined roles and tasks within a sociocultural and physical environment

WHO—International Classification of Impairments, Disabilities, and Handicaps (ICIDH)(1980)

Disease	Impairment	Disability	Handicap
The intrinsic pathology or disorder	Loss or abnormality of psychological, physiological, or anatomical structure or function at organ level	Restriction or lack of ability to perform an activity in normal manner	Disadvantage due to impairment or disability that limits or prevents fulfillment of a normal role—depending on age, sex, sociocultural factors—for the person

National Center for Medical Rehabilitation Research Classification (1992)

Pathophysiology	Impairment	Functional Limitation	Disability	Societal Limitation
Interruption with normal physiological developmental processes or structures	Loss or abnormality of cognitive, emotional, physiological, or anatomical structure or function	Restriction or lack of ability to perform an action in the manner or range consistent with the purpose of an organ or organ system	Limitation or inability in performing tasks, activities, and roles to levels expected within physical and social contexts	Restriction attributable to social policy or barriers that limit fulfillment of roles

[a]*Adapted with permission of the American Physical Therapy Association from Jette AM. Physical disablement concepts for physical therapy research and practice.* Phys Ther. *1994;74:381.*

in an efficient, typically expected, or competent manner at the level of the whole organism or person; and *disability* is the inability to perform or a limitation in the performance of actions, tasks, and activities usually expected in specific social roles that are customary for the individual or expected for the person's status or role in a specific sociocultural context and physical environment.

In 1980, the World Health Organization (WHO) developed an alternative disablement model. In WHO's *International Classification of Impairments, Disabilities, and Handicaps (ICIDH),*[9] *disease* was defined as a pathological change that manifests itself as a health condition that is an alteration or attribute of an individual's health status and that may lead to distress, interference with daily activities, or contact with health services. *Impairment* was defined as abnormal changes at the molecular, cellular, and tissue levels through abnormal structure or function at the organ level; *disability*, as the restriction in or lack of ability to perform common activities in a manner or within a range considered normal; and *handicap*, as the inability to function at the person-to-person level or person-to-environment level. Handicap indicated the social disadvantages related to impairment or disability that limit or prevent fulfillment of a normal role. WHO revised its original formulation of the disablement model and in November 2001 released the *ICF: International Classification of Functioning, Disability, and Health.*[10]

In 1992, the National Center for Medical Rehabilitation and Research (NCMRR) published a disablement model that was derived from both the Nagi and WHO models and that used the classifications of pathophysiology, impairment, functional limitation, disability, and societal limitation.[11] The NCMRR model rejected the negative connotation of the term "handicap" and suggested replacing it with the term "societal limitations" to account for the restrictions—imposed by society—that limit people's ability to participate independently in tasks, activities, and roles. In 1991, the Institute of Medicine (IOM) put forth its

Figure 2. Scope of Physical Therapist Practice Within the Continuum of Health Care Services and the Context of the Disablement Model[a]

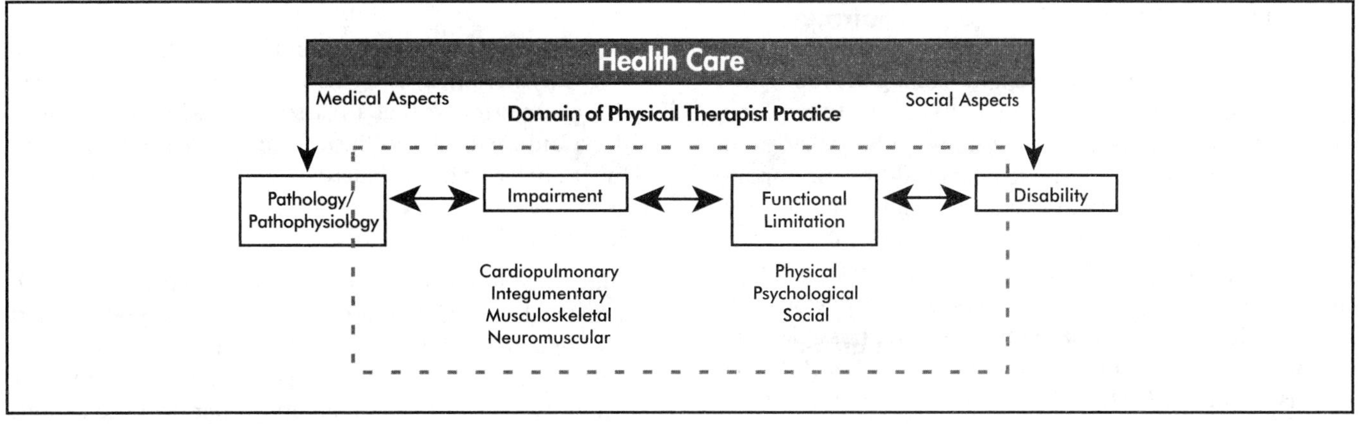

[a]*Adapted with permission of the American Physical Therapy Association from Guccione AA. Physical therapy diagnosis and the relationship between impairments and function.* Phys Ther. *1991;71:499-504.*

own disablement model to emphasize prevention, suggesting that disability may be prevented through the control of physical and social environmental risk factors in addition to biological and lifestyle risk factors.[12]

Although the various disablement models may seem to be quite different, the concepts in each of them can be "cross-walked" to describe an entire spectrum of experience of illness and disablement.

Guide Terminology

The terminology selected for the Guide framework is based on the disablement terms developed initially by Nagi (pathology/pathophysiology, impairment, functional limitation, disability) and incorporates the broadest possible interpretation of those terms. Figure 2 shows the scope of physical therapist practice both within the context of the Nagi model and within the continuum of health care services.[4]

Pathology/Pathophysiology (Disease, Disorder, or Condition)

Pathology/pathophysiology (disease, disorder, or condition) refers to an ongoing pathological/pathophysiological state that is (1) characterized by a particular cluster of signs and symptoms and (2) recognized by either the patient/client or the practitioner as "abnormal." Pathology/pathophysiology (disease, disorder, or condition) is primarily identified at the cellular level and usually is the physician's medical diagnosis. Disease may be the result of infection, trauma, metabolic imbalance, degenerative processes, or other etiologies. Any single disorder may disrupt the anatomical structures and physiological processes of one or more systems. The Guide uses a broad definition of pathology/pathophysiology to include the interruption of normal processes and to include other health threats, injury, and conditions produced by pathological or pathophysiological states.

Many of the signs and symptoms that are important to the physical therapist—and many of the conditions that affect a person's ability to function—are not associated with a single active pathology/pathophysiology, nor are they always found to have an impact exclusively on a single system or the system of origin. For example, a patient may have a medical diagnosis that indicates the presence of fixed lesions from previous insults to a body part or organ, but these lesions may not be associated with any current active pathological/pathophysiologic processes. Signs and symptoms also may exist as long-term adaptations to the original disorder or injury.

Using the disablement model as a theoretical framework to describe physical therapist practice does not negate the importance of the traditional medical diagnosis (eg, pathology/pathophysiology, injury) in patient/client management by physical therapists. In fact, changes at the cellular, tissue, and organ levels that are associated with disease and injury often may predict the range and severity of impairments at the system level. The diagnosis of multiple sclerosis, for instance, typically requires that the physical therapist understand the fatigue factors that may be associated with the disease and how those factors must be addressed both in examining the patient/client and in providing interventions. *A diagnosis of multiple sclerosis by itself, however, tells the physical therapist nothing about the impairments, functional limitations, or disabilities that would be the focus of physical therapy intervention.*

Contrast two cases involving a diagnosis of multiple sclerosis. A 79-year-old woman who needs only a posterior splint to walk efficiently and who is able to carry out all activities of daily living (ADL) and instrumental activities of daily living (IADL) with total independence has very different needs from a 36-year-old woman who is postpartum and wheelchair dependent and who is unable to take care of her family as a result of severe generalized weakness. Both patients/clients have the same medical diagnosis, but the severity of impairments, functional limitations, and disabilities are sharply different. The examination, evaluation, and subsequent diagnosis of those impairments, functional limitations, and disabilities are the key contributions of the physical therapist.

The complexity of interconnections among the four components of the disablement model is indicative of the knowledge of pathology and pathophysiology that each physical therapist must bring to bear in addressing impairments, functional limitations, and disabilities. In the case of a patient/client who is referred to a physical therapist with a general diagnosis of "shoulder pain with activity," for instance, the physical therapist has to perform an examination to differentiate among several possible conditions in order to accurately manage the patient. It therefore is important for the physical therapist to understand the many possible underlying causes for the pain. The physical therapist's knowledge that different clusters of signs and symptoms are consistent with underlying conditions—such as angina, osteoarthritis, or prior fracture—is incorporated into the examination, evaluation, and intervention processes.

If the clinical findings on examination suggest a pathological or pathophysiological condition that is inconsistent with the referring practitioner's diagnosis, or if the physical therapist notes an underlying pathology or pathophysiology that was not previously identified, the therapist responds appropriately, including returning the patient to the original referring practitioner or making a referral to another practitioner. When the underlying cause is not identified, however, the physical therapist proceeds with the examination by continually testing the signs and symptoms and by providing interventions that are justified by changes in patient/client status.

Impairments

Impairments typically are the consequence of disease, pathological processes, or lesions. They may be defined as alterations in anatomical, physiological, or psychological structures or functions that both (1) result from underlying changes in the normal state and (2) contribute to illness. Impairments occur at the tissue, organ, and system level, and they are indicated by signs and symptoms. The Guide's diagnostic classification scheme uses the definition "abnormality of structure or function" for its impairment classification.

Physical therapists most often quantify and qualify the signs and symptoms of impairment that are associated with movement. Alterations of structure and function, such as abnormal muscle strength, range of motion, or gait, would be classified and diagnosed as impairments by physical therapists.

The origin of some impairments is often unclear. Poor posture, for example, is neither a disease nor a pathological state; however, the *muscle shortening and capsular tightness* associated with poor posture are still clinically significant. The physical therapist would diagnose them as impairments that may be remedied by physical therapy intervention.

In the physical therapist's examination, impairments typically are measured using noninvasive procedures—even those impairments that are associated with disease, disorders, and medical conditions—and may predict risk for functional limitation or disability.

Functional Limitations

Functional limitations occur when impairments result in a restriction of the ability to perform a physical action, task, or activity in an efficient, typically expected, or competent manner. In other words, functional limitations occur as a result of the inability to perform the actions, tasks, and activities that constitute the "usual activities" for a given individual, such as reaching for a box on an overhead shelf. Functional limitations are measured by testing the performance of physical and mental behaviors at the level of the person and should not be confused with diseases, disorders, conditions, or impairments involving specific tissue, organ, or system abnormalities that result in signs and symptoms.

The concept of functional limitations is based on a consensus about what is "normal." The Guide uses the broad definition of functional limitations to look at the actions, tasks, or activities of that whole person during his or her usual activities.

Functional limitations include sensorimotor performance in the execution of particular actions, tasks, and activities (eg, rolling, getting out of bed, transferring, walking, climbing, bending, lifting, carrying). These sensorimotor functional abilities underlie the daily, fundamental organized patterns of behaviors that are classified as basic activities of daily living (ADL) (eg, feeding, dressing, bathing, grooming, toileting). The more complex tasks associated with independent community living (eg, use of public transportation, grocery shopping) are categorized as instrumental activities of daily living (IADL). Successful performance of complex physical functional activities, such as personal hygiene and housekeeping, typically requires integration of cognitive and affective abilities as well as physical ones.

Although physical therapists are chiefly concerned with physical function, the effects of physical therapy may go beyond improvement in physical function. For instance, physical therapists may assess patient/client mental function, including a range of such cognitive activities as telling time and calculating money transactions. Attention, concentration, memory, and judgment also may be assessed.

Figure 3. The Enabling–Disabling Process[a]

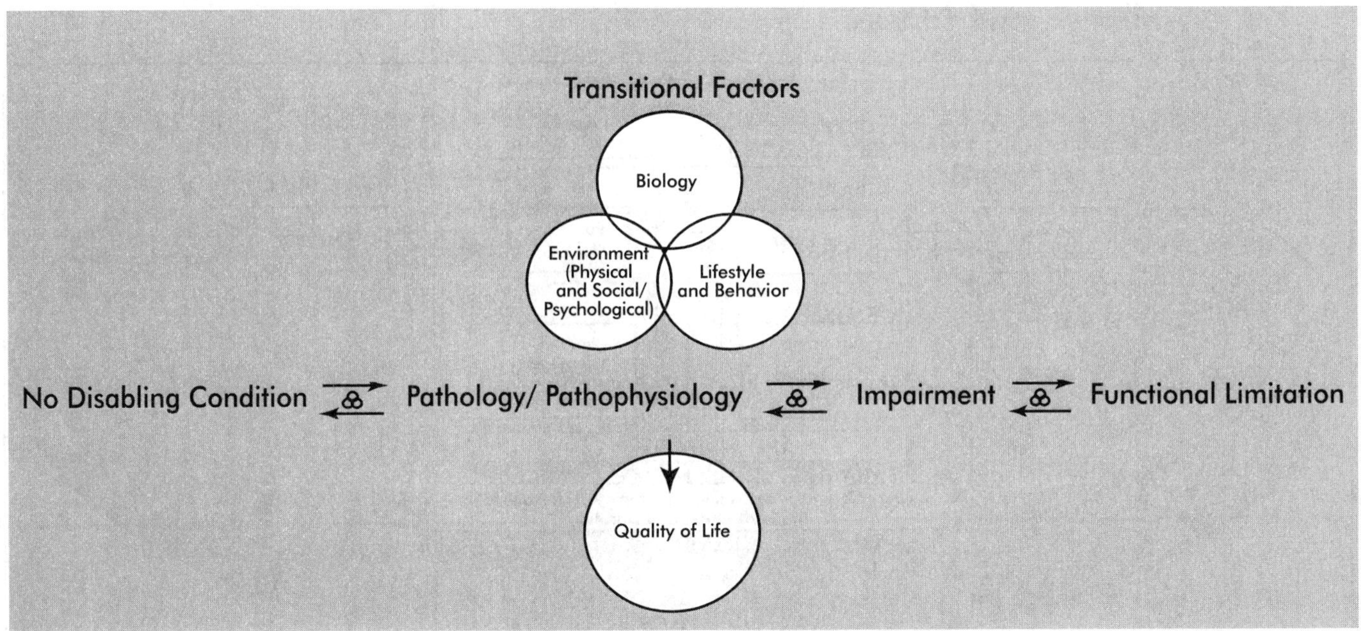

[a] *Adapted with permission of the Institute of Medicine from Brandt EN Jr, Pope AM.* Enabling America: Assessing the Role of Rehabilitation Science and Engineering. *Washington, DC: Institute of Medicine, National Academy Press; 1997:68.*

Disability

The Guide defines *disability* broadly as the inability or restricted ability to perform actions, tasks, and activities related to required self-care, home management, work (job/school/play), community, and leisure roles in the individual's sociocultural context and physical environment.

Disability refers to patterns of behavior that have emerged over periods of time during which functional limitations are severe enough that they cannot be overcome to maintain "normal" role performance. Thus, the concept of disability includes deficits in the performance of ADL and IADL that are broadly pertinent to many social roles. If a person has limited range of motion at the shoulder but bathes independently by using a shower mitt and applies the available range of motion at other joints to best mechanical advantage, that person is not "disabled," even though functional performance may be extremely limited without the use of an assistive device and altered movement patterns.

Disability is characterized by discordance between actual performance in a particular role and the expectations of the community regarding what are "normal" behaviors in that role. Labeling a person as "disabled" requires a judgment, usually by a professional, that an individual's behaviors are somehow inadequate, based on that professional's understanding of community expectations about how a given activity should be accomplished (eg, in ways that are typical for a person's age, sex, and cultural and social environment).

Disability depends on both the capacities of the individual and the expectations that are imposed on the individual by those in the immediate social environment, most often family and caregivers. Changing the expectations of a patient, family, or caregiver in a social context—for example, the physical therapist explaining to family members the level of assistance that is needed for an elder following stroke—may help to diminish disability as much as supplying the patient with assistive devices or increasing the patient's physical ability to use them.

Interrelationships Among Disease, Impairments, Functional Limitations, and Disability

When the physical therapist has determined which impairments are related to the patient's functional limitations, the therapist must determine which impairments may be remedied by physical therapy intervention. If they cannot be remedied, the physical therapist can help the patient compensate by using other abilities to accomplish the intended goal. The task or the environment also may be modified so that the task can be performed within the restrictions that the patient's condition imposes. These two approaches focus on "enablement" rather than remediation of "disablement," and they may be characterized as the classical physical therapist response to the disablement process.[3,13-17]

Disablement models have always included the concept of preventing progression toward disability. "Unidirectional," causal progression—from disease to impairment to functional limitation to disability, handicap, or societal limitation—"inexorably...without the possibility of reversal"—should not be assumed.[5] In 1997, IOM revised its disablement model to show both the interactions of the person with the environment and the "potential effects of rehabilitation and the 'enabling process'" (Fig. 3). The

Figure 4. An Expanded Disablement Model, Showing Interactions Among Individual and Environmental Factors, Prevention, and the Promotion of Health, Wellness, and Fitness[a]

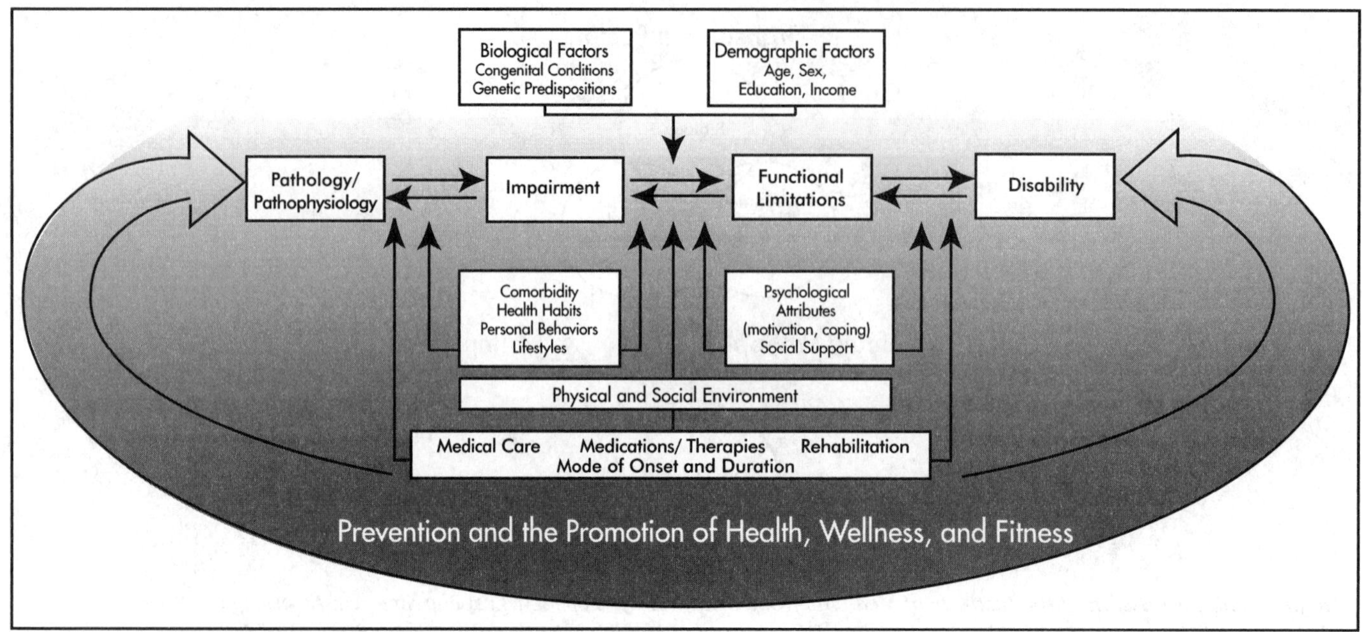

[a]*Adapted with permission of the American Physical Therapy Association from Guccione AA. Arthritis and the process of disablement.* Phys Ther. *1994;74:410.*

model suggests a bidirectional interaction among the components, in which improvement in one component has an effect on the development or progression of a preceding component. Disability was not included in the model because disability "is not inherent in the individual but, rather, a function of the interaction of the individual and the environment."[5] The "enabling-disabling process," therefore, recognizes that functional limitations and disability may be reversed.[5]

Prevention and the Promotion of Health, Wellness, and Fitness in the Context of Disablement

Progression from a healthy state to pathology—or from pathology or impairment to disability—does not have to be inevitable. The physical therapist may prevent impairments, functional limitations, or disabilities by identifying disablement risk factors during the diagnostic process and by buffering the disablement process (Fig. 4). The patient/client management described in the Guide includes three types of prevention:

- *Primary prevention.* Prevention of disease in a susceptible or potentially susceptible population through specific measures such as general health promotion efforts.
- *Secondary prevention.* Efforts to decrease duration of illness, severity of disease, and sequelae through early diagnosis and prompt intervention.
- *Tertiary prevention.* Efforts to decrease the degree of disability and promote rehabilitation and restoration of function in patients with chronic and irreversible diseases. In the diagnostic process, physical therapists identify risk factors for disability that may be independent of the disease or pathology.

The Individual, the Environment, and Health-Related Quality-of-Life Factors

Many factors may have an impact on the disablement process (Fig. 4). These factors may include individual and environmental factors that predispose or interact to create a person's disability.[2,5] Individual factors include biological factors (eg, congenital conditions, genetic predispositions) and demographic factors (eg, age, sex, education, income). Comorbidity, health habits, personal behaviors, lifestyles, psychological traits (eg, motivation, coping), and social interactions and relationships also influence the process of disablement. Furthermore, environmental factors—such as available medical or rehabilitation care, medications and other therapies, and the physical and social environment—may influence the process of disablement. Each of these factors may be modified by prevention and the promotion of health, wellness, and fitness.

Health-related quality of life (HRQL) can be said to represent the total effect of individual and environmental factors on function and health status. Three major dimensions of HRQL have been described in the literature: the *physical function component*, which includes basic activities of daily living (ADL) (eg, bathing) and instrumental activities of daily living (IADL) (eg, shopping); the *psychological component*, that is, the "various cognitive, perceptual, and personality traits" of a person; and the *social component*, which involves the interaction of the person "within a

Figure 5. Relationship Among the Disablement Model, Health-Related Quality of Life, and Quality of Life

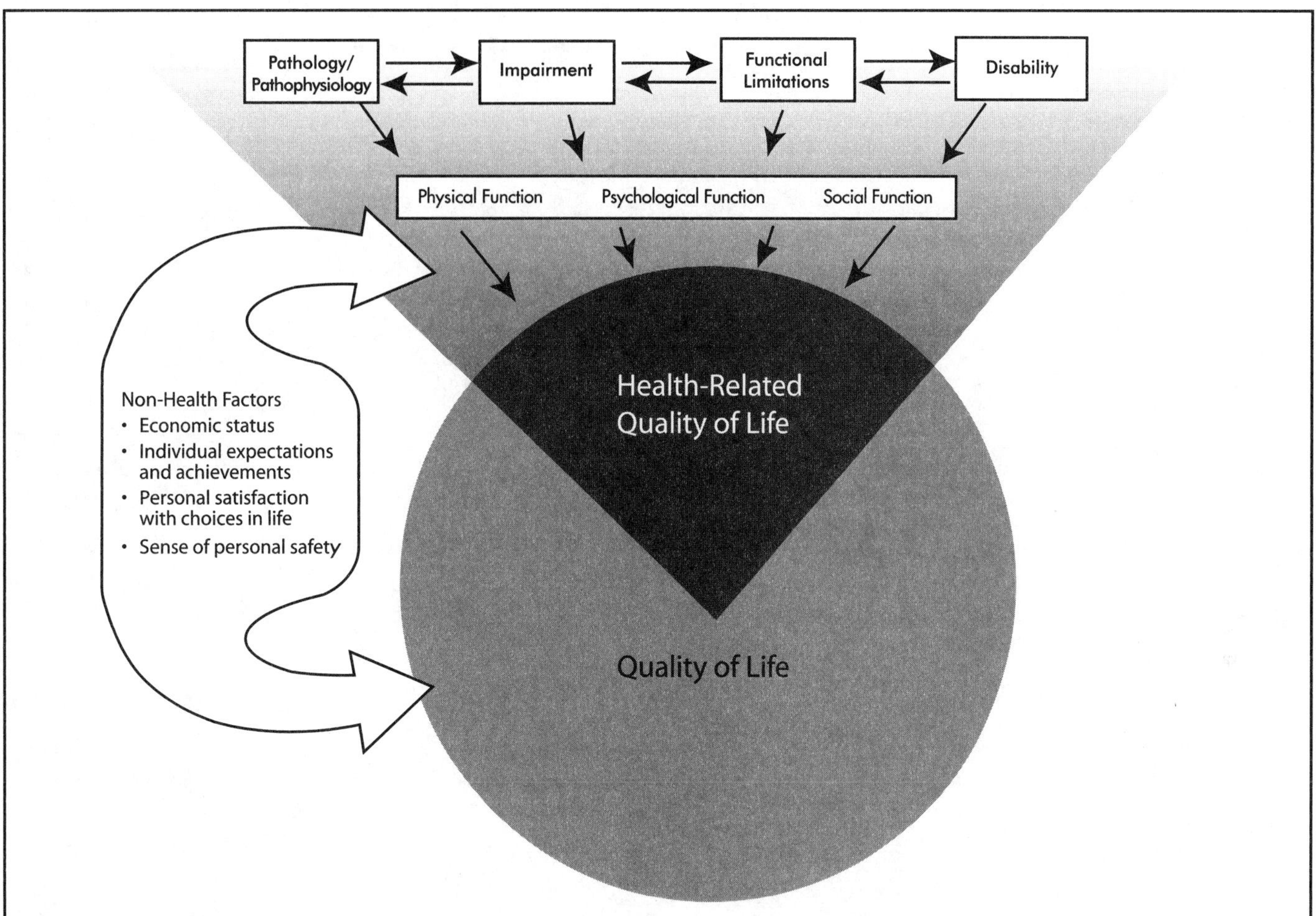

larger social context or structure."[18] As shown in Figure 5, the broad concept of HRQL encompasses the disablement model. Other "non-health" factors that typically are not included in definitions of functional limitation or disability contribute to an individual's sense of well being—and to both overall quality of life and health-related quality of life. Such factors include economic status, individual expectations and achievements, personal satisfaction with choices in life, and sense of personal safety.

References

1 Jette AM. Physical disablement concepts for physical therapy research and practice. *Phys Ther.* 1994;74:380-386.

2 Verbrugge L, Jette A. The disablement process. *Soc Sci Med.* 1994;38:1-14.

3 Guccione AA. Arthritis and the process of disablement. *Phys Ther.* 1994;74:408-414.

4 Guccione AA. Physical therapy diagnosis and the relationship between impairments and function. *Phys Ther*. 1991;71:499-504.

5 Brandt EN Jr, Pope AM, eds. *Enabling America: Assessing the Role of Rehabilitation Science and Engineering.* Washington, DC: Institute of Medicine, National Academy Press; 1997:62-80.

6 Nagi S. Some conceptual issues in disability and rehabilitation. In: Sussman M, ed. *Sociology and Rehabilitation.* Washington, DC: American Sociological Association; 1965:100-113.

7 Nagi S. *Disability and Rehabilitation.* Columbus, Ohio: Ohio State University Press; 1969.

8 Nagi S. Disability concepts revisited: implications for prevention. In: Pope A, Tarlov A, eds. *Disability in America: Toward a National Agenda for Prevention.* Washington, DC: Institute of Medicine, National Academy Press; 1991.

9 *ICIDH: International Classification of Impairments, Disabilities, and Handicaps.* Geneva, Switzerland: World Health Organization; 1980.

10 *ICF: International Classification of Functioning, Disability and Health.* Geneva, Switzerland: World Health Organization; 2001.

11 *National Advisory Board on Medical Rehabilitation Research, Draft V: Report and Plan for Medical Rehabilitation Research.* Bethesda, Md: National Institutes of Health; 1992.

12 *Disability in America: Toward a National Agenda for Prevention.* Washington, DC: Institute of Medicine, National Academy Press; 1991.

13 Craik RL. Disability following hip fracture. *Phys Ther.* 1994;74:387-398.

14 Duncan PW. Stroke disability. *Phys Ther.* 1994;74:399-407.

15 Delitto A. Are measures of function and disability important in low back care? *Phys Ther.* 1994;74:452-462.

16 Walsh M, Woodhouse LJ, Thomas SG, Finch E. Physical impairments and functional limitations: a comparison of individuals 1 year after total knee arthroplasty with control subjects. *Phys Ther.* 1998;78:248-258.

17 Gill-Body KM, Beninato M, Krebs DE. Relationship among balance impairments, functional performance, and disability in people with peripheral vestibular hypofunction. *Phys Ther.* 2000;80:748-758.

18 Jette AM. Using health-related quality of life measures in physical therapy outcomes research. *Phys Ther.* 1993;73:528-537.

What Does the Guide Contain?

Corresponds to "Content Overview" in the Interactive Guide CD-ROM

The Guide has five major components: the Introduction, which defines physical therapy, outlines the Guide's development, and describes the concepts that underlie the Guide; Part One, which delineates the physical therapist's scope of practice and describes the patient/client management that is provided by physical therapists; Part Two, which delineates preferred practice patterns (Preferred Physical Therapist Practice Patterns); Part Three, available only on CD-ROM (June 2001), which catalogs the tests and measures that are used in physical therapist practice; and the Appendixes, which include the core documents of the American Physical Therapy Association and Guide-based documentation templates. *The Guide does not contain specific treatment protocols, does not provide clinical guidelines, and does not set forth the standard of care for which a physical therapist may be legally responsible in any specific case.*

"Part One: A Description of Patient/Client Management"

Part One is an overview of physical therapists as health care professionals and their approach to patient/client management, specifically:

- Physical therapist qualifications, roles, and practice settings
- The five elements of patient/client management (examination; evaluation; diagnosis; prognosis, including plan of care; and intervention) provided by physical therapists
- Tests and measures that physical therapists frequently use, clinical indications that may prompt the use of the tests and measures, tools that may be used to gather data, and types of data that may be generated
- Interventions that physical therapists frequently provide, clinical considerations that may prompt the selection of interventions, and anticipated goals and expected outcomes of intervention

"Part Two: Preferred Physical Therapist Practice Patterns"

Part Two describes the boundaries within which the physical therapist may design and implement plans of care for patients/clients who are classified into specific practice patterns. The patterns are grouped under four categories of conditions: musculoskeletal, neuromuscular, cardiovascular/pulmonary, and integumentary. Some patients/clients may be best managed through classification in more than one pattern.

Each practice pattern describes the following:

- The specific patient/client diagnostic classification, including examples of (1) examination findings that may support inclusion of patients/clients in the pattern or exclusion of patients/clients from the pattern and (2) examination findings that may require classification of patients/clients in a different pattern or in more than one pattern
- The five elements of patient/client management for each pattern: examination (history, systems review, and tests and measures), evaluation, diagnosis, prognosis (including plan of care and expected range of number of visits), and interventions (including anticipated goals and expected outcomes)

- Reexamination
- Global outcomes (impact on pathology/pathophysiology [disease, disorder, or condition], impairments, functional limitations, and disabilities; risk reduction/prevention; impact on health, wellness, and fitness; impact on societal resources; patient/client satisfaction)
- Criteria for termination of physical therapy services

In addition, each pattern lists relevant ICD-9-CM codes. (These lists are intended as general information and are not to be used for coding purposes.)

"Part Three: Specific Tests Used in Physical Therapist Practice"

Part Three (available on CD-ROM only) contains a listing of tests and measures used in the assessment of the cardiovascular/pulmonary, integumentary, musculoskeletal, and neuromuscular systems and a listing of tests and measures of health status, health-related quality of life, and patient/client satisfaction. Citations in the peer-reviewed literature regarding the reliability and validity of specific tests are included.

Appendixes

Appendix 1 contains the Guide glossary. Appendixes 2 through 4 contain the APTA core documents on which physical therapist practice is based: *Standards of Practice for Physical Therapy and the Criteria* (Appendix 2); *Code of Ethics* and *Guide for Professional Conduct* (Appendix 3); and *Standards of Ethical Conduct for the Physical Therapist Assistant* and *Guide for Conduct of the Affiliate Member* (Appendix 4). Appendix 5 contains *Guidelines for Physical Therapy Documentation.* (Note: APTA documents are revised on a regular basis. For the most recent versions of these documents, contact APTA's Service Center, svcctr@apta.org.) Appendix 6 contains the "Documentation Templates for Physical Therapist Patient/Client Management"; Appendix 7, the "Patient/Client Satisfaction Questionnaire."

Indexes

Both numerical and alphabetical indexes of the ICD-9-CM codes cited in the Guide are provided.

PART ONE:

A Description of Patient/Client Management

- Who Are Physical Therapists, and What Do They Do?
- What Types of Tests and Measures Do Physical Therapists Use?
- What Types of Interventions Do Physical Therapists Provide?

Content in Part One corresponds to "About Physical Therapists," "Basics of Patient/Client Management," "Tests and Measures," and "Interventions" in the Interactive Guide CD-ROM

CHAPTER 1

Who Are Physical Therapists, and What Do They Do?

Corresponds to "About Physical Therapists" and "Basics of Patient/Client Management" in the Interactive Guide CD-ROM

Education and Qualifications

Physical therapists are professionally educated at the college or university level and are required to be licensed in the state or states in which they practice. Graduates from 1926 to 1959 completed physical therapy curricula approved by appropriate accreditation bodies. Graduates from 1960 to the present have successfully completed professional physical therapist education programs accredited by the Commission on Accreditation in Physical Therapy Education (CAPTE). As of January 2002, CAPTE accreditation is limited to only those professional education programs that award the postbaccalaureate degree.

Physical therapists also may be certified as clinical specialists through the American Board of Physical Therapy Specialties (ABPTS).

Practice Settings

Physical therapists practice in a broad range of inpatient, outpatient, and community-based settings, including the following:

- Hospitals (eg, critical care, intensive care, acute care, and subacute care settings)
- Outpatient clinics or offices
- Rehabilitation facilities
- Skilled nursing, extended care, or subacute facilities
- Homes
- Education or research centers
- Schools and playgrounds (preschool, primary, and secondary)
- Hospices
- Corporate or industrial health centers
- Industrial, workplace, or other occupational environments
- Athletic facilities (collegiate, amateur, and professional)
- Fitness centers and sports training facilities

Patients and Clients

Physical therapists are committed to providing necessary and high-quality services to both patients and clients. *Patients* are individuals who are the recipients of physical therapy examination, evaluation, diagnosis, prognosis, and intervention and who have a disease, disorder, condition, impairment, functional limitation, or disability. *Clients* are individuals who engage the services of a physical therapist and who can benefit from the physical therapist's consultation, interventions, professional advice, prevention services, or services promoting health, wellness, and fitness. Clients also are businesses, school systems, and others to whom physical therapists provide services. The generally accepted elements of patient/client management typically apply to both patients and clients.

Scope of Practice

Physical therapy is defined as the care and services provided by or under the direction and supervision of a physical therapist. Physical therapists are the only professionals who provide physical therapy interventions. Physical therapist assistants are the only individuals who provide selected physical therapy interventions under the direction and supervision of the physical therapist. APTA recommends that federal and state government agencies and other third-party payers require physical therapy to be provided only by physical therapists or under the direction and supervision of physical therapists. Examination, evaluation, diagnosis, and prognosis should be represented and reimbursed as physical therapy only when they are performed by a physical therapist. Intervention should be represented and reimbursed as physical therapy only when performed by a physical therapist or by a physical therapist assistant performing selected interventions under the direction and supervision of a physical therapist in accordance with APTA positions, policies, standards, codes, and guidelines.

Physical therapists:

- *Provide services to patients/clients who have impairments, functional limitations, disabilities, or changes in physical function and health status resulting from injury, disease, or other causes.* In the context of the model of disablement[1-4] on which this Guide is based, *impairment* is defined as loss or abnormality of anatomical, physiological, mental, or psychological structure or function; *functional limitation* is defined as restriction of the ability to perform, at the level of the whole person, a physical action, task, or activity in an efficient, typically expected, or competent manner; and *disability* is defined as the inability to perform or a limitation in the performance of actions, tasks, and activities usually expected in specific social roles that are customary for the individual or expected for the person's status or role in a specific sociocultural context and physical environment.

- *Interact and practice in collaboration with a variety of professionals.* The collaboration may be with physicians, dentists, nurses, educators, social workers, occupational therapists, speech-language pathologists, audiologists, and any other personnel involved with the patient/client. Physical therapists acknowledge the need to educate and inform other professionals, government agencies, third-party payers, and other health care consumers about the cost-efficient and clinically effective services that physical therapists provide.

- *Address risk.* Physical therapists identify risk factors and behaviors that may impede optimal functioning.

- *Provide prevention and promote health, wellness, and fitness.* Physical therapists provide prevention services that forestall or prevent functional decline and the need for more intense care. Through timely and appropriate screening, examination, evaluation, diagnosis, prognosis, and intervention, physical therapists frequently reduce or eliminate the need for costlier forms of care and also may shorten or even eliminate institutional stays. Physical therapists also are involved in promoting health, wellness, and fitness initiatives, including education and service provision, that stimulate the public to engage in healthy behaviors.

- *Consult, educate, engage in critical inquiry, and administrate.* Physical therapists provide consultative services to health facilities, colleagues, businesses, and community organizations and agencies. They provide education to patients/clients, students, facility staff, communities, and organizations and agencies. Physical therapists also engage in research activities, particularly those related to substantiating the outcomes of service provision. They provide administrative services in many different types of practice, research, and education settings.

- *Direct and supervise the physical therapy service, including support personnel.* Physical therapists oversee all aspects of the physical therapy service. They supervise the physical therapist assistant (PTA) when PTAs provide physical therapy interventions as selected by the physical therapist. Physical therapists also supervise any support personnel as they perform designated tasks related to the operation of the physical therapy service.

Roles in Primary Care

Physical therapists have a major role to play in the provision of *primary care*, which has been defined as

> the provision of integrated, accessible health care services by clinicians who are accountable for addressing a large majority of personal health care needs, developing a sustained partnership with patients, and practicing within the context of family and community.[5]

APTA has endorsed the concepts of primary care set forth by the Institute of Medicine's Committee on the Future of Primary Care,[5] including the following:

- Primary care can encompass myriad needs that go well beyond the capabilities and competencies of individual caregivers and that require the involvement and interaction of varied practitioners.

- Primary care is not limited to the "first contact" or point of entry into the health care system.

- The primary care program is a comprehensive one.

On a daily basis, physical therapists practicing across acute, rehabilitative, and chronic stages of care assist patients/clients in restoring health, alleviating pain, and examining, evaluating, and diagnosing impairments, functional limitations, disabilities, or changes in physical function and health status resulting from injury, disease, or other causes. Intervention, prevention, and the promotion of health, wellness, and fitness are a vital part of the practice of physical therapists. As clinicians, physical therapists are well positioned to provide services as members of primary care teams.

For acute musculoskeletal and neuromuscular conditions, triage and initial examination are appropriate physical therapist responsibilities. The primary care team may function more efficiently when it includes physical therapists, who can recognize musculoskeletal and neuromuscular disorders, perform examinations and evaluations, establish a diagnosis and prognosis, and intervene without delay. For patients/clients with low back pain, for example, physical therapists can provide immediate pain reduction through programs for pain modification, strengthening, flexibility, endurance, and postural alignment; instruction in activities of daily living (ADL); and work modification. Physical therapy intervention may result not only in more efficient and effective patient care but also in more appropriate utilization of other members of the primary care team. With physical therapists functioning in a primary care role and delivering early intervention for work-related musculoskeletal injuries, time and productivity loss due to injuries may be dramatically reduced.

For certain chronic conditions, physical therapists should be recognized as the principal providers of care within the collaborative primary care team. Physical therapists are well prepared to coordinate care related to loss of physical function as a result of musculoskeletal, neuromuscular, cardiovascular/pulmonary, or integumentary disorders. Through community-based agencies and school systems, physical therapists coordinate and integrate provision of services to patients/clients with chronic disorders.

Physical therapists also provide primary care in industrial or workplace settings, in which they manage the occupational health services provided to employees and help prevent injury by designing or redesigning the work environment. These services focus both on the individual and on the environment to ensure comprehensive and appropriate intervention.

Roles in Secondary and Tertiary Care

Physical therapists play major roles in secondary and tertiary care. Patients with musculoskeletal, neuromuscular, cardiovascular/pulmonary, or integumentary conditions may be treated initially by another practitioner and then referred to physical therapists for secondary care. Physical therapists provide secondary care in a wide range of settings, including acute care and rehabilitation hospitals, outpatient clinics, home health, and school systems.

Tertiary care is provided by physical therapists in highly specialized, complex, and technology-based settings (eg, heart and lung transplant services, burn units) or in response to other health care practitioners' requests for consultation and specialized services (eg, for patients with spinal cord lesions or closed-head trauma).

Roles in Prevention and in the Promotion of Health, Wellness, and Fitness

Physical therapists are involved in prevention; in promoting health, wellness, and fitness; and in performing screening activities. These initiatives decrease costs by helping patients/clients (1) achieve and restore optimal functional capacity; (2) minimize impairments, functional limitations, and disabilities related to congenital and acquired conditions; (3) maintain health (thereby preventing further deterioration or future illness); and (4) create appropriate environmental adaptations to enhance independent function.

There are three types of prevention in which physical therapists are involved:

- *Primary prevention.* Preventing a target condition in a susceptible or potentially susceptible population through such specific measures as general health promotion efforts.

- *Secondary prevention.* Decreasing duration of illness, severity of disease, and number of sequelae through early diagnosis and prompt intervention.

- *Tertiary prevention.* Limiting the degree of disability and promoting rehabilitation and restoration of function in patients with chronic and irreversible diseases.

Physical therapists conduct screenings to determine the need for (1) primary, secondary, or tertiary prevention services; (2) further examination, intervention, or consultation by a physical therapist; or (3) referral to another practitioner. Candidates for screening generally are not patients/clients currently receiving physical therapy services. Screening is based on a problem-focused, systematic collection and analysis of data.

Examples of the prevention screening activities in which physical therapists engage include:

- Identification of lifestyle factors (eg, amount of exercise, stress, weight) that may lead to increased risk for serious health problems

- Identification of children who may need an examination for idiopathic scoliosis

- Identification of elderly individuals in a community center or nursing home who are at high risk for falls

- Identification of risk factors for neuromusculoskeletal injuries in the workplace

- Pre-performance testing of individuals who are active in sports

Examples of prevention activities and health, wellness, and fitness promotion activities in which physical therapists engage include:

- Back schools, workplace redesign, strengthening, stretching, endurance exercise programs, and postural training to prevent and manage low back pain

- Ergonomic redesign; strengthening, stretching, and endurance exercise programs; postural training to prevent job-related disabilities, including trauma and repetitive stress injuries

- Exercise programs, including weight bearing and weight training, to increase bone mass and bone density (especially in older adults with osteoporosis)

- Exercise programs, gait training, and balance and coordination activities to reduce the risk of falls—and the risk of fractures from falls—in older adults

- Exercise programs and instruction in ADL (self-care, communication, and mobility skills required for independence in daily living) and instrumental activities of daily living (IADL) (activities that are important components of maintaining independent living, such as shopping and cooking) to decrease utilization of health care services and enhance function in patients with cardiovascular/pulmonary disorders

- Exercise programs, cardiovascular conditioning, postural training, and instruction in ADL and IADL to prevent disability and dysfunction in women who are pregnant

- Broad-based consumer education and advocacy programs to prevent problems (eg, prevent head injury by promoting the use of helmets, prevent pulmonary disease by encouraging smoking cessation)

- Exercise programs to prevent or reduce the development of sequelae in individuals with life-long conditions

The Five Elements of Patient/Client Management

The physical therapist integrates the five elements of patient/client management—examination, evaluation, diagnosis, prognosis, and intervention—in a manner designed to optimize outcomes (Fig. 1). Appendix 6 contains a template for documenting the five elements of patient/client management.

Examination, evaluation, and the establishment of a diagnosis and a prognosis are all part of the process that helps the physical therapist determine the most appropriate intervention(s) to address the outcomes that are desired by the patient/client.

Examination

Examination is required prior to the initial intervention and is performed for all patients/clients. The initial examination is a comprehensive screening and specific testing process leading to diagnostic classification or, as appropriate, to a referral to another practitioner. The examination has three components: the patient/client history, the systems review, and tests and measures.

History. The *history* is a systematic gathering of data—from both the past and the present—related to why the patient/client is seeking the services of the physical therapist. The data that are obtained (eg, through interview, through review of the patient/client record, or from other sources) include demographic information, social history, employment and work (job/school/play), growth and development, living environment, general health status, social and health habits (past and current), family history, medical/surgical history, current conditions or chief complaints, functional status and activity level, medications, and other clinical tests. While taking the history, the physical therapist also identifies health restoration and prevention needs and coexisting health problems that may have implications for intervention.

This history typically is obtained through the gathering of data from the patient/client, family, significant others, caregivers, and other interested individuals (eg, rehabilitation counselor, teacher, workers' compensation claims manager, employer); through consultation with other members of the team; and through review of the patient/client record. Figure 2 lists the types of data that may be generated from the history.

Data from the history (Fig. 2) provide the initial information that the physical therapist uses to hypothesize about the existence and origin of impairments or functional limitations that are commonly related to medical conditions, sociodemographic factors, or personal characteristics. For example, in the case of a 78-year-old woman who has a medical diagnosis of Parkinson disease and who lives alone, the medical diagnosis would suggest the *possibility* of the following impairments: loss of motor control, range-of-motion deficits, faulty posture, and decreased endurance for functional activities. Epidemiologic research that is available about functional limitations of older women, however, suggests that performance of IADL also may be problematic for that age group. Consequently, in this case, the physical therapist may use the information obtained during the history as well as the epidemiological information to create a "hypothesis" that would require further, in-depth examination during the tests-and-measures portion of the examination.

Systems review. After organizing the available history information, the physical therapist begins the "hands-on" component of the examination. The *systems review* is a brief or limited examination of (1) the anatomical and physiological status of the cardiovascular/pulmonary, integumentary, musculoskeletal, and neuromuscular systems and (2) the communication ability, affect, cognition, language, and learning style of the patient. The physical therapist especially notes how each of these last five components affects the ability to initiate, sustain, and modify purposeful movement for performance of an action, task, or activity that is pertinent to function.

The systems review includes the following:

- For the cardiovascular/pulmonary system, the assessment of heart rate, respiratory rate, blood pressure, and edema

- For the integumentary system, the assessment of pliability (texture), presence of scar formation, skin color, and skin integrity

- For the musculoskeletal system, the assessment of gross symmetry, gross range of motion, gross strength, height, and weight

- For the neuromuscular system, a general assessment of gross coordinated movement (eg, balance, gait, locomotion, transfers, and transitions) and motor function (motor control and motor learning)

Figure 1. The Elements of Patient/Client Management Leading to Optimal Outcomes

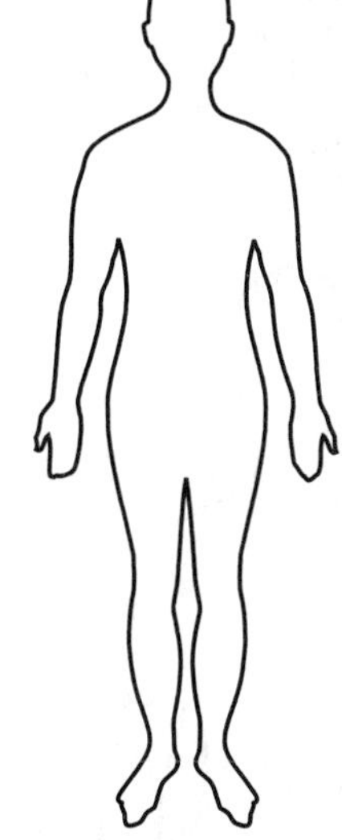

DIAGNOSIS
Both the process and the end result of evaluating examination data, which the physical therapist organizes into defined clusters, syndromes, or categories to help determine the prognosis (including the plan of care) and the most appropriate intervention strategies.

PROGNOSIS (Including Plan of Care)
Determination of the level of optimal improvement that may be attained through intervention and the amount of time required to reach that level. The plan of care specifies the interventions to be used and their timing and frequency.

INTERVENTION
Purposeful and skilled interaction of the physical therapist with the patient/client and, if appropriate, with other individuals involved in care of the patient/client, using various physical therapy procedures and techniques to produce changes in the condition that are consistent with the diagnosis and prognosis. The physical therapist conducts a reexamination to determine changes in patient/client status and to modify or redirect intervention. The decision to reexamine may be based on new clinical findings or on lack of patient/client progress. The process of reexamination also may identify the need for consultation with or referral to another provider.

OUTCOMES
Results of patient/client management, which include the impact of physical therapy interventions in the following domains: pathology/pathophysiology (disease, disorder, or condition); impairments, functional limitations, and disabilities; risk reduction/prevention; health, wellness, and fitness; societal resources; and patient/client satisfaction.

EXAMINATION
The process of obtaining a history, performing a systems review, and selecting and administering tests and measures to gather data about the patient/client. The initial examination is a comprehensive screening and specific testing process that leads to a diagnostic classification. The examination process also may identify possible problems that require consultation with or referral to another provider.

EVALUATION
A dynamic process in which the physical therapist makes clinical judgments based on data gathered during the examination. This process also may identify possible problems that require consultation with or referral to another provider.

- For communication ability, affect, cognition, language, and learning style, the assessment of the ability to make needs known; consciousness; orientation (person, place, and time); expected emotional/behavioral responses; and learning preferences (eg, learning barriers, education needs)

The systems review also assists the physical therapist in identifying possible problems that require consultation with or referral to another provider.

Tests and measures. *Tests and measures* are the means of gathering data about the patient/client. From the comprehensive identification and questioning processes of the history and systems review, the physical therapist determines patient/client needs and generates diagnostic hypotheses that may be further investigated by selecting specific tests and measures. These tests and measures are used to rule in or rule out causes of impairment and functional limitations; to establish a diagnosis, prognosis, and plan of care; and to select interventions.

The tests and measures that are performed as part of an initial examination should be only those that are necessary to (1) confirm or reject a hypothesis about the factors that contribute to making the current level of patient/client function less than optimal and (2) support the physical therapist's clinical judgments about appropriate interventions, anticipated goals, and expected outcomes.

Before, during, and after administering the tests and measures, physical therapists gauge responses, assess physical status, and obtain a more specific understanding of the condition and the diagnostic and therapeutic requirements. There are 24 tests and measures that are commonly performed by physical therapists. These tests and measures, tools used to gather data, and types of data generated are discussed in detail in Chapter 2.

Figure 2. Types of Data That May Be Generated From a Patient/Client History

General Demographics
- Age
- Sex
- Race/ethnicity
- Primary language
- Education

Social History
- Cultural beliefs and behaviors
- Family and caregiver resources
- Social interactions, social activities, and support systems

Employment/Work (Job/School/Play)
- Current and prior work (job/school/play), community, and leisure actions, tasks, or activities

Growth and Development
- Developmental history
- Hand dominance

Living Environment
- Devices and equipment (eg, assistive, adaptive, orthotic, protective, supportive, prosthetic)
- Living environment and community characteristics
- Projected discharge destinations

General Health Status (Self-Report, Family Report, Caregiver Report)
- General health perception
- Physical function (eg, mobility, sleep patterns, restricted bed days)
- Psychological function (eg, memory, reasoning ability, depression, anxiety)
- Role function (eg, community, leisure, social, work)
- Social function (eg, social activity, social interaction, social support)

Social/Health Habits (Past and Current)
- Behavioral health risks (eg, smoking, drug abuse)
- Level of physical fitness

Family History
- Familial health risks

Medical/Surgical History
- Cardiovascular
- Endocrine/metabolic
- Gastrointestinal
- Genitourinary
- Gynecological
- Integumentary
- Musculoskeletal
- Neuromuscular
- Obstetrical
- Prior hospitalizations, surgeries, and preexisting medical and other health-related conditions
- Psychological
- Pulmonary

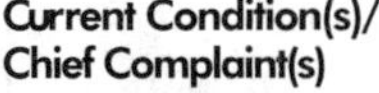

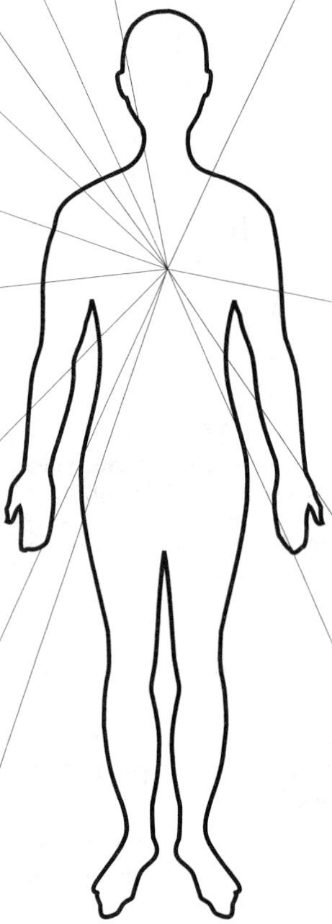

Current Condition(s)/ Chief Complaint(s)
- Concerns that led the patient/client to seek the services of a physical therapist
- Concerns or needs of patient/client who requires the services of a physical therapist
- Current therapeutic interventions
- Mechanisms of injury or disease, including date of onset and course of events
- Onset and pattern of symptoms
- Patient/client, family, significant other, and caregiver expectations and goals for the therapeutic intervention
- Patient/client, family, significant other, and caregiver perceptions of patient's/client's emotional response to the current clinical situation
- Previous occurrence of chief complaint(s)
- Prior therapeutic interventions

Functional Status and Activity Level
- Current and prior functional status in self-care and home management, including activities of daily living (ADL) and instrumental activities of daily living (IADL)
- Current and prior functional status in work (job/school/play), community, and leisure actions, tasks, or activities

Medications
- Medications for current condition
- Medications previously taken for current condition
- Medications for other conditions

Other Clinical Tests
- Laboratory and diagnostic tests
- Review of available records (eg, medical, education, surgical)
- Review of other clinical findings (eg, nutrition and hydration)

The physical therapist may decide to use one, more than one, or portions of several specific tests and measures as part of the examination, based on the purpose of the visit, the complexity of the condition, and the directions taken in the clinical decision-making process.

As the examination progresses, the physical therapist may identify additional problems that were not uncovered by the history and systems review and may conclude that other specific tests and measures or portions of other specific tests and measures are required to obtain sufficient data to perform an evaluation, establish a diagnosis and a prognosis, and select interventions. The examination therefore may be as brief or as lengthy as necessary. The physical therapist may decide that a full examination is necessary and then select appropriate tests and measures. Conversely, the physical therapist may conclude from the history and systems review that further examination and intervention are not required, that the patient/client should be referred to another practitioner, or both.

Tests and measures vary in the precision of their measurements; however, useful data may be generated through various means. For instance, data generated from either a gross muscle test of a group of muscles or from a very precise manual muscle test could be used to reject the hypothesis that muscle performance is contributing to a functional deficit. Similarly, even though a functional assessment instrument may quantify a large number of ADL or IADL, it may fail to detect the inability to perform a particular task and activity that is most important to the patient.

The tests and measures that are selected by the physical therapist should yield data that are sufficiently accurate and precise to allow the therapist to make a correct inference about the patient's/client's condition. The selection of specific tests and measures and the depth of the examination vary based on the age of the patient/client; severity of the problem; stage of recovery (acute, subacute, or chronic); phase of rehabilitation (early, intermediate, late, return to activity); home, community, or work (job/school/play) situation; and other relevant factors.

Evaluation

Physical therapists perform *evaluations* (make clinical judgments) based on the data gathered from the examination. They synthesize all of the findings from the history, systems review, and tests and measures to establish the diagnosis, prognosis, and plan of care. Factors that influence the complexity of the evaluation process include the clinical findings, the extent of loss of function, social considerations, and overall physical function and health status. The evaluation reflects the chronicity or severity of the current problem, the possibility of multisite or multisystem involvement, the presence of preexisting systemic conditions or diseases, and the stability of the condition. Physical therapists also consider the severity and complexity of the current impairments and the probability of prolonged impairment, functional limitation, and disability; the living environment; potential discharge destinations; and social support.

Diagnosis

Diagnostic labels may be used to describe multiple dimensions of the patient/client, ranging from the most basic cellular level to the highest level of functioning—as a person in society. Although physicians typically use labels that identify disease, disorder, or condition at the level of the cell, tissue, organ, or system, physical therapists use labels that identify the *impact of a condition on function at the level of the system (especially the movement system) and at the level of the whole person.*

The assigning of a diagnostic label through the classification of a patient/client within a specific practice pattern is a decision reached as a result of a systematic process. This process includes integrating and evaluating the data that are obtained during the examination (history, systems review, and tests and measures) to describe the patient/client condition in terms that will guide the physical therapist in determining the prognosis, plan of care, and intervention strategies. Thus the diagnostic label indicates the primary dysfunctions toward which the physical therapist directs interventions. The diagnostic process enables the physical therapist to verify the individual needs of each patient/client relative to similar individuals who are classified in the same pattern while also capturing the unique concerns of the patient/client in meeting those needs in a particular sociocultural and physical environment.

If the diagnostic process does not yield an identifiable cluster (eg, of signs or symptoms, impairments, functional limitations, or disabilities), syndrome, or category, the physical therapist may administer interventions for the alleviation of symptoms and remediation of impairments. As in all other cases, the physical therapist is guided by patient/client responses to those interventions and may determine that a reexamination is in order and proceed accordingly.

The objective of the physical therapist's diagnostic process is the identification of discrepancies that exist between the level of function that is desired by the patient/client and the capacity of the patient/client to achieve that level. In carrying out the diagnostic process, physical therapists may need to obtain additional information (including diagnostic labels) from other professionals. In addition, as the diagnostic process continues, physical therapists may identify findings that should be shared with other professionals (including referral sources) to ensure optimal care. If the diagnostic process reveals findings that are outside the scope of the physical therapist's knowledge, experience, or expertise, the physical therapist refers the patient/client to an appropriate practitioner.

Making a diagnosis requires the clinician to collect and sort data into categories according to a classification scheme relevant to the clinician who is making the diagnosis. These classification schemes should meet the following criteria:[6]

1. Classification schemes must be consistent with the boundaries placed on the profession by law (which may regulate the application of certain types of diagnostic categories) and by society (which grants approval for managing specific types of problems and conditions).
2. The tests and measures necessary for confirming the diagnosis must be within the legal purview of the health care professional.
3. The label used to categorize a condition should describe the problem in a way that directs the selection of interventions toward those interventions that are within the legal purview of the health care professional who is making the diagnosis.

The preferred practice patterns in Part Two of the Guide describe the management of patients who are grouped by clusters of impairments that commonly occur together, some of which are associated with health conditions that impede optimal function. Each pattern represents a diagnostic classification. The pattern title therefore reflects the diagnosis—or impairment classification—made by the physical therapist. The diagnosis may or may not be associated with a health condition for patients/clients who are classified into that pattern.

The physical therapist uses the classification scheme of the preferred practice patterns to complete a diagnostic process that begins with the collection of data (examination), proceeds through the organization and interpretation of data (evaluation), and culminates in the application of a label (diagnosis).

Prognosis (Including the Plan of Care)

Once the diagnosis has been established, the physical therapist determines the prognosis and develops the plan of care. The *prognosis* is the determination of the predicted optimal level of improvement in function and the amount of time needed to reach that level, and also may include a prediction of levels of improvement that may be reached at various intervals during the course of therapy.

The *plan of care* consists of statements that specify the anticipated goals and the expected outcomes, predicted level of optimal improvement, specific interventions to be used, and proposed duration and frequency of the interventions that are required to reach the anticipated goals and expected outcomes. The plan of care therefore describes the specific patient/client management and the timing for patient/client management for the episode of physical therapy care.

The plan of care is the culmination of the examination, diagnostic, and prognostic processes. It is established in collaboration with the patient/client and is based on the data gathered from the history, systems review, and tests and measures and on the diagnosis determined by the physical therapist. In designing the plan of care, the physical therapist analyzes and integrates the clinical implications of the severity, complexity, and acuity of the pathology/pathophysiology (disease, disorder, or condition), the impairments, the functional limitations, and the disabilities to establish the prognosis and predictions about the likelihood of achieving the anticipated goals and expected outcomes.

The plan of care identifies anticipated goals and expected outcomes, taking into consideration the expectations of the patient/client and appropriate others. (If required, the anticipated goals and expected outcomes may be expressed as short-term and long-term goals.) *Anticipated goals and expected outcomes* are the intended results of patient/client management and indicate the changes in impairments, functional limitations, and disabilities and the changes in health, wellness, and fitness needs that are expected as the result of implementing the plan of care. The anticipated goals and expected outcomes also address risk reduction, prevention, impact on societal resources, and patient/client satisfaction. The anticipated goals and expected outcomes in the plan should be measurable and time limited.

The plan of care includes the anticipated discharge plans. In consultation with appropriate individuals, the physical therapist plans for discharge and provides for appropriate follow-up or referral. The primary criterion for discharge is the achievement of the anticipated goals and expected outcomes. When physical therapy services are terminated prior to achievement of anticipated goals and expected outcomes, patient/client status and the rationale for termination are documented. For patients/clients who require multiple episodes of care, periodic follow-up is needed over the life span to ensure safety and effective adaptation following changes in physical status, caregivers, environment, or task demands.

Note: In the course of examining the patient/client and establishing the diagnosis and the prognosis, the physical therapist may find evidence of physical abuse or domestic violence. Universal screening for domestic violence is increasingly becoming a statutory requirement.

Intervention

Intervention is the purposeful interaction of the physical therapist with the patient/client and, when appropriate, with other individuals involved in patient/client care, using various physical therapy procedures and techniques to produce changes in the condition that are consistent with the diagnosis and prognosis. Decisions about interventions are contingent on the timely monitoring of patient/client response and the progress made toward achieving the anticipated goals and expected outcomes. Physical therapist interventions consist of the following components:

- Coordination, communication, and documentation
- Patient/client-related instruction
- Procedural interventions, including
  - therapeutic exercise
  - functional training in self-care and home management (including ADL and IADL)
  - functional training in work (job/school/play), community, and leisure integration and reintegration (including IADL, work hardening, and work conditioning)
  - manual therapy techniques (including mobilization/manipulation)
  - prescription, application, and, as appropriate, fabrication of devices and equipment (assistive, adaptive, orthotic, protective, supportive, and prosthetic)
  - airway clearance techniques
  - integumentary repair and protection techniques
  - electrotherapeutic modalities
  - physical agents and mechanical modalities

Coordination, communication, and documentation. These administrative and supportive processes are intended to ensure that patients/clients receive appropriate, comprehensive, efficient, and effective quality of care from admission through discharge. *Coordination* is the working together of all parties involved with the patient/client. *Communication* is the exchange of information. *Documentation* is any entry into the patient/client record—such as consultation reports, initial examination reports, progress notes, flow sheets, checklists, reexamination reports, or summations of care—that identifies the care or service provided. *Physical therapists are responsible for coordination, communication, and documentation across all settings for all patients/clients.*

Administrative and support processes may include addressing required functions, such as advanced care directives, individualized educational plans (IEPs) or individualized family service plans (IFSPs), informed consent, and mandatory communication and reporting (eg, patient advocacy and abuse reporting); admission and discharge planning; case management; collaboration and coordination with agencies; communication across settings; cost-effective resource utilization; data collection, analysis, and reporting; documentation across settings; interdisciplinary teamwork; and referrals to other professionals or resources. Documentation should follow APTA's *Guidelines for Physical Therapy Documentation* (Appendix 5).

Patient/client-related instruction. The process of informing, educating, or training patients/clients, families, significant others, and caregivers is intended to promote and optimize physical therapy services. Instruction may be related to the current condition; specific impairments, functional limitations, or disabilities; plan of care; need for enhanced performance; transition to a different role or setting; risk factors for developing a problem or dysfunction; or need for health, wellness, or fitness programs. *Physical therapists are responsible for patient/client-related instruction across all settings for all patients/clients.*

Procedural interventions. The physical therapist selects, applies, or modifies these interventions (listed above) based on examination data, the evaluation, the diagnosis and the prognosis, and the anticipated goals and expected outcomes for a particular patient in a specific patient/client practice pattern. Based on patient/client response to interventions, the physical therapist may decide that reexamination is necessary, a decision that may lead to the use of different interventions or, alternatively, the discontinuation of care.

Chapter 3 details the nine types of procedural interventions commonly selected by the physical therapist. Forming the core of most physical therapy plans of care are: therapeutic exercise, including aerobic conditioning; functional training in self-care and home management activities, including ADL and IADL; and functional training in work (job/school/play), community, and leisure integration or reintegration, including IADL, work hardening, and work conditioning.

Factors that influence the complexity, frequency, and duration of the intervention and the decision-making process may include the following: accessibility and availability of resources; adherence to the intervention program; age; anatomical and physiological changes related to growth and development; caregiver consistency or expertise; chronicity or severity of the current condition; cognitive status; comorbidities, complications, or secondary impairments; concurrent medical, surgical, and therapeutic interventions; decline in functional independence; level of impairment; level of physical function; living environment; multisite or multisystem involvement; nutritional status; overall health status; potential discharge destinations; premorbid conditions; probability of prolonged impairment, functional limitation, or disability; psychosocial and socioeconomic factors; psychomotor abilities; social support; and stability of the condition.

Reexamination

Reexamination is the process of performing selected tests and measures after the initial examination to evaluate progress and to modify or redirect interventions. Reexamination may be indicated more than once during a single episode of care. It also may be performed over the course of a disease, disorder, or condition, which for some patients/clients may be over the life span. Indications for reexamination include new clinical findings or failure to respond to physical therapy interventions.

Outcomes

Throughout the entire episode of care, the physical therapist determines the anticipated goals and expected outcomes for each intervention. Beginning with the history, the physical therapist identifies patient/client expectations, perceived need for physical therapy services, personal goals, and desired outcomes. The physical therapist then considers whether these goals and outcomes are realistic in the context of the examination data and the evaluation. In establishing a diagnosis and a prognosis and selecting interventions, the physical therapist asks the question, "What outcome is likely, given the diagnosis? " The physical therapist may use reexamination to determine whether predicted outcomes are reasonable and then modify them as necessary.

As the patient/client reaches the termination of physical therapy services and the end of the episode of care, the physical therapist measures the global outcomes of the physical therapy services by characterizing or quantifying the impact of the physical therapy interventions on the following domains:

- Pathology/pathophysiology (disease, disorder, or condition)
- Impairments
- Functional limitations
- Disabilities
- Risk reduction/prevention
- Health, wellness, and fitness
- Societal resources
- Patient/client satisfaction

The physical therapist engages in outcomes data collection and analysis—that is, the systematic review of outcomes of care in relation to selected variables (eg, age, sex, diagnosis, interventions performed)—and develops statistical reports for internal or external use.

Episode of Care, Maintenance, or Prevention

An *episode of physical therapy care* consists of all physical therapy services that are (1) provided by a physical therapist, (2) provided in an unbroken sequence, and (3) related to the physical therapy interventions for a given condition or problem or related to a request from the patient/client, family, or other provider. A defined number or identified range of number of visits will be established for an episode of care. A visit consists of all physical therapy services provided in a 24-hour period. The episode of care may include transfers between sites within or across settings or reclassification of the patient/client from one preferred practice pattern to another. Reclassification may alter the expected range of number of visits and therefore may shorten or lengthen the episode of care. If reclassification involves a condition, problem, or request that is not related to the initial episode of care, a new episode of care may be initiated.

A single episode of care should not be confused with multiple episodes of care that may be required by certain individuals who are classified in particular patterns. For these patients/clients, periodic follow-up is needed over a lifetime to ensure optimal function and safety following changes in physical status, caregivers, the environment, or task demands.

An *episode of physical therapy maintenance* is a series of occasional clinical, educational, and administrative services related to maintenance of current function. No defined number or range of number of visits is established for this type of episode.

An *episode of physical therapy prevention* is a series of occasional clinical, educational, and administrative services related to prevention, to the promotion of health, wellness, and fitness, and to the preservation of optimal function. Prevention services; programs that promote health, wellness, and fitness; and programs for maintenance of function are a vital part of the practice of physical therapy. No defined number or range of number of visits is established for this type of episode.

Criteria for Termination of Physical Therapy Services

Two processes are used for terminating physical therapy services: discharge and discontinuation.

Discharge

Discharge is the process of ending physical therapy services that have been provided during a single episode of care, when the anticipated goals and expected outcomes have been achieved. Discharge does not occur with a transfer, that is, it does not occur when the patient is moved from one site to another site within the same setting or across settings during a single episode of care. There may be facility-specific or payer-specific requirements for documentation regarding the conclusion of physical therapy services as the patient moves between sites or across settings during the episode of care; however, discharge occurs based on the physical therapist's analysis of the achievement of anticipated goals and expected outcomes.

For patients/clients who require multiple episodes of care, periodic follow-up is needed over the life span to ensure safety and effective adaptation following changes in physical status, caregivers, environment, or task demands.

In consultation with appropriate individuals, and in consideration of the anticipated goals and expected outcomes, the physical therapist plans for discharge and provides for appropriate follow-up or referral.

Discontinuation

Discontinuation is the process of ending physical therapy services that have been provided during a single episode of care when (1) the patient/client, caregiver, or legal guardian declines to continue intervention; (2) the patient/client is unable to continue to progress toward anticipated goals and expected outcomes because of medical or psychosocial complications or because financial/insurance resources have been expended; or (3) the physical therapist determines that the patient/client will no longer benefit from physical therapy. When termination of physical therapy service occurs prior to achievement of anticipated goals and expected outcomes, patient/client status and the rationale for discontinuation are documented.

In consultation with appropriate individuals, and in consideration of the anticipated goals and expected outcomes, the physical therapist plans for discontinuation and provides for appropriate follow-up or referral.

Other Professional Roles of the Physical Therapist

Consultation

Consultation is the rendering of professional or expert opinion or advice by a physical therapist. The consulting physical therapist applies highly specialized knowledge and skills to identify problems, recommend solutions, or produce a specified outcome or product in a given amount of time on behalf of a patient/client.

Patient-related consultation is a service provided by a physical therapist at the request of a patient, another practitioner, or an organization either to recommend physical therapy services that are needed or to evaluate the quality of physical therapy services being provided. Such consultation usually does not involve actual intervention.

Client-related consultation is a service provided by a physical therapist at the request of an individual, business, school, government agency, or other organization.

Examples of consultation activities in which physical therapists may engage include:

- Advising a referring practitioner about the indications for intervention
- Advising employers about the requirements of the Americans with Disabilities Act (ADA)
- Conducting a program to determine the suitability of employees for specific job assignments
- Developing programs that evaluate the effectiveness of an intervention plan in reducing work-related injuries
- Educating other health care practitioners (eg, in injury prevention)
- Examining school environments and recommending changes to improve accessibility for students with disabilities
- Instructing employers about job preplacement in accordance with provisions of the ADA
- Participating at the local, state, and federal levels in policymaking for physical therapy services
- Performing environmental assessments to minimize the risk of falls
- Providing peer review and utilization review services
- Responding to a request for a second opinion
- Serving as an expert witness in legal proceedings
- Working with employees, labor unions, and government agencies to develop injury reduction and safety programs

Education

Education is the process of imparting information or skills and instructing by precept, example, and experience so that individuals acquire knowledge, master skills, or develop competence. In addition to instructing patients/clients as an element of intervention, physical therapists may engage in education activities such as the following:

- Planning and conducting academic education, clinical education, and continuing education programs for physical therapists, other providers, and students
- Planning and conducting education programs for local, state, and federal agencies
- Planning and conducting programs for the public to increase awareness of issues in which physical therapists have expertise

Critical Inquiry

Critical inquiry is the process of applying the principles of scientific methods to read and interpret professional literature; participate in, plan, and conduct research; evaluate outcomes data; and assess new concepts and technologies.

Examples of critical inquiry activities in which physical therapists may engage include:

- Analyzing and applying research findings to physical therapy practice and education
- Disseminating the results of research
- Evaluating the efficacy and effectiveness of both new and established interventions and technologies
- Participating in, planning, and conducting clinical, basic, or applied research

Administration

Administration is the skilled process of planning, directing, organizing, and managing human, technical, environmental, and financial resources effectively and efficiently. Administration includes the management, by individual physical therapists, of resources for patient/client management and for organizational operations.

Examples of administration activities in which physical therapists engage include:

- Ensuring fiscally sound reimbursement for services rendered
- Budgeting for physical therapy services
- Managing staff resources, including the acquisition and development of clinical expertise and leadership abilities
- Monitoring quality of care and clinical productivity
- Negotiating and managing contracts
- Supervising physical therapist assistants, physical therapy aides, and other support personnel

The Physical Therapy Service: Direction and Supervision of Personnel

Physical therapy is provided by a physical therapist or by a physical therapist assistant under the direction and supervision of a physical therapist in accordance with APTA policies, positions, guidelines, standards, and ethical principles and standards.

Direction and supervision are essential to the provision of high-quality physical therapy. The degree of direction and supervision necessary for ensuring high-quality physical therapy depends on many factors, including the education, experience, and responsibilities of the parties involved; the organizational structure in which the physical therapy is provided; and applicable state law. In any case, supervision should be readily available to the individual being supervised.

The director of a physical therapy service is a physical therapist who has demonstrated qualifications based on education and experience in the field of physical therapy and who has accepted the inherent responsibilities of the role. The director of a physical therapy service must:

- Establish guidelines and procedures that will delineate the functions and responsibilities of all levels of physical therapy personnel in the service and the supervisory relationships inherent to the functions of the service and the organization
- Ensure that the objectives of the service are efficiently and effectively achieved within the framework of the stated purpose of the organization and in accordance with safe physical therapist practice
- Ensure that services provided are in accordance with established policies and procedures
- Ensure compliance with local, state, and federal regulation
- Ensure compliance with APTA policies, positions, guidelines, standards, and ethical principles and standards, including *Standards of Practice for Physical Therapy and the Criteria*, *Guide to Physical Therapist Practice*, *Code of Ethics*, *Guide for Professional Conduct*, *Standards of Ethical Conduct for the Physical Therapist Assistant*, and *Guide for Conduct of the Affiliate Member*
- Foster the professional growth of the staff

Written practice and performance criteria should be available for all levels of personnel in a physical therapy service. Regularly scheduled performance appraisals should be conducted by the supervisor based on applicable standards of practice and performance criteria.

Responsibilities should be commensurate with the qualifications—including experience, education, and training—of the individuals to whom the responsibilities are assigned. When the physical therapist of record directs and supervises physical therapist assistants to perform specific components of physical therapy interventions, that physical therapist remains responsible for supervision of the plan of care. Regardless of the setting in which the services are given, the following responsibilities must be borne solely by the physical therapist:

- Interpretation of referrals when available
- Initial examination, evaluation, diagnosis, and prognosis
- Development or modification of a plan of care that is based on the initial examination or the reexamination and that includes physical therapy anticipated goals and expected outcomes
- Determination of (1) when the expertise and decision-making capability of the physical therapist requires the physical therapist to personally render physical therapy interventions and (2) when it may be appropriate to utilize the physical therapist assistant. A physical therapist determines the most appropriate utilization of the physical therapist assistant that will ensure the delivery of service that is safe, effective, and efficient.
- Provision of physical therapy interventions
- Reexamination of the patient/client in light of the anticipated goals and expected outcomes, and revision of the plan of care when indicated
- Establishment of the discharge plan and documentation of discharge summary/status
- Oversight of all documentation for services rendered to each patient

References

1 Nagi S. Some conceptual issues in disability and rehabilitation. In: Sussman M, ed. *Sociology and Rehabilitation*. Washington, DC: American Sociological Association; 1965:100-113.

2 Nagi S. *Disability and Rehabilitation*. Columbus, Ohio: Ohio State University Press; 1969.

3 Nagi S. Disability concepts revisited: implications for prevention. In: Pope A, Tarlov A, eds. *Disability in America: Toward a National Agenda for Prevention*. Washington, DC: Institute of Medicine, National Academy Press; 1991.

4 Guccione AA. Physical therapy diagnosis and the relationship between impairments and function. *Phys Ther.* 1991;71:499-504.

5 Defining *Primary Care: An Interim Report*. Washington, DC: Institute of Medicine, National Academy Press; 1995.

6 Guccione AA. *Geriatric Physical Therapy, 2nd ed.* St Louis, Mo: Mosby; 2000.

CHAPTER 2

Corresponds to "Tests/Measures" in the Interactive Guide CD-ROM

What Types of Tests and Measures Do Physical Therapists Use?

Introduction

Tests and measures are the means of gathering information about the patient/client. Depending on the data generated during the history and systems review, the physical therapist may use one or more tests and measures, in whole or in part:

- To help identify and characterize signs and symptoms of pathology/pathophysiology, impairments, functional limitations, and disabilities
- To establish the diagnosis and the prognosis, to select interventions, and to document changes in patient/client status
- To indicate achievement of the outcomes that are the end points of care and thereby ensure timely and appropriate discharge. Physical therapists may perform more than one test or obtain more than one measurement at a time.

Physical therapists individualize the selection of tests and measures based on the history they take and systems review they perform, rather than basing their selection on a previously determined medical diagnosis. When examining a patient/client with impairments, functional limitations, or disabilities resulting from brain injury, for instance, the physical therapist may decide to perform part or all of several tests and measures, based on the signs and symptoms of that particular patient.

What Is Measurement?

Obtaining measurements is an everyday part of physical therapist practice. APTA's *Standards for Tests and Measurements in Physical Therapy Practice*[1] state that a measurement is the "numeral assigned to an object, event, or person or the class (category) to which an object, event, or person is assigned according to rules." Physical therapists obtain many different types of measurements. Assessing the magnitude of a patient's report of pain, quantifying muscle performance or range of motion, describing the various characteristics of a patient's gait pattern, categorizing the assistance that a patient requires to dress—all of these are *measurements*.

The physical therapist collects data through many different methods, such as interviewing; observation; questionnaires; palpation; auscultation; conducting performance-based assessments; electrophysiological testing; taking photographs and making other videographic recordings; recording data using scales, indexes, and inventories; obtaining data through the use of technology-assisted devices; administering patient/client self-assessment tests; and reviewing patient/client diaries and logs.

Physical therapists use tests and measures to obtain measurements, which they then interpret to identify:

- *Signs and symptoms of pathology/pathophysiology (disease, disorder, or condition)*, such as joint tenderness, pain, elevated blood pressure with activity, numbness and tingling, and edema
- *Impairments*, such as aerobic capacity; anthropometric characteristics; arousal, attention, and cognition; circulation; cranial and peripheral nerve integrity; ergonomics and body mechanics; gait, locomotion, and balance; integumentary integrity; joint integrity and mobility; motor function; muscle performance; neuromotor development and sensory integration; posture; range of motion; reflex integrity; sensory integrity; and ventilation and respiration/gas exchange
- *Functional limitations*, such as work (job/school/play), community, and leisure integration or reintegration (including instrumental activities of daily living), ergonomics and body mechanics, and self-care and home management (including activities of daily living and instrumental activities of daily living)
- *Disabilities*, such as inability to engage in community, leisure, social, and work roles
- *Device and equipment need and use*, such as assistive and adaptive devices; orthotic, protective, and supportive devices; and prosthetic devices
- *Barriers*, such as environmental, home, and work (job/school/play) barriers

In the evaluation process, the physical therapist synthesizes the examination data to establish the diagnosis and prognosis (including the plan of care). The data gathered through the use of tests and measures during initial examination provide information used for determining anticipated goals and expected outcomes. These data may indicate initial abilities in performing actions, tasks, and activities; establish criteria for placement decisions; and identify level of safety in performing a particular task or risk of injury with continued performance with or without devices and equipment. Reexamination at regular intervals during an episode of care enables the physical therapist to measure and document changes in patient/client status and the progress that the patient/client is making toward the anticipated goals and expected outcomes.

Whenever possible, physical therapists should use measurements whose reliability and validity have been documented in the peer-reviewed literature. Reliable and valid measurements enable physical therapists to gauge the certainty of their examination data and the appropriate scope of inferences that may be drawn from those data. Reliability and validity are properties of a measurement, not of the test or measure that is used to obtain the measurement. A measurement is reliable only under certain conditions and for certain types of patients/clients and is valid only for a particular purpose.

Reliability and validity have not yet been reported for every measurement used by physical therapists. Use of measurements without established reliability and validity may be appropriate, however, especially when there are no alternatives—and provided that the physical therapist is aware that those measurements may be prone to error and that, therefore, decisions made using those measurements may be less certain.

Reliability of Measurements

Assessing a measurement's reliability is an attempt to identify sources of error.[2(p73-74)] A measurement is said to be reliable when it is consistent time after time, with as little variation as possible. Because all measurements have *some* error, however, the clinician must determine whether a measurement is useful or whether there is so much error that the measurement is rendered useless for a particular purpose.

Two major types of reliability—test-retest and intratester/intertester—help determine how much error exists in a measurement. *Test-retest reliability* is the consistency of repeated measurements that are separated in time when there is no change in what is being measured; test-retest reliability indicates the stability of a measurement. *Intrarater reliability* indicates the degree to which measurements that are obtained by the same physical therapist at different times will be consistent. *Interrater reliability* indicates the degree to which measurements obtained by multiple therapists will be consistent.[1] Interrater reliability is especially important—if different physical therapists obtain different measurements when measuring the same phenomenon, the usefulness of the measurements is limited.

There are two other forms of reliability: *parallel-form reliability*, which relates to measurements that are obtained by using different versions of the same test or measure, and *internal consistency*, or homogeneity, which relates to measurements that are obtained by using tests or measures with multiple items or parts, where each part is supposed to measure one, and only one, concept.[1]

Validity of Measurements

Validity is the "degree to which a useful (meaningful) interpretation can be inferred from a measurement."[1]

There are many forms of validity, including face validity, content validity, construct validity, concurrent validity, and predictive validity.

Face validity exists when the measurement seems to reflect what is supposed to be measured—but it does not depend on evidence. Goniometric measurements, for instance, have face validity as measurements of joint position.

Content validity establishes the degree to which a measurement reflects the domain of interest. For example, an instrument that is used to assess joint pain might generate data only regarding pain on motion, not pain at rest or factors that aggravate or alleviate pain.

Construct validity is a theoretical form of validity that is established on the basis of evidence that a measurement represents the underlying concept of what is to be measured.[1] For example, the overall concept of "motor function" is the construct that underlies any particular test or measure of motor function. There are no direct tests of construct validity. Theoretical evidence of construct validity is often provided by demonstrating *convergence* if tests or measures believed to represent the same construct are highly related. For example, a test of motor function, based on a particular concept of what "motor function" means, should correlate highly with other tests or measures based on similar conceptions of "motor function" or on concepts that are closely related to "motor function," such as "dexterity" and "coordination." Evidence of construct validity is also found when there is a low association, or *divergence*, between a test or measure of one particular construct and other tests or measures reflecting distinctly different, or even unrelated, constructs. For example, there should be a low association between a test or measure of "motor function" and tests and measures that are based on the concepts of "aerobic conditioning" or "range of motion."

Concurrent validity exists when "an inferred interpretation is justified by comparing a measurement with supporting evidence that was obtained at approximately the same time as the measurement being validated."[1] The developers of a new balance test might compare the measurements obtained using the new test to those obtained using an established balance test involving one-legged stance. The comparative method of establishing concurrent validity is particularly relevant for self-assessment instruments.

Predictive validity exists when "an inferred interpretation is justified by comparing a measurement with supporting evidence that is obtained at a later point in time" and "examines the justification of using a measurement to say something about future events or conditions."[1] The predictive validity of a measurement of functional capacity might be established by verifying whether the measurement indicates the likelihood of return to work. Knowing the predictive validity of a measurement may facilitate the identification of achievable outcomes and increase the efficiency of discharge planning.

Predictive validity also may provide the physical therapist with several kinds of information about the value of selecting particular tests or measures for the examination. The *sensitivity* of a measurement indicates the proportion of individuals with a positive finding who already have or will have a particular characteristic or outcome.[1,3,4] In other words, sensitivity is the positive predictive validity of the measurement. In contrast, the *specificity* of a measurement indicates the proportion of people who have a negative finding on a test or measure who truly do not or will not have a particular characteristic or outcome.[1,3,4] Thus, specificity is the negative predictive validity of the test or measure.

Clinical Utility

In addition to reliability and validity of the measurements obtained with a given test or measure, a physical therapist considers the clinical utility of the test or measure for a particular purpose. Physical therapists should consider the precision of the data yielded by a test or measure and whether it will meet the needs of the situation. Some measurements are only gross measurements. Gross measurements may be useful for a population screen but may not be useful for identifying a small change in patient/client status after intervention. The measurements used by the physical therapist should always be sensitive enough to detect the degree of change expected as a result of intervention. The physical therapist also should consider the time involved in administering a test or measure, the cost of administering it, and such patient/client factors as tolerance of testing positions and suitability of the test or measure to a particular population.

Guide Categories for Tests and Measures

This chapter contains 24 categories of tests and measures (Figure) that the physical therapist may decide to use during an examination. Tests and measures are listed in alphabetical order. In Part Two, each preferred practice pattern contains a list of tests and measures that are used in the examination of patients/clients who are classified in the diagnostic group for that pattern. Part Three of the Guide, available on CD-ROM, provides available information on tests and measures used by physical therapists, including the reliability and validity of measurements that are obtained using those tests and measures. Physical therapists may decide to use other tests and measures that are not described in the Guide, following the principles stated in the *Standards for Tests and Measurements in Physical Therapy Practice*.[1]

Each categorization of tests and measures includes:

- *General definition and purpose of the test and measure*. A definition and purpose of the test and measure is provided. All tests and measures produce information used to identify the possible or actual causes of difficulties during performance of essential everyday activities, work tasks, and leisure pursuits. Selection of tests and measures depends on the findings of the history and systems review. The examination findings may indicate, for instance, that tests should be conducted while the patient/client performs specific activities. In all cases, the purpose of tests and measures is to ensure the gathering of information that will lead to evaluation, diagnosis, prognosis, and selection of appropriate interventions.
- *Clinical indications*. Examples of clinical indications that are identified during the history and systems review are provided to indicate the use of tests and measures. Special requirements may prompt the phys-

The patient/client management elements of examination, evaluation, diagnosis, and prognosis should be represented and reimbursed as physical therapy only when they are performed by a physical therapist. The patient/client management element of intervention should be represented and reimbursed as physical therapy only when performed by a physical therapist or by a physical therapist assistant performing selected interventions under the direction and supervision of a physical therapist in accordance with APTA positions, policies, standards, codes, and guidelines. Physical therapists are the only professionals who provide physical therapy interventions. Physical therapist assistants are the only individuals who provide selected physical therapy interventions under the direction and supervision of the physical therapist. Note: The terms "physical therapy" and "physiotherapy," and the terms "physical therapist" and "physiotherapist," are synonymous.

Figure. Guide Categories for Tests and Measures

Aerobic Capacity/Endurance
Anthropometric Characteristics
Arousal, Attention, and Cognition
Assistive and Adaptive Devices
Circulation (Arterial, Venous, Lymphatic)
Cranial and Peripheral Nerve Integrity
Environmental, Home, and Work (Job/School/Play) Barriers
Ergonomics and Body Mechanics
Gait, Locomotion, and Balance
Integumentary Integrity
Joint Integrity and Mobility
Motor Function (Motor Control and Motor Learning)
Muscle Performance (Including Strength, Power, and Endurance)
Neuromotor Development and Sensory Integration
Orthotic, Protective, and Supportive Devices
Pain
Posture
Prosthetic Requirements
Range of Motion (Including Muscle Length)
Reflex Integrity
Self-Care and Home Management (Including Activities of Daily Living and Instrumental Activities of Daily Living)
Sensory Integrity
Ventilation and Respiration/Gas Exchange
Work (Job/School/Play), Community, and Leisure Integration or Reintegration (Including Instrumental Activities of Daily Living)

ical therapist to perform tests and measures. All tests and measures are appropriate in the presence of:

- impairment, functional limitation, disability, developmental delay, injury, or suspected or identified pathology that prevents or alters performance of daily activities, including self-care, home management, work (job/school/play), community, and leisure actions, tasks, or activities
- requirements of employment that specify minimum capacity for performance
- identified risk factors
- need to initiate programs that promote health, wellness, or fitness

• *Tests and measures* (methods and techniques). Examples of specific tests and measures are provided.

• *Tools used for gathering data.* A listing of tools used for collecting data is provided.

• *Data generated.* Types of data that may be generated from the tests and measures are listed.

Other information that may be required for the examination includes findings of other professionals; results of diagnostic imaging, clinical laboratory, and electrophysiological studies; federal, state, and local work surveillance and safety reports and announcements; and the reported observations of family members, significant others, caregivers, and other interested people.

References

1 American Physical Therapy Association. Standards for Tests and Measurements in Physical Therapy Practice. *Phys Ther*. 1991;71:589-622.

2 Rothstein JM, Echternach JL. *Primer on Measurement: An Introductory Guide to Measurement Issues.* Alexandria, Va: American Physical Therapy Association; 1993.

3 Jaeschke R, Guyatt GH, Sackett DL. Users' guides to the medical literature. III. How to use an article about a diagnostic test. B. What are the results and how will they help me in caring for my patients? The Evidence-Based Medicine Working Group. *JAMA*. 1994;271:703-707.

4 Sackett DL, Straus SE, Richardson WS, et al. *Evidence-Based Medicine: How to Practice and Teach EBM.* 2nd ed. New York, NY: Churchill Livingstone Inc; 2000.

Tests and Measures

Aerobic Capacity/Endurance

Aerobic capacity/endurance is the ability to perform work or participate in activity over time using the body's oxygen uptake, delivery, and energy release mechanisms. During activity, the physical therapist uses tests and measures ranging from simple measurements to complex calculations to determine the appropriateness of patient/client responses to increased oxygen demand. Responses that are monitored both at rest and during and after activity may indicate the degree of severity of the impairment, functional limitation, or disability. Results of tests and measures of aerobic capacity/endurance are integrated with the history and systems review findings and the results of other tests and measures. All of these data are then synthesized during the evaluation process to establish the diagnosis, the prognosis, and the plan of care, which includes the selection of interventions. The results of these tests and measures may indicate the need to use or recommend other tests and measures or the need to consult with, or refer the patient/client to, another professional.

Clinical Indications

Clinical indications for the use of tests and measures are predicated on the history and systems review findings (eg, information provided by the patient/client, family, significant other, or caregiver; symptoms described by the patient/client; signs observed and documented during the systems review; and information derived from other sources and records). The findings may indicate the presence of or risk for pathology/pathophysiology (disease, disorder, or condition), impairments, functional limitations, or disabilities that require a more definitive examination through the selection of tests and measures of aerobic capacity/endurance. Clinical indications for these tests and measures may include:

- *Pathology/pathophysiology (disease, disorder, or condition) in the following systems:*
  - cardiovascular (eg, cerebral vascular accident, coronary artery disease, peripheral vascular disease)
  - endocrine/metabolic (eg, osteoporosis)
  - multiple systems (eg, AIDS, trauma)
  - musculoskeletal (eg, arthritis)
  - neuromuscular (eg, cerebral palsy, Parkinson disease)
  - pulmonary (eg, emphysema, pulmonary fibrosis)
- *Impairments in the following categories:*
  - circulation (eg, abnormal heart rate, rhythm, blood pressure)
  - muscle performance (eg, generalized muscle weakness, decreased muscle endurance)
  - posture (eg, abnormal body alignment)
  - range of motion (eg, asymmetrical chest wall motion, thorax tightness)
  - ventilation and respiration/gas exchange (eg, abnormal respiratory pattern, rate, rhythm)
- *Functional limitations in the ability to perform actions, tasks, and activities in the following categories:*
  - self-care (eg, inability to perform shower or overhead activities because of shortness of breath)
  - home management (eg, inability to vacuum or make the bed because of chest discomfort)
  - work (job/school/play) (eg, inability to keep up with peers during recess, inability as a parent to carry a child up the stairs because of increasing sense of fatigue, inability to perform overhead lifting tasks because of shortness of breath)
  - community/leisure (eg, inability to walk to religious activities because of shortness of breath, difficulty with gardening because of chest discomfort)
- *Disability—that is, the inability or the restricted ability to perform actions, tasks, or activities of required roles within the individual's sociocultural context—in the following categories:*
  - self-care
  - home management
  - work (job/school/play)
  - community/leisure
- *Risk factors for impaired aerobic capacity:*
  - family history of cardiovascular or pulmonary disease
  - obesity
  - sedentary lifestyle
  - smoking history
- *Health, wellness, and fitness needs:*
  - fitness, including physical performance (eg, submaximal oxygen uptake for age and sex, submaximal running efficiency for sprint)
  - health and wellness (eg, incomplete understanding of role of aerobic capacity/endurance during activities)

Aerobic Capacity/Endurance continued

Tests and Measures

Tests and measures may include those that characterize or quantify:

- Aerobic capacity during functional activities (eg, activities of daily living [ADL] scales, indexes, instrumental activities of daily living [IADL] scales, observations)
- Aerobic capacity during standardized exercise test protocols (eg, ergometry, step tests, time/distance walk/run tests, treadmill tests, wheelchair tests)
- Cardiovascular signs and symptoms in response to increased oxygen demand with exercise or activity, including pressures and flow; heart rate, rhythm, and sounds; and superficial vascular responses (eg, angina, claudication and exertion scales; electrocardiography; observations; palpation; sphygmomanometry)
- Pulmonary signs and symptoms in response to increased oxygen demand with exercise or activity, including breath and voice sounds; cyanosis; gas exchange; respiratory pattern, rate, and rhythm; and ventilatory flow, force, and volume (eg, auscultation, dyspnea and exertion scales, gas analyses, observations, oximetry, palpation, pulmonary function tests)

Tools Used for Gathering Data

Tools for gathering data may include:

- Devices for gas analysis
- Electrocardiographs
- Ergometers
- Force meters
- Indexes
- Measured walkways
- Nomograms
- Observations
- Palpation
- Pulse oximeters
- Scales
- Sphygmomanometers
- Spirometers
- Steps
- Stethoscopes
- Stop watches
- Treadmills

Data Generated

Data are used in providing documentation and may include:

- Cardiovascular and pulmonary signs, symptoms, and responses per unit of work
- Gas volume, concentration, and flow per unit of work
- Heart rate, rhythm, and sounds per unit of work
- Oxygen uptake during functional activity
- Oxygen uptake, time and distance walked or bicycled, and maximum aerobic performance
- Peripheral vascular responses per unit of work
- Respiratory rate, rhythm, pattern, and breath sounds per unit of work

Tests and Measures

Anthropometric Characteristics

Anthropometric characteristics are those traits that describe body dimensions, such as height, weight, girth, and body fat composition. The physical therapist uses tests and measures to quantify these traits. Results of tests and measures of anthropometric characteristics are integrated with the history and systems review findings and the results of other tests and measures. All of these data are then synthesized during the evaluation process to establish the diagnosis, the prognosis, and the plan of care, which includes the selection of interventions. The results of these tests and measures may indicate the need to use or recommend other tests and measures or the need to consult with, or refer the patient/client to, another professional.

Clinical Indications

Clinical indications for tests and measures are predicated on the history and systems review findings (eg, information provided by the patient/client, family, significant other, or caregiver; symptoms described by the patient/client; signs observed and documented during the systems review; and information derived from other sources and records). The findings may indicate the presence of or risk for pathology/pathophysiology (disease, disorder, or condition), impairments, functional limitations, or disabilities that require a more definitive examination through the selection of tests and measures of anthropometric characteristics. Clinical indications for these tests and measures may include:

- *Pathology/pathophysiology (disease, disorder, or condition) in the following systems:*
  - cardiovascular (eg, ascites, lymphedema)
  - genitourinary (eg, pregnancy)
  - multiple systems (eg, AIDS, cancer)
  - musculoskeletal (eg, amputation, muscular dystrophy)
  - neuromuscular (eg, prematurity, spinal cord injury)
  - pulmonary (eg, cystic fibrosis)

- *Impairments in the following categories:*
  - circulation (eg, abnormal blood pressure, abnormal fluid distribution)
  - muscle performance (eg, generalized muscle weakness)
  - neuromotor development (eg, abnormal growth rate)
  - range of motion (eg, abnormal fluid distribution)
  - ventilation and respiration (eg, abnormal rate and rhythm)

- *Functional limitations in the ability to perform actions, tasks, or fixed activities in the following categories:*
  - self-care (eg, inability to dress and reach because of abnormal fat or fluid distribution)
  - home management (eg, inability to get down on knees to clean floor because of weight abnormality)
  - work (job/school/play) (eg, inability to assume parenting role because of impaired fluid distribution from pregnancy, inability to gain access to classroom environment because of delayed growth, inability to perform filing tasks because of decreased range of motion and muscle weakness)
  - community/leisure (eg, inability to fish because of generalized muscle weakness, inability to participate in amateur sports because of edema, inability to participate in social activities because of perceived body image as a result of impaired fluid distribution)

- *Disability—that is, the inability or the restricted ability to perform actions, tasks, or activities of required roles within the individual's sociocultural context—in the following categories:*
  - self-care
  - home management
  - work (job/school/play)
  - community/leisure

- *Risk factors for impaired anthropometric characteristics:*
  - anorexia
  - obesity

- *Health, wellness, and fitness needs:*
  - fitness, including physical performance (eg, inefficient sprinting because of excess body fat, limited endurance for long-distance hiking because of inappropriate body composition)
  - health and wellness (eg, incomplete understanding of the relationship between nutrition and body composition)

Anthropometric Characteristics continued

Tests and Measures

Tests and measures may include those that characterize or quantify:

- Body composition (eg, body mass index, impedance measurement, skinfold thickness measurement)
- Body dimensions (eg, girth measurement, length measurement)
- Edema (eg, girth measurement, palpation, scales, volume measurement)

Tools Used for Gathering Data

Tools for gathering data may include:

- Body mass index
- Calipers
- Cameras and photographs
- Impedance devices
- Nomograms
- Palpation
- Rulers
- Scales
- Tape measures
- Volumometers
- Weight scales

Data Generated

Data are used in providing documentation and may include:

- Height and weight
- Presence and severity of abnormal body fluid distribution

Arousal, Attention, and Cognition

Arousal is a state of responsiveness to stimulation or action or of physiological readiness for activity. *Attention* is the selective awareness of the environment or selective responsiveness to stimuli. *Cognition* is the act or process of knowing, including both awareness and judgment. The physical therapist uses tests and measures to characterize the patient's/client's responsiveness. Results of tests and measures of arousal, attention, and cognition are integrated with the history and systems review findings and the results of other tests and measures. All of these data are then synthesized during the evaluation process to establish the diagnosis, the prognosis, and the plan of care, which includes the selection of interventions. The results of these tests and measures may indicate the need to use or recommend other tests and measures or the need to consult with, or refer the patient/client to, another professional.

Clinical Indications

Clinical indications for the use of tests and measures are predicated on the history and systems review findings (eg, information provided by the patient/client, family, significant other, or caregiver; symptoms described by the patient/client; signs observed and documented during the systems review; and information derived from other sources and records). The findings may indicate the presence of or risk for pathology/pathophysiology (disease, disorder, or condition), impairments, functional limitations, or disabilities that require a more definitive examination through the selection of tests and measures of arousal, attention, and cognition. Clinical indications for these tests and measures may include:

- *Pathology/pathophysiology (disease, disorder, or condition) in the following systems:*
  - cardiovascular (eg, malignant hypertension, cerebral vascular accident)
  - multiple systems (eg, Down syndrome)
  - neuromuscular (eg, hydrocephalus, traumatic brain injury)
  - pulmonary (eg, end-stage chronic obstructive pulmonary disease)
- *Impairments in the following categories:*
  - arousal (eg, lack of response to stimulation)
  - circulation (eg, abnormal blood pressure in shock)
  - cognition (eg, inability to follow instructions)
  - motor function (eg, inability to plan and carry out movement)
  - ventilation and respiration (eg, hypoventilation, somnolence)
- *Functional limitations in the ability to perform actions, tasks, or activities in the following categories:*
  - self-care (eg, inability to perform bathroom transfers because of lack of safety awareness)
  - home management (eg, decreased environmental mobility in the home because of lack of safety awareness)
  - work (job/school/play) (eg, inability to perform bricklaying because of inability to recall steps of task, inability to play at age-appropriate level because of lack of internal desire to move)
  - community/leisure (eg, inability to participate as volunteer at child's school because of inattention, inability to participate in routine exercise program because of lack of interest)
- *Disability—that is, the inability or the restricted ability to perform actions, tasks, or activities of required roles within the individual's sociocultural context—in the following categories:*
  - self-care
  - home management
  - work (job/school/play)
  - community/leisure
- *Risk factors for impaired arousal, attention, and cognition*
  - inability to manage stress
  - lack of motivation
  - poor attitude
- *Health, wellness, and fitness needs:*
  - fitness, including physical performance (eg, impaired judgment during workout, ineffective attention and recall for complete training regimen)
  - health and wellness (eg, incomplete understanding of the role of attention to safety during activities)

Arousal, Attention, and Cognition continued

Tests and Measures

Tests and measures may include those that characterize or quantify:

- Arousal and attention (eg, adaptability tests, arousal and awareness scales, indexes, profiles, questionnaires)
- Cognition, including ability to process commands (eg, developmental inventories, indexes, interviews, mental state scales, observations, questionnaires, safety checklists)
- Communication (eg, functional communication profiles, interviews, inventories, observations, questionnaires)
- Consciousness, including agitation and coma (eg, scales)
- Motivation (eg, adaptive behavior scales)
- Orientation to time, person, place, and situation (eg, attention tests, learning profiles, mental state scales)
- Recall, including memory and retention (eg, assessment scales, interviews, questionnaires)

Tools Use for Data Collection

Tools for gathering data may include:

- Adaptability tests
- Attention tests
- Indexes
- Interviews
- Inventories
- Observations
- Profiles
- Questionnaires
- Safety checklists
- Scales
- Screening tests

Data Generated

Data are used in providing documentation and may include:

- Descriptions of short-term and long-term memory
- Presence and severity of:
  - cognitive impairment
  - coma
  - communication deficits
  - depression or impaired motivation
  - impaired consciousness
- Quantifications or characterization of:
  - ability to attend to task or to participate
  - ability to recognize time, person, place, and situation

Assistive and Adaptive Devices

Assistive and *adaptive devices* are implements and equipment used to aid patients/clients in performing tasks or movements. Assistive devices include crutches, canes, walkers, wheelchairs, power devices, long-handled reachers, percussors, static and dynamic splints, and vibrators. *Adaptive devices* include raised toilet seats, seating systems, and environmental controls. The physical therapist uses tests and measures to determine whether a patient/client might benefit from such a device or, when such a device already is in use, to assess how well the patient/client performs with it. Results of tests and measures of assistive and adaptive devices are integrated with the history and systems review findings and the results of other tests and measures. All of these data are then synthesized during the evaluation process to establish the diagnosis, the prognosis, and the plan of care, which includes the selection of interventions. The results of these tests and measures may indicate the need to use or recommend other tests and measures or the need to consult with, or refer the patient/client to, another professional.

Clinical Indications

Clinical indications for the use of tests and measures are predicated on the history and systems review findings (eg, information provided by the patient/client, family, significant other, or caregiver; symptoms described by the patient/client; signs observed and documented during the systems review; and information derived from other sources and records). The findings may indicate the presence of or risk for pathology/pathophysiology (disease, disorder, or condition), impairments, functional limitations, or disabilities that require a more definitive examination through the selection of tests and measures of assistive and adaptive devices. Clinical indications for these tests and measures may include:

- *Pathology/pathophysiology (disease, disorder, or condition) in the following systems:*
  - cardiovascular (eg, cerebral vascular accident, coronary artery disease)
  - endocrine/metabolic (eg, diabetes)
  - integumentary (eg, surgical wound, vascular ulcer)
  - multiple systems (eg, sarcoidosis, trauma)
  - musculoskeletal (eg, arthritis, sprain, strain)
  - neuromuscular (eg, cerebral palsy, spina bifida, spinal cord injury)
  - pulmonary (eg, amyotrophic lateral sclerosis, respiratory failure)
- *Impairments in the following categories:*
  - aerobic capacity (eg, decreased endurance)
  - gait, locomotion, and balance (eg, frequent falls)
  - motor function (eg, inability to sit)
  - muscle performance (eg, weakness)
  - range of motion (eg, pain on reaching)
- *Functional limitations in the ability to perform actions, tasks, or activities in following categories:*
  - self-care (eg, inability to dress because of difficulty with sitting)
  - home management (eg, inability to remove items from closet shelf because of limited range of motion)
  - work (job/school/play) (eg, difficulty with keyboarding because of pain, inability to attend school because of lack of endurance, inability to get to work because of distance that must be traveled to work site)
  - community/leisure (eg, inability to walk on uneven surfaces because of altered balance)
- *Disability—that is, the inability or the restricted ability to perform actions, tasks, or activities of required roles within the individual's sociocultural context—in the following categories:*
  - self-care
  - home management
  - work (job/school/play)
  - community/leisure
- *Risk factor for improper use or lack of use of assistive and adaptive devices*
  - inactivity
- *Health, wellness, and fitness needs:*
  - fitness, including physical performance (eg, inability to participate in wheelchair sports, poor wheelchair tolerance because of inadequate fit)
  - health and wellness (eg, in adequate knowledge of how to regularly assess devices)

Assistive and Adaptive Devices continued

Tests and Measures

Tests and measures may include those that characterize or quantify:

- Assistive or adaptive devices and equipment use during functional activities (eg, activities of daily living [ADL], functional scales, instrumental activities of daily living [IADL] scales, interviews, observations)
- Components, alignment, fit, and ability to care for the assistive or adaptive devices and equipment (eg, interviews, logs, observations, pressure-sensing maps, reports)
- Remediation of impairments, functional limitations, or disabilities with use of assistive or adaptive devices and equipment (eg, activity status indexes, ADL scales, aerobic capacity tests, functional performance inventories, health assessment questionnaires, IADL scales, pain scales, play scales, videographic assessments)
- Safety during use of assistive or adaptive devices and equipment (eg, diaries, fall scales, interviews, logs, observations, reports)

Tools Used for Gathering Data

Tools for gathering data may include:

- Activity status indexes
- Aerobic capacity tests
- Diaries
- Functional performance inventories
- Health assessment questionnaires
- Interviews
- Logs
- Observations
- Pressure-sensing devices
- Reports
- Scales
- Video cameras and videotapes

Data Generated

Data are used in providing documentation and may include:

- Descriptions of:
  - alignment and fit of devices and equipment
  - ability to use and care for devices and equipment
  - components of assistive and adaptive devices and equipment
  - level of safety with devices and equipment
  - practicality of devices and equipment
  - remediation of impairment, functional limitation, or disability with devices and equipment
- Quantifications of:
  - movement patterns with or without devices and equipment
  - physiological and functional effect and benefit of devices and equipment

Circulation (Arterial, Venous, Lymphatic)

Circulation is the movement of blood through organs and tissues to deliver oxygen and to remove carbon dioxide and the passive movement (drainage) of lymph through channels, organs, and tissues for removal of cellular byproducts and inflammatory wastes. The physical therapist uses the results of circulation tests and measures to determine whether the patient/client has adequate cardiovascular pump, circulation, oxygen delivery, and lymphatic drainage systems to meet the body's demands at rest and with activity. Results of tests and measures of circulation (arterial, venous, lymphatic) are integrated with the history and systems review findings and the results of other tests and measures. All of these data are then synthesized during the evaluation process to establish the diagnosis, the prognosis, and the plan of care, which includes the selection of interventions. The results of these tests and measures may indicate the need to use or recommend other tests and measures or the need to consult with, or refer the patient/client to, another professional.

Clinical Indications

Clinical indications for the use of tests and measures are predicated on the history and systems review findings (eg, information provided by the patient/client, family, significant other, or caregiver; symptoms described by the patient/client; signs observed and documented during the systems review; and information derived from other sources and records). The findings may indicate the presence of or risk for pathology/pathophysiology (disease, disorder, or condition), impairments, functional limitations, or disabilities that require a more definitive examination through the selection of tests and measures of circulation (arterial, venous, lymphatic). Clinical indications for these tests and measures may include:

- *Pathology/pathophysiology (disease, disorder, or condition) in the following systems:*
  - cardiovascular (eg, atherosclerosis, coronary artery bypass graft, lymphedema)
  - endocrine/metabolic (eg, diabetes, reflex sympathetic dystrophy)
  - genitourinary (eg, renal failure)
  - integumentary (eg, cellulitis, lymphadenitis)
  - multiple systems (eg, cancer, trauma)
  - musculoskeletal (eg, fracture)
  - neuromuscular (eg, multiple sclerosis, spinal cord injury)
- *Impairments in the following categories:*
  - aerobic capacity (eg, shortness of breath)
  - circulation (eg, swollen feet)
  - gait, locomotion, and balance (eg, dizziness on rising from sitting to standing position)
  - muscle performance (eg, palpitations on stair climb)
  - ventilation and respiration (eg, shortness of breath at night)
- *Functional limitations in the ability to perform actions, tasks, or activities in the following categories:*
  - self-care (eg, difficulty with eating because of indigestion)
  - home management (eg, inability to mow lawn because of leg cramps)
  - work (job/school/play) (eg, difficulty with loading cargo because of shortness of breath, inability to support family financially because of shortness of breath with manual labor)
  - community/leisure (eg, inability to play tennis because of chest and shoulder pain, inability to walk to the senior center because of leg pain)
- *Disability—that is, the inability or the restricted ability to perform actions, tasks, or activities of required roles within the individual's sociocultural context—in the following categories:*
  - self-care
  - home management
  - work (job/school/play)
  - community/leisure
- *Risk factors for impaired circulation:*
  - obesity
  - positive family history of cardiovascular disease
  - sedentary lifestyle
  - smoking history
- *Health, wellness, and fitness needs:*
  - fitness, including physical performance (eg, inadequate circulation for cross-country skiing, inadequate protection of extremities during extended activities in cold weather)
  - health and wellness (eg, incomplete understanding of importance of motion to circulation)

Circulation (Arterial, Venous, Lymphatic) continued

Tests and Measures

Tests and measures may include those that characterize or quantify:

- Cardiovascular signs, including heart rate, rhythm, and sounds; pressures and flow; and superficial vascular responses (eg, auscultation, electrocardiography, girth measurement, observations, palpation, sphygmomanometry, thermography)
- Cardiovascular symptoms (eg, angina, claudication, and perceived exertion scales)
- Physiological responses to position change, including autonomic responses, central and peripheral pressures, heart rate and rhythm, respiratory rate and rhythm, ventilatory pattern (eg, auscultation, electrocardiography, observations, palpation, sphygmomanometry)

Tools Used for Gathering Data

Tools for gathering data may include:

- Doppler ultrasonographs
- Electrocardiographs
- Observations
- Palpation
- Scales
- Sphygmomanometers
- Stethoscopes
- Tape measures
- Thermographs
- Tilt tables

Data Generated

Data are used in providing documentation and may include:

- Characterizations of:
  - central pressure and volume
  - intracranial pressure responses
  - physiological responses to position change
- Descriptions of:
  - peripheral arterial circulation
  - peripheral lymphatic circulation
  - peripheral venous circulation
  - skin color
  - nail changes
- Presence of bruits
- Presence and severity of:
  - abnormal heart sounds
  - abnormal heart rate or rhythm at rest
  - cardiovascular signs and symptoms
  - edema
- Quantifications of cardiovascular pump demand
- Vital signs at rest

Cranial and Peripheral Nerve Integrity

Cranial nerve integrity is the intactness of the twelve pairs of nerves connected with the brain, including their somatic, visceral, and afferent and efferent components. *Peripheral nerve integrity* is the intactness of the spinal nerves, including their afferent and efferent components. The physical therapist uses tests and measures to assess the cranial and peripheral nerves. Results of tests and measures of cranial and peripheral nerve integrity are integrated with the history and systems review findings and the results of other tests and measures. All of these data are then synthesized during the evaluation process to establish the diagnosis, the prognosis, and the plan of care, which includes the selection of interventions. The results of these tests and measures may indicate the need to use or recommend other tests and measures or the need to consult with, or refer the patient/client to, another professional.

Clinical Indications

Clinical indications for the use of tests and measures are predicated on the history and systems review findings (eg, information provided by the patient/client, family, significant other, or caregiver; symptoms described by the patient/client; signs observed and documented during the systems review; and information derived from other sources and records). The findings may indicate the presence of or risk for pathology/pathophysiology (disease, disorder, or condition), impairments, functional limitations, or disabilities that require a more definitive examination through the selection of tests and measures of cranial and peripheral nerve integrity. Clinical indications for these tests and measures may include:

- *Pathology/pathophysiology (disease, disorder, or condition) in the following systems:*
  - cardiovascular (eg, cerebral vascular accident)
  - endocrine/metabolic (eg, Ménière disease, viral encephalitis)
  - integumentary disease/disorder (eg, neuropathic ulcer)
  - multiple systems (eg, Guillain-Barré syndrome)
  - neuromuscular (eg, Erb palsy, labyrinthitis)
  - pulmonary (eg, amyotrophic lateral sclerosis)
- *Impairments in the following categories:*
  - cranial nerve and peripheral nerve integrity (eg, numb and tingling fingers)
  - gait, locomotion, and balance (eg, staggering gait)
  - motor function (eg, numbness of foot leading to falls)
  - muscle performance (eg, weakness of upper extremity)
  - ventilation (eg, decreased expansion and excursion)
- *Functional limitations in the ability to perform actions, tasks, or activities in the following categories:*
  - self-care (eg, difficulty with eating because of swallowing difficulties)
  - home management (eg, decreased environmental mobility in the home because of unsteadiness)
  - work (job/school/play) (eg, inability to perform activities as a stuntperson because of difficulty with coordination, inability to perform electrical wiring and circuitry because of numbness of fingers)
  - community/leisure (eg, inability to play cards because of proprioceptive deficit, inability to sing in choir because of inadequate phonation control)
- *Disability—that is, the inability or the restricted ability to perform actions, tasks, or activities of required roles within the individual's sociocultural context—in the following categories:*
  - self-care
  - home management
  - work (job/school/play)
  - community/leisure
- *Risk factors for impaired cranial and peripheral nerve integrity:*
  - habitual suboptimal posture
  - increased risk for falls
- *Health, wellness, and fitness needs:*
  - fitness, including physical performance (eg, inadequate hand control in school child, limited neuromuscular control of jumping)
  - health and wellness (eg, incomplete comprehension of value of sensation in gross motor activities)

Cranial and Peripheral Nerve Integrity continued

Tests and Measures

Tests and measures may include those that characterize or quantify:

- Electrophysiological integrity (eg, electroneuromyography)
- Motor distribution of the cranial nerves (eg, dynamometry, muscle tests, observations)
- Motor distribution of the peripheral nerves (eg, dynamometry, muscle tests, observations, thoracic outlet tests)
- Response to neural provocation (eg, tension tests, vertebral artery compression tests)
- Response to stimuli, including auditory, gustatory, olfactory, pharyngeal, vestibular, and visual (eg, observations, provocation tests)
- Sensory distribution of the cranial nerves (eg, discrimination tests; tactile tests, including coarse and light touch, cold and heat, pain, pressure, and vibration)
- Sensory distribution of the peripheral nerves (eg, discrimination tests; tactile tests, including coarse and light touch, cold and heat, pain, pressure, and vibration; thoracic outlet tests)

Tools Used for Gathering Data

Tools for gathering data may include:

- Dynamometers
- Electroneuromyographs
- Muscle tests
- Observations
- Palpation
- Provocation tests
- Scales
- Sensory tests

Data Generated

Data are used in providing documentation and may include:

- Descriptions and quantification of:
  - sensory responses to provocation of cranial and peripheral nerves
  - vestibular responses
- Descriptions of ability to swallow
- Presence or absence of gag reflex
- Quantifications of electrophysiological response to stimulation
- Response to neural provocation

Environmental, Home, and Work (Job/School/Play) Barriers

Environmental, home, and work (job/school/play) barriers are the physical impediments that keep patients/clients from functioning optimally in their surroundings. The physical therapist uses the results of tests and measures to identify any of a variety of possible impediments, including safety hazards (eg, throw rugs, slippery surfaces), access problems (eg, narrow doors, thresholds, high steps, absence of power doors or elevators), and home or office design barriers (eg, excessive distances to negotiate, multistory environments, sinks, bathrooms, counters, placement of controls or switches). The physical therapist also uses the results to suggest modifications to the environment (eg, grab bars in the shower, ramps, raised toilet seats, increased lighting) that will allow the patient/client to improve functioning in the home, workplace, and other settings.

Results of tests and measures of environmental, home, and work (job/school/play) barriers are integrated with the history and systems review findings and the results of other tests and measures. All of these data are then synthesized during the evaluation process to establish the diagnosis, the prognosis, and the plan of care, which includes the selection of interventions. The results of these tests and measures may indicate the need to use or recommend other tests and measures or the need to consult with, or refer the patient/client to, another professional.

Clinical Indications

Clinical indications for the use of tests and measures are predicated on the history and systems review findings (eg, information provided by the patient/client, family, significant other, or caregiver; symptoms described by the patient/client; signs observed and documented during the systems review; and information derived from other sources and records). The findings may indicate the presence of or risk for pathology/pathophysiology (disease, disorder, or condition), impairments, functional limitations, or disabilities that require a more definitive examination through the selection of tests and measures of environmental, home, and work (job/school/play) barriers. Clinical indications for these tests and measures may include:

- *Pathology/pathophysiology (disease, disorder, or condition) in the following systems:*
  - cardiovascular (eg, congestive heart failure)
  - multiple systems (eg, trauma)
  - musculoskeletal (eg, amputation, joint replacement, muscular dystrophy)
  - neuromuscular (eg, cerebral palsy, multiple sclerosis, traumatic brain injury)
  - pulmonary (eg, chronic obstructive pulmonary disease)
- *Impairments in the following categories:*
  - circulation (eg, calf cramps with walking)
  - gait, locomotion, and balance (eg, ataxic gait)
  - muscle performance (eg, decreased muscle strength and endurance)
  - ventilation (eg, increased respiratory rate)
- *Functional limitations in the ability to perform actions, tasks, or activities in the following categories:*
  - self-care (eg, inability to get into bathtub because of decreased muscle strength)
  - home management (eg, inability to climb stairs to bathroom because of decreased muscle endurance)
  - work (job/school/play) (eg, inability as a student to gain wheelchair access to science station in school because of station height, inability to enter building because no ramp is available)
  - community/leisure (eg, inability to join friends on sailboat because of dock instability, inability to walk on beach because of ataxic gait)
- *Disability—that is, the inability or the restricted ability to perform actions, tasks, or activities of required roles within the individual's sociocultural context—in the following categories:*
  - self-care
  - home management
  - work (job/school/play)
  - community/leisure
- *Risk factors for environmental, home, and work barriers:*
  - decreased accessibility to home, work (job/school/play), community, and leisure environments
  - increased risk for falls
  - lack of emergency evacuation plan
- *Health, wellness, and fitness needs:*
  - fitness, including physical performance (eg, inability to negotiate uneven terrains, limited ability to gain access to outdoor trails)
  - health and wellness (eg, incomplete understanding of how to assess terrains for more efficient functioning)

Environmental, Home, and Work (Job/School/Play) Barriers continued

Tests and Measures

Tests and measures may include those that characterize or quantify:

- Current and potential barriers (eg, checklists, interviews, observations, questionnaires)
- Physical space and environment (eg, compliance standards, observations, photographic assessments, questionnaires, structural specifications, technology-assisted assessments, videographic assessments)

Tools Used for Gathering Data

Tools for gathering data include:

- Cameras and photographs
- Checklists
- Interviews
- Observations
- Questionnaires
- Structural specifications
- Technology-assisted analysis systems
- Video cameras and videotapes

Data Generated

Data are used in providing documentation and may include:

- Descriptions of:
  - barriers
  - environment
- Documentation and description of compliance with regulatory standards
- Observations of environment
- Quantifications of physical space

Ergonomics and Body Mechanics

Ergonomics is the relationship among the worker; the work that is done; the actions, tasks, or activities inherent in that work (job/school/play); and the environment in which the work (job/school/play) is performed. Ergonomics uses scientific and engineering principles to improve safety, efficiency, and quality of movement involved in work (job/school/play). *Body mechanics* are the interrelationships of the muscles and joints as they maintain or adjust posture in response to forces placed on or generated by the body. The physical therapist uses these tests and measures in examining both the worker and the work (job/school/play) environment and in determining the potential for trauma or repetitive stress injuries from inappropriate workplace design.These tests and measures may be conducted after a work injury or as a preventive step. The physical therapist may conduct tests and measures as part of work hardening or work conditioning programs and may use the results of tests and measures to develop such programs.

Results of tests and measures of ergonomics and body mechanics are integrated with the history and systems review findings and the results of other tests and measures. All of these data are then synthesized during the evaluation process to establish the diagnosis, the prognosis, and the plan of care, which includes the selection of interventions. The results of these tests and measures may indicate the need to use or recommend other tests and measures or the need to consult with, or refer the patient/client to, another professional.

Clinical Indications

Clinical indications for the use of tests and measures are predicated on the history and systems review findings (eg, information provided by the patient/client, family, significant other, or caregiver; symptoms described by the patient/client; signs observed and documented during the systems review; and information derived from other sources and records). The findings may indicate the presence of or risk for pathology/pathophysiology (disease, disorder, or condition), impairments, functional limitations, or disabilities that require a more definitive examination through the selection of tests and measures of ergonomics and body mechanics. Clinical indications for these tests and measures may include:

- *Pathology/pathophysiology (disease, disorder, or condition) in the following systems:*
  - cardiovascular (eg, coronary artery disease)
  - endocrine/metabolic (eg, pregnancy)
  - multiple systems (eg, deconditioning)
  - musculoskeletal (eg, repetitive strain injury, scoliosis, spinal stenosis)
  - neuromuscular (eg, paroxysmal positional vertigo, spina bifida)
  - pulmonary (eg, ventilatory pump disorders)
- *Impairments in the following categories:*
  - aerobic capacity (eg, decreased endurance and shortness of breath)
  - circulation (eg, abnormal heart rate and rhythm)
  - gait, locomotion, and balance (eg, dizziness)
  - muscle performance (eg, decreased power)
  - range of motion (eg, decreased range of motion)
- *Functional limitations in the ability to perform actions, tasks, or activities in the following categories:*
  - home management (eg, inability to lift laundry basket because of decreased range of motion)
  - community/leisure (eg, inability to bowl because of decreased muscle power, inability to deliver meals-on-wheels because of poor sitting tolerance)
  - self-care (eg, inability to tie shoes because of dizziness)
  - work (job/school/play) (eg, inability to carry school back pack because of pain, inability to rotate trunk at assembly line because of pain)
- *Disability—that is, the inability or the restricted ability to perform actions, tasks, or activities of required roles within the individual's sociocultural context—in the following categories:*
  - self-care
  - home management
  - work (job/school/play)
  - community/leisure
- *Risk factors for inefficient ergonomics and impaired body mechanics:*
  - habitual suboptimal posture
  - hazardous work environment
  - lack of safety awareness in all environments
  - risk-prone behaviors (eg, lack of use of safety gear, performance of tasks requiring repetitive motion)
- *Health, wellness, and fitness needs:*
  - fitness, including physical performance (eg, inability to perform all workplace tasks, use of inappropriate body mechanics for pushing)
  - health and wellness (incomplete understanding of importance of correct body mechanics during work tasks)

Ergonomics and Body Mechanics continued

Tests and Measures

Tests and measures may include those that characterize or quantify:

Ergonomics

- Dexterity and coordination during work (job/school/play) (eg, hand function tests, impairment rating scales, manipulative ability tests)
- Functional capacity and performance during work actions, tasks, or activities (eg, accelerometry, dynamometry, electroneuromyography, endurance tests, force platform tests, goniometry, interviews, observations, photographic assessments, physical capacity tests, postural loading analyses, technology-assisted assessments, videographic assessments, work analyses)
- Safety in work environments (eg, hazard identification checklists, job severity indexes, lifting standards, risk assessment scales, standards for exposure limits)
- Specific work conditions or activities (eg, handling checklists, job simulations, lifting models, preemployment screenings, task analysis checklists, workstation checklists)
- Tools, devices, equipment, and workstations related to work actions, tasks, or activities (eg,observations, tool analysis checklists, vibration assessments)

Body mechanics

- Body mechanics during self-care, home management, work, community, or leisure actions, tasks, or activities (eg, activities of daily living [ADL] and instrumental activities of daily living [IADL] scales, observations, photographic assessments, technology-assisted assessments, videographic assessments)

Tools Used for Gathering Data

Tools for gathering data may include:

- Accelerometers
- Cameras and photographs
- Checklists for exposure standards, hazards, lifting standards
- Dynamometers
- Electroneuromyographs
- Environmental tests
- Force platforms
- Functional capacity evaluations
- Goniometers
- Hand function tests
- Indexes
- Interviews
- Muscle tests
- Observations
- Physical capacity and endurance tests
- Postural loading tests
- Questionnaires
- Scales
- Screenings
- Technology-assisted analysis systems
- Video cameras and videotapes
- Work analyses

Data Generated

Data are used in providing documentation and may include:

Ergonomics

- Characterizations of efficiency and effectiveness of use of tools, devices, and workstations
- Characterizations of environmental hazards, health risks, and safety risks
- Descriptions of tools, devices, equipment, and workstations
- Descriptions and quantification of:
  - abnormal movement patterns associated with work actions, tasks, or activities
  - dexterity and coordination
  - functional capacity
  - repetition and work/rest cycle in work actions, tasks, or activities
  - work actions, tasks, or activities
- Presence or absence of actual, potential, or repetitive trauma in the work environment

Body mechanics

- Characterizations of abnormal or unsafe body mechanics
- Descriptions and quantification of limitations in self-care, home management, work, community, and leisure actions, tasks, or activities

Gait, Locomotion, and Balance

Gait is the manner in which a person walks, characterized by rhythm, cadence, step, stride, and speed. *Locomotion* is the ability to move from one place to another. *Balance* is the ability to maintain the body in equilibrium with gravity both statically (ie, while stationary) and dynamically (ie, while moving). The physical therapist uses these tests and measures to assess disturbances in gait, locomotion, and balance and assess the risk for falling. The physical therapist also uses these tests and measures to determine whether the patient/client is a candidate for assistive, adaptive, orthotic, protective, supportive, or prosthetic devices or equipment. Gait, locomotion, and balance problems often involve difficulty in integrating sensory, motor, and neural processes. Results of tests and measures of gait, locomotion, and balance are integrated with the history and systems review findings and the results of other tests and measures. All of these data are then synthesized during the evaluation process to establish the diagnosis, the prognosis, and the plan of care, which includes the selection of interventions. The results of these tests and measures may indicate the need to use or recommend other tests and measures or the need to consult with, or refer the patient/client to, another professional.

Clinical Indications

Clinical indications for the use of tests and measures are predicated on the history and systems review findings (eg, information provided by the patient/client, family, significant other, or caregiver; symptoms described by the patient/client; signs observed and documented during the systems review; and information derived from other sources and records). The findings may indicate the presence of or risk for pathology/pathophysiology (disease, disorder, or condition), impairments, functional limitations, or disabilities that require a more definitive examination through the selection of tests and measures of gait, locomotion, and balance. Clinical indications for these tests and measures may include:

- *Pathology/pathophysiology (disease, disorder, or condition) in the following systems:*
  - cardiovascular (eg, peripheral vascular disease)
  - endocrine/metabolic (eg, cellulitis)
  - multiple systems (eg, Down syndrome)
  - musculoskeletal (eg, arthropathy; disorders of muscle, ligament, and fascia; osteoarthrosis)
  - neuromuscular (eg, central vestibular disorders, peripheral neuropathy)
  - pulmonary (eg, emphysema)
- *Impairments in the following categories:*
  - circulation (eg, claudication pain)
  - joint integrity and mobility (eg, hip pain with mobility)
  - motor function (eg, abnormal movement pattern)
  - muscle performance (eg, decreased power and endurance)
  - range of motion (eg, abnormal range with gait)
  - ventilation (eg, paradoxical breathing pattern on ambulation)
- *Functional limitations in the ability to perform actions, tasks, or activities in the following categories:*
  - self-care (eg, difficulty with dressing because of abnormal sitting balance)
  - home management (eg, inability to perform yardwork because of decreased power)
  - work (job/school/play) (eg, inability to do shopping as household manager because of painful ambulation, inability as a parent to climb the stairs carrying a child because of decreased power)
  - community/leisure (eg, inability to coach a Little League team because of hip pain, inability to play shuffleboard because of dizziness)
- *Disability—that is, the inability or the restricted ability to perform actions, tasks, or activities of required roles within the individual's sociocultural context—in the following categories:*
  - self-care
  - home management
  - work (job/school/play)
  - community/leisure
- *Risk factors for impaired gait, locomotion, and balance:*
  - increased risk for falls
  - risk-prone behaviors (eg, scatter rugs, unclearly marked steps)
- *Health, wellness, and fitness needs:*
  - fitness, including physical performance (eg, inadequate dynamic balance for climbing, limited leg strength for squatting)
  - health and wellness (eg, incomplete understanding of need for dynamic balance in all functional actions)

Gait, Locomotion, and Balance continued

Tests and Measures

Tests and measures may include those that characterize or quantify:

- Balance during functional activities with or without the use of assistive, adaptive, orthotic, protective, supportive, or prosthetic devices or equipment (eg, activities of daily living [ADL] scales, instrumental activities of daily living [IADL] scales, observations, videographic assessments)
- Balance (dynamic and static) with or without the use of assistive, adaptive, orthotic, protective, supportive, or prosthetic devices or equipment (eg, balance scales, dizziness inventories, dynamic posturography, fall scales, motor impairment tests, observations, photographic assessments, postural control tests)
- Gait and locomotion during functional activities with or without the use of assistive, adaptive, orthotic, protective, supportive, or prosthetic devices or equipment (eg, ADL scales, gait indexes, IADL scales, mobility skill profiles, observations, videographic assessments)
- Gait and locomotion with or without the use of assistive, adaptive, orthotic, protective, supportive, or prosthetic devices or equipment (eg, dynamometry, electroneuromyography, footprint analyses, gait indexes, mobility skill profiles, observations, photographic assessments, technology-assisted assessments, videographic assessments, weight-bearing scales, wheelchair mobility tests)
- Safety during gait, locomotion, and balance (eg, confidence scales, diaries, fall scales, functional assessment profiles, logs, reports)

Tools Used for Gathering Data

Tools for gathering data may include:

- Batteries of tests
- Cameras and photographs
- Diaries
- Dynamometers
- Electroneuromyographs
- Force platforms
- Goniometers
- Indexes
- Inventories
- Logs
- Motion analysis systems
- Observations
- Postural control tests
- Profiles
- Rating scales
- Reports
- Scales
- Technology-assisted analysis systems
- Video cameras and videotapes

Data Generated

Data are used in providing documentation and may include:

- Descriptions of:
  - gait and locomotion
  - gait, locomotion, and balance characteristics with or without use of devices or equipment
  - gait, locomotion, and balance on and in different physical environments
  - level of safety during gait, locomotion, and balance
  - static and dynamic balance
  - wheelchair maneuverability and mobility

Integumentary Integrity

Integumentary integrity is the intactness of the skin, including the ability of the skin to serve as a barrier to environmental threats (eg, bacteria, parasites).The physical therapist uses these tests and measures to assess the effects of a wide variety of disorders that result in skin and subcutaneous changes, including pressure and vascular, venous, arterial, diabetic, and necropathic ulcers; burns and other traumas; and a number of diseases (eg, soft tissue disorders). Results of tests and measures of integumentary integrity are integrated with the history and systems review findings and the results of other tests and measures. All of these data are then synthesized during the evaluation process to establish the diagnosis, the prognosis, and the plan of care, which includes the selection of interventions.The results of these tests and measures may indicate the need to use or recommend other tests and measures or the need to consult with, or refer the patient/client to, another professional.

Clinical Indications

Clinical indications for the use of tests and measures are predicated on the history and systems review findings (eg, information provided by the patient/client, family, significant other, or caregiver; symptoms described by the patient/client; signs observed and documented during the systems review; and information derived from other sources and records). The findings may indicate the presence of or risk for pathology/pathophysiology (disease, disorder, or condition), impairments, functional limitations, or disabilities that require a more definitive examination through the selection of tests and measures of integumentary integrity. Clinical indications for these tests and measures may include:

- *Pathology/pathophysiology (disease, disorder, or condition) in the following systems:*
  - cardiovascular (eg, deep vein thrombosis, peripheral vascular disease)
  - endocrine/metabolic (eg, diabetes, frostbite)
  - integumentary (eg, burn, frostbite, laceration, surgical wound)
  - multiple systems (eg, trauma)
  - musculoskeletal (eg, fracture, osteomyelitis)
  - neuromuscular (eg, coma, spinal cord injury)
  - pulmonary (eg, respiratory failure)
- *Impairments in the following categories:*
  - aerobic capacity (eg, deconditioning)
  - circulation (eg, abnormal fluid distribution)
  - integumentary integrity (eg, burn eschar)
  - sensory integrity (eg, loss of sensation)
- *Functional limitations in the ability to perform actions, tasks, or activities in the following categories:*
  - self-care (eg, inability to bathe because of burn)
  - home management (eg, inability to wash dishes because of hand blisters)
  - work (job/school/play) (eg, inability to do construction work because of lower-extremity cellulitis, inability to hold a job because of pressure sore)
  - community/leisure (eg, inability to play organ at religious center because of loss of finger sensation, inability to skate because of frostbite)
- *Disability—that is, the inability or the restricted ability to perform actions, tasks, or activities of required roles within the individual's sociocultural context—in the following categories:*
  - self-care
  - home management
  - work (job/school/play)
  - community/leisure
- *Risk factors for impaired integumentary integrity:*
  - obesity
  - risk-prone behaviors (eg, excessive exposure to sun or cold)
  - sedentary lifestyle
  - smoking history
- *Health, wellness, and fitness needs:*
  - fitness, including physical performance (eg, inadequate protection from sun during outdoor activities)
  - health and wellness (eg, limited comprehension of value of skin monitoring and protection)

Integumentary Integrity continued

Tests and Measures

Tests and measures may include those that characterize or quantify:

Associated skin

- Activities, positioning, and postures that produce or relieve trauma to the skin (eg, observations, pressure-sensing maps, scales)
- Assistive, adaptive, orthotic, protective, supportive, or prosthetic devices and equipment that may produce or relieve trauma to the skin (eg, observations, pressure-sensing maps, risk assessment scales)
- Skin characteristics, including blistering, continuity of skin color, dermatitis, hair growth, mobility, nail growth, sensation, temperature, texture, and turgor (eg, observations, palpation, photographic assessments, thermography)

Wound

- Activities, positioning, and postures that aggravate the wound or scar or that produce or relieve trauma (eg, observations, pressure-sensing maps)
- Burn (body charting, planimetry)
- Signs of infection (eg, cultures, observations, palpation)
- Wound characteristics, including bleeding, contraction, depth, drainage, exposed anatomical structures, location, odor, pigment, shape, size, staging and progression, tunneling, and undermining (eg, digital and grid measurement, grading of sores and ulcers, observations, palpation, photographic assessments, wound tracing)
- Wound scar tissue characteristics, including banding, pliability, sensation, and texture (eg, observations, scar-rating scales)

Tools Used for Gathering Data

Tools for gathering data may include:

- Cameras and photographs
- Charts
- Culture kits
- Grids
- Observations
- Palpation
- Planimeters
- Pressure-sensing devices
- Rulers
- Scales
- Thermographs
- Tracings, maps, graphs

Data Generated

Data are used in providing documentation and may include:

Associated skin

- Descriptions of activities and postures that aggravate or relieve skin trauma
- Descriptions and quantifications of skin characteristics
- Descriptions of:
  - blister
  - devices and equipment that may produce skin trauma
  - hair pattern
  - skin color and continuity

Wound

- Descriptions of activities and postures that aggravate or relieve wound or scar trauma
- Descriptions of signs of infection
- Descriptions and quantifications of:
  - burn (eg, size, type, depth)
  - wound characteristics
  - wound scar tissue characteristics

Joint Integrity and Mobility

Joint integrity is the intactness of the structure and shape of the joint, including its osteokinematic and arthrokinematic characteristics. The tests and measures of joint integrity assess the anatomic and biomechanical components of the joint. *Joint mobility* is the capacity of the joint to be moved passively, taking into account the structure and shape of the joint surface in addition to characteristics of the tissue surrounding the joint. The tests and measures of joint mobility assess the performance of accessory joint movements, which are not under voluntary control. The physical therapist uses these tests and measures to assess whether there is excessive motion (hypermobility) or limited motion (hypomobility) of the joint. Results of tests and measures of joint integrity and mobility are integrated with the history and systems review findings and the results of other tests and measures. All of these data are then synthesized during the evaluation process to establish the diagnosis, the prognosis, and the plan of care, which includes the selection of interventions. The results of these tests and measures may indicate the need to use or recommend other tests and measures or the need to consult with, or refer the patient/client to, another professional.

Clinical Indications

Clinical indications for the use of tests and measures are predicated on the history and systems review findings (eg, information provided by the patient/client, family, significant other, or caregiver; symptoms described by the patient/client; signs observed and documented during the systems review; and information derived from other sources and records). The findings may indicate the presence of or risk for pathology/pathophysiology (disease, disorder, or condition), impairments, functional limitations, or disabilities that require a more definitive examination through the selection of tests and measures of joint integrity and mobility. Clinical indications for these tests and measures may include:

- *Pathology/pathophysiology (disease, disorder, or condition) in the following systems:*
  - endocrine/metabolic (eg, gout, osteoporosis)
  - multiple systems (eg, vehicular trauma)
  - musculoskeletal (eg, fracture, osteoarthritis, rheumatoid arthritis, sprain)
  - neuromuscular (eg, cerebral palsy, Parkinson disease)
  - pulmonary (eg, restrictive lung disease)

- *Impairments in the following categories:*
  - anthropometric characteristics (eg, abnormal girth of limb at the knee)
  - ergonomics and body mechanics (eg, decreased dexterity and coordination)
  - gait, locomotion, and balance (eg, uneven step length)
  - posture (eg, abnormal spinal alignment)
  - range of motion (eg, decreased muscle length)
  - ventilation (eg, abnormal breathing pattern)

- *Functional limitations in the ability to perform actions, tasks, or activities in the following categories:*
  - self-care (eg, inability to fasten garments because of limited range of motion)
  - home management (eg, inability to sew on a button because of finger joint pain)
  - work (job/school/play) (eg, inability to clean teeth as a dental hygienist because of joint stiffness, inability to climb a ladder because of joint tightness)
  - community/leisure (eg, inability as a student to attend driver's education because of limited range of motion in neck, inability to play golf because of shoulder joint pain)

- *Disability—that is, the inability or the restricted ability to perform actions, tasks, or activities of required roles within the individual's sociocultural context—in the following categories:*
  - self-care
  - home management
  - work (job/school/play)
  - community/leisure

- *Risk factors for impaired joint integrity and mobility:*
  - increased risk for falls
  - performance of tasks requiring repetitive motion

- *Health, wellness, and fitness needs:*
  - fitness, including physical performance (eg, reduced shoulder mobility for weight lifting)
  - health and wellness (eg, insufficient awareness of impact of mobility exercises on ability to lift weight)

Joint Integrity and Mobility continued

Tests and Measures

Tests and measures may include those that characterize or quantify:

- Joint integrity and mobility (eg, apprehension, compression and distraction, drawer, glide, impingement, shear, and valgus/varus stress tests; arthrometry; palpation)
- Joint play movements, including end feel (all joints of the axial and appendicular skeletal system) (eg, palpation)

Tools Used for Gathering Data

Tools for gathering data may include:

- Arthrometers
- Apprehension tests
- Compression and distraction tests
- Drawer tests
- Glide tests
- Impingement tests
- Palpation
- Shear tests
- Valgus/varus stress tests

Data Generated

Data are used in providing documentation and may include:

- Descriptions of:
  - accessory motion
  - bony and soft tissue restrictions during movement
- Descriptions or quantifications of joint hypomobility or hypermobility
- Presence of:
  - apprehension
  - joint impingement
- Presence and severity of abnormal joint articulation

Motor Function (Motor Control and Motor Learning)

Motor function is the ability to learn or demonstrate the skillful and efficient assumption, maintenance, modification, and control of voluntary postures and movement patterns. The physical therapist uses these tests and measures in the assessment of weakness, paralysis, dysfunctional movement patterns, abnormal timing, poor coordination, clumsiness, atypical movements, or dysfunctional postures. Results of tests and measures of motor function (motor control and motor learning) are integrated with the history and systems review findings and the results of other tests and measures. All of these data are then synthesized during the evaluation process to establish the diagnosis, the prognosis, and the plan of care, which includes the selection of interventions. The results of these tests and measures may indicate the need to use or recommend other tests and measures or the need to consult with, or refer the patient/client to, another professional.

Clinical Indications

Clinical indications for the use of tests and measures are predicated on the history and systems review findings (eg, information provided by the patient/client, family, significant other, or caregiver; symptoms described by the patient/client; signs observed and documented during the systems review; and information derived from other sources and records). The findings may indicate the presence of or risk for pathology/pathophysiology (disease, disorder, or condition), impairments, functional limitations, or disabilities that require a more definitive examination through the selection of tests and measures of motor function (motor control and motor learning). Clinical indications for these tests and measures may include:

- *Pathology/pathophysiology (disease, disorder, or condition) in the following systems:*
  - cardiovascular (eg, cerebral vascular accident, congenital heart anomalies)
  - multiple systems (eg, encephalitis, meningitis, seizures)
  - musculoskeletal (eg, muscular dystrophy)
  - neuromuscular (eg, cerebral palsy, multiple sclerosis, Parkinson disease, spinal cord injury, traumatic brain injury, vestibular disorders)
  - pulmonary (eg, hyaline membrane disease)
- *Impairments in the following categories:*
  - circulation (eg, increased heart rate with activities)
  - motor function (eg, irregular movement pattern)
  - muscle performance (eg, weakness)
  - orthotic, protective, and supportive devices (eg, dropfoot requiring an ankle-foot orthosis)
  - range of motion (eg, limited)
  - sensory integrity (eg, altered position sense)
- *Functional limitations in the ability to perform actions, tasks, or activities in the following categories:*
  - self-care (eg, difficulty with combing hair because of weakness)
  - home management (eg, inability to clean the shower because of dysfunctional movement pattern)
  - work (job/school/play) (eg, inability to perform functions as toll collector because of dizziness, inability to sort mail because of clumsiness)
  - community/leisure (eg, inability to play softball because of poor coordination, inability to serve as greeter at senior citizen center because of muscle weakness and decreased endurance)
- *Disability—that is, the inability or the restricted ability to perform actions, tasks, or activities of required roles within the individual's sociocultural context—in the following categories:*
  - self-care
  - home management
  - work (job/school/play)
  - community/leisure
- *Risk factors for impaired motor function:*
  - increased risk for falls
  - lack of safety in all environments
- *Health, wellness, and fitness needs:*
  - fitness, including physical performance (eg, inability to control throwing motion, inadequate eye-hand coordination in sports)
  - health and wellness (eg, incomplete understanding of importance of value of motor planning and practice in task performance)

Motor Function (Motor Control and Motor Learning) continued

Tests and Measures

Tests and measures may include those that characterize or quantify:

- Dexterity, coordination, and agility (eg, coordination screens, motor impairment tests, motor proficiency tests, observations, videographic assessments)
- Electrophysiological integrity (eg, electroneuromyography)
- Hand function (eg, fine and gross motor control tests, finger dexterity tests, manipulative ability tests, observations)
- Initiation, modification, and control of movement patterns and voluntary postures (eg, activity indexes, developmental scales, gross motor function profiles, motor scales, movement assessment batteries, neuromotor tests, observations, physical performance tests, postural challenge tests, videographic assessments)

Tools Used for Gathering Data

Tools for gathering data may include:

- Batteries of tests
- Dexterity tests
- Electroneuromyographs
- Function tests
- Hand manipulation tests
- Indexes
- Motor performance tests
- Observations
- Postural challenge tests
- Profiles
- Scales
- Screens
- Tilt boards
- Video cameras and videotapes

Data Generated

Data are used in providing documentation and may include:

- Descriptions and quantifications of:
  - dexterity, coordination, and agility
  - hand movements
  - head, trunk, and limb movements
  - sensorimotor integration
  - voluntary, age-appropriate postures and movement patterns
- Observations and descriptions of atypical movements
- Quantifications of electrophysiological responses to stimulation

Muscle Performance (Including Strength, Power, and Endurance)

Muscle performance is the capacity of a muscle or a group of muscles to generate forces. *Strength* is the muscle force exerted by a muscle or a group of muscles to overcome a resistance under a specific set of circumstances. *Power* is the work produced per unit of time or the product of strength and speed. *Endurance* is the ability of muscle to sustain forces repeatedly or to generate forces over a period of time. The muscle force that can be measured depends on the interrelationships among such factors as the length of the muscle, the velocity of the muscle contraction, and the mechanical advantage. Recruitment of motor units, fuel storage, and fuel delivery, in addition to balance, timing, and sequencing of contraction, mediate integrated muscle performance. The physical therapist uses these tests and measures to determine the ability to produce, maintain, sustain, and modify movements that are prerequisite to functional activity.

Results of tests and measures of muscle performance (including strength, power, and endurance) are integrated with the history and systems review findings and the results of other tests and measures. All of these data are then synthesized during the evaluation process to establish the diagnosis, the prognosis, and the plan of care, which includes the selection of interventions. The results of these tests and measures may indicate the need to use or recommend other tests and measures or the need to consult with, or refer the patient/client to, another professional.

Clinical Indications

Clinical indications for the use of tests and measures are predicated on the history and systems review findings (eg, information provided by the patient/client, family, significant other, or caregiver; symptoms described by the patient/client; signs observed and documented during the systems review; and information derived from other sources and records). The findings may indicate the presence of or risk for pathology/pathophysiology (disease, disorder, or condition), impairments, functional limitations, or disabilities that require a more definitive examination through the selection of tests and measures of muscle performance (including strength, power, and endurance). Clinical indications for these tests and measures may include:

- *Pathology/pathophysiology (disease, disorder, or condition) in the following systems:*
  - cardiovascular (eg, congestive heart failure, vascular insufficiency)
  - endocrine/metabolic (eg, diabetes, Down syndrome, osteoporosis)
  - integumentary (eg, post-mastectomy lymphedema, scar)
  - multiple systems (eg, AIDS)
  - musculoskeletal (eg, amputation, muscular dystrophy, osteoarthritis, spinal stenosis, synovitis, tenosynovitis)
  - neuromuscular (eg, cerebral palsy, Guillain-Barré, multiple sclerosis)
  - pulmonary (eg, cystic fibrosis, emphysema, pneumonia)
- *Impairments in the following categories:*
  - aerobic capacity (eg, decreased endurance)
  - gait, locomotion, and balance (eg, frequent falls, decreased stance phase)
  - muscle performance (eg, decreased gross strength, generalized muscle weakness)
  - posture (eg, abnormal body alignment)
  - ventilation (eg, abnormal breathing pattern)
- *Functional limitations in the ability to perform actions, tasks, or activities in the following categories:*
  - self-care (eg, inability to don and doff clothing because of proximal instability)
  - home management (eg, inability to squat to pick up laundry because of muscle weakness)
  - work (job/school/play) (eg, inability as an airline baggage handler to handle baggage because of inability to lift heavy objects, inability to carry objects because of decreased muscle endurance, inability to keep up with peers on playground because of decreased muscle endurance)
  - community/leisure (eg, inability to hike because of ankle weakness)
- *Disability—that is, the inability or the restricted ability to perform actions, tasks, or activities of required roles within the individual's sociocultural context—in the following categories:*
  - self-care
  - home management
  - work (job/school/play)
  - community/leisure
- *Risk factors for impaired muscle performance:*
  - increased risk for falls
  - sedentary lifestyle
- *Health, wellness, and fitness needs:*
  - fitness, including physical performance (eg, inadequate muscle strength for aquatic sports, insufficient muscle endurance for long distance running)
  - health and wellness (eg, incomplete understanding of the need for strength before power)

Muscle Performance (Including Strength, Power, and Endurance) continued

Tests and Measures

Tests and measures may include those that characterize or quantify:

- Electrophysiological integrity (eg, electroneuromyography)
- Muscle strength, power, and endurance (eg, dynamometry, manual muscle tests, muscle performance tests, physical capacity tests, technology-assisted assessments, timed activity tests)
- Muscle strength, power, and endurance during functional activities (eg, activities of daily living [ADL] scales, functional muscle tests, instrumental activities of daily living [IADL] scales, observations, videographic assessments)
- Muscle tension (eg, palpation)

Tools Used for Gathering Data

Tools for gathering data may include:

- Dynamometers
- Electroneuromyographs
- Functional muscle tests
- Manual muscle tests
- Muscle performance tests
- Observations
- Palpation
- Physical capacity tests
- Scales
- Sphygmomanometers
- Technology-assisted analysis systems
- Timed activity tests
- Video cameras and videotapes

Data Generated

Data are used in providing documentation and may include:

- Characterizations of:
  - electrophysiological responses to stimulation
  - muscle strength, power, and endurance
- Presence and severity of pelvic-floor muscle weakness
- Quantifications of:
  - levels of excitability of muscle
  - muscle strength, work, and power

Neuromotor Development and Sensory Integration

Neuromotor development is the acquisition and evolution of movement skills throughout the life span. *Sensory integration* is the ability to integrate information that is derived from the environment and that relates to movement. The physical therapist uses tests and measures to characterize movement skills in infants, children, and adults. The physical therapist also uses tests and measures to assess mobility; achievement of motor milestones; postural control; voluntary and involuntary movement; balance; righting and equilibrium reactions; eye-hand coordination; and other movement skills. Results of tests and measures of neuromotor development and sensory integration are integrated with the history and systems review findings and the results of other tests and measures. All of these data are then synthesized during the evaluation process to establish the diagnosis, the prognosis, and the plan of care, which includes the selection of interventions. The results of these tests and measures may indicate the need to use or recommend other tests and measures or the need to consult with, or refer the patient/client to, another professional.

Clinical Indications

Clinical indications for the use of tests and measures are predicated on the history and systems review findings (eg, information provided by the patient/client, family, significant other, or caregiver; symptoms described by the patient/client; signs observed and documented during the systems review; and information derived from other sources and records). The findings may indicate the presence of or risk for pathology/pathophysiology (disease, disorder, or condition), impairments, functional limitations, or disabilities that require a more definitive examination through the selection of tests and measures of neuromotor development and sensory integration. Clinical indications for these tests and measures may include:

- *Pathology/pathophysiology (disease, disorder, or condition) in the following systems:*
  - cardiovascular (eg, cardiac or associated vessel disorders)
  - endocrine/metabolic (eg, fetal alcohol syndrome, lead poisoning)
  - multiple systems (eg, autism, birth prematurity, seizure disorder)
  - musculoskeletal (eg, congenital amputation)
  - neuromuscular (eg, hearing loss, visual deficit)
  - pulmonary (eg, anoxia, hypoxia)
- *Impairments in the following categories:*
  - circulation (eg, abnormal heart rhythm)
  - gait, locomotion, and balance (eg, poor sitting posture)
  - motor function (eg, presence of involuntary movements)
  - muscle performance (eg, muscle weakness)
  - neuromotor development (eg, delayed motor skills)
  - posture (eg, lack of postural control)
  - prosthetic requirements (eg, poor balance with prosthesis)
  - ventilation (eg, asymmetrical expansion)
- *Functional limitations in the ability to perform actions, tasks, or activities in the following categories:*
  - self-care (eg, inability to grasp bottle for feeding because of weakness)
  - home management (eg, inability to dust because of poor sensory integration)
  - work (job/school/play) (eg, inability to do assembly piecework because of poor eye-hand coordination, inability to play with peers in day care because of inability to crawl)
  - community/leisure (eg, inability to knit because of poor movement initiation, inability to vote in standing ballot booth because of inability to stand)
- *Disability—that is, the inability or the restricted ability to perform actions, tasks, or activities of required roles within the individual's sociocultural context—in the following categories:*
  - self-care
  - home management
  - work (job/school/play)
  - community/leisure
- *Risk factors for impaired neuromotor development and sensory integration:*
  - increased risk for falls
  - poor nutritional status during gestation
  - substance abuse
- *Health, wellness, and fitness needs:*
  - fitness, including physical performance (eg, inappropriate timing or sequencing for skipping, limited ability to participate in organized play programs)
  - health and wellness (eg, lack of understanding of need for developmental screening)

Neuromotor Development and Sensory Integration continued

Tests and Measures

Tests and measures may include those that characterize or quantify:

- Acquisition and evolution of motor skills, including age-appropriate development (eg, activity indexes, developmental inventories and questionnaires, infant and toddler motor assessments, learning profiles, motor function tests, motor proficiency assessments, neuromotor assessments, reflex tests, screens, videographic assessments)
- Oral motor function, phonation, and speech production (eg, interviews, observations)
- Sensorimotor integration, including postural, equilibrium, and righting reactions (eg, behavioral assessment scales, motor and processing skill tests, observations, postural challenge tests, reflex tests, sensory profiles, visual perceptual skill tests)

Tools Used for Gathering Data

Tools for gathering data may include:

- Batteries of tests
- Behavioral assessment scales
- Electrophysiological tests
- Indexes
- Interviews
- Inventories
- Motor assessment tests
- Motor function tests
- Neuromotor assessments
- Observations
- Postural challenge tests
- Proficiency assessments
- Profiles
- Questionnaires
- Reflex tests
- Scales
- Screens
- Skill tests
- Video cameras and videotapes

Data Generated

Data are used in providing documentation and may include:

- Descriptions and quantifications of:
  - behavioral response to stimulation
  - dexterity, coordination, and agility
  - movement skills, including age-appropriate development, gross and fine motor skills, reflex development
  - oral motor function, phonation, and speech production
  - sensorimotor integration, including postural, equilibrium, and righting reactions
- Observations and description of atypical movement

Orthotic, Protective, and Supportive Devices

Orthotic, protective, and supportive devices are implements and equipment used to support or protect weak or ineffective joints or muscles and serve to enhance performance. *Orthotic devices* include braces, casts, shoe inserts, and splints. *Protective devices* include braces, cushions, helmets, and protective taping. *Supportive devices* include compression garments, corsets, elastic wraps, mechanical ventilators, neck collars, serial casts, slings, supplemental oxygen, and supportive taping. The physical therapist uses these tests and measures to assess the need for devices in patients/clients not currently using them and to evaluate the appropriateness and fit of those devices already in use. Results of tests and measures of orthotic, protective, and supportive devices are integrated with the history and systems review findings and the results of other tests and measures. All of these data are then synthesized during the evaluation process to establish the diagnosis, the prognosis, and the plan of care, which includes the selection of interventions.The results of these tests and measures may indicate the need to use or recommend other tests and measures or the need to consult with, or refer the patient/client to, another professional.

Clinical Indications

Clinical indications for the use of tests and measures are predicated on the history and systems review findings (eg, information provided by the patient/client, family, significant other, or caregiver; symptoms described by the patient/client; signs observed and documented during the systems review; and information derived from other sources and records).The findings may indicate the presence of or risk for pathology/pathophysiology (disease, disorder, or condition), impairments, functional limitations, or disabilities that require a more definitive examination through the selection of tests and measures of orthotic, protective, and supportive devices. Clinical indications for these tests and measures may include:

- *Pathology/pathophysiology (disease, disorder, or condition) in the following systems:*
  - cardiovascular (eg, cerebral vascular accident, congestive heart failure, peripheral vascular disease)
  - endocrine/metabolic (eg, rheumatological disease)
  - multiple systems (eg, AIDS, trauma)
  - musculoskeletal (eg, amputation, status post joint replacement)
  - neuromuscular (eg, cerebellar ataxia, cerebral palsy)
  - pulmonary (eg, asthma, cystic fibrosis, reactive airways disease)
- *Impairments in the following categories:*
  - anthropometric characteristics (eg, girth, height)
  - gait, locomotion, and balance (eg, impaired motor function)
  - integumentary integrity (eg, impaired sensation)
  - joint integrity and mobility (eg, joint hypermobility)
  - muscle performance (eg, weakness)
- *Functional limitations in the ability to perform actions, tasks, or activities in the following categories:*
  - self-care (eg, inability to wash hair because of upper-extremity lymphedema)
  - home management (eg, inability to walk on uneven terrain because of ankle instability)
  - work (job/school/play) (eg, inability as a factory worker to lift repetitively on assembly line because of pain, inability to maintain head position in classroom because of poor motor function, inability to stand because of low back pain)
  - community/leisure (eg, inability to bowl because of wrist pain and weakness)
- *Disability—that is, the inability or the restricted ability to perform actions, tasks, or activities of required roles within the individual's sociocultural context—in the following categories:*
  - self-care
  - home management
  - work (job/school/play)
  - community/leisure
- Risk factor for improper use or lack of use of orthotic, protective, and supportive devices:
  - lack of safety awareness
  - lack of use of adequate protective devices during activity
- Health, wellness, and fitness needs:
  - fitness, including physical performance (eg, inadequate control of skis without orthotic device for ski boot)
  - health and wellness (eg, incomplete understanding of importance of orthotic evaluation and compliance with program)

Orthotic, Protective, and Supportive Devices continued

Tests and Measures

Tests and measures may include those that characterize or quantify:

- Components, alignment, fit, and ability to care for the orthotic, protective, and supportive devices and equipment (eg, interviews, logs, observations, pressure-sensing maps, reports)
- Orthotic, protective, and supportive devices and equipment use during functional activities (eg, activities of daily living [ADL] scales, functional scales, instrumental activities of daily living [IADL] scales, interviews, observations, profiles)
- Remediation of impairments, functional limitations, or disabilities with use of orthotic, protective, and supportive devices and equipment (eg, activity status indexes, ADL scales, aerobic capacity tests, functional performance inventories, health assessment questionnaires, IADL scales, pain scales, play scales, videographic assessments)
- Safety during use of orthotic, protective, and supportive devices and equipment (eg, diaries, fall scales, interviews, logs, observations, reports)

Tools Used for Gathering Data

Tools for gathering data may include:

- Aerobic capacity tests
- Diaries
- Indexes
- Interviews
- Inventories
- Logs
- Observations
- Play scales
- Pressure-sensing devices
- Profiles
- Questionnaires
- Reports
- Scales
- Video cameras and videotapes

Data Generated

Data are used in providing documentation and may include:

- Descriptions of:
  - ability to use and care for devices and equipment
  - alignment and fit of the devices and equipment
  - components of orthotic, protective, or supportive devices and equipment
  - level of safety with devices and equipment
  - practicality of devices and equipment
  - remediation of impairment, functional limitation, or disability with devices and equipment
- Quantifications of:
  - movement patterns with or without devices
  - physiological and functional effect and benefit of devices and equipment

Pain

Pain is a disturbed sensation that causes suffering or distress. The physical therapist uses these tests and measures to determine a cause or a mechanism for the pain and to assess the intensity, quality, and temporal and physical characteristics of any pain that is important to the patient and that may result in impairments, functional limitations, or disabilities. Results of tests and measures of pain are integrated with the history and systems review findings and the results of other tests and measures. All of these data are then synthesized during the evaluation process to establish the diagnosis, the prognosis, and the plan of care, which includes the selection of interventions. The results of these tests and measures may indicate the need to use or recommend other tests and measures or the need to consult with, or refer the patient/client to, another professional.

Clinical Indications

Clinical indications for the use of tests and measures are predicated on the history and systems review findings (eg, information provided by the patient/client, family, significant other, or caregiver; symptoms described by the patient/client; signs observed and documented during the systems review; and information derived from other sources and records). The findings may indicate the presence of or risk for pathology/pathophysiology (disease, disorder, or condition), impairments, functional limitations, or disabilities that require a more definitive examination through the selection of tests and measures of pain. Clinical indications for these tests and measures may include:

- *Pathology/pathophysiology (disease, disorder, or condition) in the following systems:*
  - cardiovascular (eg, coronary artery disease, myocardial infarction)
  - endocrine/metabolic (eg, osteoporosis, rheumatological disease)
  - integumentary (eg, burn, incision, ulcer, wound)
  - multiple systems (eg, vehicular trauma)
  - musculoskeletal (eg, amputation, cumulative trauma, fracture, spinal stenosis, temporomandibular joint dysfunction)
  - neuromuscular (eg, nerve compression, spinal cord injury)
  - pulmonary (eg, lung cancer, status post thoracotomy)
- *Impairments in the following categories:*
  - circulation (eg, decreased ability to walk because of chest discomfort)
  - integumentary (eg, limited range of motion because of painful rash)
  - joint integrity (eg, decreased range of motion because of finger ache)
  - muscle performance (eg, weakness because of muscle burning)
  - pain (eg, decreased movement of spine because of stabbing back pain)
  - posture (eg, forward head position because of upper-back discomfort)
  - ventilation (eg, decreased expansion because of splinting of painful chest wall)
- *Functional limitations in the ability to perform actions, tasks, or activities in the following categories:*
  - self-care (eg, difficulty with eating because of jaw pain)
  - home management (eg, inability to shovel snow because of shoulder soreness)
  - work (job/school/play) (eg, inability as a parent to carry infant because of shooting knee pain, inability to mop floor because of chest pressure)
  - community/leisure (eg, inability to canoe because of backache, inability to keep up with grandchildren because legs ache while walking)
- *Disability—that is, the inability or the restricted ability to perform actions, tasks, or activities of required roles within the individual's sociocultural context—in the following categories:*
  - self-care
  - home management
  - work (job/school/play)
  - community/leisure
- *Risk factors for pain:*
  - habitual suboptimal posture
  - risk-prone behaviors (eg, lack of use of safety gear, performance of tasks requiring repetitive motion)
  - sedentary lifestyle
  - smoking history
- *Health, wellness, and fitness needs:*
  - fitness, including physical performance (eg, decreased ability to tolerate strength training because of pain, limited participation in leisure sports because of pain)
  - health and wellness (eg, limited information about living with pain)

Pain continued

Tests and Measures

Tests and measures may include those that characterize or quantify:

- Pain, soreness, and nociception (eg, angina scales, analog scales, discrimination tests, pain drawings and maps, provocation tests, verbal and pictorial descriptor tests)
- Pain in specific body parts (eg, pain indexes, pain questionnaires, structural provocation tests)

Tools Used for Gathering Data

Tools for gathering data may include:

- Descriptor tests (verbal and pictorial)
- Discrimination tests
- Indexes
- Pain drawings and maps
- Provocation and structural provocation tests
- Questionnaires
- Scales

Data Generated

Data are used in providing documentation and may include:

- Characterizations of activities or postures that aggravate or relieve pain
- Descriptions and quantifications of pain according to specific body part
- Localization of pain
- Sensory and temporal qualities of pain
- Severity of pain, soreness, and discomfort
- Somatic distribution of pain

Posture

Posture is the alignment and positioning of the body in relation to gravity, center of mass, or base of support. The physical therapist uses these tests and measures to assess structural alignment. *Good posture* is a state of musculoskeletal balance that protects the supporting structures of the body against injury or progressive deformity. Results of tests and measures of posture are integrated with the history and systems review findings and the results of other tests and measures. All of these data are then synthesized during the evaluation process to establish the diagnosis, the prognosis, and the plan of care, which includes the selection of interventions. The results of these tests and measures may indicate the need to use or recommend other tests and measures or the need to consult with, or refer the patient/client to, another professional.

Clinical Indications

Clinical indications for the use of tests and measures are predicated on the history and systems review findings (eg, information provided by the patient/client, family, significant other, or caregiver; symptoms described by the patient/client; signs observed and documented during the systems review; and information derived from other sources and records). The findings may indicate the presence of or risk for pathology/pathophysiology (disease, disorder, or condition), impairments, functional limitations, or disabilities that require a more definitive examination through the selection of tests and measures of posture. Clinical indications for these tests and measures may include:

- *Pathology/pathophysiology (disease, disorder, or condition) in the following systems:*
  - cardiovascular (eg, cerebral vascular accident)
  - endocrine/metabolic (eg, rheumatological disease)
  - genitourinary (eg, pelvic floor dysfunction, pregnancy)
  - multiple systems (eg, trauma)
  - musculoskeletal (eg, amputation, intervertebral disk disorders, scoliosis, joint replacement)
  - neuromuscular (eg, cerebral palsy, neurofibromatosis, spina bifida)
  - pulmonary (eg, pneumonectomy, restrictive lung disease)
- *Impairments in the following categories:*
  - circulation (eg, decreased endurance)
  - orthotic, protective, and supportive devices (eg, swollen malaligned knee)
  - muscle performance (eg, weakness, imbalance)
  - pain (eg, decreased range of motion of lumbar spine)
  - posture (eg, leg length discrepancies)
  - range of motion (eg, decreased cervical range of motion)
  - ventilation (eg, asymmetrical expansion)
- *Functional limitations in the ability to perform actions, tasks, or activities in the following categories:*
  - self-care (eg, difficulty with donning and doffing shoes and socks because of limited painful spinal range of motion)
  - home management (eg, inability to do laundry because of shortness of breath)
  - work (job/school/play) (eg, inability to bake because of painful upper-extremity postures, inability to compete on soccer team because of scoliosis)
  - community/leisure (eg, inability as a scout leader to camp and hike because of hip pain, inability to walk dog because of leg pain)
- *Disability—that is, the inability or the restricted ability to perform actions, tasks, or activities of required roles within the individual's sociocultural context—in the following categories:*
  - self-care
  - home management
  - work (job/school/play)
  - community/leisure
- *Risk factors for impaired posture:*
  - habitual suboptimal posture
  - smoking history
- *Health, wellness, and fitness needs:*
  - fitness, including physical performance (eg, inability to serve tennis ball with required speed, poor posture that limits time at computer workstation)
  - health and wellness (eg, inadequate information about need for posture stretching)

Posture continued

Tests and Measures

Tests and measures may include those that characterize or quantify:

- Postural alignment and position (static and dynamic), including symmetry and deviation from midline (eg, grid measurement, observations, photographic assessments, technology-assisted assessments, videographic assessments)
- Specific body parts (eg, angle assessments, forward-bending test, goniometry, observations, palpation, positional tests)

Tools Used for Gathering Data

Tools for gathering data may include:

- Angle assessments
- Cameras and photographs
- Goniometers
- Grids
- Observations
- Palpation
- Positional tests
- Plumb lines
- Tape measures
- Technology-assisted analysis systems
- Video cameras and videotapes

Data Generated

Data are used in providing documentation and may include:

- Quantifications of:
    - dynamic alignment, symmetry, and deviation during movement
    - postural alignment using posture grids
    - static alignment, symmetry, and deviation

Prosthetic Requirements

Prosthetic requirements are the biomechanical elements necessitated by the loss of a body part. A *prosthesis* is an artificial device used to replace a missing part of the body. The physical therapist uses these tests and measures to assess the effects and benefits, components, alignment and fit, and safe use of the prosthesis. Results of tests and measures of prosthetic requirements are integrated with the history and systems review findings and the results of other tests and measures. All of these data are then synthesized during the evaluation process to establish the diagnosis, the prognosis, and the plan of care, which includes the selection of interventions. The results of these tests and measures may indicate the need to use or recommend other tests and measures or the need to consult with, or refer the patient/client to, another professional.

Clinical Indications

Clinical indications for the use of tests and measures are predicated on the history and systems review findings (eg, information provided by the patient/client, family, significant other, or caregiver; symptoms described by the patient/client; signs observed and documented during the systems review; and information derived from other sources and records). The findings may indicate the presence of or risk for pathology/pathophysiology (disease, disorder, or condition), impairments, functional limitations, or disabilities that require a more definitive examination through the selection of tests and measures of prosthetic requirements. Clinical indications for these tests and measures may include:

- *Pathology/pathophysiology (disease, disorder, or condition) in the following systems:*
  - cardiovascular (eg, peripheral vascular disease)
  - endocrine/metabolic (eg, diabetes)
  - integumentary (eg, burn, frostbite)
  - multiple systems (eg, congenital anomalies, gangrene)
  - musculoskeletal (eg, amputation, compartment syndrome)

- *Impairments in the following categories:*
  - aerobic capacity (eg, decreased endurance)
  - circulation (eg, decreased ankle motion)
  - gait, locomotion, and balance (eg, altered stride length)
  - muscle performance (eg, decreased muscle endurance)
  - pain (eg, claudication)
  - prosthetic requirements (eg, residual limb pain)

- *Functional limitations in the ability to perform actions, tasks, or activities in the following categories:*
  - self-care (eg, inability to put on shoes because of edema)
  - home management (eg, inability to climb stairs because of leg pain)
  - work (job/school/play) (eg, inability to use a keyboard because of loss of fingers, inability to walk child to school because of distal limb ache)
  - community/leisure (eg, inability to engage in bird watching because of residual limb discomfort on uneven terrain, inability to ride bicycle to school because of poor prosthetic fit)

- *Disability—that is, the inability or the restricted ability to perform actions, tasks, or activities of required roles within the individual's sociocultural context—in the following categories:*
  - self-care
  - home management
  - work (job/school/play)
  - community/leisure

- *Risk factors for improper use or lack of use of prosthesis:*
  - obesity
  - risk of skin breakdown
  - sedentary lifestyle

- *Health, wellness, and fitness needs:*
  - fitness, including physical performance (eg, inability to participate in endurance activities with current prosthesis, inadequate prosthetic components or fit for running)
  - health and wellness (eg, inadequate knowledge about importance of prosthetic fit)

Prosthetic Requirements continued

Tests and Measures

Tests and measures may include those that characterize or quantify:

- Components, alignment, fit, and ability to care for the prosthetic device (eg, interviews, logs, observations, pressure-sensing maps, reports)
- Prosthetic device use during functional activities (eg, activities of daily living [ADL] scales, functional scales, instrumental activities of daily living [IADL] scales, interviews, observations)
- Remediation of impairments, functional limitations, or disabilities with use of the prosthetic device (eg, aerobic capacity tests, activity status indexes, ADL scales, functional performance inventories, health assessment questionnaires, IADL scales, pain scales, play scales, technology-assisted assessments, videographic assessments)
- Residual limb or adjacent segment, including edema, range of motion, skin integrity, and strength (eg, goniometry, muscle tests, observations, palpation, photographic assessments, skin integrity tests, technology-assisted assessments, videographic assessments, volume measurement)
- Safety during use of the prosthetic device (eg, diaries, fall scales, interviews, logs, observations, reports)

Tools Used for Gathering Data

Tools for gathering data may include:

- Aerobic capacity tests
- Cameras and photographs
- Diaries
- Goniometers
- Indexes
- Interviews
- Inventories
- Logs
- Muscle tests
- Observations
- Palpation
- Pressure-sensing devices
- Profiles
- Questionnaires
- Reports
- Scales
- Skin integrity tests
- Technology-assisted analysis systems
- Video cameras and videotapes
- Volumometers

Data Generated

Data are used in providing documentation and may include:

- Descriptions and quantifications of:
  - ability to use and care for device and practicality of device
  - components of prosthetic devices
  - level of safety with device
  - residual limb or adjacent segment
- Descriptions and quantifications of:
  - alignment and fit of the device
  - remediation of impairment, functional limitation, or disability with device
- Quantifications of:
  - movement patterns with or without device
  - physiological and functional effects and benefits of device

Range of Motion (Including Muscle Length)

Range of motion (ROM) is the arc through which movement occurs at a joint or a series of joints. *Muscle length* is the maximum extensibility of a muscle-tendon unit. Muscle length, in conjunction with joint integrity and soft tissue extensibility, determines flexibility. The physical therapist uses these tests and measures to assess the range of motion of a joint. Results of tests and measures of range of motion (including muscle length) are integrated with the history and systems review findings and the results of other tests and measures. All of these data are then synthesized during the evaluation process to establish the diagnosis, the prognosis, and the plan of care, which includes the selection of interventions. The results of these tests and measures may indicate the need to use or recommend other tests and measures or the need to consult with, or refer the patient/client to, another professional.

Clinical Indications

Clinical indications for the use of tests and measures are predicated on the history and systems review findings (eg, information provided by the patient/client, family, significant other, or caregiver; symptoms described by the patient/client; signs observed and documented during the systems review; and information derived from other sources and records). The findings may indicate the presence of or risk for pathology/pathophysiology (disease, disorder, or condition), impairments, functional limitations, or disabilities that require a more definitive examination through the selection of tests and measures of range of motion (including muscle length). Clinical indications for these tests and measures may include:

- *Pathology/pathophysiology (disease, disorder, or condition) in the following systems:*
  - endocrine/metabolic (eg, rheumatological disease)
  - genitourinary (eg, pregnancy)
  - multiple systems (eg, trauma)
  - musculoskeletal (eg, avulsion of tendon; disorders of muscle, ligament, and fascia; fracture; osteoarthritis; scoliosis; spinal stenosis; sprain; strain)
  - neuromuscular (eg, Parkinson disease)
  - ventilation (eg, restrictive lung disease)
- *Impairments in the following categories:*
  - assistive and adaptive devices (eg, swollen knee)
  - cranial and peripheral nerve integrity (eg, radiating leg pain)
  - gait, locomotion, and balance (eg, limp)
  - muscle performance (eg, muscle weakness)
  - range of motion (eg, limited elbow range of motion)
  - ventilation (eg, shortness of breath)
- *Functional limitations in the ability to perform actions, tasks, or activities in the following categories:*
  - self-care (eg, inability to put on stockings because of weakness)
  - home management (eg, inability to load dishwasher because of difficulty bending)
  - work (job/school/play) (eg, inability to cut hair because of painful swollen fingers, inability as a professional dancer to assume en pointe position because of painful arch)
  - community/leisure (eg, inability to roller blade because of ankle swelling, inability to serve as volunteer in hospital gift shop because of pain on standing)
- *Disability—that is, the inability or the restricted ability to perform actions, tasks, or activities of required roles within the individual's sociocultural context—in the following categories:*
  - self-care
  - home management
  - work (job/school/play)
  - community/leisure
- *Risk factors for impaired range of motion:*
  - increased risk for falls
  - habitual suboptimal posture
  - smoking history
- *Health, wellness, and fitness needs:*
  - fitness, including physical performance (eg, inadequate flexibility to participate in gymnastics, limited range of motion in shoulders for mural painting)
  - health and wellness (eg, incomplete understanding of relationship between mobility and pain-free functional activities)

Range of Motion (Including Muscle Length) continued

Tests and Measures

Tests and measures may include those that characterize or quantify:

- Functional ROM (eg, observations, squat testing, toe touch tests)
- Joint active and passive movement (eg, goniometry, inclinometry, observations, photographic assessments, technology-assisted assessments, videographic assessments)
- Muscle length, soft tissue extensibility, and flexibility (eg, contracture tests, goniometry, inclinometry, ligamentous tests, linear measurement, multisegment flexibility tests, palpation)

Tools Used for Gathering Data

Tools for gathering data may include:

- Back ROM devices
- Camera and photographs
- Cervical protractors
- Flexible rulers
- Functional tests
- Goniometers
- Inclinometers
- Ligamentous stress tests
- Multisegment flexibility tests
- Observations
- Palpation
- Scoliometers
- Tape measures
- Technology-assisted analysis systems
- Video cameras and videotapes

Data Generated

Data are used in providing documentation and may include:

- Descriptions of muscle, joint, and soft tissue characteristics
- Observations and descriptions of functional or multisegmental movement
- Quantifications of:
  - musculotendinous extensibility ROM

Reflex Integrity

Reflex integrity is the intactness of the neural path involved in a reflex. A *reflex* is a stereotypic, involuntary reaction to any of a variety of sensory stimuli. The physical therapist uses these tests and measures to determine the excitability of the nervous system and the integrity of the neuromuscular system. Results of tests and measures of reflex integrity are integrated with the history and systems review findings and the results of other tests and measures. All of these data are then synthesized during the evaluation process to establish the diagnosis, the prognosis, and the plan of care, which includes the selection of interventions. The results of these tests and measures may indicate the need to use or recommend other tests and measures or the need to consult with, or refer the patient/client to, another professional.

Clinical Indications

Clinical indications for the use of tests and measures are predicated on the history and systems review findings (eg, information provided by the patient/client, family, significant other, or caregiver; symptoms described by the patient/client; signs observed and documented during the systems review; and information derived from other sources and records). The findings may indicate the presence of or risk for pathology/pathophysiology (disease, disorder, or condition), impairments, functional limitations, or disabilities that require a more definitive examination through the selection of tests and measures of reflex integrity. Clinical indications for these tests and measures may include:

- *Pathology/pathophysiology (disease, disorder, or condition) in the following systems:*
  - cardiovascular (eg, cerebral vascular accident)
  - multiple systems (eg, Guillain-Barré syndrome)
  - neuromuscular (eg, amyotrophic lateral sclerosis, cerebral palsy, coma, prematurity, traumatic brain injury)
  - pulmonary (eg, anoxia)

- *Impairments in the following categories:*
  - assistive and adaptive devices (eg, limited mobility)
  - gait, locomotion, and balance (eg, poor balance)
  - integumentary integrity (eg, pressure sore)
  - motor function (eg, poor coordination)
  - muscle performance (eg, weakness)
  - neuromotor development and sensory integration (eg, delayed gross motor skills)
  - posture (eg, asymmetrical alignment)
  - range of motion (eg, hypermobility)

- *Functional limitations in the ability to perform actions, tasks, and activities in the following categories:*
  - self-care (eg, difficulty with eating because of jaw pain with chewing)
  - home management (eg, inability to take trash cans out because of poor coordination)
  - work (job/school/play) (eg, inability to reach to restock shelves because of poor coordination)
  - community/leisure (eg, inability to hike with friends because of poor coordination and weakness, inability to obtain driver's license because of startle reflex, inability to run because of hypermobility)

- *Disability—that is, the inability or the restricted ability to perform actions, tasks, or activities of required roles within the individual's sociocultural context—in the following categories:*
  - self-care
  - home management
  - work (job/school/play)
  - community/leisure

- *Risk factors for impaired reflex integrity:*
  - habitual suboptimal posture
  - increased risk for falls

- *Health, wellness, and fitness needs:*
  - fitness, including physical performance (eg, inability to participate in leisure activities that involve jumping and hopping, inadequate knowledge of proper stretch techniques for sports participation)
  - health and wellness (eg, inadequate knowledge of relaxation)

Reflex Integrity continued

Tests and Measures

Tests and measures may include those that characterize or quantify:

- Deep reflexes (eg, myotatic reflex scale, observations, reflex tests)
- Electrophysiological integrity (eg, electroneuromyography)
- Postural reflexes and reactions, including righting, equilibrium, and protective reactions (eg, observations, postural challenge tests, reflex profiles, videographic assessments)
- Primitive reflexes and reactions, including developmental (eg, reflex profiles, screening tests)
- Resistance to passive stretch (eg, tone scales)
- Superficial reflexes and reactions (eg, observations, provocation tests)

Tools Used for Gathering Data

Tools for gathering data may include:

- Electroneuromyographs
- Myotatic reflex scales
- Observations
- Postural challenge tests
- Provocation tests
- Reflex profiles
- Reflex tests
- Scales
- Screens
- Video cameras and videotapes

Data Generated

Data are used in providing documentation and may include:

- Characterizations and quantifications of:
  - age-appropriate reflexes
  - deep reflexes
  - electrophysiological responses to stimulation
  - postural reflexes and righting reactions
  - superficial reflexes

Self-Care and Home Management (Including Activities of Daily Living and Instrumental Activities of Daily Living)

Self-care management is the ability to perform activities of daily living (ADL), such as bed mobility, transfers, dressing, grooming, bathing, eating, and toileting. *Home management* is the ability to perform the more complex instrumental activities of daily living (IADL), such as structured play (for infants and children), maintaining a home, shopping, performing household chores, caring for dependents, and performing yard work. The physical therapist uses the results of these tests and measures to assess the level of performance of tasks necessary for independent living; the need for assistive, adaptive, orthotic, protective, supportive, or prosthetic devices or equipment; and the need for body mechanics training, organized functional training programs, or therapeutic exercise. Results of tests and measures of self-care and home management (including ADL and IADL) are integrated with the history and systems review findings and the results of other tests and measures. All of these data are then synthesized during the evaluation process to establish the diagnosis, the prognosis, and the plan of care, which includes the selection of interventions. The results of these tests and measures may indicate the need to use or recommend other tests and measures or the need to consult with, or refer the patient/client to, another professional.

Clinical Indications

Clinical indications for the use of tests and measures are predicated on the history and systems review findings (eg, information provided by the patient/client, family, significant other, or caregiver; symptoms described by the patient/client; signs observed and documented during the systems review; and information derived from other sources and records). The findings may indicate the presence of or risk for pathology/pathophysiology (disease, disorder, or condition), impairments, functional limitations, or disabilities that require a more definitive examination through the selection of tests and measures of self-care and home management (including ADL and IADL). Clinical indications for these tests and measures may include:

- *Pathology/pathophysiology (disease, disorder, or condition) in the following systems:*
  - cardiovascular (eg, cerebral vascular accident, congestive heart failure, peripheral vascular disease)
  - endocrine/metabolic (eg, rheumatological disease)
  - genitourinary (eg, pelvic floor dysfunction)
  - multiple systems (eg, AIDS, trauma)
  - musculoskeletal (eg, amputation, joint replacement, spinal stenosis, spinal surgery)
  - neuromuscular (eg, cerebellar ataxia, cerebral palsy, multiple sclerosis, post-polio syndrome, spinal cord injury, traumatic brain injury)
  - pulmonary (eg, asthma, chronic obstructive pulmonary disease, cystic fibrosis, reactive airways disease)

- *Impairments in the following categories:*
  - aerobic capacity (eg, decreased endurance, shortness of breath)
  - arousal, attention, cognition (eg, lack of safety awareness)
  - circulation (eg, abnormal heart rate and rhythm)
  - gait, locomotion, and balance (eg, falls)
  - muscle performance (eg, decreased power)
  - neuromotor development (eg, abnormal movement patterns)
  - orthotic, protective, and supportive devices (eg, wearing a corset)
  - posture (eg, severe kyphosis)
  - prosthetic requirements (eg, use of prosthesis)
  - range of motion (eg, decreased muscle length)
  - ventilation (eg, accessory muscle use)

- *Functional limitations in the ability to perform actions, tasks, or activities in the following categories:*
  - self-care (eg, inability to dress because of abnormal range of motion, inability to tie shoes as a first grader because of poor coordination)
  - home management (eg, inability to shop because of decreased endurance)
  - community/leisure (eg, inability to garden because of shortness of breath, inability to travel to visit relatives because of lack of safety awareness)

- *Disability—that is, the inability or the restricted ability to perform actions, tasks, or activities of required roles within the individual's sociocultural context—in the following categories:*
  - self-care
  - home management
  - work (job/school/play)
  - community/leisure

- *Risk factors for limitations in self-care and home management:*
  - habitual suboptimal posture
  - lack of safety awareness in all environments
  - risk-prone behaviors (eg, performance of tasks requiring repetitive motion, lack of use of safety gear)
  - sedentary lifestyle

- *Health, wellness, and fitness needs:*
  - fitness, including physical performance (eg, inadequate endurance to perform heavy chores)
  - health and wellness (eg, limited knowledge of adaptations to allow independent function)

Self-Care and Home Management continued

Tests and Measures

Tests and measures may include those that characterize or quantify:

- Ability to gain access to home environments (eg, barrier identification, observations, physical performance tests)
- Ability to perform self-care and home management activities with or without assistive, adaptive, orthotic, protective, supportive, or prosthetic devices and equipment (eg, ADL scales, aerobic capacity tests, IADL scales, interviews, observations, profiles)
- Safety in self-care and home management activities and environments (eg, diaries, fall scales, interviews, logs, observations, reports, videographic assessments)

Tools Used for Gathering Data

Tools for gathering data may include:

- Aerobic capacity tests
- Barrier identification checklists
- Diaries
- Fall scales
- Indexes
- Interviews
- Inventories
- Logs
- Observations
- Physical performance tests
- Profiles
- Reports
- Questionnaires
- Scales
- Video cameras and videotapes

Data Generated

Data are used in providing documentation and may include:

- Descriptions and quantifications of:
  - ability to participate in variety of environments
  - functional capacity
  - level of safety in self-care and home management activities
  - need for devices or equipment
  - physiological responses to activity

Sensory Integrity

Sensory integrity is the intactness of cortical sensory processing, including proprioception, pallesthesia, stereognosis, and topognosis. *Proprioception* is the reception of stimuli from within the body (eg, from muscles and tendons) and includes position sense (the awareness of joint position) and kinesthesia (the awareness of movement). *Pallesthesia* is the ability to sense mechanical vibration. *Stereognosis* is the ability to perceive, recognize, and name familiar objects. *Topognosis* is the ability to localize exactly a cutaneous sensation. The physical therapist uses the results of tests and measures to determine the integrity of the sensory, perceptual, and somatosensory processes. Results of tests and measures of sensory integrity are integrated with the history and systems review findings and the results of other tests and measures. All of these data are then synthesized during the evaluation process to establish the diagnosis, the prognosis, and the plan of care, which includes the selection of interventions. The results of these tests and measures may indicate the need to use or recommend other tests and measures or the need to consult with, or refer the patient/client to, another professional.

Clinical Indications

Clinical indications for the use of tests and measures are predicated on the history and systems review findings (eg, information provided by the patient/client, family, significant other, or caregiver; symptoms described by the patient/client; signs observed and documented during the systems review; and information derived from other sources and records). The findings may indicate the presence of or risk for pathology/pathophysiology (disease, disorder, or condition), impairments, functional limitations, or disabilities that require a more definitive examination through the selection of tests and measures of sensory integrity. Clinical indications for these tests and measures may include:

- *Pathology/pathophysiology (disease, disorder, or condition) in the following systems:*
  - cardiovascular (eg, cerebral vascular accident, peripheral vascular disease)
  - endocrine/metabolic (eg, diabetes, rheumatological disease)
  - integumentary (eg, burn, frostbite, lymphedema)
  - multiple systems (eg, AIDS, Guillain-Barré syndrome, trauma)
  - musculoskeletal (eg, derangement of joint; disorders of bursa, synovia, and tendon)
  - neuromuscular (eg, cerebral palsy, developmental delay, spinal cord injury, traumatic brain injury)
  - pulmonary (eg, respiratory failure, ventilatory pump failure)
- *Impairments in the following categories:*
  - circulation (eg, numb feet)
  - integumentary integrity (eg, redness under orthotic)
  - muscle performance (eg, decreased grip strength)
  - orthotic, protective, and supportive devices (eg, wears ankle foot orthosis)
  - posture (eg, forward head)
- *Functional limitations in the ability to perform actions, tasks, or activities in the following categories:*
  - self-care (eg, inability to put on trousers while standing because of loss of feeling in foot)
  - home management (eg, difficulty with sorting change because of numbness)
  - work (job/school/play) (eg, inability as a day care provider to change child's diaper because of loss of finger sensation, inability to operate cash register because of clumsiness)
  - community/leisure (eg, inability to drive car because of loss of spatial awareness, inability to play guitar because of hyperesthesia)
- *Disability—that is, the inability or the restricted ability to perform actions, tasks, or activities of required roles within the individual's sociocultural context—in the following categories:*
  - self-care
  - home management
  - work (job/school/play)
  - community/leisure
- *Risk factors for impaired sensory integrity:*
  - lack of safety awareness in all environments
  - risk-prone behaviors (eg, working without protective gloves)
  - smoking history
  - substance abuse
- *Health, wellness, and fitness needs:*
  - fitness, including physical performance (eg, inadequate balance to compete in dancing competition, limited perception of arms and legs in space during ballroom dancing)
  - health and wellness (eg, inadequate understanding of role of proprioception in balance)

Sensory Integrity continued

Tests and Measures

Tests and measures may include those that characterize or quantify:

- Combined/cortical sensations (eg, stereognosis tests, tactile discrimination tests)
- Deep sensations (eg, kinesthesiometry, observations, photographic assessments, vibration tests)
- Electrophysiological integrity (eg, electroneuromyography)

Tools Used for Gathering Data

Tools for gathering data may include:

- Cameras and photographs
- Esthesiometers
- Electroneuromyographs
- Filaments
- Kinesthesiometers
- Observations
- Palpation
- Pressure scales
- Sensory tests
- Tuning forks

Data Generated

Data are used in providing documentation and may include:

- Characterizations and quantifications of:
  - electrophysiological responses to stimulation
  - position and movement sense
  - sensory processing
  - sensory responses to provocation

Ventilation and Respiration/Gas Exchange

Ventilation is the movement of a volume of gas into and out of the lungs. *Respiration* is the exchange of oxygen and carbon dioxide across a membrane either in the lungs or at the cellular level. The physical therapist uses these tests and measures to determine whether the patient has an adequate ventilatory pump and oxygen uptake/carbon dioxide elimination system to meet the oxygen demands at rest, during aerobic exercise, and during the performance of activities of daily living. Results of tests and measures of ventilation and respiration/gas exchange are integrated with the history and systems review findings and the results of other tests and measures. All of these data are then synthesized during the evaluation process to establish the diagnosis, the prognosis, and the plan of care, which includes the selection of interventions. The results of these tests and measures may indicate the need to use or recommend other tests and measures or the need to consult with, or refer the patient/client to, another professional.

Clinical Indications

Clinical indications for the use of tests and measures are predicated on the history and systems review findings (eg, information provided by the patient/client, family, significant other, or caregiver; symptoms described by the patient/client; signs observed and documented during the systems review; and information derived from other sources and records). The findings may indicate the presence of or risk for pathology/pathophysiology (disease, disorder, or condition), impairments, functional limitations, or disabilities that require a more definitive examination through the selection of tests and measures of ventilation and respiration/gas exchange. Clinical indications for these tests and measures may include:

- *Pathology/pathophysiology (disease, disorder, or condition) in the following systems:*
  - cardiovascular (eg, cerebral vascular accident, congestive heart failure, coronary artery disease)
  - endocrine/metabolic (eg, diabetes, rheumatological disease)
  - genitourinary (eg, pelvic floor dysfunction)
  - multiple systems (eg, AIDS, deconditioning, trauma)
  - musculoskeletal (eg, kyphoscoliosis, muscular dystrophy)
  - neuromuscular (eg, coma, cerebral palsy, Parkinson disease, spinal cord injury, traumatic brain injury)
  - pulmonary (eg, asthma, cystic fibrosis, chronic obstructive pulmonary disease, hyaline membrane disease, pneumonia, pulmonary edema, reactive airways disease, respiratory failure, restrictive lung disease, status post thoracotomy)
- *Impairments in the following categories:*
  - aerobic capacity (eg, shortness of breath)
  - anthropometric characteristics (eg, pedal edema)
  - circulation (eg, abnormal heart rate, calf cramps with walking)
  - muscle performance (eg, decreased endurance)
  - posture (eg, scoliosis)
  - prosthetic requirements (eg, dyspnea on exertion while wearing prosthesis)
  - ventilation (eg, accessory muscle use)
- *Functional limitations in the ability to perform actions, tasks, or activities in the following categories:*
  - self-care (eg, inability to put on socks because of shortness of breath)
  - home management (eg, inability to do yard work because of decreased power)
  - work (job/school/play) (eg, inability to preach sermons because of uncontrolled breathing pattern, inability to suck as neonate because of rapid respiratory rate)
  - community/leisure (eg, inability to participate in community gardening events because of dyspnea on exertion, inability to swim because of dyspnea and chest tightness)
- *Disability—that is, the inability or the restricted ability to perform actions, tasks, or activities of required roles within the individual's sociocultural context—in the following categories:*
  - self-care
  - home management
  - work (job/school/play)
  - community/leisure
- *Risk factors for impaired ventilation and respiration/gas exchange:*
  - risk-prone behaviors (eg, exercise in high-pollution environments, lack of understanding of the need for flu shot)
  - sedentary lifestyle
  - smoking history
- *Health, wellness, and fitness needs:*
  - fitness, including physical performance (eg, inadequate oxygen consumption for participating in marathon running, inadequate peripheral response for running)
  - health and wellness (eg, incomplete understanding of necessity for paced breathing during activity)

Ventilation and Respiration/Gas Exchange continued

Tests and Measures

Tests and measures may include those that characterize or quantify:

- Pulmonary signs of respiration/gas exchange, including breath sounds (eg, gas analyses, observations, oximetry)
- Pulmonary signs of ventilatory function, including airway protection; breath and voice sounds; respiratory rate, rhythm, and pattern; ventilatory flow, forces, and volumes (eg, airway clearance tests, observations, palpation, pulmonary function tests, ventilatory muscle force tests)
- Pulmonary symptoms (eg, dyspnea and perceived exertion indexes and scales)

Tools Used for Gathering Data

Tools for gathering data may include:

- Airway clearance tests
- Force meters
- Gas analyses
- Indexes
- Observations
- Palpation
- Pulse oximeters
- Spirometers
- Stethoscopes

Data Generated

Data are used in providing documentation and may include:

- Descriptions and characterization of:
  - breath and voice sounds
  - chest wall and related structures
  - phonation
  - pulmonary-related symptoms
  - pulmonary vital signs
  - thoracoabdominal ventilatory patterns
- Observations and descriptions of nail beds
- Presence and level of cyanosis
- Quantifications of:
  - ability to clear and protect airway
  - gas exchange and oxygen transport
  - pulmonary function and ventilatory mechanics

Work (Job/School/Play), Community, and Leisure Integration or Reintegration (Including Instrumental Activities of Daily Living)

Work (job/school/play) integration or reintegration is the process of assuming or resuming roles and functions at work (job/school/play), such as negotiating school environments, gaining access to work (job/school/play) environments and workstations, and participating in age-appropriate play activities. *Community integration or reintegration* is the process of assuming or resuming roles and functions in the community, such as gaining access to transportation (eg, driving a car, boarding a bus, negotiating a neighborhood), to community businesses and services (eg, bank, shops, parks), and to public facilities (eg, attending theaters, town hal meetings, and places of worship). *Leisure integration or reintegration* is the process of assuming or resuming roles and functions of avocational and enjoyable pastimes, such as recreational activities (eg, playing a sport) and age-appropriate hobbies (eg, collecting antiques, gardening, or making crafts). The physical therapist uses the results of work, community, and leisure integration or reintegration tests and measures to (1) make judgments as to whether a patient/client is currently prepared to assume or resume community or work (job/school/play) roles, including all instrumental activities of daily living (IADL), (2) determine when and how such integration or reintegration might occur, or (3) assess the need for assistive, adaptive, orthotic, protective, supportive, or prosthetic devices or equipment. The physical therapist also uses the results of these tests and measures to determine whether the patient/client is a candidate for a work hardening or work conditioning program.

Results of tests and measures of work (job/school/play), community, and leisure integration or reintegration are integrated with the history and systems review findings and the results of other tests and measures. All of the data are then synthesized during the evaluation process to establish the diagnosis, the prognosis, and the plan of care, which includes the selection of interventions. The results of these tests and measures may indicate the need to use or recommend other tests and measures or the need to consult with, or refer the patient/client to, another professional.

Clinical Indications

Clinical indications for the use of tests and measures are predicated on the history and systems review findings (eg, information provided by the patient/client, family, significant other, or caregiver; symptoms described by the patient/client; signs observed and documented during the systems review; and information derived from other sources and records). The findings may indicate the presence of or risk for pathology/pathophysiology (disease, disorder, or condition), impairments, functional limitations, or disabilities that require a more definitive examination through the selection of tests and measures of work (job/school/play), community, and leisure integration or reintegration. Clinical indications for these tests and measures may include:

- *Pathology/pathophysiology (disease, disorder, or condition) in the following systems:*
  - cardiovascular (eg, cerebral vascular accident, peripheral vascular disease)
  - endocrine/metabolic (eg, rheumatological disease)
  - genitourinary (eg, pelvic floor dysfunction)
  - multiple systems (eg, AIDS, trauma)
  - musculoskeletal (eg, amputation, status post joint replacement)
  - neuromuscular (eg, cerebellar ataxia, cerebral palsy)
  - pulmonary (eg, asthma, cystic fibrosis)
- *Impairments in the following categories:*
  - circulation (eg, calf cramps with walking)
  - muscle performance (eg, decreased strength)
  - neuromotor development (eg, abnormal movement control)
  - posture (eg, pain on sitting)
  - range of motion (eg, decreased muscle length)
  - ventilation (eg, abnormal breathing pattern)
- *Functional limitations in the ability to perform actions, tasks, and activities in the following categories:*
  - work (job/school/play) (eg, inability to sit at desk because of pain)
  - community/leisure (eg, inability to attend a concert because of incontinence, inability to board a bus because of muscle weakness, inability to gain access to recreational facilities because of abnormal movement control, inability to visit friends in neighborhood because of decreased endurance)
- *Disability—that is, the inability or the restricted ability to perform actions, tasks, or activities of required roles within the individual's sociocultural context—in the following categories:*
  - self-care
  - home management
  - work (job/school/play)
  - community/leisure
- *Risk factors for limitations in work (job/school/play), community, and leisure integration and reintegration:*
  - lack of safety awareness in all environments
- *Health, wellness, and fitness needs:*
  - fitness, including physical performance (eg, inadequate motor skill to perform repeated lifting activities as part of job, inadequate muscle strength for lifting boxes to and from shelves)
  - health and wellness (eg, incomplete understanding of need for community support during reintegration)

Work (Job/School/Play), Community, and Leisure Integration or Reintegration continued

Tests and Measures

Tests and measures may include those that characterize or quantify:

- Ability to assume or resume work (job/school/play), community, and leisure activities with or without assistive, adaptive, orthotic, protective, supportive, or prosthetic devices and equipment (eg, activity profiles, disability indexes, functional status questionnaires, IADL scales, observations, physical capacity tests)
- Ability to gain access to work (job/school/play), community, and leisure environments (eg, barrier identification, interviews, observations, physical capacity tests, transportation assessments)
- Safety in work (job/school/play), community, and leisure activities and environments (eg, diaries, fall scales, interviews, logs, observations, videographic assessments)

Tools Used for Gathering Data

Tools for gathering data may include:

- Diaries
- Indexes
- Interviews
- Logs
- Observations
- Physical capacity tests
- Profiles
- Questionnaires
- Transportation assessments
- Scales
- Video cameras and videotapes

Data Generated

Data are used in providing documentation and may include:

- Descriptions of:
  - level of safety in work (job/school/play), community, and leisure activities
  - physiological responses to activity
- Quantifications of:
  - ability to participate in variety of environments
  - functional capacity
  - need for devices or equipment

Chapter 3

Corresponds to "Interventions" in the Interactive Guide CD-ROM

What Types of Interventions Do Physical Therapists Provide?

Introduction

In its broadest sense, *intervention* is the purposeful interaction of the physical therapist with the patient/client—and, when appropriate, with other individuals involved in patient/client care—using various methods and techniques to produce changes that are consistent with the examination and reexamination findings, the evaluation, the diagnosis, and the prognosis. Decisions about intervention are contingent on the timely monitoring of patient/client responses to interventions and on the progress made toward anticipated goals and expected outcomes.

Physical therapist intervention consists of three major components (Figure):

- Coordination, communication, and documentation
- Patient/client-related instruction
- Procedural interventions

Coordination, communication, and documentation and patient/client-related instruction are provided as part of intervention for all patients/clients. The use of procedural interventions varies, however, because those interventions are selected, applied, or modified according to examination and reexamination findings and the anticipated goals and expected outcomes for a particular patient/client in a specific diagnostic group.

Physical therapist intervention encourages functional independence, emphasizes patient/client-related instruction, and promotes proactive, wellness-oriented lifestyles. Through appropriate education and instruction, the patient/client is encouraged to develop habits that will maintain or improve function, prevent recurrence of problems, and promote health, wellness, and fitness.

Selection of Procedural Interventions

Physical therapists select interventions based on the complexity and severity of the clinical problems. In determining the prognosis, the interventions to be used, and the likelihood of an intervention's success, physical therapists also must consider the differences between the highest level of function of which the individual is *capable* and the highest level of function that is likely to be *habitual* for that individual. Patients/clients are more likely to achieve the anticipated goals and expected outcomes that are determined with the physical therapist if they perceive a need to function at the highest level of their ability—and if they are *motivated* to function habitually at that level. Thus understanding the difference between what a person currently does and what that person *potentially* could do is essential in making a prognosis and identifying realistic, achievable goals and outcomes. Physical therapists ultimately must abide by the decisions of the patient/client regarding actions, tasks, and activities that will be incorporated into a daily routine and regarding what constitutes a meaningful level of function.

The physical therapist's selection of procedural interventions should be based on:

- Examination findings (including those of the history, systems review, and tests and measures), an evaluation, and a diagnosis that supports physical therapy intervention
- A prognosis that is associated with improved or maintained health status through risk reduction; health, wellness, and fitness programs; or the remediation of impairments, functional limitations, or disabilities
- A plan of care designed to improve, enhance, and maximize function through interventions of appropriate intensity, frequency, and duration to achieve anticipated goals and expected outcomes efficiently using available resources

The physical therapist selects, applies, or modifies one or more procedural interventions based on anticipated goals and expected outcomes that have been developed *with the patient/client.* Anticipated goals and expected outcomes relate to specific impairments, functional limitations, or disabilities; signs or symptoms; risk reduction/prevention; and health, wellness, or fitness needs. The anticipated goals and expected outcomes listed in the plan of care should be measurable and time-specific.

In conjunction with coordination, communication, and documentation and patient/client-related instruction, three categories of procedural interventions form the core of most physical therapy plans of care: therapeutic exercise, functional training in self-care and home man-

Figure. The Three Components of Physical Therapy Intervention

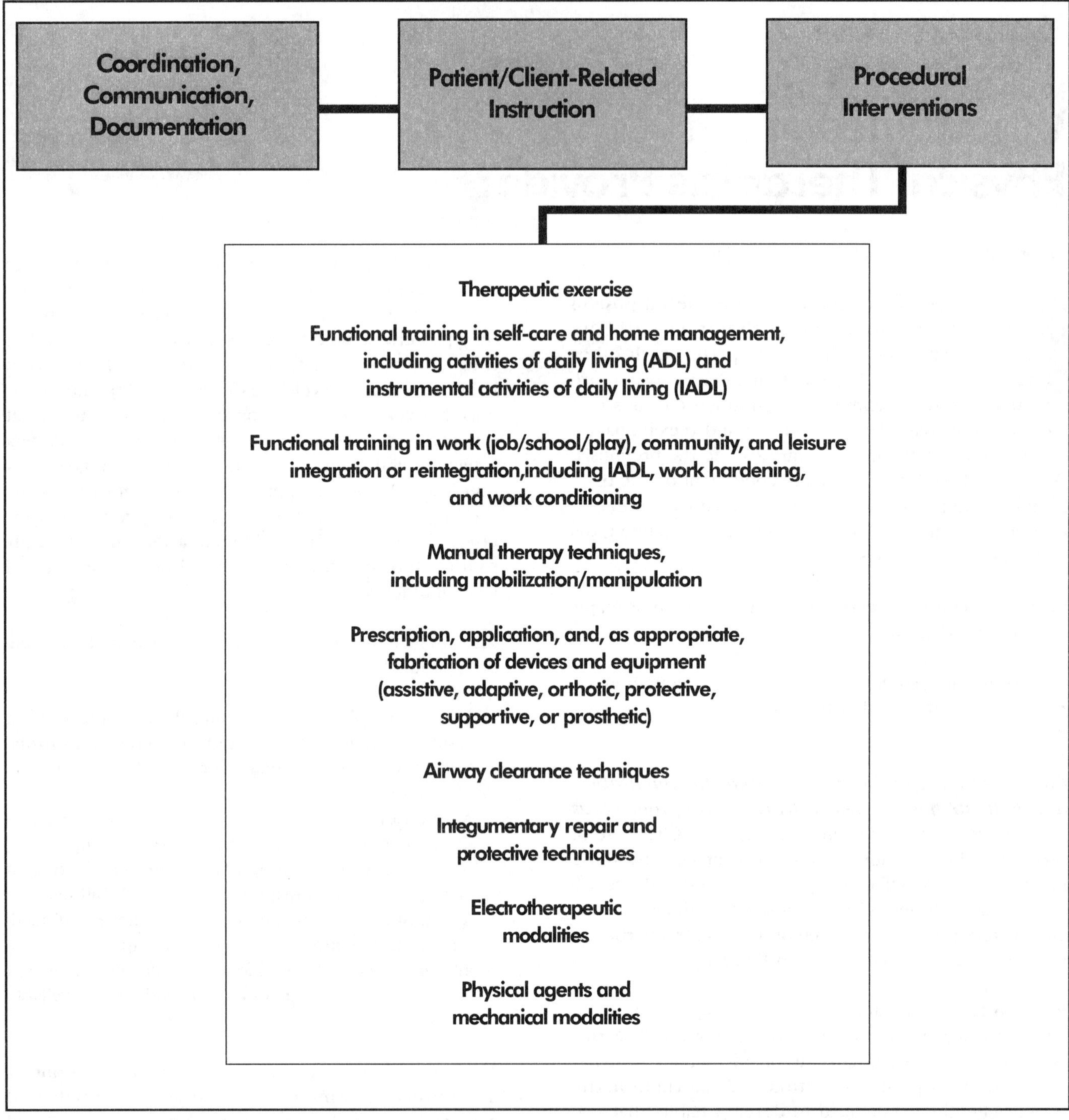

agement, and functional training in work (job/school/play), community, and leisure integration or reintegration. The other categories of procedural interventions may be used when the examination, evaluation, diagnosis, and prognosis indicate their necessity.

Factors that influence the complexity of both the examination process and the selection of interventions may include chronicity or severity of current condition; level of current impairment and probability of prolonged impairment, functional limitation, or disability; living environment; multisite or multisystem involvement; overall physical function and health status; potential discharge destinations; preexisting systemic conditions or diseases; social supports; and stability of the condition.

Through routine monitoring and reexamination, the physical therapist determines the need for any alteration in an intervention or in the plan of care. The interventions used, including their frequency and duration, are consistent with patient/client needs and physiological and cognitive status, anticipated goals and expected outcomes, and resource constraints. The independent performance of the procedure or technique by the patient/client (or significant other, family, or caregiver) is encouraged following instruction in safe and effective application.

Failing to intervene appropriately to prevent illness or to habilitate or rehabilitate patients/clients with impairments, functional limitations, and disabilities leads to greater costs for both the person and society. The Guide provides administrators and policy makers with the information they need to make decisions about the cost-effectiveness of physical therapist intervention.

Criteria for Termination of Physical Therapy Services

Two processes are used for terminating physical therapy services: discharge and discontinuation.

Discharge

Discharge is the process of ending physical therapy services that have been provided during a single episode of care, when the anticipated goals and expected outcomes have been achieved. Discharge does not occur with a transfer, that is, it does not occur when the patient is moved from one site to another site within the same setting or across settings during a single episode of care. There may be facility-specific or payer-specific requirements for documentation regarding the conclusion of physical therapy services as the patient moves between sites or across settings during the episode of care; however, discharge occurs based on the physical therapist's analysis of the achievement of anticipated goals and expected outcomes.

For patients/clients who require multiple episodes of care, periodic follow-up is needed over the life span to ensure safety and effective adaptation following changes in physical status, caregivers, environment, or task demands.

In consultation with appropriate individuals, and in consideration of the anticipated goals and expected outcomes, the physical therapist plans for discharge and provides for appropriate follow-up or referral.

Discontinuation

Discontinuation is the process of ending physical therapy services that have been provided during a single episode of care when (1) the patient/client, caregiver, or legal guardian declines to continue intervention; (2) the patient/client is unable to continue to progress toward anticipated goals and expected outcomes because of medical or psychosocial complications or because financial/insurance resources have been expended; or (3) the physical therapist determines that the patient/client will no longer benefit from physical therapy. When termination of physical therapy service occurs prior to achievement of anticipated goals and expected outcomes, patient/client status and the rationale for discontinuation are documented.

In consultation with appropriate individuals, and in consideration of the anticipated goals and expected outcomes, the physical therapist plans for discontinuation and provides for appropriate follow-up or referral.

In this chapter, each component of physical therapist intervention—coordination, communication, and documentation; patient/client-related instruction; and procedural interventions—is described, including:

- *General definitions.* General definitions of each category of intervention are provided.
- *Clinical considerations.* Clinical considerations for selection of interventions are provided. For procedural interventions, examples are given of the types of examination and diagnostic findings that may indicate that a procedural intervention may be appropriate for a given patient/client. Findings may include pathology/pathophysiology (disease, disorder, or condition); impairments; functional limitations; disabilities; risk reduction/prevention needs; and health, wellness, and fitness needs.
- *Interventions.* Examples of methods, procedures, or techniques that may be used are provided.
- *Anticipated goals and expected outcomes.* Anticipated goals and expected outcomes are categorized according to a procedural intervention's impact on pathology/ pathophysiology; impairments; functional limitations; disabilities; risk reduction/prevention; health, wellness, and fitness; impact on societal resources; and patient/client satisfaction.

The patient/client management elements of examination, evaluation, diagnosis, and prognosis should be represented and reimbursed as physical therapy only when they are performed by a physical therapist. The patient/client management element of intervention should be represented and reimbursed as physical therapy only when performed by a physical therapist or by a physical therapist assistant performing selected interventions under the direction and supervision of a physical therapist in accordance with APTA positions, policies, standards, codes, and guidelines. Physical therapists are the only professionals who provide physical therapy interventions. Physical therapist assistants are the only individuals who provide selected physical therapy interventions under the direction and supervision of the physical therapist. Note: The terms "physical therapy" and "physiotherapy," and the terms "physical therapist" and "physiotherapist," are synonymous.

Coordination, communication, and documentation are administrative and supportive processes that are intended to ensure that patients/clients receive appropriate, comprehensive, efficient, effective, and high-quality care from admission through discharge. *Coordination* is the working together of all parties involved with the patient/client. *Communication* is the exchange of information. *Documentation* is any entry into the patient/client record—such as consultation reports, initial examination reports, progress notes, flow sheets, checklists, reexamination reports, or summations of care—that identifies the care or service provided.

Administrative and support processes may include the addressing of such required functions as advance directives, individualized education plans (IEPs), individualized family service plans (IFSPs), informed consent, and mandatory communication and reporting (eg, patient advocacy and abuse reporting); admission and discharge planning; case management; collaboration and coordination with agencies; communication across settings; cost-effective resource utilization; data collection, analysis, and reporting; documentation across settings; interdisciplinary teamwork; and referrals to other professionals or resources.

Physical therapists are responsible for coordination, communication, and documentation across all settings for all patients/clients.

Clinical Considerations

Considerations that may direct the type and specificity of interventions for coordination, communication, and documentation may include:

- Patient/client seeks physical therapy services.
- Patient/client is referred to physical therapy services.
- Patient/client condition indicates need for referral to physical therapy services.
- Patient/client requires referral from the physical therapist to another service or provider.
- Physical therapist obtains informed consent from patient/client in accordance with jurisdictional law.
- Patient/client has signs or symptoms of physical abuse that must be reported in accordance with jurisdictional law.
- Patient/client is admitted to or transferred across patient care settings.
- Physical therapy services are terminated (through discharge or discontinuation).
- Patient/client experiences changes in pathology/pathophysiology (disease, disorder, or condition), impairments, functional limitations, disabilities, or overall health status.
- Patient/client is managed by interdisciplinary team.
- Physical therapist's plan of care for patient/client requires coordination of resources.
- Patient/client, family, significant other, or caregiver requests physical therapist participation in coordination, communication, and documentation activities.
- Physical therapist is contacted by internal communities or external agencies related to patient/client.

Interventions

Coordination, communication, and documentation may include:

- Addressing required functions
  - advance directives
  - IFSPs or IEPs
  - informed consent
  - mandatory communication and reporting (eg, patient advocacy and abuse reporting)
- Admission and discharge planning
- Case management
- Collaboration and coordination with agencies, including:
  - equipment suppliers
  - home care agencies
  - payer groups
  - schools
  - transportation agencies
- Communication across settings, including:
  - case conferences
  - documentation
  - education plans
- Cost-effective resource utilization
- Data collection, analysis, and reporting
  - outcome data
  - peer review findings
  - record reviews
- Documentation across settings, following APTA's *Guidelines for Physical Therapy Documentation* (Appendix 5), including:
  - changes in impairments, functional limitations, and disabilities
  - changes in interventions
  - elements of patient/client management (examination, evaluation, diagnosis, prognosis, intervention)
  - outcomes of intervention
- Interdisciplinary teamwork
  - case conferences
  - patient care rounds
  - patient/client family meetings
- Referrals to other professionals or resources

Anticipated Goals and Expected Outcomes

Anticipated goals and expected outcomes related to interventions for coordination, communication, and documentation may include:

- Accountability for services is increased.
- Admission data and discharge planning are completed.
- Advance directives, IFSPs or IEPs, informed consent, and mandatory communication and reporting (eg, patient advocacy and abuse reporting) are obtained or completed.
- Available resources are maximally utilized.
- Care is coordinated with patient/client, family, significant other, caregiver, and other professionals.
- Case is managed throughout the episode of care.
- Collaboration and coordination occurs with agencies, including equipment suppliers, home care agencies, payer groups, schools, and transportation agencies.
- Communication enhances risk reduction and prevention.
- Communication occurs across settings through case conferences, education plans, and documentation.
- Data are collected, analyzed, and reported, including outcome data, peer review findings, and record reviews.
- Decision making is enhanced regarding health, wellness, and fitness needs.
- Decision making is enhanced regarding patient/client health and the use of health care resources by patient/client, family, significant others, and caregivers.
- Documentation occurs throughout patient/client management and across settings and follows APTA's *Guidelines for Physical Therapy Documentation* (Appendix 5).
- Interdisciplinary collaboration occurs through case conferences, patient care rounds, and patient/client family meetings.
- Patient/client, family, significant other, and caregiver understanding of anticipated goals and expected outcomes is increased.
- Placement needs are determined.
- Referrals are made to other professionals or resources whenever necessary and appropriate.
- Resources are utilized in a cost-effective way.

Patient/Client-Related Instruction

Patient/client-related instruction is the process of informing, educating, or training patients/clients, families, significant others, and caregivers with the intent to promote and optimize physical therapy services. Instruction may be related to the current condition (eg, specific impairments, functional limitations, or disabilities); the plan of care; the need to enhance performance; transition to a different role or setting; risk factors for developing a problem or dysfunction; or the need for health, wellness, and fitness programs.

Physical therapists are responsible for patient/client-related instruction across all settings for all patients/clients.

Clinical Considerations

Considerations that may direct the type and specificity of interventions for patient/client-related instruction may include:

- Patient/client requires instruction to optimize interventions that are designed to decrease impairments, functional limitations, or disabilities.
- Patient/client requires instruction to reduce risk factors for pathology/pathophysiology (disease, disorder, or condition), impairments, functional limitations, or disabilities.
- Patient/client requires instruction that is appropriate for impaired arousal, attention, and cognition that may have an impact on learning and memory.
- Patient/client requires instruction that is appropriate for sensory impairment (eg, vision, hearing) that may affect learning and skill acquisition.
- Patient/client requires instructional or educational assistive technology (eg, large print cards) or environmental accommodations or modifications (eg, enhanced lighting, signage) that may be required for effective learning and skill acquisition.
- Physical therapist identifies potential learning barriers (eg, beliefs, cultural expectations, and language) that must be addressed prior to and throughout patient/client-related instruction and education.
- Physical therapist identifies patient/client impairments, functional limitations, or disabilities that indicate assistance (eg, caregiver, family member, equipment) is required for effective learning and skill acquisition.
- Physical therapist provides instruction and education to patient/client and patient/client support system regarding the plan of care.
- Physical therapist provides instruction when patient/client has identified personal goals for enhanced performance.
- Physical therapist provides instruction when patient/client is transitioning across care settings or performing in a new role that will require an increased or decreased level of service.
- Physical therapist provides instruction when patient/client will benefit from health, wellness, and fitness programs.

Interventions

Patient/client-related instruction may include:

- Instruction, education, and training of patients/clients and caregivers regarding
  - current condition (pathology/pathophysiology [disease, disorder, or condition], impairments, functional limitations, or disabilities)
  - enhancement of performance
  - health, wellness, and fitness programs
  - plan of care
  - risk factors for pathology/pathophysiology (disease, disorder, or condition), impairments, functional limitations, or disabilities
  - transitions across settings
  - transitions to new roles

Anticipated Goals and Expected Outcomes

Anticipated goals and expected outcomes related to patient/client-related instruction may include:

- Ability to perform physical actions, tasks, or activities is improved.
- Awareness and use of community resources are improved.
- Behaviors that foster healthy habits, wellness, and prevention are acquired.
- Decision making is enhanced regarding patient/client health and the use of health care resources by patient/client, family, significant others, and caregivers.
- Disability associated with acute or chronic illnesses is reduced.
- Functional independence in activities of daily living (ADL) and instrumental activities of daily living (IADL) is increased.
- Health status is improved.
- Intensity of care is decreased.
- Level of supervision required for task performance is decreased.
- Patient/client, family, significant other, and caregiver knowledge and awareness of the diagnosis, prognosis, interventions, and anticipated goals and expected outcomes are increased.
- Patient/client knowledge of personal and environmental factors associated with the condition is increased.
- Performance levels in self-care, home management, work (job/school/play), community or leisure actions, tasks, or activities are improved.
- Physical function is improved.
- Risk of recurrence of condition is reduced.
- Risk of secondary impairment is reduced.
- Safety of patient/client, family, significant others, and caregivers is improved.
- Self-management of symptoms is increased.
- Utilization and cost of health care services are decreased.

Procedural Interventions

Therapeutic Exercise

Therapeutic exercise is the systematic performance or execution of planned physical movements, postures, or activities intended to enable the patient/client to (1) remediate or prevent impairments, (2) enhance function, (3) reduce risk, (4) optimize overall health, and (5) enhance fitness and well-being. Therapeutic exercise may include aerobic and endurance conditioning and reconditioning; agility training; balance training, both static and dynamic; body mechanics training; breathing exercises; coordination exercises; developmental activities training; gait and locomotion training; motor training; muscle lengthening; movement pattern training; neuromotor development activities training; neuromuscular education or reeducation; perceptual training; postural stabilization and training; range-of-motion exercises and soft tissue stretching; relaxation exercises; and strength, power, and endurance exercises.

Physical therapists select, prescribe, and implement exercise activities when the examination findings, diagnosis, and prognosis indicate the use of therapeutic exercise to enhance bone density; enhance breathing; enhance or maintain physical performance; enhance performance in activities of daily living (ADL) and instrumental activities of daily living (IADL); improve safety; increase aerobic capacity/endurance; increase muscle strength, power, and endurance; enhance postural control and relaxation; increase sensory awareness; increase tolerance to activity; prevent or remediate impairments, functional limitations, or disabilities to improve physical function; enhance health, wellness, and fitness; reduce complications, pain, restriction, and swelling; or reduce risk and increase safety during activity performance.

Clinical Considerations

Examination findings that may direct the type and specificity of the procedural intervention may include:

- *Pathology/pathophysiology (disease, disorder, or condition), history (including risk factors) of medical/surgical conditions, or signs and symptoms (eg, pain, shortness of breath, stress) in the following systems:*
  - cardiovascular
  - endocrine/metabolic
  - genitourinary
  - integumentary
  - multiple systems
  - musculoskeletal
  - neuromuscular
  - pulmonary

- *Impairments in the following categories:*
  - aerobic capacity/endurance (eg, decreased walk distance)
  - anthropometric characteristics (eg, increased body mass index)
  - arousal, attention, and cognition (eg, decreased motivation to participate in fitness activities)
  - circulation (eg, abnormal elevation in heart rate with activity)
  - cranial and peripheral nerve integrity (eg, difficulty with swallowing, risk of aspiration, positive neural provocation response)
  - ergonomics and body mechanics (eg, inability to squat because of weakness in gluteus maximus and quadriceps femoris muscles)
  - gait, locomotion, and balance (eg, inability to perform ankle dorsiflexion)
  - integumentary integrity (eg, limited finger flexion as a result of dorsal burn scar)
  - joint integrity and mobility (eg, limited range of motion in the shoulder)
  - motor function (eg, uncoordinated limb movements)
  - muscle performance (eg, weakness of lumbar stabilizers)
  - neuromotor development and sensory integration (eg, delayed development)
  - posture (eg, forward head, kyphosis)
  - range of motion (eg, increased laxity in patellofemoral joint)
  - reflex integrity (eg, poor balance in standing)
  - sensory integrity (eg, lack of position sense)
  - ventilation and respiration/gas exchange (eg, abnormal breathing patterns)

- *Functional limitations in the ability to perform actions, tasks, and activities in the following categories:*
  - self-care (eg, difficulty with dressing, bathing)
  - home management (eg, difficulty with raking, shoveling, making bed)
  - work (job/school/play) (eg, difficulty with keyboarding, pushing, or pulling, difficulty with play activities)
  - community/leisure (eg, inability to negotiate steps and curbs)

- *Disability—that is, the inability or the restricted ability to perform actions, tasks, or activities of required roles within the individual's sociocultural context—in the following categories:*
  - work (eg, inability to assume parenting role, inability to care for elderly relatives, inability to return to work as a police officer)
  - community/leisure (eg, difficulty with jogging or playing golf, inability to attend religious services)

- *Risk reduction/prevention in the following areas:*
  - risk factors (eg, need to decrease body fat composition)
  - recurrence of condition (eg, need to increase mobility and postural control for work [job/school/play] actions, tasks, and activities)
  - secondary impairments (eg, need to improve strength and balance for fall risk reduction)

- *Health, wellness, and fitness needs:*
  - fitness, including physical performance (eg, need to improve golf-swing timing, need to maximize gymnastic performance, need to maximize pelvic-floor muscle function)
  - health and wellness (eg, need to improve balance for recreation, need to increase muscle strength to help maintain bone density)

Therapeutic Exercise continued

Interventions

Therapeutic exercise may include:

- Aerobic capacity/endurance conditioning or reconditioning
  - aquatic programs
  - gait and locomotor training
  - increased workload over time
  - movement efficiency and energy conservation training
  - walking and wheelchair propulsion programs
- Balance, coordination, and agility training
  - developmental activities training
  - motor function (motor control and motor learning) training or retraining
  - neuromuscular education or reeducation
  - perceptual training
  - posture awareness training
  - sensory training or retraining
  - standardized, programmatic, complementary exercise approaches
  - task-specific performance training
  - vestibular training
- Body mechanics and postural stabilization
  - body mechanics training
  - postural control training
  - postural stabilization activities
  - posture awareness training
- Flexibility exercises
  - muscle lengthening
  - range of motion
  - stretching
- Gait and locomotion training
  - developmental activities training
  - gait training
  - implement and device training
  - perceptual training
  - standardized, programmatic, complementary exercise approaches
  - wheelchair training
- Neuromotor development training
  - developmental activities training
  - motor training
  - movement pattern training
  - neuromuscular education or reeducation
- Relaxation
  - breathing strategies
  - movement strategies
  - relaxation techniques
  - standardized, programmatic, complementary exercise approaches
- Strength, power, and endurance training for head, neck, limb, pelvic-floor, trunk, and ventilatory muscles
  - active assistive, active, and resistive exercises (including concentric, dynamic/isotonic, eccentric, isokinetic, isometric, and plyometric)
  - aquatic programs
  - standardized, programmatic, complementary exercise approaches
  - task-specific performance training

Anticipated Goals and Expected Outcomes

Anticipated goals and expected outcomes related to therapeutic exercise may include:

- Impact on pathology/pathophysiology (disease, disorder, or condition)
  - Atelectasis is decreased.
  - Joint swelling, inflammation, or restriction is reduced.
  - Nutrient delivery to tissue is increased.
  - Osteogenic effects of exercise are maximized.
  - Pain is decreased.
  - Physiological response to increased oxygen demand is improved.
  - Soft tissue swelling, inflammation, or restriction is reduced.
  - Symptoms associated with increased oxygen demand are decreased.
  - Tissue perfusion and oxygenation are enhanced.
- Impact on impairments
  - Aerobic capacity is increased.
  - Airway clearance is improved.
  - Balance is improved.
  - Endurance is increased.
  - Energy expenditure per unit of work is decreased.
  - Gait, locomotion, and balance are improved.
  - Integumentary integrity is improved.
  - Joint integrity and mobility are improved.
  - Motor function (motor control and motor learning) is improved.
  - Muscle performance (strength, power, and endurance) is increased.
  - Postural control is improved.
  - Quality and quantity of movement between and across body segments are improved.
  - Range of motion is improved.
  - Relaxation is increased.
  - Sensory awareness is increased.
  - Ventilation and respiration/gas exchange are improved.
  - Weight-bearing status is improved.
  - Work of breathing is decreased.
- Impact on functional limitations
  - Ability to perform physical actions, tasks, or activities related to self-care, home management, work (job/school/play), community, and leisure is improved.
  - Level of supervision required for task performance is decreased.
  - Performance of and independence in ADL and IADL with or without devices and equipment are increased.
  - Tolerance of positions and activities is increased.
- Impact on disabilities
  - Ability to assume or resume required self-care, home management, work (job/school/play), community, and leisure roles is improved.
- Risk reduction/prevention
  - Preoperative and postoperative complications are reduced.
  - Risk factors are reduced.
  - Risk of recurrence of condition is reduced.
  - Risk of secondary impairment is reduced.
  - Safety is improved.
  - Self-management of symptoms is improved.
- Impact on health, wellness, and fitness
  - Fitness is improved.
  - Health status is improved.
  - Physical capacity is increased.
  - Physical function is improved.
- Impact on societal resources
  - Utilization of physical therapy services is optimized.
  - Utilization of physical therapy services results in efficient use of health care dollars.
- Patient/client satisfaction
  - Access, availability, and services provided are acceptable to patient/client.
  - Administrative management of practice is acceptable to patient/client.
  - Clinical proficiency of physical therapist is acceptable to patient/client.
  - Coordination of care is acceptable to patient/client.
  - Cost of health care services is decreased.
  - Intensity of care is decreased.
  - Interpersonal skills of physical therapist are acceptable to patient/client, family, and significant others.
  - Sense of well-being is improved.
  - Stressors are decreased.

Functional Training in Self-Care and Home Management (Including Activities of Daily Living and Instrumental Activities of Daily Living)

Functional training in self-care and home management is the education and training of patients/clients in activities of daily living (ADL) and instrumental activities of daily living (IADL). Functional training in self-care and home management is intended to improve the ability to perform physical actions, tasks, or activities in an efficient, typically expected, or competent manner. *Self-care* includes ADL such as bed mobility, transfers, dressing, grooming, bathing, eating, and toileting. *Home management* includes more complex IADL, such as caring for dependents, maintaining a home, performing household chores and yard work, shopping, and structured play (for infants and children). Activities may include accommodation to or modification of environmental and home barriers; ADL and IADL training; guidance and instruction in injury prevention or reduction; functional training programs; training in the use of assistive, adaptive, orthotic, protective, supportive, or prosthetic devices and equipment during self-care and home management activities; task simulation and adaptation; and travel training.

Physical therapists select, prescribe, and implement specific training activities when the examination findings, diagnosis, and prognosis indicate the use of functional training in self-care and home management to enhance health, wellness, and fitness; enhance musculoskeletal, neuromuscular, and cardiovascular/pulmonary capabilities; improve body mechanics; increase assumption or resumption of self-care or home management in a safe and efficient manner; increase postural awareness; prevent or remediate impairments, functional limitations, or disabilities to improve physical function; or reduce risk and increase safety during activity performance.

Clinical Considerations

Examination findings that may direct the type and specificity of the procedural intervention may include:

- *Pathology/pathophysiology (disease, disorder, or condition), history (including risk factors) of medical/surgical conditions, or signs and symptoms (eg, pain, shortness of breath, stress) in the following systems:*
  - cardiovascular
  - endocrine/metabolic
  - genitourinary
  - integumentary
  - multiple systems
  - musculoskeletal
  - neuromuscular
  - pulmonary

- *Impairments that have an impact on function in self-care and home management actions, tasks, and activities in the following categories:*
  - aerobic capacity/endurance (eg, shortness of breath interferes with raking, shoveling, mopping)
  - anthropometric characteristics (eg, swollen arm interferes with grooming)
  - arousal, attention and cognition (eg, inability to recall sequence of daily routine interferes with dressing)
  - circulation (eg, heart rate increases during hair drying)
  - cranial and peripheral nerve integrity (eg, paresthesia interferes with bathing)
  - ergonomics and body mechanics (eg, pain increases during vacuuming)
  - gait, locomotion, and balance (eg, dizziness interferes with climbing stairs into home)
  - integumentary integrity (eg, decreased sensation as a result of second degree burns of hand interferes with personal hygiene)
  - joint integrity and mobility (eg, hip and knee pain interferes with taking out trash)
  - motor function (eg, loss of finger dexterity interferes with use of utensils)
  - muscle performance (eg, decreased lower-extremity strength interferes with bathroom transfers)
  - neuromotor development and sensory integration (eg, delayed development interferes with self-care)
  - posture (eg, cervical posture interferes with desk work)
  - range of motion (eg, decreased shoulder range of motion interferes with reaching behind the back to fasten buttons)
  - reflex integrity (eg, primitive reflexes interfere with positioning for feeding)
  - sensory integrity (eg, altered proprioception interferes with yard work)
  - ventilation and respiration (eg, decreased oxygen saturation interferes with showering)

- *Functional limitations in the ability to perform actions, tasks, or activities in the following categories:*
  - self-care (eg, inability to bottle feed independently, inability to dress and bathe)
  - home management (eg, inability to perform meal preparation tasks)

- *Disability—that is, the inability or the restricted ability to perform actions, tasks, or activities of required roles within the individual's sociocultural context—in the following categories:*
  - work (eg, inability to assume parenting roles)
  - community/leisure (eg, inability to serve as volunteer in hospital coffee shop)

- *Risk reduction/prevention needs in the following areas:*
  - risk factors (eg, need to learn correct biomechanics of lifting for daily activities)
  - recurrence of condition (eg, need to use assistive device or equipment to perform tasks that are likely to cause reinjury)
  - secondary impairments (eg, need to relearn adaptive skills for self-care and home management)

- *Health, wellness, and fitness needs:*
  - fitness, including physical performance (eg, need to increase endurance to complete self-care tasks, need to maximize independence in self-care, need to maximize safety in home management)
  - health and wellness (eg, need to improve physical ability to paint landscapes, need to increase ability to travel)

Functional Training in Self-Care and Home Management continued

Interventions

Functional training in self-care and home management may include:

- ADL training
  - bathing
  - bed mobility and transfer training
  - developmental activities
  - dressing
  - eating
  - grooming
  - toileting
- Barrier accommodations or modifications
- Device and equipment use and training
  - assistive and adaptive device or equipment training during ADL and IADL
  - orthotic, protective, or supportive device or equipment training during self-care and home management
  - prosthetic device or equipment training during ADL and IADL
- Functional training programs
  - back schools
  - simulated environments and tasks
  - task adaptation
  - travel training
- IADL training
  - caring for dependents
  - home maintenance
  - household chores
  - shopping
  - structured play for infants and children
  - yard work
- Injury prevention or reduction
  - injury prevention education during self-care and home management
  - injury prevention or reduction with use of devices and equipment
  - safety awareness training during self-care and home management

Anticipated Goals and Expected Outcomes

Anticipated goals and expected outcomes related to functional training in self-care and home management may include:

- Impact on pathology/pathophysiology (disease, disorder, or condition)
  - Pain is decreased.
  - Physiological response to increased oxygen demand is improved.
  - Symptoms associated with increased oxygen demand are decreased.
- Impact on impairments
  - Balance is improved.
  - Endurance is increased.
  - Energy expenditure per unit of work is decreased.
  - Motor function (motor control and motor learning) is improved.
  - Muscle performance (strength, power, and endurance) is increased.
  - Postural control is improved.
  - Sensory awareness is increased.
  - Weight-bearing status is improved.
  - Work of breathing is decreased.
- Impact on functional limitations
  - Ability to perform physical actions, tasks, or activities related to self-care and home management is improved.
  - Level of supervision required for task performance is decreased.
  - Performance of and independence in ADL and IADL with or without devices and equipment are increased.
  - Tolerance of positions and activities is increased.
- Impact on disabilities
  - Ability to assume or resume required self-care and home management roles is improved.
- Risk reduction/prevention
  - Risk factors are reduced.
  - Risk of secondary impairment is reduced.
  - Safety is improved.
  - Self-management of symptoms is improved.
- Impact on health, wellness, and fitness
  - Fitness is improved.
  - Health status is improved.
  - Physical capacity is increased.
  - Physical function is improved.
- Impact on societal resources
  - Utilization of physical therapy services is optimized.
  - Utilization of physical therapy services results in efficient use of health care dollars.
- Patient/client satisfaction
  - Access, availability, and services provided are acceptable to patient/client.
  - Administrative management of practice is acceptable to patient/client.
  - Clinical proficiency of physical therapist is acceptable to patient/client.
  - Coordination of care is acceptable to patient/client.
  - Cost of health care services is decreased.
  - Intensity of care is decreased.
  - Interpersonal skills of physical therapist are acceptable to patient/client, family, and significant others.
  - Sense of well-being is improved.
  - Stressors are decreased.

Functional Training in Work (Job/School/Play), Community, and Leisure Integration or Reintegration (Including Instrumental Activities of Daily Living, Work Hardening, and Work Conditioning)

Functional training in work (job/school/play), community, and leisure integration or reintegration is the education and training of patients/clients in assumption and resumption of roles and functions in the work environment, in the community, and during leisure activities so that (1) the physical actions or activities required for these roles and functions are performed in an efficient, typically expected, or competent manner and (2) the expectations of work (job/school/play), community, and leisure roles are fulfilled.

Work integration or reintegration into roles may include functions such as gaining access to work (job/school/play) environments and workstations, participating in work hardening or work conditioning programs, negotiating school environments, and participating in age-appropriate play activities. Activities may include accommodations to or modifications of environmental and work barriers; functional training programs (eg, work hardening or conditioning programs); guidance and instruction in injury prevention or reduction; job coaching; leisure and play activity training; training in instrumental activities of daily living (IADL); task simulation and adaptation; training in the use of assistive, adaptive, orthotic, protective, supportive, or prosthetic devices and equipment during work (job/school/play), community, and leisure activities; and travel training. *Community integration or reintegration* into roles may include activities such as gaining access to transportation (eg, driving a car, boarding a bus), a neighborhood (eg, negotiating curbs, crossing streets), community businesses and services (eg, banking, shopping), and public facilities (eg, attending theaters, town hall meetings, and places of worship). *Leisure integration or reintegration* is the process of assuming or resuming roles and functions of avocational and enjoyable pastimes, such as recreational activities (eg, playing a sport) and age-appropriate hobbies (eg, collecting antiques, gardening, or making crafts)

Physical therapists select, prescribe, and implement specific training activities when the examination findings, diagnosis, and prognosis indicate the use of functional training in work (job/school/play), community, and leisure integration or reintegration to enhance health, wellness, and fitness; improve body mechanics; improve safety and efficiency of performance of work (job/school/play), community, and leisure actions, tasks, and activities; increase independence in work and community environments; increase postural awareness; prevent or remediate impairments, functional limitations, or disabilities to improve physical function; or reduce risk.

Clinical Considerations

Examination findings that may direct the type and specificity of the procedural intervention may include:,

- *Pathology/pathophysiology (disease, disorder, or condition), history (including risk factors) of medical/surgical conditions, or signs and symptoms (eg, pain, shortness of breath, stress) in the following systems:*
  - cardiovascular
  - endocrine/metabolic
  - genitourinary
  - integumentary
  - multiple systems
  - musculoskeletal
  - neuromuscular
  - pulmonary

- *Impairments that have an impact on function in work (job/school/play), community, and leisure integration or reintegration actions, tasks, and activities in the following categories:*
  - aerobic capacity/endurance (eg, shortness of breath interferes with loading delivery van)
  - anthropometric characteristics (eg, obesity interferes with accessing transportation)
  - arousal, attention, and cognition (eg, inability to recall sequencing in assembly-line processing interferes with job)
  - circulation (eg, chest pain interferes with walking during cold weather to catch bus)
  - cranial and peripheral nerve integrity (eg, tingling of the feet interferes with pushing cart up ramp)
  - ergonomics and body mechanics (eg, pain increases with squatting and reaching to stock shelves)
  - gait, locomotion, and balance (eg, unsteady gait interferes with walking in the park)
  - integumentary integrity (eg, finger numbness interferes with manipulative skills)
  - joint integrity and mobility (eg, elbow hypomobility interferes with driving a bus)
  - motor function (eg, ataxic movements interfere with keyboarding)
  - muscle performance (eg, decreased trunk strength interferes with participation in school physical education activities)
  - neuromotor development and sensory integration (eg, inability to go from sitting position to standing position interferes with office activities)
  - posture (eg, leg length discrepancy interferes with standing during food preparation)
  - range of motion (eg, decreased shoulder and elbow range of motion interferes with tennis swing)
  - reflex integrity (eg, decreased postural reflexes or reactions interfere with walking in a crowd)
  - sensory integrity (eg, altered proprioception interferes with stadium stair climbing)
  - ventilation and respiration (eg, shortness of breath interferes with postal carrier's mail delivery)

- *Functional limitations in the ability to perform actions, tasks, or activities in the following categories:*
  - work (job/school/play) integration or reintegration (eg, inability to perform manual labor)
  - community/leisure integration or reintegration (eg, inability to get on and off a train, difficulty with sports activities)

- *Disability—that is, the inability or the restricted ability to perform actions, tasks, or activities of required roles within the individual's sociocultural context—in the following categories:*
  - work (eg, inability to practice as a surgeon)
  - community/leisure (eg,inability to participate in League of Women Voters, inability to participate in local park cleanup, inability to participate as member of community soccer team)

- *Risk reduction/prevention needs in the following areas:*
  - risk factors (eg, need to use correct protective equipment for a given task)
  - recurrence of condition (eg, need to learn correct balance of work, rest, and stretching)
  secondary impairments (eg, need to correctly train for each new task)

- *Health, wellness, and fitness needs:*
  - fitness, including physical performance (eg, need to maximize independence or safety in work [job/school/ play]), community, and leisure; need to increase endurance to complete work [job/school/play], community, and leisure tasks)
  - health and wellness (eg, need to improve breathing efficiency for singing in choir, need to increase strength for community environmental work)

Functional Training in Work (Job/School/Play), Community, and Leisure continued

Interventions

Functional training in work (job/school/play), community, and leisure integration or reintegration may include:

- Barrier accommodations or modifications
- Device and equipment use and training
  - assistive and adaptive device or equipment training during IADL
  - orthotic, protective, or supportive device or equipment training during IADL
  - prosthetic device or equipment training during IADL
- Functional training programs
  - back schools
  - job coaching
  - simulated environments and tasks
  - task adaptation
  - task training
  - travel training
  - work conditioning
  - work hardening
- IADL training
  - community service training involving instruments
  - school and play activities training including tools and instruments
  - work training with tools
- Injury prevention or reduction
  - injury prevention education during work (job/school/play), community, and leisure integration or reintegration
  - injury prevention education with use of devices and equipment
  - safety awareness training during work (job/school/play), community, and leisure integration or reintegration
- Leisure and play activities and training

Anticipated Goals and Expected Outcomes

Anticipated goals and expected outcomes related to functional training in work (job/school/play), community, and leisure integration or reintegration may include:

- Impact on pathology/pathophysiology (disease, disorder, or condition)
  - Pain is decreased.
  - Physiological response to increased oxygen demand is improved.
  - Symptoms associated with increased oxygen demand are decreased.
- Impact on impairments
  - Balance is improved.
  - Endurance is increased.
  - Energy expenditure per unit of work is decreased.
  - Motor function (motor control and motor learning) is improved.
  - Muscle performance (strength, power, and endurance) is increased.
  - Postural control is improved.
  - Sensory awareness is increased.
  - Weight-bearing status is improved.
  - Work of breathing is decreased.
- Impact on functional limitations
  - Ability to perform physical actions, tasks, or activities related to work (job/school/play), community, and leisure integration or reintegration is improved.
  - Level of supervision required for task performance is decreased.
  - Performance of and independence in IADL with or without devices and equipment are increased.
  - Tolerance of positions and activities is increased.
- Impact on disabilities
  - Ability to assume or resume required work (job/school/play), community, and leisure roles is improved.
- Risk reduction/prevention
  - Risk factors are reduced.
  - Risk of secondary impairment is reduced.
  - Safety is improved.
  - Self-management of symptoms is improved.
- Impact on health, wellness, and fitness
  - Fitness is improved.
  - Health status is improved.
  - Physical capacity is increased.
  - Physical function is improved.
- Impact on societal resources
  - Costs of work-related injury or disability are reduced.
  - Utilization of physical therapy services is optimized.
  - Utilization of physical therapy services results in efficient use of health care dollars.
- Patient/client satisfaction
  - Access, availability, and services provided are acceptable to patient/client.
  - Administrative management of practice is acceptable to patient/client.
  - Clinical proficiency of physical therapist is acceptable to patient/client.
  - Coordination of care is acceptable to patient/client.
  - Cost of health care services is decreased.
  - Intensity of care is decreased.
  - Interpersonal skills of physical therapist are acceptable to patient/client, family, and significant others.
  - Sense of well-being is improved.
  - Stressors are decreased.

Procedural Interventions

Manual Therapy Techniques (Including Mobilization/Manipulation)

Manual therapy techniques are skilled hand movements intended to improve tissue extensibility; increase range of motion; induce relaxation; mobilize or manipulate soft tissue and joints; modulate pain; and reduce soft tissue swelling, inflammation, or restriction. Procedures and modalities may include manual lymphatic drainage, manual traction, massage, mobilization/manipulation, and passive range of motion.

Physical therapists select, prescribe, and implement manual techniques when the examination findings, diagnosis, and prognosis indicate use of manual therapy to decrease edema, pain, spasm, or swelling; enhance health, wellness, and fitness; enhance or maintain physical performance; increase the ability to move; or prevent or remediate impairments, functional limitations, or disabilities to improve physical function.

Clinical Considerations

Examination findings that may direct the type and specificity of the procedural intervention may include:

- *Pathology/pathophysiology (disease, disorder, or condition), history (including risk factors) of medical/surgical conditions, or signs and symptoms (eg, pain, shortness of breath, stress) in the following systems:*
  - endocrine/metabolic
  - genitourinary
  - integumentary
  - multiple systems
  - musculoskeletal
  - neuromuscular
  - pulmonary
  - vascular

- *Impairments in the following categories:*
  - anthropometric characteristics (eg, increased limb girth)
  - cranial and peripheral nerve integrity (eg, pain on forward bending)
  - ergonomics and body mechanics (eg, inability to flex knee)
  - gait, locomotion, and balance (eg, inability to flex hip)
  - integumentary integrity (eg, decreased skin extensibility)
  - joint integrity and mobility (eg, decreased joint play)
  - motor function (eg, decreased agility)
  - muscle performance (eg, decreased muscle strength)
  - posture (eg, forward head)
  - range of motion (eg, inability to flex, abduct, and externally rotate hip)
  - ventilation and respiration (eg, decreased rib cage mobility)

- *Functional limitations in the ability to perform actions, tasks, or activities in the following categories:*
  - self-care (eg, difficulty with brushing teeth, combing hair, sit-to-stand activities)
  - home management (eg, difficulty with carrying loads, painting, shoveling)
  - work (job/school/play) (eg, difficulty with typing, driving a car)
  - community/leisure (eg, inability to ride bicycle)

- *Disability—that is, the inability or the restricted ability to perform actions, tasks, or activities of required roles within the individual's sociocultural context—in the following categories:*
  - work (job/school/play) (eg, inability to assume role as family caregiver, inability to resume job as first violinist in orchestra)
  - community/leisure (eg, difficulty with varsity swimming, inability to volunteer at neighborhood school)

- *Risk reduction/prevention needs in the following areas:*
  - risk factors (eg, need to perform preventive stretching)
  - recurrence of condition (eg, need to learn cycle of dependent position/elevation for edema control)
  - secondary impairments (eg, need to continue home traction and massage to maintain mobility)

- *Health, wellness, and fitness needs:*
  - fitness, including physical performance (eg,need to increase muscle length to optimize fitness, need to maximize flexibility for ballet)
  - health and wellness (eg, need to improve relaxation, need to increase flexiblity for yoga)

Manual Therapy Techniques continued

Interventions

Manual therapy techniques may include:

- Manual lymphatic drainage
- Manual traction
- Massage
  - connective tissue massage
  - therapeutic massage
- Mobilization/manipulation
  - soft tissue
  - spinal and peripheral joints
- Passive range of motion

Anticipated Goals and Expected Outcomes

Anticipated goals and expected outcomes related to manual therapy techniques may include:

- Impact on pathology/pathophysiology (disease, disorder, or condition)
  - Edema, lymphedema, or effusion is decreased.
  - Joint swelling, inflammation, or restriction is reduced.
  - Neural compression is decreased
  - Pain is decreased.
  - Soft tissue swelling, inflammation, or restriction is reduced.
- Impact on impairments
  - Airway clearance is improved.
  - Balance is improved.
  - Energy expenditure per unit of work is decreased.
  - Gait, locomotion, and balance are improved.
  - Integumentary integrity is improved.
  - Joint integrity and mobility are improved.
  - Muscle performance (strength, power, and endurance) is increased.
  - Postural control is improved.
  - Quality and quantity of movement between and across body segments are improved.
  - Range of motion is improved.
  - Relaxation is increased.
  - Sensory awareness is increased.
  - Weight-bearing status is improved.
  - Work of breathing is decreased.
- Impact on functional limitations
  - Ability to perform movement tasks is improved.
  - Ability to perform physical actions, tasks, or activities related to self-care, home management, work (job/school/play), community, and leisure is improved.
  - Tolerance of positions and activities is increased.
- Impact on disabilities
  - Ability to assume or resume required self-care, home management, work (job/school/play), community, and leisure roles is improved.
- Risk reduction/prevention
  - Preoperative and postoperative complications are reduced.
  - Risk factors are reduced.
  - Risk of recurrence of condition is reduced.
  - Risk of secondary impairment is reduced.
  - Self-management of symptoms is improved.
- Impact on health, wellness, and fitness
  - Fitness is improved.
  - Physical capacity is increased.
  - Physical function is improved.
- Impact on societal resources
  - Utilization of physical therapy services is optimized.
  - Utilization of physical therapy services results in efficient use of health care dollars.
- Patient/client satisfaction
  - Access, availability, and services provided are acceptable to patient/client.
  - Administrative management of practice is acceptable to patient/client.
  - Clinical proficiency of physical therapist is acceptable to patient/client.
  - Coordination of care is acceptable to patient/client.
  - Cost of health care services is decreased.
  - Intensity of care is decreased.
  - Interpersonal skills of physical therapist are acceptable to patient/client, family, and significant others.
  - Sense of well-being is improved.

Procedural Interventions

Prescription, Application, and, as Appropriate, Fabrication of Devices and Equipment (Assistive, Adaptive, Orthotic, Protective, Supportive, and Prosthetic)

Prescription, application, and, as appropriate, fabrication of assistive, adaptive, orthotic, protective, supportive, and prosthetic devices and equipment are processes to select, provide, and train for utilization of therapeutic implements and equipment that are intended to (1) aid patients/clients in performing tasks or movements, (2) support weak or ineffective joints or muscles and serve to enhance performance, (3) replace a missing part of the body, or (4) adapt the environment to facilitate functional performance of activities related to self-care, home management, work, community, and leisure. These devices and equipment may include adaptive, assistive, orthotic, protective, supportive, and prosthetic devices.

Physical therapists prescribe, apply, and, as appropriate, fabricate devices and equipment when the examination findings, diagnosis, and prognosis indicate the use of devices and equipment to decrease edema and swelling; enhance health, wellness, and fitness; enhance performance and independence in activities of daily living (ADL) and instrumental activities of daily living (IADL); enhance or maintain physical performance; increase alignment, mobility, or stability; prevent or remediate impairments, functional limitations, or disabilities to improve physical function; protect body parts; or reduce risk factors and complications.

Clinical Considerations

Examination findings that may direct the type and specificity of the procedural intervention may include:

- *Pathology/pathophysiology (disease, disorder, or condition), history (including risk factors) of medical/surgical conditions, or signs and symptoms (eg, pain, shortness of breath, stress) in the following systems:*
  - cardiovascular
  - endocrine/metabolic
  - genitourinary
  - integumentary
  - multiple systems
  - musculoskeletal
  - neuromuscular
  - pulmonary

- *Impairments in the following categories:*
  - aerobic capacity/endurance (eg, increased shortness of breath during ambulation with prosthesis)
  - anthropometric characteristics (eg, weight gain interferes with orthotic fit)
  - arousal, attention, and cognition (eg, decreased attention interferes with safety)
  - circulation (eg, decreased peripheral circulation alters venous return)
  - cranial and peripheral nerve integrity (eg, loss of sensation)
  - ergonomics and body mechanics (eg, back pain)
  - gait, locomotion, and balance (eg, footdrop)
  - integumentary integrity (eg, pressure ulcer)
  - joint integrity and mobility (eg, joint hypermobility)
  - motor function (eg, loss of coordination)
  - muscle performance (eg, decreased lower-extremity strength)
  - neuromotor development and sensory integration (eg, delayed development)
  - posture (eg, abnormal foot alignment)
  - range of motion (eg, increased hallux adduction)
  - reflex integrity (eg, decreased protective reactions)
  - sensory integrity (eg, altered proprioception)
  - ventilation and respiration/gas exchange (eg, paradoxical breathing)

- *Functional limitations in the ability to perform actions, tasks, or activities in the following categories:*
  - self-care (eg, difficulty with entering bathtub)
  - home management (eg, difficulty with keyboarding while ordering groceries)
  - work (job/school/play) (eg, difficulty with violin playing)
  - community/leisure (eg, difficulty with answering hotline telephones without headset, inability to gain access to playground)

- *Disability—that is, the inability or the restricted ability to perform actions, tasks, or activities of required roles within the individual's sociocultural context—in the following categories:*
  - work (eg, inability to lift child without back support, inability to stand comfortably without orthotics while waitressing)
  - community/leisure (eg, difficulty with jogging without pregnancy sling, inability to attend dancing lessons without prosthesis)

- *Risk reduction/prevention needs in the following areas:*
  - risk factors (eg, need to properly monitor skin)
  - recurrence of condition (eg, need to use protective seating system)
  - secondary impairments (eg, need to continue use of prosthetic device for activity)

- *Health, wellness, and fitness needs:*
  - fitness, including physical performance (eg, need to maximize performance with knee brace at the Special Olympics, need to enhance aerobic performance with supplemental oxygen)
  - health and wellness (eg, need to enhance endurance for dancing, need to improve use of assistive, adaptive, orthotic, protective, supportive, or prosthetic device during violin practice)

Prescription, Application, and, as Appropriate, Fabrication of Devices and Equipment continued

Interventions

Prescription, application, and, as appropriate, fabrication of devices and equipment may include:

- Adaptive devices
  - environmental controls
  - hospital beds
  - raised toilet seats
  - seating systems
- Assistive devices
  - canes
  - crutches
  - long-handled reachers
  - percussors and vibrators
  - power devices
  - static and dynamic splints
  - walkers
  - wheelchairs
- Orthotic devices
  - braces
  - casts
  - shoe inserts
  - splints
- Prosthetic devices (lower-extremity and upper-extremity)
- Protective devices
  - braces
  - cushions
  - helmets
  - protective taping
- Supportive devices
  - compression garments
  - corsets
  - elastic wraps
  - mechanical ventilators
  - neck collars
  - serial casts
  - slings
  - supplemental oxygen
  - supportive taping

Anticipated Goals and Expected Outcomes

Anticipated goals and expected outcomes related to prescription, application, and, as appropriate, fabrication of devices and equipment may include:

- Impact on pathology/pathophysiology (disease, disorder, or condition)
  - Edema, lymphedema, or effusion is reduced.
  - Joint swelling, inflammation, or restriction is reduced.
  - Pain is decreased.
  - Physiological response to increased oxygen demand is improved.
  - Soft tissue swelling, inflammation, or restriction is reduced.
  - Symptoms associated with increased oxygen demand are decreased.
- Impact on impairments
  - Airway clearance is improved.
  - Balance is improved.
  - Endurance is increased.
  - Energy expenditure per unit of work is decreased.
  - Gait, locomotion, and balance are improved.
  - Integumentary integrity is improved.
  - Joint stability is improved.
  - Motor function (motor control and motor learning) is improved.
  - Muscle performance (strength, power, and endurance) is increased.
  - Optimal joint alignment is achieved.
  - Optimal loading on a body part is achieved.
  - Postural control is improved.
  - Prosthetic fit is achieved.
  - Quality and quantity of movement between and across body segments are improved.
  - Range of motion is improved.
  - Ventilation and respiration/gas exchange are improved.
  - Weight-bearing status is improved.
  - Work of breathing is decreased.
- Impact on functional limitations
  - Ability to perform physical actions, tasks, or activities related to self-care, home management, work (job/school/ play), community, and leisure is improved.
  - Level of supervision required for task performance is decreased.
  - Performance of and independence in ADL and IADL with or without devices and equipment are increased.
  - Tolerance of positions and activities is increased.
- Impact on disabilities
  - Ability to assume or resume required self-care, home management, work (job/school/play), community, and leisure roles is improved.
- Risk reduction/prevention
  - Pressure on body tissues is reduced.
  - Protection of body parts is increased.
  - Risk factors are reduced.
  - Risk of recurrence of condition is reduced.
  - Risk of secondary impairment is reduced.
  - Safety is improved.
  - Self-management of symptoms is improved.
  - Stresses precipitating injury are decreased.
- Impact on health, wellness, and fitness
  - Fitness is improved.
  - Health status is improved.
  - Physical capacity is increased.
  - Physical function is improved.
- Impact on societal resources
  - Utilization of physical therapy services is optimized.
  - Utilization of physical therapy services results in efficient use of health care dollars.
- Patient/client satisfaction
  - Access, availability, and services provided are acceptable to patient/client.
  - Administrative management of practice is acceptable to patient/client.
  - Clinical proficiency of physical therapist is acceptable to patient/client.
  - Coordination of care is acceptable to patient/client.
  - Cost of health care services is decreased.
  - Intensity of care is decreased.
  - Interpersonal skills of physical therapist are acceptable to patient/client, family, and significant others.
  - Sense of well-being is improved.
  - Stressors are decreased.

Procedural Interventions

Airway Clearance Techniques

Airway clearance techniques are a group of therapeutic activities intended to manage or prevent the consequences of impaired mucociliary transport or the inability to protect the airway (eg, impaired cough). Techniques may include breathing strategies for airway clearance, manual/mechanical techniques for airway clearance, positioning, and pulmonary postural drainage.

Physical therapists select, prescribe, and implement airway clearance activities when the examination findings, diagnosis, and prognosis indicate the use of airway clearance techniques to enhance exercise performance; enhance health, wellness, or fitness; enhance or maintain physical performance; improve cough; improve ventilation; prevent or remediate impairments, functional limitations, or disabilities to improve physical function; or reduce risk factors and complications.

Clinical Considerations

Examination findings that may direct the type and specificity of the procedural intervention may include:

- *Pathology/pathophysiology (disease, disorder, or condition), history (including risk factors) of medical/surgical conditions, or signs and symptoms (eg, pain, shortness of breath, stress) in the following systems:*
  - *cardiovascular*
  - endocrine/metabolic
  - genitourinary
  - integumentary
  - multiple systems
  - musculoskeletal
  - neuromuscular
  - pulmonary

- *Impairments in the following categories:*
  - aerobic capacity/endurance (eg, persistent coughing)
  - anthropometric characteristics (eg, decreased cough because of obesity)
  - arousal, attention, and cognition (eg, inability to understand directions)
  - circulation (eg, bilateral pedal edema)
  - cranial and peripheral nerve integrity (eg, decreased gag/cough reflex)
  - joint integrity and mobility (eg, decreased thoracic mobility)
  - muscle performance (eg, decreased ventilatory muscle strength)
  - neuromotor development and sensory integration (eg, coughing on change of position)
  - posture (eg, decreased thoracic mobility because of scoliosis)
  - ventilation and respiration (eg, increased secretions)

- *Functional limitations in the ability to perform actions, tasks, or activities in the following categories:*
  - self-care (eg, difficulty with dressing and bathing because of increased wheezing)
  - home management (eg, difficulty with vacuuming because of persistent coughing)
  - work (job/school/play) (eg, difficulty with repetitive overhead activities because of shortness of breath)
  - community/leisure (eg, inability to negotiate steps because of shortness of breath)

- *Disability—that is, the inability or the restricted ability to perform actions, tasks, or activities of required roles within the individual's sociocultural context—in the following categories:*
  - work (eg, inability to assume role as caregiver of spouse, inability to return to work at a construction site)
  - community/leisure (eg, difficulty with walking to post office, inability to attend a theater performance)

- *Risk reduction/prevention needs in the following areas:*
  - risk factors (eg, need to pursue smoking cessation)
  - recurrence of condition (eg, need to continue home airway clearance techniques)
  - secondary impairments (eg, need to strengthen muscles of breathing)

- *Health, wellness, and fitness needs:*
  - fitness, including physical performance (eg,need to increase diaphragmatic muscle strength, need to maximize breathing capabilities during aerobic class)
  - health and wellness (eg, need to increase relaxation for breathing control during speaking, need to optimize oxygen use while providing elder services)

Airway Clearance Techniques continued

Interventions

Airway clearance techniques may include:

- Breathing strategies
  - active cycle of breathing or forced expiratory techniques
  - assisted cough/huff techniques
  - autogenic drainage
  - paced breathing
  - pursed lip breathing
  - techniques to maximize ventilation (eg, maximum inspiratory hold, stair case breathing, manual hyperinflation)
- Manual/mechanical techniques
  - assistive devices
  - chest percussion, vibration, and shaking
  - chest wall manipulation
  - suctioning
  - ventilatory aids
- Positioning
  - positioning to alter work of breathing
  - positioning to maximize ventilation and perfusion
  - pulmonary postural drainage

Anticipated Goals and Expected Outcomes

Anticipated goals and expected outcomes related to airway clearance techniques may include:

- Impact on pathology/pathophysiology (disease, disorder, or condition)
  - Atelectasis is decreased.
  - Nutrient delivery to tissue is increased.
  - Physiological response to increased oxygen demand is improved.
  - Symptoms associated with increased oxygen demand are decreased.
  - Tissue perfusion and oxygenation are enhanced.
- Impact on impairments
  - Airway clearance is improved.
  - Cough is improved.
  - Endurance is increased.
  - Energy expenditure per unit of work is decreased.
  - Exercise tolerance is improved.
  - Muscle performance (strength, power, and endurance) is increased.
  - Ventilation and respiration/gas exchange are improved.
  - Work of breathing is decreased.
- Impact on functional limitations
  - Ability to perform physical actions, tasks, or activities related to self-care, home management, work (job/school/play), community, and leisure is improved.
  - Performance of and independence in activities of daily living (ADL) and instrumental activities of daily living (IADL) with or without devices and equipment are increased.
  - Tolerance of positions and activities is increased.
- Impact on disabilities
  - Ability to assume or resume required self-care, home management, work (job/school/play), community, and leisure roles is improved.
- Risk reduction/prevention
  - Preoperative and postoperative complications are reduced.
  - Risk factors are reduced.
  - Risk of recurrence of condition is reduced.
  - Risk of secondary impairment is reduced.
  - Safety is improved.
  - Self-management of symptoms is improved.
- Impact on health, wellness, and fitness
  - Fitness is improved.
  - Health status is improved.
  - Physical capacity is increased.
  - Physical function is improved.
- Impact on societal resources
  - Utilization of physical therapy services is optimized.
  - Utilization of physical therapy services results in efficient use of health care dollars.
- Patient/client satisfaction
  - Access, availability, and services provided are acceptable to patient/client.
  - Administrative management of practice is acceptable to patient/client.
  - Clinical proficiency of physical therapist is acceptable to patient/client.
  - Coordination of care is acceptable to patient/client.
  - Cost of health care services is decreased.
  - Intensity of care is decreased.
  - Interpersonal skills of physical therapist are acceptable to patient/client, family, and significant others.
  - Sense of well-being is improved.
  - Stressors are decreased.

Procedural Interventions

Integumentary Repair and Protection Techniques

Integumentary repair and protection techniques involve the application of therapeutic procedures and modalities that are intended to enhance wound perfusion, manage scar, promote an optimal wound environment, remove excess exudate from a wound complex, and eliminate nonviable tissue from a wound bed. Procedures and modalities may include debridement; dressings; orthotic, protective, and supportive devices; physical agents and mechanical and electrotherapeutic modalities; and topical agents.

Physical therapists select, prescribe, and implement procedures and modalities when the examination findings, diagnosis, and prognosis indicate the use of integumentary repair and protection techniques to enhance tissue perfusion; enhance wound and soft tissue healing; prevent or remediate impairments, functional limitations, or disabilities to improve physical function; or reduce risk factors and complications.

Clinical Considerations

Examination findings that may direct the type and specificity of the procedural intervention may include:

- *Pathology/pathophysiology (disease, disorder, or condition), history (including risk factors) of medical/surgical conditions, or signs and symptoms (eg, pain, shortness of breath, stress) in the following systems:*
  - *cardiovascular*
  - endocrine/metabolic
  - genitourinary
  - integumentary
  - multiple systems
  - musculoskeletal
  - neuromuscular
  - pulmonary

- *Impairments in the following categories:*
  - anthropometric characteristics (eg, increased limb girth)
  - circulation (eg, decreased peripheral perfusion)
  - cranial and peripheral nerve integrity (eg, decreased hand sensation as a result of burn)
  - gait, locomotion, and balance (eg, decreased balance as a result of foot ulcer pain)
  - integumentary integrity (eg, open wound)
  - joint integrity and mobility (eg, limited elbow range of motion because of scar)
  - muscle performance (eg, limited strength because of wound pain)
  - neuromotor development and sensory integration (eg, knee abrasions because of creeping)
  - posture (eg, pressure ulcer because of prolonged sitting)
  - range of motion (eg, decreased range of thorax motion as a result of surgical wound)
  - reflex integrity (eg, altered withdrawal response)
  - sensory integrity (eg, decreased proprioception)
  - ventilation and respiration/gas exchange (eg, delayed wound healing because of impaired tissue oxygenation)

- *Functional limitations in the ability to perform actions, tasks, or activities in the following categories:*
  - self-care (eg, difficulty with wearing shoes as a result of edematous wound)
  - home management (eg, difficulty with dish washing as a result of dermatitis)
  - work (job/school/play) (eg, difficulty with lifting and bending because of burn scars, inability to sit in school because of sacral decubitus ulcer)
  - community/leisure (eg, inability to go to bank because of residual limb pressure ulcer)

- *Disability—that is, the inability or the restricted ability to perform actions, tasks, or activities of required roles within the individual's sociocultural context—in the following categories:*
  - work (eg, inability to assume role as parent because of infected wound, inability to return to work as a toll taker because of sensation loss in fingers)
  - community/leisure (eg, inability to swim competitively because of skin breakdown, inability to attend school social events because of low self-esteem associated with facial scarring)

- *Risk reduction/prevention needs in the following areas:*
  - risk factors (eg, need to properly monitor skin)
  - recurrence of condition (eg, need to protect skin surfaces)
  - secondary impairments (eg, need to maintain scar mobility)

- *Health, wellness, and fitness needs:*
  - fitness, including physical performance (eg, need to limit sun exposure during gardening, need to promote foot skin protection during marathon training)
  - health and wellness (eg, need to improve nutrition and hydration, need to understand personal and environmental factors that promote optimal health status)

Interventions

Integumentary repair and protection techniques may include:

- Debridement—nonselective
  - enzymatic debridement
  - wet dressings
  - wet-to-dry dressings
  - wet-to-moist dressings
- Debridement—selective
  - debridement with other agents (eg, autolysis)
  - enzymatic debridement
  - sharp debridement
- Dressings
  - hydrogels
  - vacuum-assisted closure
  - wound coverings
- Oxygen therapy
  - supplemental
  - topical
- Topical agents
  - cleansers
  - creams
  - moisturizers
  - ointments
  - sealants

Anticipated Goals and Expected Outcomes

Anticipated goals and expected outcomes related to integumentary repair and protection techniques may include:

- Impact on pathology/pathophysiology (disease, disorder, or condition)
  - Debridement of nonviable tissue is achieved.
  - Joint swelling, inflammation, or restriction is reduced.
  - Nutrient delivery to tissue is increased.
  - Pain is decreased.
  - Physiological response to increased oxygen demand is improved.
  - Soft tissue or wound healing is enhanced.
  - Soft tissue swelling, inflammation, or restriction is reduced.
  - Tissue perfusion and oxygenation are enhanced.
  - Wound size is reduced.
- Impact on impairments
  - Gait, locomotion, and balance are improved.
  - Integumentary integrity is improved.
  - Joint integrity and mobility are improved.
  - Muscle performance (strength, power, and endurance) is increased.
  - Postural control is improved.
  - Range of motion is improved.
  - Sensory awareness is increased.
  - Weight-bearing status is improved.
- Impact on functional limitations
  - Ability to perform physical actions, tasks, or activities related to self-care, home management, work (job/school/play), community, and leisure is improved.
  - Level of supervision required for task performance is decreased.
  - Performance of and independence in activities of daily living (ADL) and instrumental activities of daily living (IADL) with or without devices and equipment are increased.
  - Tolerance of positions and activities is increased.
- Impact on disabilities
  - Ability to assume or resume required self-care, home management, work (job/school/play), community, and leisure roles is improved.
- Risk reduction/prevention
  - Preoperative and postoperative complications are reduced.
  - Risk factors are reduced.
  - Risk of recurrence of condition is reduced.
  - Risk of secondary impairment is reduced.
  - Safety is improved.
  - Self-management of symptoms is improved.
- Impact on health, wellness, and fitness
  - Fitness is improved.
  - Health status is improved.
  - Physical capacity is increased.
  - Physical function is improved.
- Impact on societal resources
  - Utilization of physical therapy services is optimized.
  - Utilization of physical therapy services results in efficient use of health care dollars.
- Patient/client satisfaction
  - Access, availability, and services provided are acceptable to patient/client.
  - Administrative management of practice is acceptable to patient/client.
  - Clinical proficiency of physical therapist is acceptable to patient/client.
  - Coordination of care is acceptable to patient/client.
  - Cost of health care services is decreased.
  - Intensity of care is decreased.
  - Interpersonal skills of physical therapist are acceptable to patient/client, family, and significant others.
  - Sense of well-being is improved.
  - Stressors are decreased.

Procedural Interventions

Electrotherapeutic Modalities

Electrotherapeutic modalities are a broad group of agents that use electricity and are intended to assist functional training; assist muscle force generation and contraction; decrease unwanted muscular activity; increase the rate of healing of open wounds and soft tissue; maintain strength after injury or surgery; modulate or decrease pain; or reduce or eliminate soft tissue swelling, inflammation, or restriction. Modalities may include biofeedback, electrical stimulation (muscle and nerve), and electrotherapeutic delivery of medication.

Physical therapists select, prescribe, and implement these modalities when the examination findings, diagnosis, and prognosis indicate the use of electrotherapeutic modalities to decrease edema and swelling; enhance activity and task performance; enhance health, wellness, or fitness; enhance or maintain physical performance; enhance wound healing; increase joint mobility, muscle performance, and neuromuscular performance; increase tissue perfusion; prevent or remediate impairments, functional limitations, or disabilities to improve physical function; or reduce risk factors and complications.

The use of electrotherapeutic modalities in the absence of other interventions should not be considered physical therapy unless there is documentation that justifies the necessity of their exclusive use.

Clinical Considerations

Examination findings that may direct the type and specificity of the procedural intervention may include:

- *Pathology/pathophysiology (disease, disorder, or condition), history (including risk factors) of medical/surgical conditions, or signs and symptoms (eg, pain, shortness of breath, stress) in the following systems:*
  - cardiovascular
  - endocrine/metabolic
  - genitourinary
  - integumentary
  - multiple systems
  - musculoskeletal
  - neuromuscular
  - pulmonary
- *Impairments in the following categories:*
  - aerobic capacity/endurance (eg, increased pain with activity)
  - anthropometric characteristics (eg, edema)
  - circulation (eg, increased limb girth)
  - cranial and peripheral nerve integrity (eg, decreased muscle activity because of peripheral nerve compression)
  - ergonomics and body mechanics (eg, abnormal sequencing of muscle activation)
  - gait, locomotion, and balance (eg, incoordination in gait)
  - integumentary integrity (eg, open wound)
  - joint integrity and mobility (eg, increased joint play)
  - motor function (eg, muscle hypertonicity)
  - muscle performance (eg, increased muscle spasm)
  - neuromotor development and sensory integration (eg, atypical movement patterns)
  - posture (eg, static deviation from midline)
  - range of motion (eg, increased joint laxity)
  - ventilation and respiration/gas exchange (eg, decreased rib cage symmetry)
- *Functional limitations in the ability to perform actions, tasks, or activities in the following categories:*
  - self-care (eg, difficulty with rolling, sitting, reaching; inability to dress and bathe)
  - home management (eg, difficulty with cleaning, cooking, vacuuming)
  - work (job/school/play) tasks (eg, difficulty with manual handling, shoveling)
  - community/leisure (eg, difficulty with walking, lifting)
- *Disability—that is, the inability or the restricted ability to perform actions, tasks, or activities of required roles within the individual's sociocultural context—in the following categories:*
  - work (eg, inability to return to work as court stenographer because of lack of coordination in upper extremities, inability to take care of child because of loss of strength)
  - community/leisure (eg, difficulty with card playing because of loss of dexterity, inability to visit friends because of wound)
- *Risk reduction/prevention needs in the following areas:*
  - risk factors (eg, need to learn stress management)
  - recurrence of condition (eg, need to continue strengthening program)
  - secondary impairments (eg, need to appropriately use transcutaneous electrical nerve stimulation [TENS] for pain management)
- *Health, wellness, and fitness needs:*
  - fitness, including physical performance (eg, need to routinely use functional electrical stimulation [FES] to maximize muscle contraction)
  - health and wellness (eg, need to increase muscle force to optimize bone density, need to modulate pain during hospital volunteering)

Electrotherapeutic Modalities continued

Interventions

Electrotherapeutic modalities may include:

- Biofeedback
- Electrotherapeutic delivery of medications
  - iontophoresis
- Electrical stimulation
  - electrical muscle stimulation (EMS)
  - electrical stimulation for tissue repair (ESTR)
  - functional electrical stimulation (FES)
  - high voltage pulsed current (HVPC)
  - neuromuscular electrical stimulation (NMES)
  - transcutaneous electrical nerve stimulation (TENS)

Anticipated Goals and Expected Outcomes

Anticipated goals and expected outcomes related to electrotherapeutic modalities may include:

- Impact on pathology/pathophysiology (disease, disorder, or condition)
  - Edema, lymphedema, or effusion is decreased.
  - Joint swelling, inflammation, or restriction is reduced.
  - Nutrient delivery to tissue is increased.
  - Osteogenic effects are enhanced.
  - Pain is decreased.
  - Soft tissue or wound healing is enhanced.
  - Soft tissue swelling, inflammation, or restriction is reduced.
  - Tissue perfusion and oxygenation are enhanced.
- Impact on impairments
  - Integumentary integrity is improved.
  - Motor function (motor control and motor learning) is improved.
  - Muscle performance (strength, power, and endurance) is increased.
  - Postural control is improved.
  - Quality and quantity of movement between and across body segments are improved.
  - Range of motion is improved.
  - Relaxation is increased.
  - Sensory awareness is increased.
  - Weight-bearing status is improved.
  - Work of breathing is decreased.
- Impact on functional limitations
  - Ability to perform physical actions, tasks, or activities related to self-care, home management, work (job/school/play), community, and leisure is improved.
  - Level of supervision required for task performance is decreased.
  - Performance of and independence in activities of daily living (ADL) and instrumental activities of daily living (IADL) with or without devices and equipment are increased.
  - Tolerance of positions and activities is increased.
- Impact on disabilities
  - Ability to assume or resume required self-care, home management, work (job/school/play), community, and leisure roles is improved.
- Risk reduction/prevention
  - Complications of immobility are reduced.
  - Preoperative and postoperative complications are reduced.
  - Risk factors are reduced.
  - Risk of recurrence of condition is reduced.
  - Risk of secondary impairment is reduced.
  - Self-management of symptoms is improved.
- Impact on health, wellness, and fitness
  - Fitness is improved.
  - Health status is improved.
  - Physical capacity is increased.
  - Physical function is improved.
- Impact on societal resources
  - Utilization of physical therapy services is optimized.
  - Utilization of physical therapy services results in efficient use of health care dollars.
- Patient/client satisfaction
  - Access, availability, and services provided are acceptable to patient/client.
  - Administrative management of practice is acceptable to patient/client.
  - Clinical proficiency of physical therapist is acceptable to patient/client.
  - Coordination of care is acceptable to patient/client.
  - Interpersonal skills of physical therapist are acceptable to patient/client, family, and significant others.
  - Sense of well-being is improved.
  - Stressors are decreased.

Procedural Interventions

Physical Agents and Mechanical Modalities

Physical agents are a broad group of procedures using various forms of energy that are applied to tissues in a systematic manner and that are intended to increase connective tissue extensibility; increase the healing rate of open wounds and soft tissue; modulate pain; reduce or eliminate soft tissue swelling, inflammation, or restriction associated with musculoskeletal injury or circulatory dysfunction; remodel scar tissue; or treat skin conditions. These agents may include athermal, cryotherapy, hydrotherapy, light, sound, and thermotherapy agents. *Mechanical modalities* are a group of devices that use forces such as approximation, compression, and distraction and that are intended to improve circulation, increase range of motion, modulate pain, or stabilize an area that requires temporary support. These modalities may include compression therapies, gravity-assisted compression devices, mechanical motion devices, and traction devices.

Physical therapists select, prescribe, and implement use of these agents and modalities when the examination findings, diagnosis, and prognosis indicate the use of physical agents or mechanical modalities to decrease neural compression; decrease pain and swelling; decrease soft tissue and circulatory disorders; enhance airway clearance; enhance movement performance; enhance or maintain physical performance; improve joint mobility; improve tissue perfusion; prevent or remediate impairments, functional limitations, or disabilities to improve physical function; reduce edema; or reduce risk factors and complications.

The use of physical agents or mechanical modalities in the absence of other interventions should not be considered physical therapy unless there is documentation that justifies the necessity of their exclusive use.

Clinical Considerations

Examination findings that may direct the type and specificity of the procedural intervention may include:

- *Pathology/pathophysiology (disease, disorder, or condition), history (including risk factors) of medical/surgical conditions, or signs and symptoms (eg, pain, shortness of breath, stress) in the following systems:*
  - cardiovascular
  - endocrine/metabolic
  - genitourinary
  - integumentary
  - multiple systems
  - musculoskeletal
  - neuromuscular
  - pulmonary

- *Impairments in the following categories:*
  - aerobic capacity/endurance (eg, decreased muscle endurance)
  - anthropometric characteristics (eg, increased edema)
  - circulation (eg, decreased peripheral circulation)
  - cranial and peripheral nerve integrity (eg, neural compression)
  - ergonomics and body mechanics (eg, segment instability)
  - gait, locomotion, and balance (eg, antalgic gait)
  - integumentary integrity (eg, skin condition irritated by device)
  - joint integrity and mobility (eg, increased joint compression)
  - muscle performance (eg, incontinence because of decreased muscle strength)
  - neuromotor development and sensory integration (eg, limited tolerance to upright position)
  - posture (eg, abnormal postural alignment)
  - range of motion (eg, postoperative limitation of motion)
  - reflex integrity (eg, decreased deep reflex response)
  - sensory integrity (eg, altered proprioception)
  - ventilation and respiration (eg, small airway congestion)

- *Functional limitations in the ability to perform actions, tasks, or activities in the following categories:*
  - self-care (eg, difficulty with hair care and ironing, inability to maintain positions)
  - work (job/school/play) (eg, difficulty with operating heavy machinery, difficulty with washing windows)
  - community/leisure (eg, difficulty with serving in soup kitchen)

- *Disability—that is, the inability or the restricted ability to perform actions, tasks, or activities of required roles within the individual's sociocultural context—in the following categories:*
  - work (eg, inability to return to work as a taxi driver because of neck pain, inability to put child in car seat because of back pain)
  - community/leisure (eg, difficulty with jogging with baby stroller because of Achilles tendinitis, inability to go to the movies as a result of incontinence)

- *Risk reduction/prevention needs in the following areas:*
  - risk factors (eg, need to learn how to use proper lower-limb compressive garments)
  - recurrence of condition (eg, need to continue daily standing program)
  - secondary impairments (eg, need to participate in continuous exercise program)

- *Health, wellness, and fitness needs:*
  - fitness, including physical performance (eg, need to increase muscle length for aquatics, need to maximize pelvic-floor muscle function)
  - health and wellness (eg, need to increase circulation during skating, need to modulate pain during shopping)

Physical Agents and Mechanical Modalities continued

Interventions

Physical agents may include:

- Athermal agents
  - pulsed electromagnetic fields
- Cryotherapy
  - cold packs
  - ice massage
  - vapocoolant spray
- Hydrotherapy
  - contrast bath
  - pools
  - pulsatile lavage
  - whirlpool tanks
- Light agents
  - infrared
  - laser
  - ultraviolet
- Sound agents
  - phonophoresis
  - ultrasound
- Thermotherapy
  - diathermy
  - dry heat
  - hot packs
  - paraffin baths

Mechanical modalities may include:

- Compression therapies
  - compression bandaging
  - compression garments
  - taping
  - total contact casting
  - vasopneumatic compression devices
- Gravity-assisted compression devices
  - standing frame
  - tilt table
- Mechanical motion devices
  - continuous passive motion (CPM)
- Traction devices
  - intermittent
  - positional
  - sustained

Anticipated Goals and Expected Outcomes

Anticipated goals and expected outcomes related to physical agents and mechanical modalities may include:

- Impact on pathology/pathophysiology (disease, disorder, or condition)
  - Atelectasis is decreased.
  - Debridement of nonviable tissue is achieved.
  - Edema, lymphedema, or effusion is reduced.
  - Joint swelling, inflammation, or restriction is reduced.
  - Neural compression is decreased.
  - Nutrient delivery to tissue is increased.
  - Osteogenic effects are enhanced.
  - Pain is decreased.
  - Soft tissue swelling, inflammation, or restriction is reduced.
  - Tissue perfusion and oxygenation are enhanced.
- Impact on impairments
  - Airway clearance is improved.
  - Integumentary integrity is improved.
  - Muscle performance (strength, power, and endurance) is increased.
  - Range of motion is improved.
  - Relaxation is increased.
  - Weight-bearing status is improved.
- Impact on functional limitations
  - Ability to perform physical actions, tasks, or activities related to self-care, home management, work (job/school/play), community, and leisure is improved.
  - Performance of and independence in activities of daily living (ADL) and instrumental activities of daily living (IADL) with or without devices and equipment are increased.
  - Tolerance of positions and activities is increased.
- Impact on disabilities
  - Ability to assume or resume required self-care, home management, work (job/school/play), community, and leisure roles is improved.
- Risk reduction/prevention
  - Complications of soft tissue and circulatory disorders are decreased.
  - Risk of secondary impairment is reduced.
  - Self-management of symptoms is improved.
  - Stresses precipitating injury are decreased.
- Impact on health, wellness, and fitness
  - Fitness is improved.
  - Physical capacity is increased.
  - Physical function is improved.
- Impact on societal resources
  - Utilization of physical therapy services is optimized.
- Patient/client satisfaction
  - Access, availability, and services provided are acceptable to patient/client.
  - Administrative management of practice is acceptable to patient/client.
  - Clinical proficiency of physical therapist is acceptable to patient/client.
  - Coordination of care is acceptable to patient/client.
  - Interpersonal skills of physical therapist are acceptable to patient/client, family, and significant others.
  - Sense of well-being is improved.
  - Stressors are decreased.

PART TWO:

Preferred Physical Therapist Practice Patterns

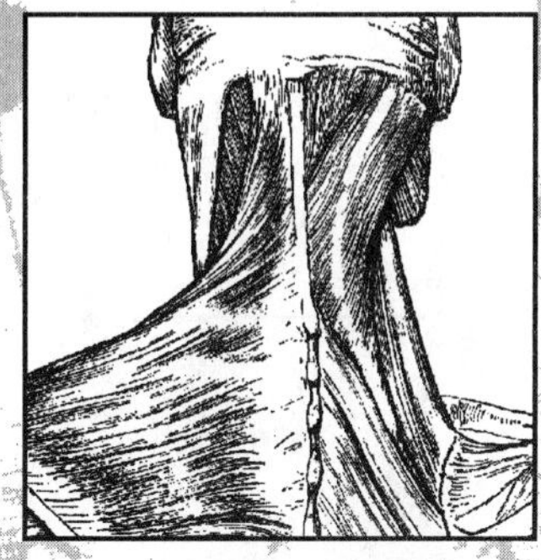

Musculoskeletal

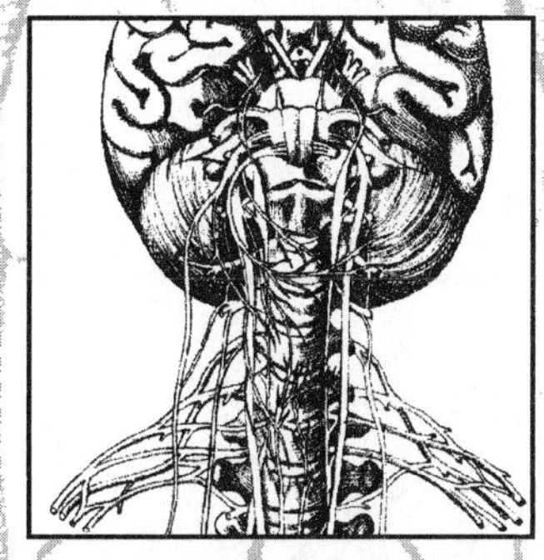

Neuromuscular

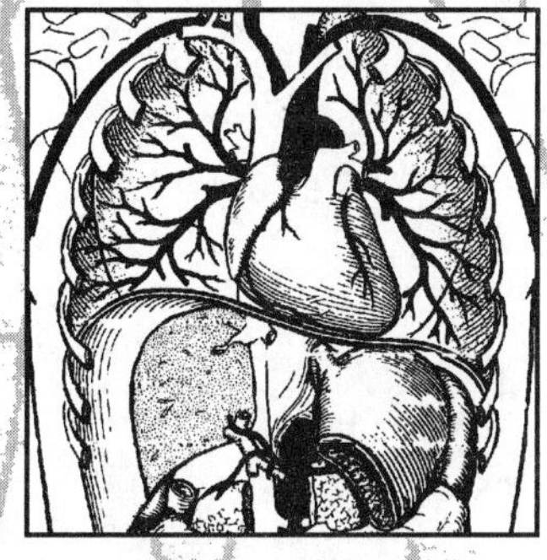

Cardiovascular/ Pulmonary

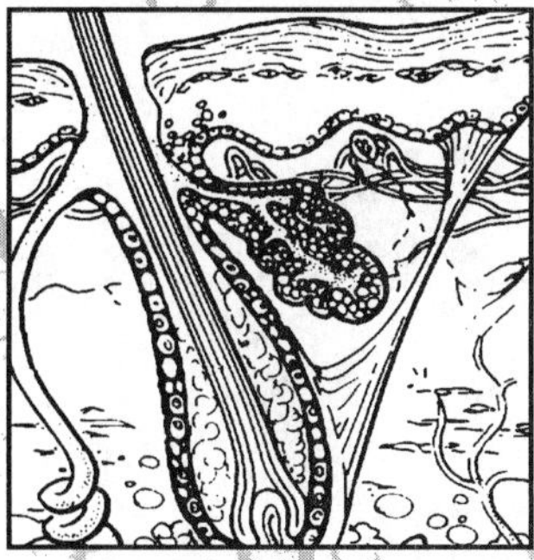

Integumentary

How to Use the Preferred Practice Patterns

Corresponds to "How to Use the Patterns" in the Interactive Guide CD-ROM

Part Two contains the preferred practice patterns, which are grouped under four categories of conditions: Musculoskeletal (Chapter 4), Neuromuscular (Chapter 5), Cardiovascular/Pulmonary (Chapter 6), and Integumentary (Chapter 7). A table of contents preceding each set of patterns lists the pattern titles for that set. Below is an at-a-glance depiction of the contents of each pattern; on the following pages, take a walk through one example of how physical therapists may use Part Two in the management of patients/clients.

Contents of Each Pattern at a Glance

1 Patient/Client Diagnostic Classification

- Criteria for inclusion (based on examination findings regarding risk factors or consequences of pathology/pathophysiology [disease, disorder, or condition], impairments, functional limitations, or disabilities)
- Criteria for exclusion from pattern or for multiple-pattern classification (based on examination findings)

2 ICD-9-CM Codes

Codes that may relate to the practice pattern—intended only for information purposes, not for coding purposes

The Five Elements of Patient/Client Management

3 Examination

Description of the history, systems review, and tests and measures that generate data that help the physical therapist confirm classification of the patients/clients in the pattern

4 Evaluation, Diagnosis, and Prognosis (Including Plan of Care)

Description of the evaluation, diagnostic, and prognostic processes, including the expected range of number of visits and factors that may require a new episode of care or that may modify frequency of visits and duration of the episode

5 Intervention

A listing of the interventions that may be used for patients/clients who are classified in the pattern

6 Reexamination, Global Outcomes, and Criteria for Termination of Physical Therapy Services

Description of when reexamination is indicated; measurement of global outcomes of physical therapy services in 8 domains; the 2 ways in which physical therapy services are terminated

Examination

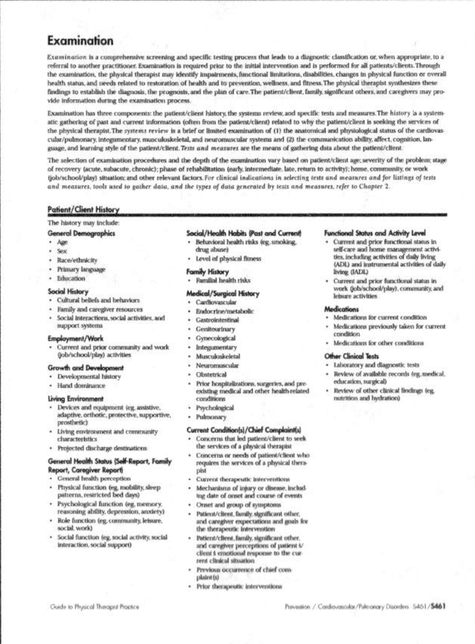

Examination

Examination is a comprehensive screening and specific testing process that leads to a diagnostic classification or, when appropriate, to a referral to another practitioner. Examination is required prior to the initial intervention and is performed for all patients/clients. Through the examination, the physical therapist may identify impairments, functional limitations, disabilities, changes in physical function or overall health status, and needs related to restoration of health and to prevention, wellness, and fitness. The physical therapist synthesizes these findings to establish the diagnosis, the prognosis, and the plan of care. The patient/client, family, significant others, and caregivers may provide information during the examination process.

Examination has three components: the patient/client history, the systems review, and specific tests and measures. The *history* is a systematic gathering of past and current information (often from the patient/client) related to why the patient/client is seeking the services of the physical therapist. The *systems review* is a brief or limited examination of (1) the anatomical and physiological status of the cardiovascular/pulmonary, integumentary, musculoskeletal, and neuromuscular systems and (2) the communication ability, affect, cognition, language, and learning style of the patient/client. *Tests and measures* are the means of gathering data about the patient/client.

The selection of examination procedures and the depth of the examination vary based on patient/client age; severity of the problem; stage of recovery (acute, subacute, chronic); phase of rehabilitation (early, intermediate, late, return to activity); home, community, or work (job/school/play) situation; and other relevant factors. *For clinical indications in selecting tests and measures and for listings of tests and measures, tools used to gather data, and the types of data generated by tests and measures, refer to Chapter 2.*

Patient/Client History

The history may include:

General Demographics
- Age
- Sex
- Race/ethnicity
- Primary language
- Education

Social History
- Cultural beliefs and behaviors
- Family and caregiver resources
- Social interactions, social activities, and support systems

Employment/Work
- Current and prior community and work (job/school/play) activities

Growth and Development
- Developmental history
- Hand dominance

Living Environment
- Devices and equipment (eg, assistive, adaptive, orthotic, protective, supportive, prosthetic)
- Living environment and community characteristics
- Projected discharge destinations

General Health Status (Self-Report, Family Report, Caregiver Report)
- General health perception
- Physical function (eg, mobility, sleep patterns, restricted bed days)
- Psychological function (eg, memory, reasoning ability, depression, anxiety)
- Role function (eg, community, leisure, social, work)
- Social function (eg, social activity, social interaction, social support)

Social/Health Habits (Past and Current)
- Behavioral health risks (eg, smoking, drug abuse)
- Level of physical fitness

Family History
- Familial health risks

Medical/Surgical History
- Cardiovascular
- Endocrine/metabolic
- Gastrointestinal
- Genitourinary
- Gynecological
- Integumentary
- Musculoskeletal
- Neuromuscular
- Obstetrical
- Prior hospitalizations, surgeries, and preexisting medical and other health-related conditions
- Psychological
- Pulmonary

Current Condition(s)/Chief Complaint(s)
- Concerns that led patient/client to seek the services of a physical therapist
- Concerns or needs of patient/client who requires the services of a physical therapist
- Current therapeutic interventions
- Mechanisms of injury or disease, including date of onset and course of events
- Onset and group of symptoms
- Patient/client, family, significant other, and caregiver expectations and goals for the therapeutic intervention
- Patient/client, family, significant other, and caregiver perceptions of patient's/client's emotional response to the current clinical situation
- Previous occurrence of chief complaint(s)
- Prior therapeutic interventions

Functional Status and Activity Level
- Current and prior functional status in self-care and home management activities, including activities of daily living (ADL) and instrumental activities of daily living (IADL)
- Current and prior functional status in work (job/school/play), community, and leisure activities

Medications
- Medications for current condition
- Medications previously taken for current condition
- Medications for other conditions

Other Clinical Tests
- Laboratory and diagnostic tests
- Review of available records (eg, medical, education, surgical)
- Review of other clinical findings (eg, nutrition and hydration)

Guide to Physical Therapist Practice   Prevention / Cardiovascular/Pulmonary Disorders S461/S461

First, the patient/client provides a *history*. Through the history, the physical therapist gathers data—from both the past and the present—related to why the patient/client is seeking physical therapy services. Through the history, the physical therapist learns the chief complaints of the patient/client—in this example, the inability to walk without pain and a sensation of "buckling" in both knees and the inability to participate in recreational sports.

Systems Review

The systems review may include:

Physiological and anatomical status
- Cardiovascular/Pulmonary
  - Blood pressure
  - Edema
  - Heart rate
  - Respiratory rate
- Integumentary
  - Presence of scar formation
  - Skin color
  - Skin integrity
- Musculoskeletal
  - Gross range of motion
  - Gross strength
  - Gross symmetry
  - Height
  - Weight
- Neuromuscular
  - Gross coordinated movements (eg, balance, locomotion, transfers, transitions)

Communication, affect, cognition, language, and learning style
- Ability to make needs known
- Consciousness
- Expected emotional/behavioral responses
- Learning preferences (eg, education needs, learning barriers)
- Orientation (person, place, time)

Next, the physical therapist performs a *systems review*, which is a brief examination of the anatomical and physiological status of the cardiovascular/pulmonary, integumentary, musculoskeletal, and neuromuscular systems. The systems review not only helps focus the examination, it indicates whether the patient/client should be referred for other health care services in addition to physical therapy. In this example, the systems review findings indicate that the patient/client has impairments in the cardiovascular/pulmonary system (high blood pressure at rest), musculoskeletal system (impaired gross range of motion, impaired gross strength, disproportionate weight for height), and neuromuscular system (impaired gait, impaired balance). The systems review suggests there are no current impairments in the integumentary system; however, the history shows the presence of diabetes, which is a risk factor for cardiovascular/pulmonary, neuromuscular, and integumentary conditions. There are no limitations in communication, affect, cognition, language, and learning style.

Tests and Measures

Tests and measures for this pattern may include those that characterize or quantify:

Aerobic Capacity and Endurance
- Aerobic capacity during functional activities (eg, activities of daily living [ADL] scales, indexes, instrumental activities of daily living [IADL] scales, observations)
- Aerobic capacity during standardized exercise test protocols (eg, ergometry, step tests, time/distance walk/run tests, treadmill tests, wheelchair tests)

Anthropometric Characteristics
- Edema (eg, girth measurement, palpation, scales, volume measurement)

Assistive and Adaptive Devices
- Assistive or adaptive devices and equipment use during functional activities (eg, ADL scales, functional scales, IADL scales, interviews, observations)
- Components, alignment, fit, and ability to care for the assistive or adaptive devices and equipment (eg, interviews, logs, observations, pressure-sensing maps, reports)
- Remediation of impairments, functional limitations, or disabilities with use of assistive or adaptive devices and equipment (eg, ADL scales, IADL scales, pain scales, play scales)
- Safety during use of assistive or adaptive devices and equipment (eg, diaries, fall scales, interviews, logs, observations, reports)

Community and Work (Job/School/Play) Integration or Reintegration (Including IADL)
- Ability to assume or resume community, work (job/school/play), and leisure activities with or without assistive, adaptive, orthotic, protective, supportive, or prosthetic devices and equipment (eg, activity profiles, disability indexes, functional status questionnaires, IADL scales, observations, physical capacity tests)
- Ability to gain access to community, work (job/school/play), and leisure environments (eg, barrier identification, interviews, observations, physical capacity tests, transportation assessments)
- Safety in community, work (job/school/play), and leisure activities and environments (eg, diaries, fall scales, interviews, logs, observations, videographic assessments)

Cranial and Peripheral Nerve Integrity
- Electrophysiological integrity (eg, electroneuromyography)
- Motor distribution of the cranial nerves (eg, dynamometry, muscle tests, observations)
- Motor distribution of the peripheral nerves (eg, dynamometry, muscle tests, observations, thoracic outlet tests)
- Response to neural provocation (eg, tension tests, vertebral artery compression tests)
- Sensory distribution of the cranial nerves (eg, discrimination tests; tactile tests, including coarse and light touch, cold and heat, pain, pressure, and vibration)
- Sensory distribution of the peripheral nerves (eg, discrimination tests; tactile tests, including coarse and light touch, cold and heat, pain, pressure, and vibration; thoracic outlet tests)

Environmental, Home, and Work (Job/School/Play) Barriers
- Current and potential barriers (eg, checklists, interviews, observations, questionnaires)

S200/S200 Guide to Physical Therapist Practice   Physical Therapy • Volume 81 • Number 1 • January 2001

Based on the history and systems review findings, the physical therapist notes key *clinical indications* for the use of particular tests and measures during the in-depth portion of the examination. (For examples of clinical indications for the use of tests and measures, refer to Chapter 2.) The key clinical indications in this case example: impaired gait; impaired joint integrity and mobility; impaired muscle performance; and a history of diabetes, hypertension, and morbid obesity. Based on these key clinical indications, the physical therapist decides to examine the following test-and-measure categories in detail: aerobic capacity/endurance, circulation (arterial, venous, and lymphatic), community and work (job/school/play) integration or reintegration (including instrumental activities of daily living [IADL]); environmental, home, and work (job/school/play) barriers; gait, locomotion, and balance; joint integrity and mobility; muscle performance (strength, power, and endurance); pain; range of motion (including muscle length); self-care and home management (including activities of daily living [ADL] and IADL), and ventilation and respiration/gas exchange. Due to the presence of cardiovascular/pulmonary risk factors such as hypertension, the monitoring of vital signs during ambulation will be an important part of the in-depth examination.

Evaluation, Diagnosis, and Prognosis (Including Plan of Care)

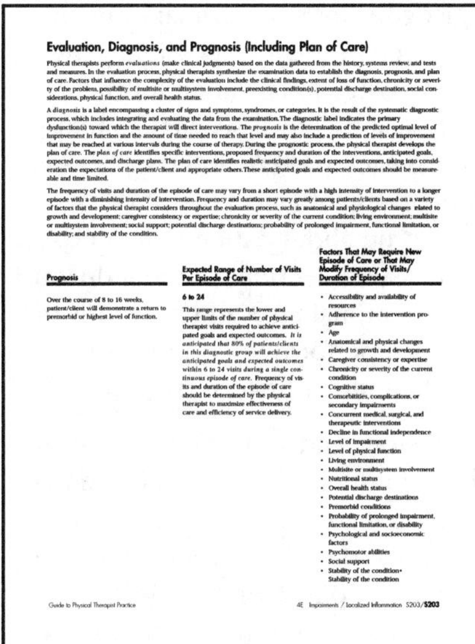

Evaluation, Diagnosis, and Prognosis (Including Plan of Care)

Physical therapists perform *evaluations* (make clinical judgments) based on the data gathered from the history, systems review, and tests and measures. In the evaluation process, physical therapists synthesize the examination data to establish the diagnosis, prognosis, and plan of care. Factors that influence the complexity of the evaluation include the clinical findings, extent of loss of function, chronicity or severity of the problem, possibility of multisite or multisystem involvement, preexisting condition(s), potential discharge destination, social considerations, physical function, and overall health status.

A *diagnosis* is a label encompassing a cluster of signs and symptoms, syndromes, or categories. It is the result of the systematic diagnostic process, which includes integrating and evaluating the data from the examination. The diagnostic label indicates the primary dysfunction(s) toward which the therapist will direct interventions. The *prognosis* is the determination of the predicted optimal level of improvement in function and the amount of time needed to reach that level and may also include a prediction of levels of improvement that may be reached at various intervals during the course of therapy. During the prognostic process, the physical therapist develops the plan of care. The *plan of care* identifies specific interventions, proposed frequency and duration of the interventions, anticipated goals, expected outcomes, and discharge plans. The plan of care identifies realistic anticipated goals and expected outcomes, taking into consideration the expectations of the patient/client and appropriate others. These anticipated goals and expected outcomes should be measureable and time limited.

The frequency of visits and duration of the episode of care may vary from a short episode with a high intensity of intervention to a longer episode with a diminishing intensity of intervention. Frequency and duration may vary greatly among patients/clients based on a variety of factors that the physical therapist considers throughout the evaluation process, such as anatomical and physiological changes elated to growth and development; caregiver consistency or expertise; chronicity or severity of the current condition; living environment; multisite or multisystem involvement; social support; potential discharge destinations; probability of prolonged impairment, functional limitation, or disability; and stability of the condition.

Prognosis	Expected Range of Number of Visits Per Episode of Care	Factors That May Require New Episode of Care or That May Modify Frequency of Visits/ Duration of Episode
Over the course of 8 to 16 weeks, patient/client will demonstrate a return to premorbid or highest level of function.	**6 to 24** This range represents the lower and upper limits of the number of physical therapist visits required to achieve anticipated goals and expected outcomes. *It is anticipated that 80% of patients/clients in this diagnostic group will achieve the anticipated goals and expected outcomes within 6 to 24 visits during a single continuous episode of care.* Frequency of visits and duration of the episode of care should be determined by the physical therapist to maximize effectiveness of care and efficiency of service delivery.	• Accessibility and availability of resources • Adherence to the intervention program • Age • Anatomical and physical changes related to growth and development • Caregiver consistency or expertise • Chronicity or severity of the current condition • Cognitive status • Comorbidities, complications, or secondary impairments • Concurrent medical, surgical, and therapeutic interventions • Decline in functional independence • Level of impairment • Level of physical function • Living environment • Multisite or multisystem involvement • Nutritional status • Overall health status • Potential discharge destinations • Premorbid conditions • Probability of prolonged impairment, functional limitation, or disability • Psychological and socioeconomic factors • Psychomotor abilities • Social support • Stability of the condition• Stability of the condition

Guide to Physical Therapist Practice　4E Impairments / Localized Inflammation S203/**S203**

During the *evaluation* process, all data from the history, systems review, and tests and measures are synthesized to establish the diagnosis and the prognosis, including the plan of care.

In this example, based on the evaluation of the history, systems review, and tests-and-measures data, the physical therapist determines that the patient/client has the following primary impairments: impaired joint integrity and mobility in the knees; decreased muscle performance; decreased range of motion; and decreased aerobic capacity/endurance with ambulation. The physical therapist hypothesizes that the morbid obesity may be contributing to the knee pain as well as to the decrease in aerobic capacity/endurance.

The physical therapist notes the following functional limitations: difficulty in performing ADL and IADL, inability to run bases during softball league games, and inability to perform heavy household chores. Disability is noted in the following roles: community/leisure (inability to participate on the league softball team), work (job/school/play) (inability to walk to different work sites within the same plant), and home management (inability to perform as homemaker).

Even though patients/clients may be referred to physical therapy services with a medical diagnosis, that does not tell the physical therapist how to manage the patient/client. The medical diagnosis is a diagnostic label that identifies disease at the level of the cell, tissue, organ, or system. In this case, for instance, the medical diagnosis may be osteoarthritis of the knees. The physical therapist's diagnosis, however, is a diagnostic label that identifies the impact of a condition on function *at the level of the system* (especially the movement system) and *at the level of the whole person*. The physical therapist's goal is to restore function, and therefore the physical therapist's examination, evaluation, and interventions focus on impairments, functional limitations, disabilities, risk factor reduction, and prevention.

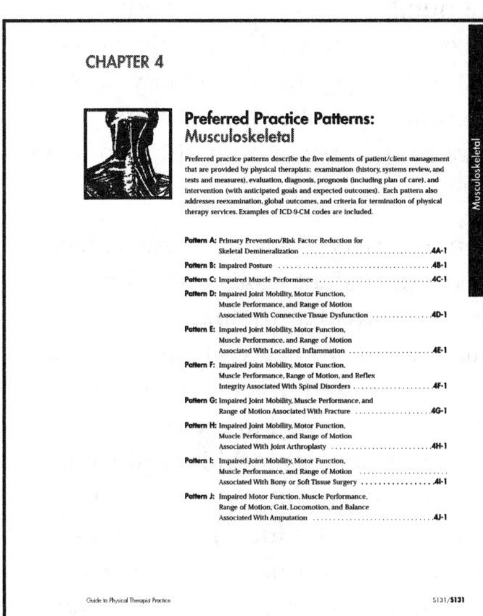

CHAPTER 4

Preferred Practice Patterns: Musculoskeletal

Musculoskeletal

Preferred practice patterns describe the five elements of patient/client management that are provided by physical therapists: examination (history, systems review, and tests and measures), evaluation, diagnosis, prognosis (including plan of care), and intervention (with anticipated goals and expected outcomes). Each pattern also addresses reexamination, global outcomes, and criteria for termination of physical therapy services. Examples of ICD-9-CM codes are included.

Guide to Physical Therapist Practice　S131/**S131**

In this example, the physical therapist determines that decreased muscle performance, decreased range of motion, and pain are the primary contributors to the identified functional limitations. The physical therapist also has noted that the patient/client has decreased aerobic/capacity endurance. The physical therapist therefore focuses on four preferred practice patterns: "Impaired Muscle Performance" (Pattern 4C) "Impaired Joint Mobility, Motor Function, Muscle Performance, and Range of Motion Associated With Connective Tissue Dysfunction" (Pattern 4D) "Impaired Joint Mobility, Motor Function, Muscle Performance, and Range of Motion Associated With Localized Inflammation" (Pattern 4E) and "Impaired Aerobic Capacity/Endurance Associated With Deconditioning" (Pattern 6B).

Evaluation continued

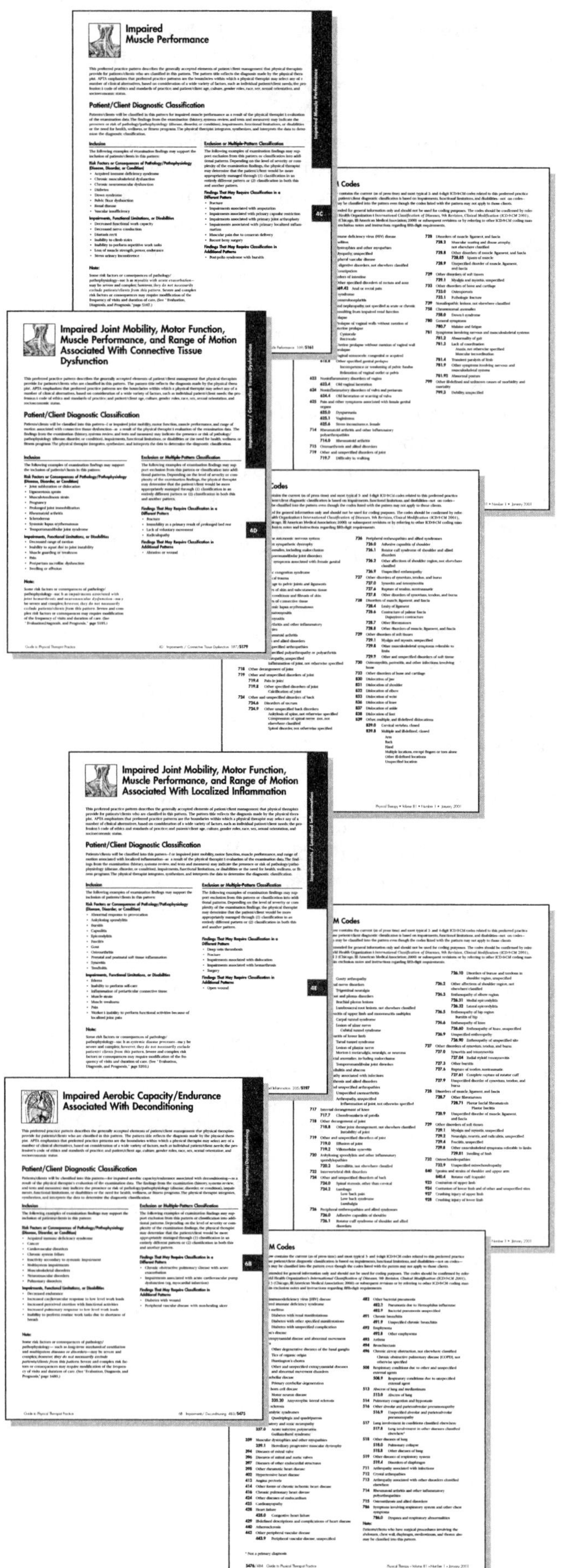

Impaired Muscle Performance

Patient/Client Diagnostic Classification

ICD-9-CM Codes

Impaired Joint Mobility, Motor Function, Muscle Performance, and Range of Motion Associated With Connective Tissue Dysfunction

Patient/Client Diagnostic Classification

ICD-9-CM Codes

Impaired Joint Mobility, Motor Function, Muscle Performance, and Range of Motion Associated With Localized Inflammation

Patient/Client Diagnostic Classification

ICD-9-CM Codes

Impaired Aerobic Capacity/Endurance Associated With Deconditioning

Patient/Client Diagnostic Classification

ICD-9-CM Codes

The physical therapist considers the primary impairments to determine which of the four possible patterns may be the most appropriate classification for the patient/client. The physical therapist scans the inclusions and exclusions for each pattern and the ICD-9-CM codes that are listed in each pattern. If the physical therapist remains uncertain about patient/client classification, the tests-and-measures sections of the individual patterns may suggest additional tests and measures that the physical therapist can perform to confirm placement of the patient/client into a pattern.

In this example, the history and systems review show signs and symptoms of joint effusion but indicate that joint integrity and mobility are not contributing factors. The physical therapist therefore classifies the patient/ client in "Impaired Joint Mobility, Motor Function, Muscle Performance, and Range of Motion Associated With Localized Inflammation" (Pattern 4E). The patient/client also has a history of diabetes. If the physical therapist determines that patient/client monitoring for primary prevention of lower-extremity vascular problems and the need to increase aerobic capacity are high priorities, the physical therapist may place the patient/client in an additional pattern: "Primary Prevention/Risk Reduction for Cardiovascular/Pulmonary Disorders" (Pattern 6A).

Based on the evaluation, the physical therapist makes the prognosis—that is, determines the predicted optimal level of improvement in function and the amount of time needed to reach that level. The physical therapist refers to the evaluation section of the selected pattern to ascertain whether the therapist's prediction of improvement, frequency of visits, and duration of episode of care are consistent with the expected prognosis and range of number of visits for patients/clients who are classified in that pattern. The physical therapist also notes any factors (eg, age, chronicity or severity of the current condition, adherence to the intervention program) that may modify the frequency of visits or duration of the episode.

In this example, on the basis of such modifying factors as extremely high patient/client motivation, the physical therapist may determine that the patient/client will require fewer visits than are expected to achieve the anticipated goals and expected outcomes for 80% of patients/clients who are classified in the pattern. On the other hand, the presence of morbid obesity may indicate that the patient/client may not be able to improve aerobic capacity/endurance at an expected rate. In addition, if the hypertension and diabetes become uncontrolled, the ability of the patient/client to participate in physical therapy may be affected.

Intervention

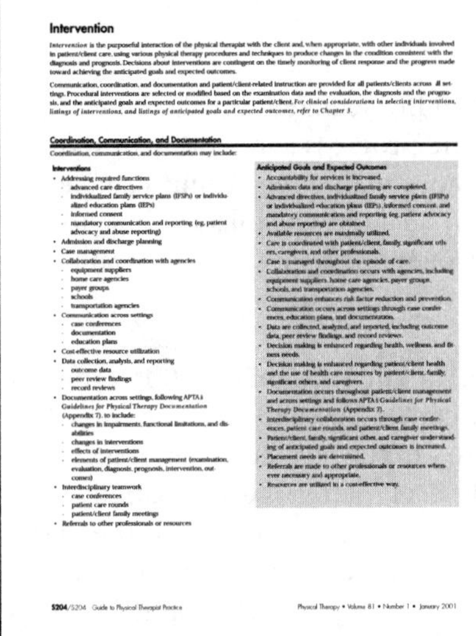

Intervention

Intervention is the purposeful interaction of the physical therapist with the client and, when appropriate, with other individuals involved in patient/client care, using various physical therapy procedures and techniques to produce changes in the condition consistent with the diagnosis and prognosis. Decisions about interventions are contingent on the timely monitoring of client response and the progress made toward achieving the anticipated goals and expected outcomes.

Communication, coordination, and documentation and patient/client-related instruction are provided for all patients/clients across all settings. Procedural interventions are selected or modified based on the examination data and the evaluation, the diagnosis and the prognosis, and the anticipated goals and expected outcomes for a particular patient/client. *For clinical considerations in selecting interventions, listings of interventions, and listings of anticipated goals and expected outcomes, refer to Chapter 3.*

Coordination, Communication, and Documentation

Coordination, communication, and documentation may include:

Interventions

- Addressing required functions
  - advanced care directives
  - individualized family service plans (IFSPs) or individualized education plans (IEPs)
  - informed consent
  - mandatory communication and reporting (eg, patient advocacy and abuse reporting)
- Admission and discharge planning
- Case management
- Collaboration and coordination with agencies
  - equipment suppliers
  - home care agencies
  - payer groups
  - schools
  - transportation agencies
- Communication across settings
  - case conferences
  - documentation
  - education plans
- Cost-effective resource utilization
- Data collection, analysis, and reporting
  - outcome data
  - peer review findings
  - record reviews
- Documentation across settings, following APTA's *Guidelines for Physical Therapy Documentation* (Appendix 7), to include:
  - changes in impairments, functional limitations, and disabilities
  - changes in interventions
  - effects of interventions
  - elements of patient/client management (examination, evaluation, diagnosis, prognosis, intervention, outcomes)
- Interdisciplinary teamwork
  - case conferences
  - patient care rounds
  - patient/client family meetings
- Referrals to other professionals or resources

Anticipated Goals and Expected Outcomes

- Accountability for services is increased.
- Admission data and discharge planning are completed.
- Advanced directives, individualized family service plans (IFSPs) or individualized education plans (IEPs), informed consent, and mandatory communication and reporting (eg, patient advocacy and abuse reporting) are obtained.
- Available resources are maximally utilized.
- Care is coordinated with patient/client, family, significant others, caregivers, and other professionals.
- Case is managed throughout the episode of care.
- Collaboration and coordination occurs with agencies, including equipment suppliers, home care agencies, payer groups, schools, and transportation agencies.
- Communication enhances risk factor reduction and prevention.
- Communication occurs across settings through case conferences, education plans, and documentation.
- Data are collected, analyzed, and reported, including outcome data, peer review findings, and record reviews.
- Decision making is enhanced regarding health, wellness, and fitness needs.
- Decision making is enhanced regarding patient/client health and the use of health care resources by patient/client, family, significant others, and caregivers.
- Documentation occurs throughout patient/client management and across settings and follows APTA's *Guidelines for Physical Therapy Documentation* (Appendix 7).
- Interdisciplinary collaboration occurs through case conferences, patient care rounds, and patient/client family meetings.
- Patient/client, family, significant other, and caregiver understanding of anticipated goals and expected outcomes is increased.
- Placement needs are determined.
- Referrals are made to other professionals or resources whenever necessary and appropriate.
- Resources are utilized in a cost-effective way.

S204/S204 Guide to Physical Therapist Practice — Physical Therapy • Volume 81 • Number 1 • January 2001

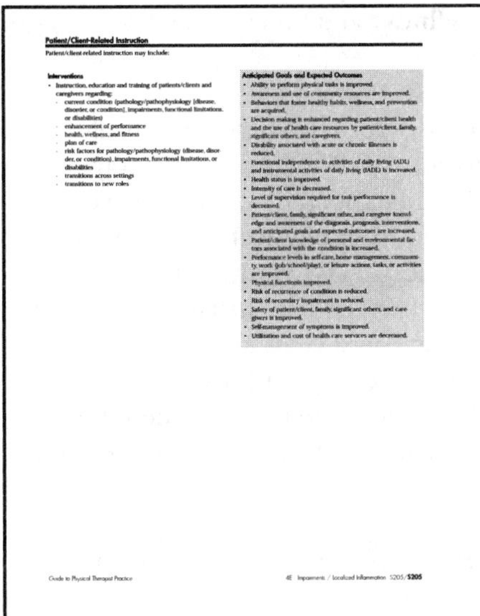

Patient/Client-Related Instruction

Patient/client-related instruction may include:

Interventions

- Instruction, education and training of patients/clients and caregivers regarding:
  - current condition (pathology/pathophysiology [disease, disorder, or condition], impairments, functional limitations, or disabilities)
  - enhancement of performance
  - health, wellness, and fitness
  - plan of care
  - risk factors for pathology/pathophysiology (disease, disorder, or condition), impairments, functional limitations, or disabilities
  - transitions across settings
  - transitions to new roles

Anticipated Goals and Expected Outcomes

- Ability to perform physical tasks is improved.
- Awareness and use of community resources are improved.
- Behaviors that foster healthy habits, wellness, and prevention are acquired.
- Decision making is enhanced regarding patient/client health and the use of health care resources by patient/client, family, significant others, and caregivers.
- Disability associated with acute or chronic illnesses is reduced.
- Functional independence in activities of daily living (ADL) and instrumental activities of daily living (IADL) is increased.
- Health status is improved.
- Intensity of care is decreased.
- Level of supervision required for task performance is decreased.
- Patient/client, family, significant other, and caregiver knowledge and awareness of the diagnosis, prognosis, interventions, and anticipated goals and expected outcomes are increased.
- Patient/client knowledge of personal and environmental factors associated with the condition is increased.
- Performance levels in self-care, home management, community, work (job/school/play), or leisure actions, tasks, or activities are improved.
- Physical function is improved.
- Risk of recurrence of condition is reduced.
- Risk of secondary impairment is reduced.
- Safety of patient/client, family, significant others, and caregivers is improved.
- Self-management of symptoms is improved.
- Utilization and cost of health care services are decreased.

Guide to Physical Therapist Practice — 4E Impairments / Localized Inflammation S205/S205

As part of the prognostic process, the physical therapist develops a plan of care. This plan delineates the types of interventions (physical therapy procedures and techniques) to be used to produce changes in the condition and in patient/client status, the frequency and duration of those interventions, anticipated goals, expected outcomes, and discharge plans. *Anticipated goals and expected outcomes should be measurable and time limited.*

Each pattern contains a listing of interventions that are likely to be used for patients/clients who are classified in the pattern. *Coordination, communication, and documentation and patient/client-related instruction are interventions that are provided to all patients/clients across all settings.* The use of procedural interventions varies for the particular patient/client in the specific pattern. (For examples of clinical considerations for the use of procedural interventions, refer to Chapter 3.) In this example, the physical therapist might select interventions that emphasize therapeutic exercise, functional training in self-care and home management (including ADL and IADL), and functional training in community and work (job/school/play) integration or reintegration (including IADL, work hardening, and work conditioning) in addition to interventions to modulate pain and diminish the effects of joint effusion.

Reexamination, Global Outcomes, and Criteria for Termination of Physical Therapy Services

Reexamination—the process of performing selected tests and measures after the initial examination to determine progress and modify or redirect interventions—may be indicated more than once during a single episode of care. In this example, the physical therapist may decide to perform a reexamination if the patient/client develops a new condition or shows no progress.

Throughout the entire episode of care, the physical therapist determines the anticipated goals and expected outcomes for each intervention. These goals and outcomes are delineated in the shaded boxes that accompany each list of interventions in each pattern. As the patient/client reaches the termination of physical therapy services and the end of the episode of care, the physical therapist measures the global outcomes (that is, the impact) of the physical therapy services in the following domains: pathology/pathophysiology (disease, disorder, or condition); impairments; functional limitations; disabilities; risk reduction/prevention; impact on health, wellness, and fitness; societal resources; and patient/client satisfaction.

The physical therapist uses two processes for terminating physical therapy services: *discharge* and *discontinuation*. If the physical therapist determines that the anticipated goals and expected outcomes have been achieved, the patient/client is discharged from physical therapy services. Physical therapy services are discontinued (1) when the patient/client declines to continue intervention, (2) when the patient/client is unable to continue to progress toward the anticipated goals and expected outcomes because of medical or psychosocial complications or because financial/insurance resources have been expended, or (3) when the physical therapist determines that the patient/client will no longer benefit from physical therapy.

A template for documenting all aspects of patient/client management, including termination of physical therapy services, is provided in Appendix 6. Patient/client satisfaction outcomes may be collected using the Patient/Client Satisfaction Questionnaire in Appendix 7.

CHAPTER 4

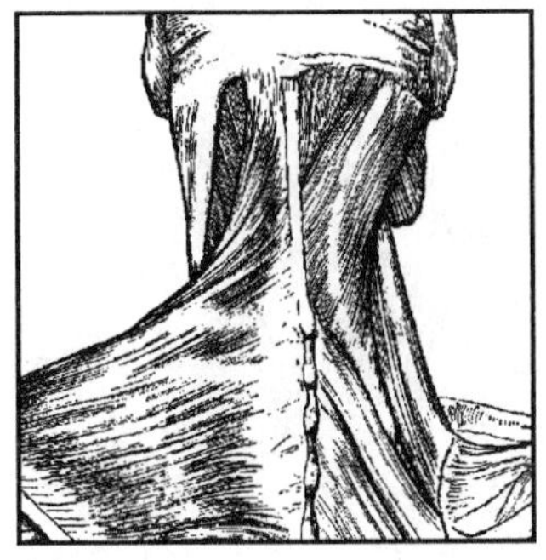

Preferred Physical Therapist Practice Patterns: Musculoskeletal

Preferred Physical Therapist Practice Patterns describe the five elements of patient/client management that are provided by physical therapists: examination (history, systems review, and tests and measures), evaluation, diagnosis, prognosis (including plan of care), and intervention (with anticipated goals and expected outcomes). Each pattern also addresses reexamination, global outcomes, and criteria for termination of physical therapy services. Examples of ICD-9-CM codes are included.

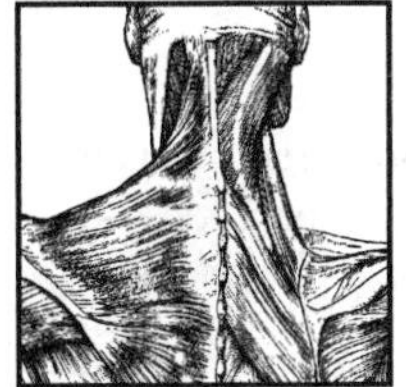

Primary Prevention/Risk Reduction for Skeletal Demineralization

This preferred practice pattern describes the generally accepted elements of patient/client management that physical therapists provide for patient/clients who are classified in this pattern. The pattern title reflects the diagnosis made by the physical therapist. APTA emphasizes that preferred practice patterns are the boundaries within which a physical therapist may select any of a number of clinical alternatives, based on consideration of a wide variety of factors, such as individual patient/client needs; the profession's code of ethics and standards of practice; and patient/client age, culture, gender roles, race, sex, sexual orientation, and socio-economic status.

Patient/Client Diagnostic Classification

Patients/clients will be classified in this primary prevention/risk reduction pattern as a result of the physical therapist's evaluation of the examination data. The findings from the examination (history, systems review, and tests and measures) may indicate the need for a prevention/risk reduction program or for health, wellness, or fitness programs. The physical therapist integrates, synthesizes, and interprets the data to determine the diagnostic classification.

Inclusion

The following examples of examination findings may support the inclusion of clients in this pattern:

Risk Factors or Consequences of Pathology/Pathophysiology (Disease, Disorder, or Condition)

- Chronic cardiovascular/pulmonary dysfunction
- Deconditioning
- Hormonal changes
- Hysterectomy
- Medications (eg, anti-epileptic medications, steroids, thyroid hormone)
- Menopause
- Nutritional deficiency
- Paget disease
- Prolonged non-weight-bearing state

Impairments, Functional Limitations, or Disabilities

- Inability to ambulate
- Joint immobilization associated with inactivity
- Prolonged muscle weakness or paralysis

Note:

Prevention and risk reduction are inherent in all practice patterns. Patients/clients included in this pattern are in need of primary prevention/risk reduction only.

ICD-9-CM Codes

The listing below contains the current (as of press time) and most typical 3- and 4-digit ICD-9-CM codes related to this preferred practice pattern. Because patient/client diagnostic classification is based on impairments, functional limitations, and disabilities—not on codes—patients/clients may be classified into the pattern even though the codes listed with the pattern may not apply to those patients/clients.

This listing is intended for general information only and should not be used for coding purposes. The codes should be confirmed by referring to the World Health Organization's *International Classification of Diseases, 9th Revision, Clinical Modification (ICD-9-CM 2001)*, Volumes 1 and 3 (Chicago, Ill: American Medical Association; 2000) or subsequent revisions or by referring to other ICD-9-CM coding manuals that contain exclusion notes and instructions regarding fifth-digit requirements.

138 Late effects of acute poliomyelitis

262 Other severe, protein-calorie malnutrition

263 Other and unspecified protein-calorie malnutrition

268 Vitamin D deficiency

269 Other nutritional deficiencies

275 Disorders of mineral metabolism

337 Disorders of the autonomic nervous system

- **337.2** Reflex sympathetic dystrophy

344 Other paralytic syndromes

- **344.0** Quadriplegia and quadriparesis
- **344.1** Paraplegia
- **344.3** Monoplegia of lower limb

588 Disorders resulting from impaired renal function

627 Menopausal and postmenopausal disorders

714 Rheumatoid arthritis and other inflammatory polyarthropathies

719 Other and unspecified disorders of joint

- **719.5** Stiffness of joint, not elsewhere classified
- **719.7** Difficulty in walking
- **719.8** Other specified disorders of joint
  - Calcification of joint

728 Disorders of muscle, ligament, and fascia

- **728.2** Muscular wasting and disuse atrophy, not elsewhere classified
- **728.3** Other specific muscle disorders
  - Arthrogryposis

729 Other disorders of soft tissues

- **729.9** Other and unspecified disorders of soft tissue

731 Osteitis deformans and osteopathies associated with other disorders classified elsewhere

- **731.0** Osteitis deformans without mention of bone tumor
  - Paget's disease of bone

732 Osteochondropathies

- **732.0** Juvenile osteochondrosis of spine

733 Other disorders of bone and cartilage

- **733.0** Osteoporosis
- **733.1** Pathologic fracture
- **733.9** Other and unspecified disorders of bone and cartilage
  - **733.90** Osteopenia

737 Curvature of spine

- **737.3** Kyphoscoliosis and scoliosis
- **737.4** Curvature of spine associated with other conditions*

756 Other congenital musculoskeletal anomalies

- **756.5** Osteodystrophies
  - **756.51** Osteogenesis imperfecta

* Not a primary diagnosis

Examination

Examination is a comprehensive screening and specific testing process that leads to a diagnostic classification or, when appropriate, to a referral to another practitioner. Examination is required prior to the initial intervention and is performed for all patients/clients. Through the examination, the physical therapist may identify impairments, functional limitations, disabilities, changes in physical function or overall health status, and needs related to restoration of health and to prevention, wellness, and fitness. The physical therapist synthesizes the examination findings to establish the diagnosis and the prognosis (including the plan of care). The patient/client, family, significant others, and caregivers may provide information during the examination process.

Examination has three components: the patient/client history, the systems review, and tests and measures. The *history* is a systematic gathering of past and current information (often from the patient/client) related to why the patient/client is seeking the services of the physical therapist. The *systems review* is a brief or limited examination of (1) the anatomical and physiological status of the cardiovascular/pulmonary, integumentary, musculoskeletal, and neuromuscular systems and (2) the communication ability, affect, cognition, language, and learning style of the patient/client. *Tests and measures* are the means of gathering data about the patient/client.

The selection of examination procedures and the depth of the examination vary based on patient/client age; severity of the problem; stage of recovery (acute, subacute, chronic); phase of rehabilitation (early, intermediate, late, return to activity); home, work (job/school/play), or community situation; and other relevant factors. *For clinical indications in selecting tests and measures and for listings of tests and measures, tools used to gather data, and the types of data generated by tests and measures, refer to Chapter 2.*

Patient/Client History

The history may include:

General Demographics
- Age
- Sex
- Race/ethnicity
- Primary language
- Education

Social History
- Cultural beliefs and behaviors
- Family and caregiver resources
- Social interactions, social activities, and support systems

Employment/Work (Job/School/Play)
- Current and prior work (job/school/play), community, and leisure actions, tasks, or activities

Growth and Development
- Developmental history
- Hand dominance

Living Environment
- Devices and equipment (eg, assistive, adaptive, orthotic, protective, supportive, prosthetic)
- Living environment and community characteristics
- Projected discharge destinations

General Health Status (Self-Report, Family Report, Caregiver Report)
- General health perception
- Physical function (eg, mobility, sleep patterns, restricted bed days)
- Psychological function (eg, memory, reasoning ability, depression, anxiety)
- Role function (eg, community, leisure, social, work)
- Social function (eg, social activity, social interaction, social support)

Social/Health Habits (Past and Current)
- Behavioral health risks (eg, smoking, drug abuse)
- Level of physical fitness

Family History
- Familial health risks

Medical/Surgical History
- Cardiovascular
- Endocrine/metabolic
- Gastrointestinal
- Genitourinary
- Gynecological
- Integumentary
- Musculoskeletal
- Neuromuscular
- Obstetrical
- Prior hospitalizations, surgeries, and preexisting medical and other health-related conditions
- Psychological
- Pulmonary

Current Condition(s)/Chief Complaint(s)
- Concerns that led patient/client to seek the services of a physical therapist
- Concerns or needs of patient/client who requires the services of a physical therapist
- Current therapeutic interventions
- Mechanisms of injury or disease, including date of onset and course of events
- Onset and pattern of symptoms
- Patient/client, family, significant other, and caregiver expectations and goals for the therapeutic intervention
- Patient/client, family, significant other, and caregiver perceptions of patient's/client's emotional response to the current clinical situation
- Previous occurrence of chief complaint(s)
- Prior therapeutic interventions

Functional Status and Activity Level
- Current and prior functional status in self-care and home management activities, including activities of daily living (ADL) and instrumental activities of daily living (IADL)
- Current and prior functional status in work (job/school/play), community, and leisure actions, tasks, or activities

Medications
- Medications for current condition
- Medications previously taken for current condition
- Medications for other conditions

Other Clinical Tests
- Laboratory and diagnostic tests
- Review of available records (eg, medical, education, surgical)
- Review of other clinical findings (eg, nutrition and hydration)

Systems Review

The systems review may include:

Anatomical and Physiological Status

- Cardiovascular/Pulmonary
  - Blood pressure
  - Edema
  - Heart rate
  - Respiratory rate
- Integumentary
  - Pliability (texture)
  - Presence of scar formation
  - Skin color
  - Skin integrity
- Musculoskeletal
  - Gross range of motion
  - Gross strength
  - Gross symmetry
  - Height
  - Weight
- Neuromuscular
  - Gross coordinated movements (eg, balance, gait, locomotion, transfers, transitions)
  - Motor function (motor control, motor learning)

Communication, Affect, Cognition, Language, and Learning Style

- Ability to make needs known
- Consciousness
- Expected emotional/behavioral responses
- Learning preferences (eg, education needs, learning barriers)
- Orientation (person, place, time)

Tests and Measures

Tests and measures for this pattern may include those that characterize or quantify:

Aerobic Capacity and Endurance

- Aerobic capacity during standardized exercise test protocols (eg, ergometry, step tests, time/distance walk/run tests, treadmill tests, wheelchair tests)

Anthropometric Characteristics

- Body composition (eg, body mass index, impedance measurement, skinfold thickness measurement)
- Body dimensions (eg, girth measurement, length measurement)

Arousal, Attention, and Cognition

- Motivation (eg, adaptive behavior scales)

Environmental, Home, and Work (Job/School/Play) Barriers

- Current and potential barriers (eg, checklists, interviews, observations, questionnaires)
- Physical space and environment (eg, compliance standards, observations, photographic assessments, questionnaires, structural specifications, technology-assisted assessments, videographic assessments)

Ergonomics and Body Mechanics

Ergonomics

- Safety in work environments (eg, hazard identification checklists, job severity indexes, lifting standards, risk assessment scales, standards for exposure limits)

Body mechanics

- Body mechanics during self-care, home management, work, community, or leisure actions, tasks, or activities (eg, activities of daily living [ADL] scales, instrumental activities of daily living [IADL] scales, observations, photographic assessments, technology-assisted assessments, videographic assessments)

Gait, Locomotion, and Balance

- Balance during functional activities with or without the use of assistive, adaptive, orthotic, protective, supportive, or prosthetic devices or equipment (eg, ADL scales, IADL scales, observations, videographic assessments)
- Gait and locomotion during functional activities with or without the use of assistive, adaptive, orthotic, protective, supportive, or prosthetic devices or equipment (eg, ADL scales, gait indexes, IADL scales, mobility skill profiles, observations, videographic assessments)
- Safety during gait, locomotion, and balance (eg, confidence scales, diaries, fall scales, functional assessment profiles, logs, reports)

Motor Function (Motor Control and Motor Learning)

- Dexterity, coordination, and agility (eg, coordination screens, motor impairment tests, motor proficiency tests, observations, videographic assessments)

Muscle Performance (Including Strength, Power, and Endurance)

- Muscle strength, power, and endurance (eg, dynamometry, manual muscle tests, muscle performance tests, physical capacity tests, technology-assisted assessments, timed activity tests)
- Muscle strength, power, and endurance during functional activities (eg, ADL scales, functional muscle tests, IADL scales, observations, videographic assessments)

Posture

- Postural alignment and position (dynamic and static), including symmetry and deviation from midline (eg, observations, grid measurement, photographic assessments, technology-assisted assessments, videographic assessments)
- Specific body parts (eg, angle assessments, forward-bending test, goniometry, observations, palpation, positional tests)

Range of Motion (ROM) (Including Muscle Length)

- Functional ROM (eg, observations, squat tests, toe touch tests)
- Joint active and passive movement (eg, goniometry, inclinometry, observations, photographic assessments, videographic assessments)
- Muscle length, soft tissue extensibility, and flexibility (eg, contracture tests, goniometry, inclinometry, ligamentous tests, linear measurement, multisegment flexibility tests, palpation)

Self-Care and Home Management (Including ADL and IADL)

- Ability to gain access to home environments (eg, barrier identification, observations, physical performance tests)
- Safety in self-care and home management activities and environments (eg, fall scales, interviews, observations)

Work (Job/School/Play), Community, and Leisure Integration or Reintegration (Including IADL)

- Ability to gain access to work (job/school/play), community, and leisure environments (eg, barrier identification, interviews, observations, physical capacity tests, transportation assessments)
- Safety in work (job/school/play), community, and leisure activities and environments (eg, diaries, fall scales, interviews, logs, observations, videographic assessments)

Evaluation, Diagnosis, and Prognosis (Including Plan of Care)

Physical therapists perform *evaluations* (make clinical judgments) based on the data gathered from the history, systems review, and tests and measures. In the evaluation process, physical therapists synthesize the examination data to establish the diagnosis and prognosis (including the plan of care). Factors that influence the complexity of the evaluation include the clinical findings, extent of loss of function, chronicity or severity of the problem, possibility of multisite or multisystem involvement, preexisting condition(s), potential discharge destination, social considerations, physical function, and overall health status.

A *diagnosis* is a label encompassing a cluster of signs and symptoms, syndromes, or categories. It is the result of the systematic diagnostic process, which includes integrating and evaluating the data from the examination.The diagnostic label indicates the primary dysfunction(s) toward which the therapist will direct interventions. The *prognosis* is the determination of the predicted optimal level of improvement in function and the amount of time needed to reach that level and may also include a prediction of levels of improvement that may be reached at various intervals during the course of therapy. During the prognostic process, the physical therapist develops the plan of care. The *plan of care* identifies specific interventions, proposed frequency and duration of the interventions, anticipated goals, expected outcomes, and discharge plans. The plan of care identifies realistic anticipated goals and expected outcomes, taking into consideration the expectations of the patient/client and appropriate others.These anticipated goals and expected outcomes should be measureable and time limited.

The frequency of visits and duration of the episode of care may vary from a short episode with a high intensity of intervention to a longer episode with a diminishing intensity of intervention. Frequency and duration may vary greatly among patients/clients based on a variety of factors that the physical therapist considers throughout the evaluation process, such as anatomical and physiological changes related to growth and development; caregiver consistency or expertise; chronicity or severity of the current condition; living environment; multisite or multisystem involvement; social support; potential discharge destinations; probability of prolonged impairment, functional limitation, or disability; and stability of the condition.

Prognosis

Patient/client will reduce the risk of skeletal demineralization through strength-training and weight-bearing therapeutic exercise programs and through lifestyle modifications.

Expected Range of Number of Visits Per Episode of Care

3 to 18

This range represents the lower and upper limits of the number of physical therapist visits required to achieve anticipated goals and expected outcomes. *It is anticipated that 80% of patients/ clients who are classified into this pattern will achieve the anticipated goals and expected outcomes within 3 to 18 visits during a single continuous episode of care.* Frequency of visits and duration of the episode of care should be determined by the physical therapist to maximize effectiveness of care and efficiency of service delivery.

Factors That May Modify Frequency of Visits

- Accessibility and availability of resources
- Adherence to the intervention program
- Age
- Anatomical and physiological changes related to growth and development
- Caregiver consistency or expertise
- Chronicity or severity of the current condition
- Cognitive status
- Comorbitities, complications, or secondary impairments
- Concurrent medical, surgical, and therapeutic interventions
- Decline in functional independence
- Level of impairment
- Level of physical function
- Living environment
- Multisite or multisystem involvement
- Nutritional status
- Overall health status
- Potential discharge destinations
- Premorbid conditions
- Probability of prolonged impairment, functional limitation, or disability
- Psychological and socioeconomic factors
- Psychomotor abilities
- Social support
- Stability of the condition

Intervention

Intervention is the purposeful interaction of the physical therapist with the patient/client and, when appropriate, with other individuals involved with the patient/client, using various physical therapy procedures and techniques to produce changes in the condition consistent with the diagnosis and prognosis. Decisions about interventions are contingent on the timely monitoring of patient/client response and the progress made toward achieving the anticipated goals and expected outcomes.

Communication, coordination, and documentation and patient/client-related instruction are provided for all patients/clients. Procedural interventions are selected or modified based on the examination data, the evaluation, the diagnosis, the prognosis, and the anticipated goals and expected outcomes for a particular patient/client. *For clinical considerations in selecting interventions, listings of interventions, and listings of anticipated goals and expected outcomes, refer to Chapter 3.*

Coordination, Communication, and Documentation

Coordination, communication, and documentation for primary prevention/risk reduction may include:

Interventions

- Addressing required functions
  - individualized family service plans (IFSPs) or individualized education plans (IEPs)
  - informed consent
  - mandatory communication and reporting (eg, patient/client advocacy and abuse reporting)
- Collaboration and coordination with agencies, including:
  - equipment suppliers
  - home care agencies
  - payer groups
  - schools
  - transportation agencies
- Communication, including:
  - education plans
  - documentation
- Data collection, analysis and reporting
  - outcome data
  - peer review findings
  - record reviews
- Documentation
  - elements of patient/client management (examination, evaluation, diagnosis, prognosis, intervention)
  - outcomes of intervention
- Referrals to other professionals or resources

Anticipated Goals and Expected Outcomes

- Accountability for services is increased.
- Individualized family service plans (IFSPs) or individualized education plans (IEPs), informed consent, and mandatory communication and reporting (eg, patient/client advocacy and abuse reporting) are obtained or completed.
- Available resources are maximally utilized.
- Collaboration and coordination occurs with agencies, including equipment suppliers, home care agencies, payer groups, schools, and transportation agencies.
- Communication occurs through education plans and documentation.
- Data are collected, analyzed, and reported, including outcome data, peer review findings, and record reviews.
- Decision making is enhanced regarding patient/client health and the use of health care resources by patient/client, family, significant others, and caregivers.
- Documentation occurs throughout patient/client management and follows APTA's *Guidelines for Physical Therapy Documentation* (Appendix 5).
- Patient/client, family, significant other, and caregiver understanding of anticipated goals and expected outcomes is increased.
- Referrals are made to other professionals or resources whenever necessary and appropriate.
- Resources are utilized in a cost-effective way.

Patient/Client-Related Instruction

Patient/client-related instruction may include:

Interventions

- Instruction, education, and training of patients/clients and caregivers regarding:
  - enhancement of performance
  - health, wellness, and fitness programs
  - plan for intervention
  - risk factors for pathology/pathophysiology (disease, disorder, or condition), impairments, functional limitations, or disabilities

Anticipated Goals and Expected Outcomes

- Ability to perform physical actions, tasks, or activities is improved.
- Awareness and use of community resources are improved.
- Behaviors that foster healthy habits, wellness, and prevention are acquired.
- Decision making is enhanced regarding patient/client health and the use of health care resources by patient/client, family, significant others, and caregivers.
- Health status is improved.
- Patient/client, family, significant other, and caregiver knowledge and awareness of the diagnosis, prognosis, interventions, and anticipated goals and expected outcomes are increased.
- Patient/client knowledge of personal and environmental factors associated with the condition is increased.
- Performance levels in self-care, home management, work (job/school/play), community, or leisure actions, tasks, or activities are improved.
- Physical function is improved.
- Risk of recurrence of condition is reduced.
- Safety of patient/client, family, significant others, and caregivers is improved.
- Utilization and cost of health care services are decreased.

Procedural Interventions

Procedural interventions for this pattern may include:

Therapeutic Exercise

Interventions

- Aerobic capacity/endurance conditioning or reconditioning
  - aquatic programs
  - gait and locomotor training
  - increased workload over time
  - walking and wheelchair propulsion programs
- Balance, coordination, and agility training
  - developmental activities training
  - motor function (motor control and motor learning) training or retraining
  - neuromuscular education or reeducation
  - posture awareness training
  - standardized, programmatic, complementary exercise approaches
  - task-specific performance training
- Body mechanics and postural stabilization
  - body mechanics training
  - posture awareness training
  - postural control training
  - postural stabilization activities
- Flexibility exercises
  - muscle lengthening
  - range of motion
  - stretching
- Gait and locomotion training
  - developmental activities training
  - gait training
  - implement and device training
  - perceptual training
  - standardized, programmatic, complementary exercise approaches
- Relaxation
  - breathing strategies
  - movement strategies
  - relaxation techniques
  - standardized, programmatic, complementary exercise approaches
- Strength, power, and endurance training for head, neck, limb, pelvic-floor, trunk, and ventilatory muscles
  - active assistive, active, and resistive exercises (including concentric, dynamic/isotonic, eccentric, isokinetic, isometric, and plyometric)
  - aquatic programs
  - standardized, programmatic, complementary exercise approaches
  - task-specific performance training

Anticipated Goals and Expected Outcomes

- Impact on pathology/pathophysiology (disease, disorder, or condition)
  - Nutrient delivery to tissue is increased.
  - Osteogenic effects of exercise are maximized.
  - Physiological response to increased oxygen demand is improved.
  - Tissue perfusion and oxygenation are enhanced.
- Impact on impairments
  - Aerobic capacity is increased.
  - Balance is improved.
  - Endurance is increased.
  - Energy expenditure per unit of work is decreased.
  - Gait, locomotion, and balance are improved.
  - Joint integrity and mobility are improved.
  - Motor function (motor control and motor learning) is improved.
  - Muscle performance (strength, power, and endurance) is increased.
  - Postural control is improved.
  - Quality and quantity of movement between and across body segments are improved.
  - Range of motion is improved.
  - Relaxation is increased.
  - Sensory awareness is increased.
  - Weight-bearing status is improved.
- Impact on functional limitations
  - Ability to perform physical actions, tasks, or activities related to self-care, home management, work (job/school/play), community, and leisure is improved.
  - Level of supervision required for task performance is decreased.
  - Performance of and independence in activities of daily living (ADL) and instrumental activities of daily living (IADL) with or without devices and equipment are increased.
  - Tolerance of positions and activities is increased.
- Impact on disabilities
  - Ability to assume or resume required self-care, home management, work (job/school/play), community, and leisure roles is improved.
- Risk reduction/prevention
  - Risk factors are reduced.
  - Risk of secondary impairment is reduced.
  - Safety is improved.
- Impact on health, wellness, and fitness
  - Fitness is improved.
  - Health status is improved.
  - Physical capacity is increased.
  - Physical function is improved.
- Impact on societal resources
  - Utilization of physical therapy services is optimized.
  - Utilization of physical therapy services results in efficient use of health care dollars.
- Patient/client satisfaction
  - Access, availability, and services provided are acceptable to patient/client.
  - Administrative management of practice is acceptable to patient/client.
  - Clinical proficiency of physical therapist is acceptable to patient/client.
  - Coordination of care is acceptable to patient/client.
  - Cost of health care services is decreased.
  - Interpersonal skills of physical therapist are acceptable to patient/client, family, and significant others.
  - Sense of well-being is improved.
  - Stressors are decreased.

Functional Training in Self-Care and Home Management (Including Activities of Daily Living [ADL] and Instrumental Activities of Daily Living [IADL])

Interventions

- Barrier accommodations or modifications
- Injury prevention or reduction
  - injury prevention education during self-care and home management
  - injury prevention or reduction with use of devices and equipment
  - safety awareness training during self-care and home management

Anticipated Goals and Expected Outcomes

- Impact on pathology/pathophysiology (disease, disorder, or condition)
  - Physiological response to increased oxygen demand is improved.
- Impact on impairments
  - Postural control is improved.
  - Weight-bearing status is improved.
- Impact on functional limitations
  - Ability to perform physical actions, tasks, or activities related to self-care and home management is improved.
  - Level of supervision required for task performance is decreased.
  - Performance of and independence in ADL and IADL with or without devices and equipment are increased.
  - Tolerance of positions and activities is increased.
- Impact on disabilities
  - Ability to assume or resume required self-care and home management roles is improved.
- Risk reduction/prevention
  - Risk factors are reduced.
  - Risk of secondary impairments is reduced.
  - Safety is improved.
- Impact on health, wellness, and fitness
  - Fitness is improved.
  - Health status is improved.
  - Physical function is improved.
- Impact on societal resources
  - Utilization of physical therapy services is optimized.
  - Utilization of physical therapy services results in efficient use of health care dollars.
- Patient/client satisfaction
  - Access, availability, and services provided are acceptable to patient/client.
  - Administrative management of practice is acceptable to patient/client.
  - Clinical proficiency of physical therapist is acceptable to patient/client.
  - Coordination of care is acceptable to patient/client.
  - Cost of health care services is decreased.
  - Interpersonal skills of physical therapist are acceptable to patient/client, family, and significant others.
  - Sense of well-being is improved.
  - Stressors are decreased.

Functional Training in Work (Job/School/Play), Community, and Leisure Integration or Reintegration (Including Instrumental Activities of Daily Living [IADL], Work Hardening, and Work Conditioning)

Interventions

- Barrier accommodations or modifications
- Injury prevention or reduction
  - injury prevention education during work (job/school/play), community, and leisure integration or reintegration
  - injury prevention or reduction with use of devices and equipment
  - safety awareness training during work (job/school/play), community, and leisure integration or reintegration

Anticipated Goals and Outcomes

- Impact on pathology/pathophysiology (disease, disorder, or condition)
  - Physiological response to increased oxygen demand is improved.
- Impact on impairments
  - Postural control is improved.
  - Weight-bearing status is improved.
- Impact on functional limitations
  - Ability to perform physical actions, tasks, or activities related to work (job/school/play), community, and leisure integration or reintegration is improved.
  - Level of supervision required for task performance is decreased.
  - Performance of and independence in IADL with or without devices and equipment are increased.
  - Tolerance of positions and activities is increased.
- Impact on disabilities
  - Ability to assume or resume required work (job/school/play), community, and leisure roles is improved.
- Risk reduction/prevention
  - Risk factors are reduced.
  - Risk of secondary impairment is reduced.
  - Safety is improved.
- Impact on health, wellness, and fitness
  - Fitness is improved.
  - Health status is improved.
  - Physical function is improved.
- Impact on societal resources
  - Costs of work-related injury or disability are reduced.
  - Utilization of physical therapy services is optimized.
  - Utilization of physical therapy services results in efficient use of health care dollars.
- Patient/client satisfaction
  - Access, availability, and services provided are acceptable to patient/client.
  - Administrative management of practice is acceptable to patient/client.
  - Clinical proficiency of physical therapist is acceptable to patient/client.
  - Coordination of care is acceptable to patient/client.
  - Cost of health care services is decreased.
  - Interpersonal skills of physical therapist are acceptable to patient/client, family, and significant others.
  - Sense of well-being is improved.
  - Stressors are decreased.

Reexamination

Reexamination is the process of performing selected tests and measures after the initial examination to evaluate progress and to modify or redirect interventions. Reexamination may be indicated more than once during a single episode of care. It also may be performed over the course of a disease, disorder, or condition, which for some patients/clients may be over the life span. Indications for reexamination include new clinical findings or failure to respond to physical therapy interventions.

Global Outcomes for Patients/Clients in This Pattern

Throughout the entire episode of care, the physical therapist determines the anticipated goals and expected outcomes for each intervention. These anticipated goals and expected outcomes are delineated in shaded boxes that accompany the lists of interventions in each preferred practice pattern. As the patient/client reaches the termination of physical therapy services and the end of the episode of care, the physical therapist measures the global outcomes of the physical therapy services by characterizing or quantifying the impact of the physical therapy interventions in the following domains:

- Pathology/pathophysiology (disease, disorder, or condition)
- Impairments
- Functional limitations
- Disabilities
- Risk reduction/prevention
- Health, wellness, and fitness
- Societal resources
- Patient/client satisfaction

In some instances, a particular anticipated goal or expected outcome is thoroughly achieved through implementation of a single form of intervention. More commonly, however, the anticipated goals and expected outcomes are achieved as a result of the combined effects of several forms of interventions, leading to enhancement of both health status and health-related quality of life.

Criteria for Termination of Physical Therapy Services

Discharge is the process of ending physical therapy services that have been provided during a single episode of care. It occurs when the anticipated goals and expected outcomes have been achieved. Discharge does *not* occur with a *transfer* (defined as the time when a patient is moved from one site to another site within the same setting or across settings during a single episode of care). Although there may be facility-specific or payer-specific requirements for documentation regarding the conclusion of physical therapy services, *discharge occurs based on the physical therapist's analysis of the achievement of anticipated goals and expected outcomes.*

Discontinuation is the process of ending physical therapy services that have been provided during a single episode of care when (1) the patient/client, caregiver, or legal guardian declines to continue intervention; (2) the patient/client is unable to continue to progress toward outcomes because of medical or psychosocial complications or because financial/insurance resources have been expended; or (3) the physical therapist determines that the patient/client will no longer benefit from physical therapy. When physical therapy services are terminated prior to achievement of anticipated goals and expected outcomes, patient/client status and the rationale for termination are documented.

For patients/clients who require multiple episodes of care, periodic follow-up is needed over the life span to ensure safety and effective adaptation following changes in physical status, caregivers, environment, or task demands. In consultation with appropriate individuals, and in consideration of the outcomes, the physical therapist plans for discharge or discontinuation and provides for appropriate follow-up or referral.

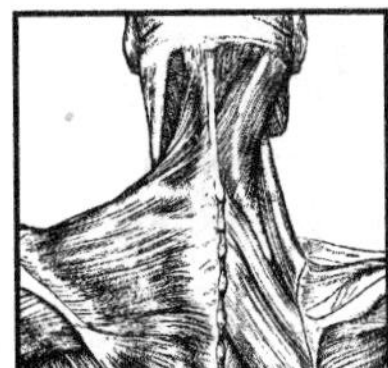

Impaired Posture

This preferred practice pattern describes the generally accepted elements of patient/client management that physical therapists provide for patients/clients who are classified in this pattern. The pattern title reflects the diagnosis made by the physical therapist. APTA emphasizes that preferred practice patterns are the boundaries within which a physical therapist may select any of a number of clinical alternatives, based on consideration of a wide variety of factors, such as individual patient/client needs; the profession's code of ethics and standards of practice; and patient/client age, culture, gender roles, race, sex, sexual orientation, and socioeconomic status.

Patient/Client Diagnostic Classification

Patients/clients will be classified in this pattern for impaired posture as a result of the physical therapist's evaluation of the examination data. The findings from the examination (history, systems review, and tests and measures) may indicate the presence or risk of pathology/pathophysiology (disease, disorder, or condition), impairments, functional limitations, or disabilities or the need for health, wellness, or fitness programs. The physical therapist integrates, synthesizes, and interprets the examination data to determine the diagnostic classification.

Inclusion

The following examples of examination findings may support the inclusion of patients/clients in this pattern:

Risk Factors or Consequences of Pathology/Pathophysiology (Disease, Disorder, or Condition)

- Congenital torticollis
- Pain
- Pregnancy
- Repetitive stress syndrome
- Scheuermann disease
- Scoliosis, kyphoscoliosis

Impairments, Functional Limitations, or Disabilities

- Impaired joint mobility
- Inability to tolerate prolonged sitting
- Leg length discrepancy
- Muscle imbalance
- Muscle weakness

Note:

Some risk factors or consequences of pathology/pathophysiology—such as *primary posture impairment associated with cerebral palsy*—may be severe and complex; however, *they do not necessarily exclude patients/clients from this pattern.* Severe and complex risk factors or consequences may require modification of the frequency of visits and duration of care (See "Evaluation, Diagnosis, and Prognosis," page 150.)

Exclusion or Multiple-Pattern Classification

The following examples of examination findings may support exclusion from this pattern or classification into additional patterns. Depending on the level of severity or complexity of the examination findings, the physical therapist may determine that the patient/client would be more appropriately managed through (1) classification in an entirely different pattern or (2) classification in both this and another pattern.

Findings That May Require Classification in a Different Pattern

- Impairments associated with chronic obstructive pulmonary disease with kyphosis
- Impairments associated with spinal stabilization surgery
- Radicular signs

Findings That May Require Classification in Additional Patterns

- Impairments associated with scoliosis, with contusion of the thigh

ICD-9-CM Codes

The listing below contains the current (as of press time) and most typical 3- and 4-digit ICD-9-CM codes related to this preferred practice pattern. Because patient/client diagnostic classification is based on impairments, functional limitations, and disabilities—not on codes—patients/clients may be classified into the pattern even though the codes listed with the pattern may not apply to those clients.

This listing is intended for general information only and should not be used for coding purposes. The codes should be confirmed by referring to the World Health Organization's *International Classification of Diseases, 9th Revision, Clinical Modification (ICD-9-CM 2001)*, Volumes 1 and 3 (Chicago, Ill: American Medical Association; 2000) or subsequent revisions or by referring to other ICD-9-CM coding manuals that contain exclusion notes and instructions regarding fifth-digit requirements.

353 Nerve root and plexus disorders
- **353.0** Brachial plexus lesions
  - Thoracic outlet syndrome

524 Dentofacial anomalies, including malocclusion
- **524.6** Temporomandibular joint disorders

568 Other disorders of peritoneum
- **568.0** Peritoneal adhesions (postoperative) (postinfection)

718 Other derangement of joint
- **718.8** Other joint derangement, not elsewhere classified

719 Other and unspecified disorders of joint
- **719.5** Stiffness of joint, not elsewhere classified
- **719.7** Difficulty in walking

722 Intervertebral disk disorders
- **722.4** Degeneration of cervical intervertebral disk
- **722.5** Degeneration of thoracic or lumbar intervertebral disk
- **722.6** Degeneration of intervertebral disk, site unspecified

723 Other disorders of cervical region
- **723.1** Cervicalgia
- **723.5** Torticollis, unspecified

724 Other and unspecified disorders of back
- **724.1** Pain in thoracic spine
- **724.2** Lumbago
  - Low back pain
  - Low back syndrome
  - Lumbalgia
- **724.6** Disorders of sacrum
- **724.9** Other unspecified back disorders
  - Ankylosis of spine, not otherwise specified
  - Compression of spinal nerve root, not elsewhere classified
  - Spinal disorders, not otherwise specified

725 Polymyalgia rheumatica

728 Disorders of muscle, ligament, and fascia
- **728.2** Muscular wasting and disuse atrophy, not elsewhere classified
- **728.8** Other disorders of muscle, ligament, and fascia
  - **728.85** Spasm of muscle

729 Other disorders of soft tissues
- **729.1** Myalgia and myositis, unspecified
- **729.9** Other and unspecified disorders of soft tissue

732 Osteochondropathies
- **732.0** Juvenile osteochondrosis of spine

733 Other disorders of bone and cartilage
- **733.0** Osteoporosis

736 Other acquired deformities of limbs
- **736.3** Acquired deformities of hip
- **736.4** Genu valgum or varum
- **736.7** Other acquired deformities of ankle and foot
- **736.8** Acquired deformities of other parts of limbs
  - **736.81** Unequal leg length (acquired)

737 Curvature of spine
- **737.1** Kyphosis (acquired)
- **737.2** Lordosis (acquired)
- **737.3** Kyphoscoliosis and scoliosis

738 Other acquired deformity
- **738.4** Acquired spondylolisthesis
- **738.6** Acquired deformity of pelvis

756 Other congenital musculoskeletal anomalies
- **756.1** Anomalies of spine

781 Symptoms involving nervous and musculoskeletal systems
- **781.2** Abnormality of gait
- **781.9** Other symptoms involving nervous and musculoskeletal systems
  - **781.92** Abnormal posture

Examination

Examination is a comprehensive screening and specific testing process that leads to a diagnostic classification or, when appropriate, to a referral to another practitioner. Examination is required prior to the initial intervention and is performed for all patients/clients. Through the examination, the physical therapist may identify impairments, functional limitations, disabilities, changes in physical function or overall health status, and needs related to restoration of health and to prevention, wellness, and fitness. The physical therapist synthesizes the examination findings to establish the diagnosis and the prognosis (including the plan of care). The patient/client, family, significant others, and caregivers may provide information during the examination process.

Examination has three components: the patient/client history, the systems review, and tests and measures. The *history* is a systematic gathering of past and current information (often from the patient/client) related to why the patient/client is seeking the services of the physical therapist. The *systems review* is a brief or limited examination of (1) the anatomical and physiological status of the cardiovascular/pulmonary, integumentary, musculoskeletal, and neuromuscular systems and (2) the communication ability, affect, cognition, language, and learning style of the patient/client. *Tests and measures* are the means of gathering data about the patient/client.

The selection of examination procedures and the depth of the examination vary based on patient/client age; severity of the problem; stage of recovery (acute, subacute, chronic); phase of rehabilitation (early, intermediate, late, return to activity); home, work (job/school/play), or community situation; and other relevant factors. *For clinical indications in selecting tests and measures and for listings of tests and measures, tools used to gather data, and the types of data generated by tests and measures, refer to Chapter 2.*

Patient/Client History

The history may include:

General Demographics
- Age
- Sex
- Race/ethnicity
- Primary language
- Education

Social History
- Cultural beliefs and behaviors
- Family and caregiver resources
- Social interactions, social activities, and support systems

Employment/Work (Job/School/Play)
- Current and prior work (job/school/play), community, and leisure actions, tasks, or activities

Growth and Development
- Developmental history
- Hand dominance

Living Environment
- Devices and equipment (eg, assistive, adaptive, orthotic, protective, supportive, prosthetic)
- Living environment and community characteristics
- Projected discharge destinations

General Health Status (Self-Report, Family Report, Caregiver Report)
- General health perception
- Physical function (eg, mobility, sleep patterns, restricted bed days)
- Psychological function (eg, memory, reasoning ability, depression, anxiety)
- Role function (eg, community, leisure, social, work)
- Social function (eg, social activity, social interaction, social support)

Social/Health Habits (Past and Current)
- Behavioral health risks (eg, smoking, drug abuse)
- Level of physical fitness

Family History
- Familial health risks

Medical/Surgical History
- Cardiovascular
- Endocrine/metabolic
- Gastrointestinal
- Genitourinary
- Gynecological
- Integumentary
- Musculoskeletal
- Neuromuscular
- Obstetrical
- Prior hospitalizations, surgeries, and preexisting medical and other health-related conditions
- Psychological
- Pulmonary

Current Condition(s)/Chief Complaint(s)
- Concerns that led patient/client to seek the services of a physical therapist
- Concerns or needs of patient/client who requires the services of a physical therapist
- Current therapeutic interventions
- Mechanisms of injury or disease, including date of onset and course of events
- Onset and pattern of symptoms
- Patient/client, family, significant other, and caregiver expectations and goals for the therapeutic intervention
- Patient/client, family, significant other, and caregiver perceptions of patient's/client's emotional response to the current clinical situation
- Previous occurrence of chief complaint(s)
- Prior therapeutic interventions

Functional Status and Activity Level
- Current and prior functional status in self-care and home management activities, including activities of daily living (ADL) and instrumental activities of daily living (IADL)
- Current and prior functional status in work (job/school/play), community, and leisure actions, tasks, or activities

Medications
- Medications for current condition
- Medications previously taken for current condition
- Medications for other conditions

Other Clinical Tests
- Laboratory and diagnostic tests
- Review of available records (eg, medical, education, surgical)
- Review of other clinical findings (eg, nutrition and hydration)

Systems Review

The systems review may include:

Anatomical and Physiological Status

- Cardiovascular/Pulmonary
  - Blood pressure
  - Edema
  - Heart rate
  - Respiratory rate
- Integumentary
  - Pliability (texture)
  - Presence of scar formation
  - Skin color
  - Skin integrity
- Musculoskeletal
  - Gross range of motion
  - Gross strength
  - Gross symmetry
  - Height
  - Weight
- Neuromuscular
  - Gross coordinated movements (eg, balance, gait, locomotion, transfers, transitions)
  - Motor function (motor control, motor learning)

Communication, Affect, Cognition, Language, and Learning Style

- Ability to make needs known
- Consciousness
- Expected emotional/behavioral responses
- Learning preferences (eg, education needs, learning barriers)
- Orientation (person, place, time)

Tests and Measures

Tests and measures for this pattern may include those that characterize or quantify:

Anthropometric Characteristics

- Body dimensions (eg, girth measurement, length measurement)

Assistive and Adaptive Devices

- Assistive or adaptive devices and equipment use during functional activities (eg, activities of daily living [ADL] scales, functional scales, instrumental activities of daily living [IADL] scales, interviews, observations)
- Safety during use of assistive or adaptive devices and equipment (eg, diaries, fall scales, interviews, logs, observations, reports)

Ergonomics and Body Mechanics

Ergonomics

- Functional capacity and performance during work actions, tasks, or activities (eg, accelerometry, dynamometry, electroneuromyography, endurance tests, force platform tests, goniometry, interviews, observations, photographic assessments, physical capacity tests, postural loading analyses, technology-assisted assessments, videographic assessments, work analyses)
- Safety in work environments (eg, hazard identification checklists, job severity indexes, lifting standards, risk assessment scales, standards for exposure limits)

Body mechanics

- Body mechanics during self-care, home management, work, community, or leisure actions, tasks, or activities (eg, ADL scales, IADL scales, observations, photographic assessments, technology-assisted assessments, videographic assessments)

Gait, Locomotion, and Balance

- Balance during functional activities with or without the use of assistive, adaptive, orthotic, protective, supportive, or prosthetic devices or equipment (eg, ADL scales, IADL scales, observations, videographic assessments)
- Balance (dynamic and static) with or without the use of assistive, adaptive, orthotic, protective, supportive, or prosthetic devices or equipment (eg, balance scales, dizziness inventories, dynamic posturography, fall scales, motor impairment tests, observations, photographic assessments, postural control tests)
- Safety during gait, locomotion, and balance (eg, confidence scales, diaries, fall scales, functional assessment profiles, logs, reports)

Motor Function (Motor Control and Motor Learning)

- Dexterity, coordination, and agility (eg, coordination screens, motor impairment tests, motor proficiency tests, observations, videographic assessments)
- Initiation, modification, and control of movement patterns and voluntary postures (eg, activity indexes)

Muscle Performance (Including Strength, Power, and Endurance)

- Electrophysiological integrity (eg, electroneuromyography)
- Muscle strength, power, and endurance (eg, dynamometry, manual muscle tests, muscle performance tests, physical capacity tests, technology-assisted assessments, timed activity tests)
- Muscle strength, power, and endurance during functional activities (eg, ADL scales, functional muscle tests, IADL scales, observations, videographic assessments)
- Muscle tension (eg, palpation)

Orthotic, Protective, and Supportive Devices

- Orthotic, protective, and supportive devices and equipment use during functional activities (eg, ADL scales, functional scales, IADL scales, interviews, observations, profiles)
- Safety during use of orthotic, protective, and supportive devices and equipment (eg, diaries, fall scales, interviews, logs, observations, reports)

Pain

- Pain, soreness, and nociception (eg, analog scales, discrimination tests, pain drawings and maps, provocation tests, verbal and pictorial descriptor tests)
- Pain in specific body parts (eg, pain indexes, pain questionnaires, structural provocation tests)

Posture

- Postural alignment and position (static and dynamic), including symmetry and deviation from midline (eg, observations, grid measurement, technology-assisted assessments, photographic assessments, videographic assessments)
- Specific body parts (eg, angle assessments, forward-bending test, goniometry, observations, palpation, positional tests)

Range of Motion (ROM) (Including Muscle Length)

- Functional ROM (eg, observations, squat tests, toe touch tests)
- Joint active and passive movement (eg, goniometry, inclinometry, observations, photographic assessments, videographic assessments)
- Muscle length, soft tissue extensibility, and flexibility (eg, contracture tests, goniometry, inclinometry, ligamentous tests, linear measurement, multisegment flexibility tests, palpation)

Self-Care and Home Management (Including ADL and IADL)

- Safety in self-care and home management activities and environments (eg, diaries, fall scales, interviews, logs, observations, reports, videographic assessments)

Sensory Integrity

- Deep sensations (eg, kinesthesiometry, observations, photographic assessments, vibration tests)

Work (Job/School/Play), Community, and Leisure Integration or Reintegration (Including IADL)

- Safety in work (job/school/play), community, and leisure activities and environments (eg, diaries, fall scales, interviews, logs, observations, videographic assessments)

Ventilation and Respiration/Gas Exchange

- Pulmonary signs of ventilatory function, including airway protection; breath and voice sounds; respiratory rate, rhythm, and pattern; ventilatory flow, forces, and volumes (eg, airway clearance tests, observations, palpation, pulmonary function tests, ventilatory muscle force tests)
- Pulmonary symptoms (eg, dyspnea and perceived exertion indexes and scales)

Evaluation, Diagnosis, and Prognosis (Including Plan of Care)

Physical therapists perform *evaluations* (make clinical judgments) based on the data gathered from the history, systems review, and tests and measures. In the evaluation process, physical therapists synthesize the examination data to establish the diagnosis and prognosis (including the plan of care). Factors that influence the complexity of the evaluation include the clinical findings, extent of loss of function, chronicity or severity of the problem, possibility of multisite or multisystem involvement, preexisting condition(s), potential discharge destination, social considerations, physical function, and overall health status.

A *diagnosis* is a label encompassing a cluster of signs and symptoms, syndromes, or categories. It is the result of the systematic diagnostic process, which includes integrating and evaluating the data from the examination.The diagnostic label indicates the primary dysfunction(s) toward which the therapist will direct interventions. The *prognosis* is the determination of the predicted optimal level of improvement in function and the amount of time needed to reach that level and may also include a prediction of levels of improvement that may be reached at various intervals during the course of therapy. During the prognostic process, the physical therapist develops the plan of care. The *plan of care* identifies specific interventions, proposed frequency and duration of the interventions, anticipated goals, expected outcomes, and discharge plans. The plan of care identifies realistic anticipated goals and expected outcomes, taking into consideration the expectations of the patient/client and appropriate others.These anticipated goals and expected outcomes should be measureable and time limited.

The frequency of visits and duration of the episode of care may vary from a short episode with a high intensity of intervention to a longer episode with a diminishing intensity of intervention. Frequency and duration may vary greatly among patients/clients based on a variety of factors that the physical therapist considers throughout the evaluation process, such as anatomical and physiological changes related to growth and development; caregiver consistency or expertise; chronicity or severity of the current condition; living environment; multisite or multisystem involvement; social support; potential discharge destinations; probability of prolonged impairment, functional limitation, or disability; and stability of the condition.

Prognosis

Over the course of 3 to 6 months, patient/client will demonstrate the ability to maintain an optimal posture and the highest level of functioning in home, work (job/school/play), community, and leisure environments.

During the episode of care, patient/client will achieve (1) the anticipated goals and expected outcomes of the interventions that are described in the plan of care and (2) the global outcomes for patients/clients who are classified in this pattern.

Expected Range of Number of Visits Per Episode of Care

6 to 20

This range represents the lower and upper limits of the number of physical therapist visits required to achieve anticipated goals and expected outcomes. *It is anticipated that 80% of patients/clients who are classified into this pattern will achieve the anticipated goals and expected outcomes within 6 to 20 visits during a single continuous episode of care.* Frequency of visits and duration of the episode of care should be determined by the physical therapist to maximize effectiveness of care and efficiency of service delivery.

Factors That May Require New Episode of Care or That May Modify Frequency of Visits/Duration of Episode

- Accessibility and availability of resources
- Adherence to the intervention program
- Age
- Anatomical and physiological changes related to growth and development
- Caregiver consistency or expertise
- Chronicity or severity of the current condition
- Cognitive status
- Comorbitities, complications, or secondary impairments
- Concurrent medical, surgical, and therapeutic interventions
- Decline in functional independence
- Level of impairment
- Level of physical function
- Living environment
- Multisite or multisystem involvement
- Nutritional status
- Overall health status
- Potential discharge destinations
- Premorbid conditions
- Probability of prolonged impairment, functional limitation, or disability
- Psychological and socioeconomic factors
- Psychomotor abilities
- Social support
- Stability of the condition

Intervention

Intervention is the purposeful interaction of the physical therapist with the patient/client and, when appropriate, with other individuals involved in patient/client care, using various physical therapy procedures and techniques to produce changes in the condition consistent with the diagnosis and prognosis. Decisions about interventions are contingent on the timely monitoring of patient/client response and the progress made toward achieving the anticipated goals and expected outcomes.

Communication, coordination, and documentation and patient/client-related instruction are provided for all patients/clients across all settings. Procedural interventions are selected or modified based on the examination data and the evaluation, the diagnosis and the prognosis, and the anticipated goals and expected outcomes for a particular patient/client. *For clinical considerations in selecting interventions, listings of interventions, and listings of anticipated goals and expected outcomes, refer to Chapter 3.*

Coordination, Communication, and Documentation

Coordination, communication, and documentation may include:

Interventions

- Addressing required functions
  - advance directives
  - individualized family service plans (IFSPs) or individualized education plans (IEPs)
  - informed consent
  - mandatory communication and reporting (eg, patient advocacy and abuse reporting)
- Admission and discharge planning
- Case management
- Collaboration and coordination with agencies, including:
  - equipment suppliers
  - home care agencies
  - payer groups
  - schools
  - transportation agencies
- Communication across settings, including:
  - case conferences
  - documentation
  - education plans
- Cost-effective resource utilization
- Data collection, analysis, and reporting
  - outcome data
  - peer review findings
  - record reviews
- Documentation across settings, following APTA's *Guidelines for Physical Therapy Documentation* (Appendix 5), including:
  - changes in impairments, functional limitations, and disabilities
  - changes in interventions
  - elements of patient/client management (examination, evaluation, diagnosis, prognosis, intervention)
  - outcomes of intervention
- Interdisciplinary teamwork
  - case conferences
  - patient care rounds
  - patient/client family meetings
- Referrals to other professionals or resources

Anticipated Goals and Expected Outcomes

- Accountability for services is increased.
- Admission data and discharge planning are completed.
- Advance directives, individualized family service plans (IFSPs) or individualized education plans (IEPs), informed consent, and mandatory communication and reporting (eg, patient advocacy and abuse reporting) are obtained or completed.
- Available resources are maximally utilized.
- Care is coordinated with patient/client, family, significant others, caregivers, and other professionals.
- Case is managed throughout the episode of care.
- Collaboration and coordination occurs with agencies, including equipment suppliers, home care agencies, payer groups, schools, and transportation agencies.
- Communication enhances risk reduction and prevention.
- Communication occurs across settings through case conferences, education plans, and documentation.
- Data are collected, analyzed, and reported, including outcome data, peer review findings, and record reviews.
- Decision making is enhanced regarding health, wellness, and fitness needs.
- Decision making is enhanced regarding patient/client health and the use of health care resources by patient/client, family, significant others, and caregivers.
- Documentation occurs throughout patient/client management and across settings and follows APTA's *Guidelines for Physical Therapy Documentation* (Appendix 5).
- Interdisciplinary collaboration occurs through case conferences, patient care rounds, and patient/client family meetings.
- Patient/client, family, significant other, and caregiver understanding of anticipated goals and expected outcomes is increased.
- Placement needs are determined.
- Referrals are made to other professionals or resources whenever necessary and appropriate.
- Resources are utilized in a cost-effective way.

Patient/Client-Related Instruction

Patient/client-related instruction may include:

Interventions

- Instruction, education, and training of patients/clients and caregivers regarding:
  - current condition (pathology/pathophysiology [disease, disorder, or condition], impairments, functional limitations, or disabilities)
  - enhancement of performance
  - health, wellness, and fitness programs
  - plan of care
  - risk factors for pathology/pathophysiology (disease, disorder, or condition), impairments, functional limitations, or disabilities
  - transitions across settings
  - transitions to new roles

Anticipated Goals and Expected Outcomes

- Ability to perform physical actions, tasks, or activities is improved.
- Awareness and use of community resources are improved.
- Behaviors that foster healthy habits, wellness, and prevention are acquired.
- Decision making is enhanced regarding patient/client health and the use of health care resources by patient/client, family, significant others, and caregivers.
- Disability associated with acute or chronic illnesses is reduced.
- Functional independence in activities of daily living (ADL) and instrumental activities of daily living (IADL) is increased.
- Health status is improved.
- Intensity of care is decreased.
- Level of supervision required for task performance is decreased.
- Patient/client, family, significant other, and caregiver knowledge and awareness of the diagnosis, prognosis, interventions, and anticipated goals and expected outcomes are increased.
- Patient/client knowledge of personal and environmental factors associated with the condition is increased.
- Performance levels in self-care, home management, work (job/school/play), community, or leisure actions, tasks, or activities are improved.
- Physical function is improved.
- Risk of recurrence of condition is reduced.
- Risk of secondary impairment is reduced.
- Safety of patient/client, family, significant others, and caregivers is improved.
- Self-management of symptoms is improved.
- Utilization and cost of health care services are decreased.

Procedural Interventions

Procedural interventions for this pattern may include:

Therapeutic Exercise

Interventions

- Aerobic capacity/endurance conditioning or reconditioning
  - aquatic programs
  - gait and locomotor training
  - increased workload over time
  - walking and wheelchair propulsion programs
- Balance, coordination, and agility training
  - developmental activities training
  - motor function (motor control and motor learning) training or retraining
  - neuromuscular education or reeducation
  - perceptual training
  - posture awareness training
  - standardized, programmatic, complementary exercise approaches
  - task-specific performance training
- Body mechanics and postural stabilization
  - body mechanics training
  - posture awareness training
  - postural control training
  - postural stabilization activities
- Flexibility exercises
  - muscle lengthening
  - range of motion
  - stretching
- Relaxation
  - breathing strategies
  - movement strategies
  - relaxation techniques
  - standardized, programmatic, complementary exercise approaches
- Strength, power, and endurance training for head, neck, limb, pelvic-floor, trunk, and ventilatory muscles
  - active assistive, active, and resistive exercises (including concentric, dynamic/isotonic, eccentric, isokinetic, isometric, and plyometric)
  - aquatic programs
  - standardized, programmatic, complementary exercise approaches
  - task-specific performance training

Anticipated Goals and Expected Outcomes

- Impact on pathology/pathophysiology (disease, disorder, or condition)
  - Joint swelling, inflammation, or restriction is reduced.
  - Nutrient delivery to tissue is increased.
  - Osteogenic effects of exercise are maximized.
  - Pain is decreased.
  - Soft tissue swelling, inflammation, or restriction is reduced.
  - Tissue perfusion and oxygenation are enhanced.
- Impact on impairments
  - Balance is improved.
  - Endurance is increased.
  - Energy expenditure per unit of work is decreased.
  - Joint integrity and mobility are improved.
  - Motor function (motor control and motor learning) is improved.
  - Muscle performance (strength, power, and endurance) is increased.
  - Postural control is improved.
  - Quality and quantity of movement between and across body segments are improved.
  - Range of motion is improved.
  - Relaxation is increased.
  - Sensory awareness is increased.
  - Weight-bearing status is improved.
- Impact on functional limitations
  - Ability to perform physical actions, tasks, or activities related to self-care, home management, work (job/school/play), community, and leisure is improved.
  - Level of supervision required for task performance is decreased.
  - Performance of and independence in activities of daily living (ADL) and instrumental activities of daily living (IADL) with or without devices and equipment are increased.
  - Tolerance of positions and activities is increased.
- Impact on disabilities
  - Ability to assume or resume required self-care, home management, work (job/school/play), community, and leisure roles is improved.
- Risk reduction/prevention
  - Risk factors are reduced.
  - Risk of recurrence of condition is reduced.
  - Risk of secondary impairment is reduced.
  - Safety is improved.
  - Self-management of symptoms is improved.
- Impact on health, wellness, and fitness
  - Fitness is improved.
  - Health status is improved.
  - Physical capacity is increased.
  - Physical function is improved.
- Impact on societal resources
  - Utilization of physical therapy services is optimized.
  - Utilization of physical therapy services results in efficient use of health care dollars.
- Patient/client satisfaction
  - Access, availability, and services provided are acceptable to patient/client.
  - Administrative management of practice is acceptable to patient/client.
  - Clinical proficiency of physical therapist is acceptable to patient/client.
  - Coordination of care is acceptable to patient/client.
  - Cost of health care services is decreased.
  - Intensity of care is decreased.
  - Interpersonal skills of physical therapist are acceptable to patient/client, family, and significant others.
  - Sense of well-being is improved.
  - Stressors are decreased.

Functional Training in Self-Care and Home Management (Including Activities of Daily Living [ADL]) and Instrumental Activities of Daily Living [IADL])

Interventions

- ADL training
  - bathing
  - bed mobility and transfer training
  - developmental activities
  - dressing
  - eating
  - grooming
  - toileting
- Devices and equipment use and training
  - assistive and adaptive device or equipment training during ADL and IADL
  - orthotic, protective, or supportive device or equipment training during ADL and IADL
- Functional training programs
  - back schools
  - simulated environments and tasks
  - task adaptation
- IADL training
  - caring for dependents
  - home maintenance
  - household chores
  - shopping
  - structured play for infants and children
  - yard work
- Injury prevention or reduction
  - injury prevention education during self-care and home management
  - injury prevention or reduction with use of devices and equipment
  - safety awareness training during self-care and home management

Anticipated Goals and Expected Outcomes

- Impact on pathology/pathophysiology (disease/disorder/condition)
  - Pain is decreased.
  - Physiological response to increased oxygen demand is improved.
- Impact on impairments
  - Balance is improved.
  - Endurance is increased.
  - Energy expenditure per unit of work is decreased.
  - Motor function (motor control and motor learning) is improved.
  - Muscle performance (strength, power, and endurance) is increased.
  - Postural control is improved.
  - Sensory awareness is increased.
  - Weight-bearing status is improved.
- Impact on functional limitations
  - Ability to perform physical actions, tasks, or activities related to self-care and home management is improved.
  - Level of supervision required for task performance is decreased.
  - Performance of and independence in ADL and IADL with or without devices and equipment are increased.
  - Tolerance of positions and activities is increased.
- Impact on disabilities
  - Ability to assume or resume required self-care and home management roles is improved.
- Risk reduction/prevention
  - Risk factors are reduced.
  - Risk of secondary impairments is reduced.
  - Safety is improved.
  - Self-management of symptoms is improved.
- Impact on health, wellness, and fitness
  - Fitness is improved.
  - Health status is improved.
  - Physical capacity is increased.
  - Physical function is improved.
- Impact on societal resources
  - Utilization of physical therapy services is optimized.
  - Utilization of physical therapy services results in efficient use of health care dollars.
- Patient/client satisfaction
  - Access, availability, and services provided are acceptable to patient/client.
  - Administrative management of practice is acceptable to patient/client.
  - Clinical proficiency of physical therapist is acceptable to patient/client.
  - Coordination of care is acceptable to patient/client.
  - Cost of health care services is decreased.
  - Intensity of care is decreased.
  - Interpersonal skills of physical therapist are acceptable to patient/client, family, and significant others.
  - Sense of well-being is improved.
  - Stressors are decreased.

Functional Training in Work (Job/School/Play), Community, and Leisure Integration or Reintegration (Including Instrumental Activities of Daily Living [IADL], Work Hardening, and Work Conditioning)

Interventions

- Devices and equipment use and training
  - assistive and adaptive device or equipment training during IADL
  - orthotic, protective, or supportive device or equipment training during IADL
- Functional training programs
  - back schools
  - job coaching
  - simulated environments
  - task simulation and adaptation
  - task training
- IADL training
  - community service training involving instruments
  - school and play activities training including tools and instruments
  - work training with tools
- Injury prevention or reduction
  - injury prevention education during work (job/school/play), community, and leisure integration or reintegration
  - injury prevention or reduction with use of devices and equipment
  - safety awareness training during work (job/school/play), community, and leisure integration or reintegration
- Leisure and play activities and training

Anticipated Goals and Expected Outcomes

- Impact on pathology/pathophysiology (disease, disorder, or condition)
  - Pain is decreased.
  - Physiological response to increased oxygen demand is improved.
- Impact on impairments
  - Balance is improved.
  - Endurance is increased.
  - Energy expenditure per unit of work is decreased.
  - Motor function (motor control and motor learning) is improved.
  - Muscle performance (strength, power, and endurance) is increased.
  - Postural control is improved.
  - Sensory awareness is increased.
  - Weight-bearing status is improved.
- Impact on functional limitations
  - Ability to perform physical actions, tasks, or activities related to work (job/school/play), community, and leisure integration or reintegration is improved.
  - Level of supervision required for task performance is decreased.
  - Performance of and independence in IADL with or without devices and equipment are increased.
  - Tolerance of positions and activities is increased.
- Impact on disabilities
  - Ability to assume or resume required work (job/school/play), community, and leisure roles is improved.
- Risk reduction/prevention
  - Risk factors are reduced.
  - Risk of secondary impairment is reduced.
  - Safety is improved.
  - Self-management of symptoms is improved.
- Impact on health, wellness, and fitness
  - Fitness is improved.
  - Health status is improved.
  - Physical capacity is increased.
  - Physical function is improved.
- Impact on societal resources
  - Costs of work-related injury or disability are reduced.
  - Utilization of physical therapy services is optimized.
  - Utilization of physical therapy services results in efficient use of health care dollars.
- Patient/client satisfaction
  - Access, availability, and services provided are acceptable to patient/client.
  - Administrative management of practice is acceptable to patient/client.
  - Clinical proficiency of physical therapist is acceptable to patient/client.
  - Coordination of care is acceptable to patient/client.
  - Cost of health care services is decreased.
  - Intensity of care is decreased.
  - Interpersonal skills of physical therapist are acceptable to patient/client, family, and significant others.
  - Sense of well-being is improved.
  - Stressors are decreased.

Manual Therapy Techniques (Including Mobilization/Manipulation)

Interventions

- Manual traction
- Massage
  - connective tissue massage
  - therapeutic massage
- Mobilization/manipulation
  - soft tissue
  - spinal and peripheral joints
- Passive range of motion

Anticipated Goals and Expected Outcomes

- Impact on pathology/pathophysiology (disease, disorder, or condition)
  - Edema, lymphedema, or effusion is reduced.
  - Joint swelling, inflammation, or restriction is reduced.
  - Pain is decreased.
  - Soft tissue swelling, inflammation, or restriction is reduced.
- Impact on impairments
  - Joint integrity and mobility are improved.
  - Muscle performance (strength, power, and endurance) is increased.
  - Postural control is improved.
  - Quality and quantity of movement between and across body segments are improved.
  - Range of motion is improved.
  - Relaxation is increased.
  - Sensory awareness is increased.
  - Weight-bearing status is improved.
  - Work of breathing is decreased.
- Impact on functional limitations
  - Ability to perform movement tasks is improved.
  - Ability to perform physical actions, tasks, or activities related to self-care, home management, work (job/school/play), community, and leisure is improved.
  - Tolerance of positions and activities is increased.
- Impact on disabilities
  - Ability to assume or resume required self-care, home management, work (job/school/play), community, and leisure roles is improved.
- Risk reduction/prevention
  - Risk factors are reduced.
  - Risk of recurrence of condition is reduced.
  - Risk of secondary impairment is reduced.
  - Self-management of symptoms is improved.
- Impact on health, wellness, and fitness
  - Fitness is improved.
  - Physical capacity is increased.
  - Physical function is improved.
- Impact on societal resources
  - Utilization of physical therapy services is optimized.
  - Utilization of physical therapy services results in efficient use of health care dollars.
- Patient/client satisfaction
  - Access, availability, and services provided are acceptable to patient/client.
  - Administrative management of practice is acceptable to patient/client.
  - Clinical proficiency of physical therapist is acceptable to patient/client.
  - Coordination of care is acceptable to patient/client.
  - Cost of health care services is decreased.
  - Intensity of care is decreased.
  - Interpersonal skills of physical therapist are acceptable to patient/client, family, and significant others.
  - Sense of well-being is improved.
  - Stressors are decreased.

Prescription, Application, and, as Appropriate, Fabrication of Devices and Equipment (Assistive, Adaptive, Orthotic, Protective, Supportive, and Prosthetic)

Interventions

- Adaptive devices
  - seating systems
- Assistive devices
  - canes
  - crutches
  - power devices
  - static and dynamic splints
  - walkers
  - wheelchairs
- Orthotic devices
  - braces
  - casts
  - shoe inserts
  - splints
- Protective devices
  - braces
  - cushions
  - protective taping
- Supportive devices
  - corsets
  - neck collars
  - serial casts
  - slings
  - supportive taping

Anticipated Goals and Expected Outcomes

- Impact on pathology/pathophysiology (disease, disorder, or condition)
  - Edema, lymphedema, or effusion is reduced.
  - Joint swelling, inflammation, or restriction is reduced.
  - Pain is decreased.
  - Soft tissue swelling, inflammation, or restriction is reduced.
- Impact on impairments
  - Balance is improved.
  - Endurance is increased.
  - Energy expenditure per unit of work is decreased.
  - Gait, locomotion, and balance are improved.
  - Joint stability is improved.
  - Motor function (motor control and motor learning) is improved.
  - Muscle performance (strength, power, and endurance) is increased.
  - Optimal joint alignment is achieved.
  - Optimal loading on a body part is achieved.
  - Postural control is improved.
  - Quality and quantity of movement between and across body segments are improved.
  - Range of motion is improved.
  - Relaxation is increased.
  - Weight-bearing status is improved.
- Impact on functional limitations
  - Ability to perform physical actions, tasks, or activities related to self-care, home management, work (job/school/play), community, and leisure is improved.
  - Level of supervision required for task performance is decreased.
  - Performance of and independence in activities of daily living (ADL) and instrumental activities of daily living (IADL) with or without devices and equipment are increased.
  - Tolerance of positions and activities is increased.
- Impact on disabilities
  - Ability to assume or resume required self-care, home management, work (job/school/play), community, and leisure roles is improved.
- Risk reduction/prevention
  - Pressure on body tissues is reduced.
  - Protection of body parts is increased.
  - Risk factors are reduced.
  - Risk of recurrence of condition is reduced.
  - Risk of secondary impairment is reduced.
  - Safety is improved.
  - Self-management of symptoms is improved.
- Impact on health, wellness, and fitness
  - Fitness is improved.
  - Health status is improved.
  - Physical capacity is increased.
  - Physical function is improved.
- Impact on societal resources
  - Utilization of physical therapy services is optimized.
  - Utilization of physical therapy services results in efficient use of health care dollars.
- Patient/client satisfaction
  - Access, availability, and services provided are acceptable to patient/client.
  - Administrative management of practice is acceptable to patient/client.
  - Clinical proficiency of physical therapist is acceptable to patient/client.
  - Coordination of care is acceptable to patient/client.
  - Cost of health care services is decreased.
  - Intensity of care is decreased.
  - Interpersonal skills of physical therapist are acceptable to patient/client, family, and significant others.
  - Sense of well-being is improved.
  - Stressors are decreased.

Electrotherapeutic Modalities

Interventions

- Biofeedback
- Electrical stimulation
  - electrical muscle stimulation (EMS)
  - functional electrical stimulation (FES)
  - transcutaneous electrical nerve stimulation (TENS)

Anticipated Goals and Expected Outcomes

- Impact on pathology/pathophysiology (disease, disorder, or condition)
  - Osteogenic effects are enhanced.
  - Pain is decreased.
- Impact on impairments
  - Motor function (motor control and motor learning) is improved.
  - Muscle performance (strength, power, and endurance) is increased.
  - Postural control is improved.
  - Quality and quantity of movement between and across body segments are improved.
  - Relaxation is increased.
  - Sensory awareness is increased.
- Impact on functional limitations
  - Ability to perform physical actions, tasks, or activities related to self-care, home management, work (job/school/play), community, and leisure is improved.
  - Level of supervision required for task performance is decreased.
  - Performance of and independence in activities of daily living (ADL) and instrumental activities of daily living (IADL) with or without devices and equipment are increased.
  - Tolerance of positions and activities is increased.
- Impact on disabilities
  - Ability to assume or resume required self-care, home management, work (job/school/play), community, and leisure roles is improved.
- Risk reduction/prevention
  - Complications of immobility are reduced.
  - Risk factors are reduced.
  - Risk of recurrence of condition is reduced.
  - Risk of secondary impairment is reduced.
  - Self-management of symptoms is improved.
- Impact on health, wellness, and fitness
  - Fitness is improved.
  - Physical capacity is increased.
  - Physical function is improved.
- Impact on societal resources
  - Utilization of physical therapy services is optimized.
  - Utilization of physical therapy services results in efficient use of health care dollars.
- Patient/client satisfaction
  - Access, availability, and services provided are acceptable to patient/client.
  - Administrative management of practice is acceptable to patient/client.
  - Clinical proficiency of physical therapist is acceptable to patient/client.
  - Coordination of care is acceptable to patient/client.
  - Interpersonal skills of physical therapist are acceptable to patient/client, family, and significant others.
  - Sense of well-being is improved.
  - Stressors are decreased.

Physical Agents and Mechanical Modalities

Interventions

Physical agents may include:

- Sound agents
  - phonophoresis
  - ultrasound
- Cryotherapy
  - cold packs
  - ice massage
  - vapocoolant spray
- Thermotherapy
  - dry heat
  - hot packs
  - paraffin baths

Mechanical modalities may include:

- Traction devices
  - intermittent
  - positional
  - sustained

Anticipated Goals and Expected Outcomes

- Impact on pathology/pathophysiology (disease, disorder, or condition)
  - Joint tissue swelling, inflammation, or restriction is reduced.
  - Neural compression is decreased.
  - Nutrient delivery to tissue is increased.
  - Pain is decreased.
  - Soft tissue swelling, inflammation, or restriction is reduced.
  - Tissue perfusion and oxygenation are enhanced.
- Impact on impairments
  - Range of motion is improved.
  - Weight-bearing status is improved.
- Impact on functional limitations
  - Ability to perform physical actions, tasks, or activities related to self-care, home management, work (job/school/play), community, and leisure is improved.
  - Performance of and independence in activities of daily living (ADL) and instrumental activities of daily living (IADL) with or without devices and equipment are increased.
  - Tolerance of positions and activities is increased.
- Impact on disabilities
  - Ability to assume or resume required self-care, home management, work (job/school/play), community, and leisure roles is improved.
- Risk reduction/prevention
  - Complications of soft tissue and circulatory disorders are decreased.
  - Risk of secondary impairment is reduced.
  - Self-management of symptoms is improved.
- Impact on health, wellness, and fitness
  - Physical capacity is increased.
  - Fitness is improved.
  - Physical function is improved.
- Impact on societal resources
  - Utilization of physical therapy services is optimized.
- Patient/client satisfaction
  - Access, availability, and services provided are acceptable to patient/client.
  - Administrative management of practice is acceptable to patient/client.
  - Clinical proficiency of physical therapist is acceptable to patient/client.
  - Coordination of care is acceptable to patient/client.
  - Interpersonal skills of physical therapist is acceptable to patient/client, family, and significant others.
  - Sense of well-being is improved.
  - Stressors are decreased.

Reexamination

Reexamination is the process of performing selected tests and measures after the initial examination to evaluate progress and to modify or redirect interventions. Reexamination may be indicated more than once during a single episode of care. It also may be performed over the course of a disease, disorder, or condition, which for some patients/clients may be over the life span. Indications for reexamination include new clinical findings or failure to respond to physical therapy interventions.

Global Outcomes for Patients/Clients in This Pattern

Throughout the entire episode of care, the physical therapist determines the anticipated goals and expected outcomes for each intervention. These anticipated goals and expected outcomes are delineated in shaded boxes that accompany the lists of interventions in each preferred practice pattern. As the patient/client reaches the termination of physical therapy services and the end of the episode of care, the physical therapist measures the global outcomes of the physical therapy services by characterizing or quantifying the impact of the physical therapy interventions in the following domains:

- Pathology/pathophysiology (disease, disorder, or condition)
- Impairments
- Functional limitations
- Disabilities
- Risk reduction/prevention
- Health, wellness, and fitness
- Societal resources
- Patient/client satisfaction

In some instances, a particular anticipated goal or expected outcome is thoroughly achieved through implementation of a single form of intervention. More commonly, however, the anticipated goals and expected outcomes are achieved as a result of the combined effects of several forms of interventions, leading to enhancement of both health status and health-related quality of life.

Criteria for Termination of Physical Therapy Services

Discharge is the process of ending physical therapy services that have been provided during a single episode of care. It occurs when the anticipated goals and expected outcomes have been achieved. Discharge does *not* occur with a *transfer* (defined as the time when a patient is moved from one site to another site within the same setting or across settings during a single episode of care). Although there may be facility-specific or payer-specific requirements for documentation regarding the conclusion of physical therapy services, *discharge occurs based on the physical therapist's analysis of the achievement of anticipated goals and expected outcomes.*

Discontinuation is the process of ending physical therapy services that have been provided during a single episode of care when (1) the patient/client, caregiver, or legal guardian declines to continue intervention; (2) the patient/client is unable to continue to progress toward outcomes because of medical or psychosocial complications or because financial/insurance resources have been expended; or (3) the physical therapist determines that the patient/client will no longer benefit from physical therapy. When physical therapy services are terminated prior to achievement of anticipated goals and expected outcomes, patient/client status and the rationale for termination are documented.

For patients/clients who require multiple episodes of care, periodic follow-up is needed over the life span to ensure safety and effective adaptation following changes in physical status, caregivers, environment, or task demands. In consultation with appropriate individuals, and in consideration of the outcomes, the physical therapist plans for discharge or discontinuation and provides for appropriate follow-up or referral.

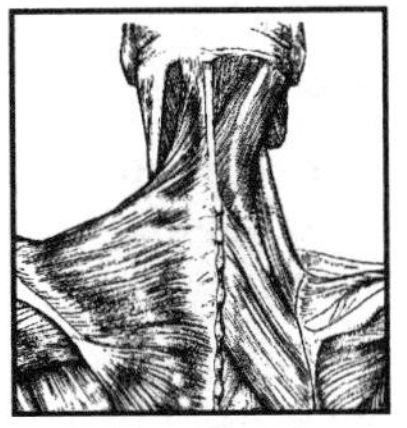

Impaired Muscle Performance

This preferred practice pattern describes the generally accepted elements of patient/client management that physical therapists provide for patients/clients who are classified in this pattern. The pattern title reflects the diagnosis made by the physical therapist. APTA emphasizes that preferred practice patterns are the boundaries within which a physical therapist may select any of a number of clinical alternatives, based on consideration of a wide variety of factors, such as individual patient/client needs; the profession's code of ethics and standards of practice; and patient/client age, culture, gender roles, race, sex, sexual orientation, and socioeconomic status.

Patient/Client Diagnostic Classification

Patients/clients will be classified in this pattern for impaired muscle performance as a result of the physical therapist's evaluation of the examination data. The findings from the examination (history, systems review, and tests and measures) may indicate the presence or risk of pathology/pathophysiology (disease, disorder, or condition), impairments, functional limitations, or disabilities or the need for health, wellness, or fitness programs. The physical therapist integrates, synthesizes, and interprets the data to determine the diagnostic classification.

Inclusion

The following examples of examination findings may support the inclusion of patients/clients in this pattern:

Risk Factors or Consequences of Pathology/Pathophysiology (Disease, Disorder, or Condition)

- Acquired immune deficiency syndrome
- Chronic musculoskeletal dysfunction
- Chronic neuromuscular dysfunction
- Diabetes
- Down syndrome
- Pelvic floor dysfunction
- Renal disease
- Vascular insufficiency

Impairments, Functional Limitations, or Disabilities

- Decreased functional work capacity
- Decreased nerve conduction
- Diastasis recti
- Inability to climb stairs
- Inability to perform repetitive work tasks
- Loss of muscle strength, power, endurance
- Stress urinary incontinence

Note:

Some risk factors or consequences of pathology/pathophysiology—such as *myositis with acute exacerbation*—may be severe and complex; however, *they do not necessarily exclude patients/clients from this pattern.* Severe and complex risk factors or consequences may require modification of the frequency of visits and duration of care. (See "Evaluation, Diagnosis, and Prognosis," page 167.)

Exclusion or Multiple-Pattern Classification

The following examples of examination findings may support exclusion from this pattern or classification into additional patterns. Depending on the level of severity or complexity of the examination findings, the physical therapist may determine that the patient/client would be more appropriately managed through (1) classification in an entirely different pattern or (2) classification in both this and another pattern.

Findings That May Require Classification in a Different Pattern

- Fracture
- Impairments associated with amputation
- Impairments associated with primary capsular restriction
- Impairments associated with primary joint arthroplasty
- Impairments associated with primary localized inflammation
- Muscular pain due to cesarean delivery
- Recent bony surgery

Findings That May Require Classification in Additional Patterns

- Post-polio syndrome with bursitis

ICD-9-CM Codes

The listing below contains the current (as of press time) and most typical 3- and 4-digit ICD-9-CM codes related to this preferred practice pattern. Because patient/client diagnostic classification is based on impairments, functional limitations, and disabilities—not on codes—patients/clients may be classified into the pattern even though the codes listed with the pattern may not apply to those clients.

This listing is intended for general information only and should not be used for coding purposes. The codes should be confirmed by referring to the World Health Organization's *International Classification of Diseases, 9th Revision, Clinical Modification (ICD-9-CM 2001)*, Volumes 1 and 3 (Chicago, Ill: American Medical Association; 2000) or subsequent revisions or by referring to other ICD-9-CM coding manuals that contain exclusion notes and instructions regarding fifth-digit requirements.

- **042** Human immunodeficiency virus [HIV] disease
- **250** Diabetes mellitus
- **359** Muscular dystrophies and other myopathies
  - **359.9** Myopathy, unspecified
- **443** Other peripheral vascular disease
- **564** Functional digestive disorders, not elsewhere classified
  - **564.0** Constipation
- **569** Other disorders of intestine
  - **569.4** Other specified disorders of rectum and anus
    - **569.42** Anal or rectal pain
- **581** Nephrotic syndrome
- **582** Chronic glomerulonephritis
- **583** Nephritis and nephropathy, not specified as acute or chronic
- **588** Disorders resulting from impaired renal function
- **618** Genital prolapse
  - **618.0** Prolapse of vaginal walls without mention of uterine prolapse
    - Cystocele
    - Rectocele
  - **618.1** Uterine prolapse without mention of vaginal wall prolapse
  - **618.6** Vaginal enterocele, congenital or acquired
  - **618.8** Other specified genital prolapse
    - Incompetence or weakening of pelvic fundus
    - Relaxation of vaginal outlet or pelvis
- **623** Noninflammatory disorders of vagina
  - **623.4** Old vaginal laceration
- **624** Noninflammatory disorders of vulva and perineum
  - **624.4** Old laceration or scarring of vulva
- **625** Pain and other symptoms associated with female genital organs
  - **625.0** Dyspareunia
  - **625.1** Vaginismus
  - **625.6** Stress incontinence, female
- **714** Rheumatoid arthritis and other inflammatory polyarthropathies
  - **714.0** Rheumatoid arthritis
- **715** Osteoarthrosis and allied disorders
- **719** Other and unspecified disorders of joint
  - **719.7** Difficulty in walking
- **728** Disorders of muscle, ligament, and fascia
  - **728.2** Muscular wasting and disuse atrophy, not elsewhere classified
  - **728.8** Other disorders of muscle, ligament, and fascia
    - **728.85** Spasm of muscle
  - **728.9** Unspecified disorder of muscle, ligament, and fascia
- **729** Other disorders of soft tissues
  - **729.1** Myalgia and myositis, unspecified
- **733** Other disorders of bone and cartilage
  - **733.0** Osteoporosis
  - **733.1** Pathologic fracture
- **739** Nonallopathic lesions, not elsewhere classified
- **758** Chromosomal anomalies
  - **758.0** Down's syndrome
- **780** General symptoms
  - **780.7** Malaise and fatigue
- **781** Symptoms involving nervous and musculoskeletal systems
  - **781.2** Abnormality of gait
  - **781.3** Lack of coordination
    - Ataxia, not otherwise specified
    - Muscular incoordination
  - **781.4** Transient paralysis of limb
  - **781.9** Other symptoms involving nervous and musculoskeletal systems
    - **781.92** Abnormal posture
- **799** Other ill-defined and unknown causes of morbidity and mortality
  - **799.3** Debility, unspecified

Examination

Examination is a comprehensive screening and specific testing process that leads to a diagnostic classification or, when appropriate, to a referral to another practitioner. Examination is required prior to the initial intervention and is performed for all patients/clients. Through the examination, the physical therapist may identify impairments, functional limitations, disabilities, changes in physical function or overall health status, and needs related to restoration of health and to prevention, wellness, and fitness. The physical therapist synthesizes the examination findings to establish the diagnosis and the prognosis (including the plan of care). The patient/client, family, significant others, and caregivers may provide information during the examination process.

Examination has three components: the patient/client history, the systems review, and tests and measures. The *history* is a systematic gathering of past and current information (often from the patient/client) related to why the patient/client is seeking the services of the physical therapist. The *systems review* is a brief or limited examination of (1) the anatomical and physiological status of the cardiovascular/pulmonary, integumentary, musculoskeletal, and neuromuscular systems and (2) the communication ability, affect, cognition, language, and learning style of the patient/client. *Tests and measures* are the means of gathering data about the patient/client.

The selection of examination procedures and the depth of the examination vary based on patient/client age; severity of the problem; stage of recovery (acute, subacute, chronic); phase of rehabilitation (early, intermediate, late, return to activity); home, work (job/school/play), or community situation; and other relevant factors. *For clinical indications in selecting tests and measures and for listings of tests and measures, tools used to gather data, and the types of data generated by tests and measures, refer to Chapter 2.*

Patient/Client History

The history may include:

General Demographics

- Age
- Sex
- Race/ethnicity
- Primary language
- Education

Social History

- Cultural beliefs and behaviors
- Family and caregiver resources
- Social interactions, social activities, and support systems

Employment/Work (Job/School/Play)

- Current and prior work (job/school/play), community, and leisure actions, tasks, or activities

Growth and Development

- Developmental history
- Hand dominance

Living Environment

- Devices and equipment (eg, assistive, adaptive, orthotic, protective, supportive, prosthetic)
- Living environment and community characteristics
- Projected discharge destinations

General Health Status (Self-Report, Family Report, Caregiver Report)

- General health perception
- Physical function (eg, mobility, sleep patterns, restricted bed days)
- Psychological function (eg, memory, reasoning ability, depression, anxiety)
- Role function (eg, community, leisure, social, work)
- Social function (eg, social activity, social interaction, social support)

Social/Health Habits (Past and Current)

- Behavioral health risks (eg, smoking, drug abuse)
- Level of physical fitness

Family History

- Familial health risks

Medical/Surgical History

- Cardiovascular
- Endocrine/metabolic
- Gastrointestinal
- Genitourinary
- Gynecological
- Integumentary
- Musculoskeletal
- Neuromuscular
- Obstetrical
- Prior hospitalizations, surgeries, and preexisting medical and other health-related conditions
- Psychological
- Pulmonary

Current Condition(s)/Chief Complaint(s)

- Concerns that led patient/client to seek the services of a physical therapist
- Concerns or needs of patient/client who requires the services of a physical therapist
- Current therapeutic interventions
- Mechanisms of injury or disease, including date of onset and course of events
- Onset and pattern of symptoms
- Patient/client, family, significant other, and caregiver expectations and goals for the therapeutic intervention
- Patient/client, family, significant other, and caregiver perceptions of patient's/client's emotional response to the current clinical situation
- Previous occurrence of chief complaint(s)
- Prior therapeutic interventions

Functional Status and Activity Level

- Current and prior functional status in self-care and home management activities, including activities of daily living (ADL) and instrumental activities of daily living (IADL)
- Current and prior functional status in work (job/school/play), community, and leisure actions, tasks, or activities

Medications

- Medications for current condition
- Medications previously taken for current condition
- Medications for other conditions

Other Clinical Tests

- Laboratory and diagnostic tests
- Review of available records (eg, medical, education, surgical)
- Review of other clinical findings (eg, nutrition and hydration)

Systems Review

The systems review may include:

Anatomical and Physiological Status

- Cardiovascular/Pulmonary
  - Blood pressure
  - Edema
  - Heart rate
  - Respiratory rate
- Integumentary
  - Pliability (texture)
  - Presence of scar formation
  - Skin color
  - Skin integrity
- Musculoskeletal
  - Gross range of motion
  - Gross strength
  - Gross symmetry
  - Height
  - Weight
- Neuromuscular
  - Gross coordinated movements (eg, balance, gait, locomotion, transfers, transitions)
  - Motor function (motor control, motor learning)

Communication, Affect, Cognition, Language, and Learning Style

- Ability to make needs known
- Consciousness
- Expected emotional/behavioral responses
- Learning preferences (eg, education needs, learning barriers)
- Orientation (person, place, time)

Tests and Measures

Tests and measures for this pattern may include those that characterize or quantify:

Aerobic Capacity and Endurance

- Aerobic capacity during functional activities (eg, activities of daily living [ADL] scales, indexes, instrumental activities of daily living [IADL] scales, observations)
- Aerobic capacity during standardized exercise test protocols (eg, ergometry, step tests, time/distance walk/run tests, treadmill tests, wheelchair tests)

Anthropometric Characteristics

- Body composition (eg, body mass index, impedance measurement, skinfold thickness measurement)
- Body dimensions (eg, girth measurement, length measurement)

Assistive and Adaptive Devices

- Assistive or adaptive devices and equipment use during functional activities (eg, ADL scales, functional scales, IADL scales, interviews, observations)
- Components, alignment, fit, and ability to care for assistive or adaptive devices and equipment (eg, interviews, logs, observations, pressure-sensing maps, reports)
- Remediation of impairments, functional limitations, or disabilities with use of assistive or adaptive devices and equipment (eg, activity status indexes, ADL scales, aerobic capacity tests, functional performance inventories, health assessment questionnaires, IADL scales, pain scales, play scales, videographic assessments)
- Safety during use of assistive or adaptive devices and equipment (eg, diaries, fall scales, interviews, logs, observations, reports)

Cranial and Peripheral Nerve Integrity

- Electrophysiological integrity (eg, electroneuromyography)
- Motor distribution of the cranial nerves (eg, dynamometry, muscle tests, observations)
- Motor distribution of the peripheral nerves (eg, dynamometry, muscle tests, observations, thoracic outlet tests)
- Sensory distribution of the cranial nerves (eg, discrimination tests; tactile tests, including coarse and light touch, cold and heat, pain, pressure, and vibration)
- Sensory distribution of the peripheral nerves (eg, discrimination tests; tactile tests, including coarse and light touch, cold and heat, pain, pressure, and vibration; thoracic outlet tests)

Environmental, Home, and Work (Job/School/Play) Barriers

- Current and potential barriers (eg, checklists, interviews, observations, questionnaires)

Ergonomics and Body Mechanics

Ergonomics

- Dexterity and coordination during work (job/school/play) (eg, hand function tests, impairment rating scales, manipulative ability tests)
- Functional capacity and performance during work actions, tasks, or activities (eg, accelerometry, dynamometry, electroneuromyography, endurance tests, force platform tests, goniometry, interviews, observations, photographic assessments, physical capacity tests, postural loading analyses, technology-assisted assessments, videographic assessments, work analyses)
- Safety in work environments (eg, hazard identification checklists, job severity indexes, lifting standards, risk assessment scales, standards for exposure limits)
- Specific work conditions or activities (eg, handling checklists, job simulations, lifting models, preemployment screenings, task analysis checklists, workstation checklists)

Body mechanics

- Body mechanics during self-care, home management, work, community, or leisure actions, tasks, or activities (eg, ADL scales, IADL scales, observations, photographic assessments, technology-assisted assessments, videographic assessments)

Gait, Locomotion, and Balance

- Balance during functional activities with or without the use of assistive, adaptive, orthotic, protective, supportive, or prosthetic devices or equipment (eg, ADL scales, IADL scales, observations, videographic assessments)
- Balance (dynamic and static) with or without the use of assistive, adaptive, orthotic, protective, supportive, or prosthetic devices or equipment (eg, balance scales, dizziness inventories, dynamic posturography, fall scales, motor impairment tests, observations, photographic assessments, postural control tests)
- Gait and locomotion during functional activities with or without the use of assistive, adaptive, orthotic, protective, supportive, or prosthetic devices or equipment (eg, ADL scales, gait indexes, IADL scales, mobility skill profiles, observations, videographic assessments)
- Gait and locomotion with or without the use of assistive, adaptive, orthotic, protective, supportive, or prosthetic devices or equipment (eg, dynamometry, electroneuromyography, footprint analyses, gait indexes, mobility skill profiles, observations, photographic assessments, technology-assisted assessments, videographic assessments, weight-bearing scales, wheelchair mobility tests)
- Safety during gait, locomotion, and balance (eg, confidence scales, diaries, fall scales, functional assessment profiles, logs, reports)

Motor Function (Motor Control and Motor Learning)

- Dexterity, coordination, and agility (eg, coordination screens, motor impairment tests, motor proficiency tests, observations, videographic assessments)
- Electrophysiological integrity (eg, electroneuromyography)
- Hand function (eg, fine and gross control tests, finger dexterity tests, manipulative ability tests, observations)
- Initiation, modification, and control of movement patterns and voluntary postures (eg, activity indexes, gross motor function profiles, movement assessment batteries, observations, physical performance tests, videographic assessments)

Muscle Performance (Including Strength, Power and Endurance)

- Electrophysiological integrity (eg, electroneuromyography)
- Muscle strength, power, and endurance (eg, dynamometry, manual muscle tests, muscle performance tests, physical capacity tests, technology-assisted assessments, timed activity tests)
- Muscle strength, power, and endurance during functional activities (eg, ADL scales, functional muscle tests, IADL scales, observations, videographic assessments)
- Muscle tension (eg, palpation)

Orthotic, Protective, and Supportive Devices

- Components, alignment, fit, and ability to care for orthotic, protective, and supportive devices and equipment (eg, interviews, logs, observations, pressure-sensing maps, reports)
- Orthotic, protective, and supportive devices and equipment use during functional activities (eg, ADL scales, functional scales, IADL scales, interviews, observations, profiles)
- Remediation of impairments, functional limitations, or disabilities with use of orthotic, protective, and supportive devices and equipment (eg, activity status indexes, ADL scales, aerobic capacity tests, functional performance inventories, health assessment questionnaires, IADL scales, pain scales, play scales, videographic assessments)
- Safety during use of orthotic, protective, and supportive devices and equipment (eg, diaries, fall scales, interviews, logs, observations, reports)

Pain

- Pain, soreness, and nociception (eg, analog scales, discrimination tests, pain drawings and maps, provocation tests, verbal and pictorial descriptor tests)
- Pain in specific body parts (eg, pain indexes, pain questionnaires, structural provocation tests)

Posture

- Postural alignment and position (static and dynamic), including symmetry and deviation from midline (eg, observations, grid measurement, photographic assessments, technology-assisted assessments, videographic assessments)
- Specific body parts (eg, angle assessments, forward-bending test, goniometry, observations, palpation, positional tests)

Range of Motion (ROM) (Including Muscle Length)

- Functional ROM (eg, observations, squat tests, toe touch tests)
- Joint active and passive movement (eg, goniometry, inclinometry, observations, photographic assessments, videographic assessments)
- Muscle length, soft tissue extensibility, and flexibility (eg, contracture tests, goniometry, inclinometry, ligamentous tests, linear measurement, multisegment flexibility tests, palpation)

Reflex Integrity

- Deep reflexes (eg, myotatic reflex scale, observations, reflex tests)
- Electrophysiological integrity (eg, electroneuromyography)

Self-Care and Home Management (Including ADL and IADL)
- Ability to gain access to home environments (eg, barrier identification, observations, physical performance tests)
- Ability to perform self-care and home management activities with or without assistive, adaptive, orthotic, protective, supportive, or prosthetic devices and equipment (eg, ADL scales, aerobic capacity tests, IADL scales, interviews, observations, profiles)
- Safety in self-care and home management activities and environments (eg, diaries, fall scales, interviews, logs, observations, reports, videographic assessments)

Sensory Integrity
- Deep sensations (eg, kinesthesiometry, observations, photographic assessments, vibration tests)
- Electrophysiological integrity (eg, electroneuromyography)

Ventilation and Respiration (Gas Exchange)
- Pulmonary signs of respiration/gas exchange, including breath sounds (eg, gas analyses, observations, oximetry)

Work (Job/School/Play), Community, and Leisure Integration or Reintegration (Including IADL)
- Ability to assume or resume work (job/school/play), community and leisure activities with or without assistive, adaptive, orthotic, protective, supportive, or prosthetic devices and equipment (eg, activity profiles, disability indexes, functional status questionnaires, IADL scales, observations, physical capacity tests)
- Ability to gain access to work (job/school/play), community, and leisure environments (eg, barrier identification, interviews, observations, physical capacity tests, transportation assessments)
- Safety in work (job/school/play), community, and leisure activities and environments (eg, diaries, fall scales, interviews, logs, observations, videographic assessments)

Evaluation, Diagnosis, and Prognosis (Including Plan of Care)

Physical therapists perform *evaluations* (make clinical judgments) based on the data gathered from the history, systems review, and tests and measures. In the evaluation process, physical therapists synthesize the examination data to establish the diagnosis and prognosis (including the plan of care). Factors that influence the complexity of the evaluation include the clinical findings, extent of loss of function, chronicity or severity of the problem, possibility of multisite or multisystem involvement, preexisting condition(s), potential discharge destination, social considerations, physical function, and overall health status.

A *diagnosis* is a label encompassing a cluster of signs and symptoms, syndromes, or categories. It is the result of the systematic diagnostic process, which includes integrating and evaluating the data from the examination. The diagnostic label indicates the primary dysfunction(s) toward which the therapist will direct interventions. The *prognosis* is the determination of the predicted optimal level of improvement in function and the amount of time needed to reach that level and may also include a prediction of levels of improvement that may be reached at various intervals during the course of therapy. During the prognostic process, the physical therapist develops the plan of care. The *plan of care* identifies specific interventions, proposed frequency and duration of the interventions, anticipated goals, expected outcomes, and discharge plans. The plan of care identifies realistic anticipated goals and expected outcomes, taking into consideration the expectations of the patient/client and appropriate others. These anticipated goals and expected outcomes should be measureable and time limited.

The frequency of visits and duration of the episode of care may vary from a short episode with a high intensity of intervention to a longer episode with a diminishing intensity of intervention. Frequency and duration may vary greatly among patients/clients based on a variety of factors that the physical therapist considers throughout the evaluation process, such as anatomical and physiological changes related to growth and development; caregiver consistency or expertise; chronicity or severity of the current condition; living environment; multisite or multisystem involvement; social support; potential discharge destinations; probability of prolonged impairment, functional limitation, or disability; and stability of the condition.

Prognosis

Over the course of 2 to 6 months, patient/client will demonstrate optimal muscle performance and the highest level of functioning in home, work (job/school/play), community, and leisure environments.

During the episode of care, patient/client will achieve (1) the anticipated goals and expected outcomes of the interventions that are described in the plan of care and (2) the global outcomes for patients/clients who are classified in this pattern.

Expected Range of Number of Visits Per Episode of Care

6 to 30

This range represents the lower and upper limits of the number of physical therapist visits required to achieve anticipated goals and expected outcomes. *It is anticipated that 80% of patients/clients who are classified into this pattern will achieve the anticipated goals and expected outcomes within 6 to 30 visits during a single continuous episode of care.* Frequency of visits and duration of the episode of care should be determined by the physical therapist to maximize effectiveness of care and efficiency of service delivery.

Factors That May Require New Episode of Care or That May Modify Frequency of Visits/Duration of Episode

- Accessibility and availability of resources
- Adherence to the intervention program
- Age
- Anatomical and physiological changes related to growth and development
- Caregiver consistency or expertise
- Chronicity or severity of the current condition
- Cognitive status
- Comorbitities, complications, or secondary impairments
- Concurrent medical, surgical, and therapeutic interventions
- Decline in functional independence
- Level of impairment
- Level of physical function
- Living environment
- Multisite or multisystem involvement
- Nutritional status
- Overall health status
- Potential discharge destinations
- Premorbid conditions
- Probability of prolonged impairment, functional limitation, or disability
- Psychological and socioeconomic factors
- Psychomotor abilities
- Social support
- Stability of the condition

Intervention

Intervention is the purposeful interaction of the physical therapist with the patient/client and, when appropriate, with other individuals involved in patient/client care, using various physical therapy procedures and techniques to produce changes in the condition consistent with the diagnosis and prognosis. Decisions about interventions are contingent on the timely monitoring of patient/client response and the progress made toward achieving the anticipated goals and expected outcomes.

Communication, coordination, and documentation and patient/client-related instruction are provided for all patients/clients across all settings. Procedural interventions are selected or modified based on the examination data and the evaluation, the diagnosis and the prognosis, and the anticipated goals and expected outcomes for a particular patient/client. *For clinical considerations in selecting interventions, listings of interventions, and listings of anticipated goals and expected outcomes, refer to Chapter 3.*

Coordination, Communication, and Documentation

Coordination, communication, and documentation may include:

Interventions

- Addressing required functions
  - advance directives
  - individualized family service plans (IFSPs) or individualized education plans (IEPs)
  - informed consent
  - mandatory communication and reporting (eg, patient advocacy and abuse reporting)
- Admission and discharge planning
- Case management
- Collaboration and coordination with agencies, including:
  - equipment suppliers
  - home care agencies
  - payer groups
  - schools
  - transportation agencies
- Communication across settings, including:
  - case conferences
  - documentation
  - education plans
- Cost-effective resource utilization
- Data collection, analysis, and reporting
  - outcome data
  - peer review findings
  - record reviews
- Documentation across settings, following APTA's *Guidelines for Physical Therapy Documentation* (Appendix 5), including:
  - changes in impairments, functional limitations, and disabilities
  - changes in interventions
  - elements of patient/client management (examination, evaluation, diagnosis, prognosis, intervention)
  - outcomes of intervention
- Interdisciplinary teamwork
  - case conferences
  - patient care rounds
  - patient/client family meetings
- Referrals to other professionals or resources

Anticipated Goals and Expected Outcomes

- Accountability for services is increased.
- Admission data and discharge planning are completed.
- Advance directives, individualized family service plans (IFSPs) or individualized education plans (IEPs), informed consent, and mandatory communication and reporting (eg, patient advocacy and abuse reporting) are obtained or completed.
- Available resources are maximally utilized.
- Care is coordinated with patient/client, family, significant others, caregivers, and other professionals.
- Case is managed throughout the episode of care.
- Collaboration and coordination occurs with agencies, including equipment suppliers, home care agencies, payer groups, schools, and transportation agencies.
- Communication enhances risk reduction and prevention.
- Communication occurs across settings through case conferences, education plans, and documentation.
- Data are collected, analyzed, and reported, including outcome data, peer review findings, and record reviews.
- Decision making is enhanced regarding health, wellness, and fitness needs.
- Decision making is enhanced regarding patient/client health and the use of health care resources by patient/client, family, significant others, and caregivers.
- Documentation occurs throughout patient/client management and across settings and follows APTA's *Guidelines for Physical Therapy Documentation* (Appendix 5).
- Interdisciplinary collaboration occurs through case conferences, patient care rounds, and patient/client family meetings.
- Patient/client, family, significant other, and caregiver understanding of anticipated goals and expected outcomes is increased.
- Placement needs are determined.
- Referrals are made to other professionals or resources whenever necessary and appropriate.
- Resources are utilized in a cost-effective way.

Patient/Client-Related Instruction

Patient/client-related instruction may include:

Interventions

- Instruction, education, and training of patients/clients and caregivers regarding:
  - current condition (pathology/pathophysiology [disease, disorder, or condition], impairments, functional limitations, or disabilities)
  - enhancement of performance
  - health, wellness, and fitness programs
  - plan of care
  - risk factors for pathology/pathophysiology (disease, disorder, or condition), impairments, functional limitations, or disabilities
  - transitions across settings
  - transitions to new roles

Anticipated Goals and Expected Outcomes

- Ability to perform physical actions, tasks, or activities is improved.
- Awareness and use of community resources are improved.
- Behaviors that foster healthy habits, wellness, and prevention are acquired.
- Decision making is enhanced regarding patient/client health and the use of health care resources by patient/client, family, significant others, and caregivers.
- Disability associated with acute or chronic illnesses is reduced.
- Functional independence in activities of daily living (ADL) and instrumental activities of daily living (IADL) is increased.
- Health status is improved.
- Intensity of care is decreased.
- Level of supervision required for task performance is decreased.
- Patient/client, family, significant other, and caregiver knowledge and awareness of the diagnosis, prognosis, interventions, and anticipated goals and expected outcomes are increased.
- Patient/client knowledge of personal and environmental factors associated with the condition is increased.
- Performance levels in self-care, home management, work (job/school/play), community, or leisure actions, tasks, or activities are improved.
- Physical function is improved.
- Risk of recurrence of condition is reduced.
- Risk of secondary impairment is reduced.
- Safety of patient/client, family, significant others, and caregivers is improved.
- Self-management of symptoms is improved.
- Utilization and cost of health care services are decreased.

Procedural Interventions

Procedural interventions for this pattern may include:

Therapeutic Exercise

Interventions

- Aerobic capacity/endurance conditioning or reconditioning
  - aquatic programs
  - gait and locomotor training
  - increased workload over time
  - walking and wheelchair propulsion programs
- Balance, coordination, and agility training
  - developmental activities training
  - motor function (motor control and motor learning) training or retraining
  - neuromuscular education or reeducation
  - perceptual training
  - posture awareness training
  - standardized, programmatic, complementary exercise approaches
  - task-specific performance training
- Body mechanics and postural stabilization
  - body mechanics training
  - posture awareness training
  - postural control training
  - postural stabilization activities
- Flexibility exercises
  - muscle lengthening
  - range of motion
  - stretching
- Gait and locomotion training
  - developmental activities training
  - gait training
  - implement and device training
  - perceptual training
  - standardized, programmatic, complementary exercise approaches
  - wheelchair training
- Relaxation
  - breathing strategies
  - movement strategies
  - relaxation techniques
  - standardized, programmatic, complementary exercise approaches
- Strength, power, and endurance training for head, neck, limb, pelvic-floor, trunk, and ventilatory muscles
  - active assistive, active, and resistive exercises (including concentric, dynamic/isotonic, eccentric, isokinetic, isometric, and plyometric)
  - aquatic programs
  - standardized, programmatic, complementary exercise approaches
  - task-specific performance training

Anticipated Goals and Expected Outcomes

- Impact on pathology/pathophysiology (disease, disorder, or condition)
  - Nutrient delivery to tissue is increased.
  - Osteogenic effects of exercise are maximized.
  - Pain is decreased.
  - Physiological response to increased oxygen demand is improved.
  - Tissue perfusion and oxygenation are enhanced.
- Impact on impairments:
  - Aerobic capacity is increased.
  - Balance is improved.
  - Endurance is increased.
  - Energy expenditure per unit of work is decreased.
  - Gait, locomotion, and balance are improved.
  - Joint integrity and mobility are increased.
  - Motor function (motor control and motor learning) is improved.
  - Muscle performance (strength, power, and endurance) is increased.
  - Postural control is improved.
  - Quality and quantity of movement between and across body segments are improved.
  - Range of motion is improved.
  - Relaxation is increased.
  - Sensory awareness is increased.
  - Weight-bearing status is improved.
- Impact on functional limitations
  - Ability to perform physical actions, tasks, or activities related to self-care, home management, work (job/school/play), community, and leisure is improved.
  - Level of supervision required for task performance is decreased.
  - Performance of and independence in activities of daily living (ADL) and instrumental activities of daily living (IADL) with or without devices and equipment are increased.
  - Tolerance of positions and activities is increased.
- Impact on disabilities
  - Ability to assume or resume required self-care, home management, work (job/school/play), community, and leisure roles is improved.
- Risk reduction/prevention
  - Risk factors are reduced.
  - Risk of recurrence of condition is reduced.
  - Risk of secondary impairments is reduced.
  - Safety is improved.
  - Self-management of symptoms is improved.
- Impact on health, wellness, and fitness
  - Fitness is improved.
  - Health status is improved.
  - Physical capacity is increased.
  - Physical function is improved.
- Impact on societal resources
  - Utilization of physical therapy services is optimized.
  - Utilization of physical therapy services results in efficient use of health care dollars.
- Patient/client satisfaction
  - Access, availability, and services provided are acceptable to patient/client.
  - Administrative management of practice is acceptable to patient/client.
  - Clinical proficiency of physical therapist is acceptable to patient/client.
  - Coordination of care is acceptable to patient/client.
  - Cost of health care services is decreased.
  - Intensity of care is decreased.
  - Interpersonal skills of physical therapist are acceptable to patient/client, family, and significant others.
  - Sense of well-being is improved.
  - Stressors are decreased.

Functional Training in Self-Care and Home Management (Including Activities of Daily Living [ADL] and Instrumental Activities of Daily Living [IADL])

Interventions

- ADL training
  - bathing
  - bed mobility and transfer training
  - developmental activities
  - dressing
  - eating
  - grooming
  - toileting
- Devices and equipment use and training
  - assistive and adaptive device or equipment training during ADL and IADL
  - orthotic, protective, or supportive device or equipment training during ADL and IADL
  - prosthetic device or equipment training during ADL and IADL
- Functional training programs
  - back schools
  - simulated environments and tasks
  - task adaptation
- IADL training
  - caring for dependents
  - home maintenance
  - household chores
  - shopping
  - structured play for infants and children
  - yard work
- Injury prevention or reduction
  - injury prevention education during self-care and home management
  - injury prevention or reduction with use of devices and equipment
  - safety awareness training during self-care and home management

Anticipated Goals and Expected Outcomes

- Impact on pathology/pathophysiology (disease, disorder, or condition)
  - Pain is decreased.
  - Physiological response to increased oxygen demand is improved.
- Impact on impairments
  - Balance is improved.
  - Endurance is increased.
  - Energy expenditure per unit of work is decreased.
  - Motor function (motor control and motor learning) is improved.
  - Muscle performance (strength, power, and endurance) is increased.
  - Postural control is improved.
  - Sensory awareness is increased.
  - Weight-bearing status is improved.
- Impact on functional limitations
  - Ability to perform physical actions, tasks, or activities related to self-care and home management is improved.
  - Level of supervision required for task performance is decreased.
  - Performance of and independence in ADL and IADL with or without devices and equipment are increased.
  - Tolerance of positions and activities are increased.
- Impact on disabilities
  - Ability to assume or resume required self-care and home management roles is improved.
- Risk reduction/prevention
  - Risk factors are reduced.
  - Risk of secondary impairments is reduced.
  - Safety is improved.
  - Self-management of symptoms is improved.
- Impact on health, wellness, and fitness
  - Fitness is improved.
  - Health status is improved.
  - Physical capacity is increased.
  - Physical function is improved.
- Impact on societal resources
  - Utilization of physical therapy services is optimized.
  - Utilization of physical therapy services results in efficient use of health care dollars.
- Patient/client satisfaction
  - Access, availability, and services provided are acceptable to patient/client.
  - Administrative management of practice is acceptable to patient/client.
  - Clinical proficiency of physical therapist is acceptable to patient/client.
  - Coordination of care is acceptable to patient/client.
  - Cost of health care services is decreased.
  - Intensity of care is decreased.
  - Interpersonal skills of physical therapist are acceptable to patient/client, family, and significant others.
  - Sense of well-being is improved.
  - Stressors are decreased.

Functional Training in Work (Job/School/Play), Community, and Leisure Integration or Reintegration (Including Instrumental Activities of Daily Living [IADL], Work Hardening, and Work Conditioning)

Interventions

- Devices and equipment use and training
  - assistive and adaptive device or equipment training during IADL
  - orthotic, protective, or supportive device or equipment training during IADL
  - prosthetic device or equipment training during IADL
- Functional training programs
  - back schools
  - job coaching
  - simulated environments and tasks
  - task adaptation
  - task training
- IADL training
  - community service training involving instruments
  - school and play activities training including tools and instruments
  - work training with tools
- Injury prevention or reduction
  - injury prevention education during work (job/school/play), community, and leisure integration or reintegration
  - injury prevention or reduction with use of devices and equipment
  - safety awareness training during work (job/school/play), community, and leisure integration or reintegration
- Leisure and play activities and training

Anticipated Goals and Expected Outcomes

- Impact on pathology/pathophysiology (disease, disorder, or condition)
  - Pain is decreased.
  - Physiological response to increased oxygen demand is improved.
- Impact on impairments
  - Balance is improved.
  - Endurance is increased.
  - Energy expenditure per unit of work is decreased.
  - Motor function (motor control and motor learning) is improved.
  - Muscle performance (strength, power, and endurance) is increased.
  - Postural control is improved.
  - Sensory awareness is increased.
  - Weight-bearing status is improved.
- Impact on functional limitations
  - Ability to perform physical actions, tasks, or activities related to work (job/school/play), community, and leisure integration or reintegration is improved.
  - Level of supervision required for task performance is decreased.
  - Performance of and independence in IADL with or without devices and equipment are increased.
  - Tolerance of positions and activities is increased.
- Impact on disabilities
  - Ability to assume or resume required work (job/school/play), community, and leisure roles is improved.
- Risk reduction/prevention
  - Risk factors are reduced.
  - Risk of secondary impairment is reduced.
  - Safety is improved.
  - Self-management of symptoms is improved.
- Impact on health, wellness, and fitness
  - Fitness is improved.
  - Health status is improved.
  - Physical capacity is increased.
  - Physical function is improved.
- Impact on societal resources
  - Costs of work-related injury or disability are reduced.
  - Utilization of physical therapy services is optimized.
  - Utilization of physical therapy services results in efficient use of health care dollars.
- Patient/client satisfaction
  - Access, availability, and services provided are acceptable to patient/client.
  - Administrative management of practice is acceptable to patient/client.
  - Clinical proficiency of physical therapist is acceptable to patient/client.
  - Coordination of care is acceptable to patient/client.
  - Cost of health care services is decreased.
  - Intensity of care is decreased.
  - Interpersonal skills of physical therapist are acceptable to patient/client, family, and significant others.
  - Sense of well-being is improved.
  - Stressors are decreased.

Manual Therapy Techniques (Including Mobilization/Manipulation)

Interventions

- Manual traction
- Massage
  - connective tissue massage
  - therapeutic massage
- Mobilization
  - soft tissue
- Passive range of motion

Anticipated Goals and Expected Outcomes

- Impact on pathology/pathophysiology (disease, disorder, or condition)
  - Pain is decreased.
  - Soft tissue swelling, inflammation, or restriction is reduced.
- Impact on impairments
  - Muscle performance (strength, power, and endurance) is increased.
  - Range of motion is improved.
  - Relaxation is increased.
- Impact on functional limitations
  - Ability to perform movement tasks is improved.
  - Ability to perform physical actions, tasks, or activities related to work (job/school/play), community, and leisure is improved.
  - Tolerance of positions and activities is increased.
- Impact on disabilities
  - Ability to assume or resume required self-care, home management, work (job/school/play), community, and leisure roles is improved.
- Risk reduction/prevention
  - Risk of secondary impairment is reduced.
  - Self-management of symptoms is improved.
- Impact on health, wellness, and fitness
  - Fitness is improved.
  - Physical capacity is increased.
  - Physical function is improved.
- Impact on societal resources
  - Utilization of physical therapy services is optimized.
  - Utilization of physical therapy services results in efficient use of health care dollars.
- Patient/client satisfaction
  - Access, availability, and services provided are acceptable to patient/client.
  - Administrative management of practice is acceptable to patient/client.
  - Clinical proficiency of physical therapist is acceptable to patient/client.
  - Coordination of care is acceptable to patient/client.
  - Cost of health care services is decreased.
  - Intensity of care is decreased.
  - Interpersonal skills of physical therapist are acceptable to patient/client, family, and significant others.
  - Sense of well-being is improved.
  - Stressors are decreased.

Prescription, Application, and, as Appropriate, Fabrication of Devices and Equipment (Assistive, Adaptive, Orthotic, Protective, Supportive, and Prosthetic)

Interventions

- Adaptive devices
  - environmental controls
  - raised toilet seats
  - seating systems
- Assistive devices
  - canes
  - crutches
  - long-handled reachers
  - power devices
  - static and dynamic splints
  - walkers
  - wheelchairs
- Orthotic devices
  - braces
  - casts
  - shoe inserts
  - splints
- Prosthetic devices (lower-extremity and upper-extremity)
- Protective devices
  - braces
  - cushions
  - protective taping
- Supportive devices
  - compression garments
  - corsets
  - elastic wraps
  - neck collars
  - serial casts
  - slings
  - supportive taping

Anticipated Goals and Expected Outcomes

- Impact on pathology/pathophysiology (disease, disorder, or condition)
  - Edema, lymphedema, or effusion is reduced.
  - Joint swelling, inflammation, or restriction is reduced.
  - Pain is decreased.
  - Soft tissue swelling, inflammation, or restriction is reduced.
- Impact on impairments
  - Balance is improved.
  - Energy expenditure per unit of work is decreased.
  - Gait, locomotion, and balance are improved.
  - Joint stability is improved.
  - Muscle performance (strength, power, and endurance) is increased.
  - Optimal joint alignment is achieved.
  - Optimal loading on a body part is achieved.
  - Postural control is improved.
  - Quality and quantity of movement between and across body segments are improved.
  - Range of motion is improved.
  - Weight-bearing status is improved.
- Impact on functional limitations
  - Ability to perform physical actions, tasks, or activities related to self-care, home management, work (job/school/play), community, and leisure is improved.
  - Level of supervision required for task performance is decreased.
  - Performance of and independence in activities of daily living (ADL) and instrumental activities of daily living (IADL) with or without devices and equipment are increased.
  - Tolerance of positions and activities is increased.
- Impact on disabilities
  - Ability to assume or resume required self-care, home management, work (job/school/play), community, and leisure roles is improved.
- Risk reduction/prevention
  - Pressure on body tissues is reduced.
  - Protection of body parts is increased.
  - Risk factors are reduced.
  - Risk of secondary impairment is reduced.
  - Safety is improved.
  - Self-management of symptoms is improved.
- Impact on health, wellness, and fitness
  - Fitness is improved.
  - Health status is improved.
  - Physical capacity is increased.
  - Physical function is improved.
- Impact on societal resources
  - Utilization of physical therapy services is optimized.
  - Utilization of physical therapy services results in efficient use of health care dollars.
- Patient/client satisfaction
  - Access, availability, and services provided are acceptable to patient/client.
  - Administrative management of practice is acceptable to patient/client.
  - Clinical proficiency of physical therapist is acceptable to patient/client.
  - Coordination of care is acceptable to patient/client.
  - Cost of health care services is decreased.
  - Intensity of care is decreased.
  - Interpersonal skills of physical therapist are acceptable to patient/client, family, and significant others.
  - Sense of well-being is improved.
  - Stressors are decreased.

Electrotherapeutic Modalities

Interventions

- Biofeedback
- Electrical stimulation
  - electrical muscle stimulation (EMS)
  - functional electrical stimulation (FES)
  - neuromuscular electrical stimulation (NMES)
  - transcutaneous electrical nerve stimulation (TENS)

Anticipated Goals and Expected Outcomes

- Impact on pathology/pathophysiology
  - Joint tissue swelling, inflammation, or restriction is reduced.
  - Nutrient delivery to tissue is increased.
  - Osteogenic effects are enhanced.
  - Pain is decreased.
  - Soft tissue swelling, inflammation, or restriction is reduced.
  - Tissue perfusion and oxygenation are enhanced.
- Impact on impairments
  - Motor function (motor control and motor learning) is improved.
  - Muscle performance (strength, power, and endurance) is increased.
  - Postural control is improved.
  - Quality and quantity of movement between and across body segments are improved.
  - Relaxation is increased.
  - Sensory awareness is increased.
- Impact on functional limitations
  - Ability to perform physical actions, tasks, or activities related to self-care, home management, community, work (job/ school/ play), and leisure is improved.
  - Level of supervision required for task performance is decreased.
  - Performance of and independence in activities of daily living (ADL) and instrumental activities of daily living (IADL) with or without devices and equipment are increased.
  - Tolerance of positions and activities is increased.
- Impact on disabilities
  - Ability to assume or resume required self-care, home management, work (job/school/play), community, and leisure roles is improved.
- Risk reduction/prevention
  - Complications of immobility are reduced.
  - Risk factors are reduced.
  - Risk of secondary impairment is reduced.
  - Self-management of symptoms is improved.
- Impact on health, wellness, and fitness
  - Fitness is improved.
  - Physical capacity is increased.
  - Physical function is improved.
- Impact on societal resources
  - Utilization of physical therapy services is optimized.
  - Utilization of physical therapy services results in efficient use of health care dollars.
- Patient/client satisfaction
  - Access, availability, and services provided are acceptable to patient/client.
  - Administrative management of practice is acceptable to patient/client.
  - Clinical proficiency of physical therapist is acceptable to patient/client.
  - Coordination of care is acceptable to patient/client.
  - Interpersonal skills of physical therapist are acceptable to patient/client, family, and significant others.
  - Sense of well-being is improved.
  - Stressors are decreased.

Physical Agents and Mechanical Modalities

Interventions

Physical agents may include:

- Cryotherapy
  - cold packs
  - ice massage
  - vapocoolant spray
- Hydrotherapy
  - pools
- Sound agents
  - phonophoresis
  - ultrasound
- Thermotherapy
  - dry heat
  - hot packs
  - paraffin baths

Mechanical modalities may include:

- Compression therapies
  - taping
- Gravity-assisted compression devices
  - standing frame
  - tilt table
- Traction devices
  - intermittent
  - positional
  - sustained

Anticipated Goals and Expected Outcomes

- Impact on pathology/pathophysiology (disease, disorder, or condition)
  - Joint swelling, inflammation, or restriction is reduced.
  - Nutrient delivery to tissue is increased.
  - Neural compression is decreased.
  - Osteogenic effects are enhanced.
  - Pain is decreased.
  - Soft tissue swelling, inflammation, or restriction is reduced.
  - Tissue perfusion and oxygenation are enhanced.
- Impact on impairments:
  - Muscle performance (strength, power, and endurance) is increased.
  - Range of motion is improved.
  - Weight-bearing status is improved.
- Impact on functional limitations
  - Ability to perform physical actions, tasks, or activities related to self-care, home management, work (job/school/play), community, and leisure is improved.
  - Performance of and independence in activities of daily living (ADL) and instrumental activities of daily living (IADL) with or without devices and equipment are increased.
  - Tolerance of positions and activities is increased.
- Impact on disabilities
  - Ability to assume or resume required self-care, home management, work (job/school/play), community, and leisure roles is improved.
- Risk reduction/prevention
  - Complications of soft tissue and circulatory disorders are decreased.
  - Risk of secondary impairments is reduced.
  - Self-management of symptoms is improved.
- Impact on health, wellness, and fitness
  - Physical function is improved.
- Impact on societal resources
  - Utilization of physical therapy services is optimized.
- Patient/client satisfaction
  - Access, availability, and services provided are acceptable to patient/client.
  - Administrative management of practice is acceptable to patient/client.
  - Clinical proficiency of physical therapist is acceptable to patient/client.
  - Coordination of care is acceptable to patient/client.
  - Interpersonal skills of physical therapist are acceptable to patient/client, family, and significant others.
  - Sense of well-being is improved.
  - Stressors are decreased.

Reexamination

Reexamination is the process of performing selected tests and measures after the initial examination to evaluate progress and to modify or redirect interventions. Reexamination may be indicated more than once during a single episode of care. It also may be performed over the course of a disease, disorder, or condition, which for some patients/clients may be over the life span. Indications for reexamination include new clinical findings or failure to respond to physical therapy interventions.

Global Outcomes for Patients/Clients in This Pattern

Throughout the entire episode of care, the physical therapist determines the anticipated goals and expected outcomes for each intervention. These anticipated goals and expected outcomes are delineated in shaded boxes that accompany the lists of interventions in each preferred practice pattern. As the patient/client reaches the termination of physical therapy services and the end of the episode of care, the physical therapist measures the global outcomes of the physical therapy services by characterizing or quantifying the impact of the physical therapy interventions in the following domains:

- Pathology/pathophysiology (disease, disorder, or condition)
- Impairments
- Functional limitations
- Disabilities
- Risk reduction/prevention
- Health, wellness, and fitness
- Societal resources
- Patient/client satisfaction

In some instances, a particular anticipated goal or expected outcome is thoroughly achieved through implementation of a single form of intervention. More commonly, however, the anticipated goals and expected outcomes are achieved as a result of the combined effects of several forms of interventions, leading to enhancement of both health status and health-related quality of life.

Criteria for Termination of Physical Therapy Services

Discharge is the process of ending physical therapy services that have been provided during a single episode of care. It occurs when the anticipated goals and expected outcomes have been achieved. Discharge does *not* occur with a *transfer* (defined as the time when a patient is moved from one site to another site within the same setting or across settings during a single episode of care). Although there may be facility-specific or payer-specific requirements for documentation regarding the conclusion of physical therapy services, *discharge occurs based on the physical therapist's analysis of the achievement of anticipated goals and expected outcomes.*

Discontinuation is the process of ending physical therapy services that have been provided during a single episode of care when (1) the patient/client, caregiver, or legal guardian declines to continue intervention; (2) the patient/client is unable to continue to progress toward outcomes because of medical or psychosocial complications or because financial/insurance resources have been expended; or (3) the physical therapist determines that the patient/client will no longer benefit from physical therapy. When physical therapy services are terminated prior to achievement of anticipated goals and expected outcomes, patient/client status and the rationale for termination are documented.

For patients/clients who require multiple episodes of care, periodic follow-up is needed over the life span to ensure safety and effective adaptation following changes in physical status, caregivers, environment, or task demands. In consultation with appropriate individuals, and in consideration of the outcomes, the physical therapist plans for discharge or discontinuation and provides for appropriate follow-up or referral.

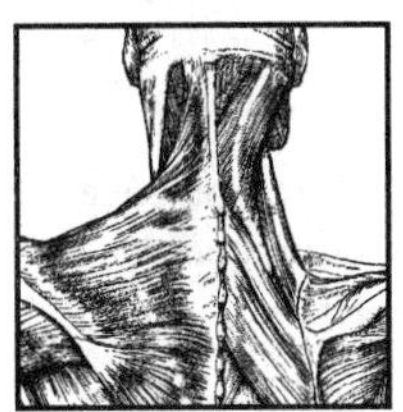

Impaired Joint Mobility, Motor Function, Muscle Performance, and Range of Motion Associated With Connective Tissue Dysfunction

This preferred practice pattern describes the generally accepted elements of patient/client management that physical therapists provide for patients/clients who are classified in this pattern. The pattern title reflects the diagnosis made by the physical therapist. APTA emphasizes that preferred practice patterns are the boundaries within which a physical therapist may select any of a number of clinical alternatives, based on consideration of a wide variety of factors, such as individual patient/client needs; the profession's code of ethics and standards of practice; and patient/client age, culture, gender roles, race, sex, sexual orientation, and socioeconomic status.

Patient/Client Diagnostic Classification

Patients/clients will be classified into this pattern—for impaired joint mobility, motor function, muscle performance, and range of motion associated with connective tissue dysfunction—as a result of the physical therapist's evaluation of the examination data. The findings from the examination (history, systems review, and tests and measures) may indicate the presence or risk of pathology/pathophysiology (disease, disorder, or condition), impairments, functional limitations, or disabilities or the need for health, wellness, or fitness programs. The physical therapist integrates, synthesizes, and interprets the data to determine the diagnostic classification.

Inclusion

The following examples of examination findings may support the inclusion of patients/clients in this pattern:

Risk Factors or Consequences of Pathology/Pathophysiology (Disease, Disorder, or Condition)

- Joint subluxation or dislocation
- Ligamentous sprain
- Musculotendinous strain
- Pregnancy
- Prolonged joint immobilization
- Rheumatoid arthritis
- Scleroderma
- Systemic lupus erythematosus
- Temporomandibular joint syndrome

Impairments, Functional Limitations, or Disabilities

- Decreased range of motion
- Inability to squat due to joint instability
- Muscle guarding or weakness
- Pain
- Postpartum sacroiliac dysfunction
- Swelling or effusion

Note:

Some risk factors or consequences of pathology/pathophysiology—such as *impairments associated with joint hemarthrosis* and *neuromuscular dysfunction*—may be severe and complex; *however, they do not necessarily exclude patients/clients from this pattern.* Severe and complex risk factors or consequences may require modification of the frequency of visits and duration of care. (See "Evaluation, Diagnosis, and Prognosis," page 185.)

Exclusion or Multiple-Pattern Classification

The following examples of examination findings may support exclusion from this pattern or classification into additional patterns. Depending on the level of severity or complexity of the examination findings, the physical therapist may determine that the patient/client would be more appropriately managed through (1) classification in an entirely different pattern or (2) classification in both this and another pattern.

Findings That May Require Classification in a Different Pattern

- Fracture
- Immobility as a primary result of prolonged bed rest
- Lack of voluntary movement
- Radiculopathy

Findings That May Require Classification in Additional Patterns

- Abrasion or wound

ICD-9-CM Codes

The listing below contains the current (as of press time) and most typical 3- and 4-digit ICD-9-CM codes related to this preferred practice pattern. Because patient/client diagnostic classification is based on impairments, functional limitations, and disabilities—not on codes—patients/clients may be classified into the pattern even though the codes listed with the pattern may not apply to those clients.

This listing is intended for general information only and should not be used for coding purposes. The codes should be confirmed by referring to the World Health Organization's *International Classification of Diseases, 9th Revision, Clinical Modification (ICD-9-CM 2001)*, Volumes 1 and 3 (Chicago, Ill: American Medical Association; 2000) or subsequent revisions or by referring to other ICD-9-CM coding manuals that contain exclusion notes and instructions regarding fifth-digit requirements.

337 Disorders of the autonomic nervous system
- **337.2** Reflex sympathetic dystrophy

524 Dentofacial anomalies, including malocclusion
- **524.6** Temporomandibular joint disorders

625 Pain and other symptoms associated with female genital organs
- **625.5** Pelvic congestion syndrome

665 Other obstetrical trauma
- **665.6** Damage to pelvic joints and ligaments

709 Other disorders of skin and subcutaneous tissue
- **709.2** Scar conditions and fibrosis of skin

710 Diffuse diseases of connective tissue
- **710.0** Systemic lupus erythematosus
- **710.3** Dermatomyositis
- **710.4** Polymyositis

714 Rheumatoid arthritis and other inflammatory polyarthropathies
- **714.0** Rheumatoid arthritis

715 Osteoarthrosis and allied disorders

716 Other and unspecified arthropathies
- **716.5** Unspecified polyarthropathy or polyarthritis
- **716.9** Arthropathy, unspecified
  - Inflammation of joint, not otherwise specified

718 Other derangement of joint

719 Other and unspecified disorders of joint
- **719.4** Pain in joint
- **719.8** Other specified disorders of joint
  - Calcification of joint

724 Other and unspecified disorders of back
- **724.6** Disorders of sacrum
- **724.9** Other unspecified back disorders
  - Ankylosis of spine, not otherwise specified
  - Compression of spinal nerve root, not elsewhere classified
  - Spinal disorder, not otherwise specified

726 Peripheral enthesopathies and allied syndromes
- **726.0** Adhesive capsulitis of shoulder
- **726.1** Rotator cuff syndrome of shoulder and allied disorders
- **726.2** Other affections of shoulder region, not elsewhere classified
- **726.9** Unspecified enthesopathy

727 Other disorders of synovium, tendon, and bursa
- **727.0** Synovitis and tenosynovitis
- **727.6** Rupture of tendon, nontraumatic
- **727.8** Other disorders of synovium, tendon, and bursa

728 Disorders of muscle, ligament, and fascia
- **728.4** Laxity of ligament
- **728.6** Contracture of palmar fascia
  - Dupuytren's contracture
- **728.7** Other fibromatoses
- **728.8** Other disorders of muscle, ligament, and fascia

729 Other disorders of soft tissues
- **729.1** Myalgia and myositis, unspecified
- **729.8** Other musculoskeletal symptoms referable to limbs
- **729.9** Other and unspecified disorders of soft tissue

730 Osteomyelitis, periostitis, and other infections involving bone

733 Other disorders of bone and cartilage

830 Dislocation of jaw

831 Dislocation of shoulder

832 Dislocation of elbow

833 Dislocation of wrist

836 Dislocation of knee

837 Dislocation of ankle

838 Dislocation of foot

839 Other, multiple, and ill-defined dislocations
- **839.0** Cervical vertebra, closed
- **839.8** Multiple and ill-defined, closed
  - Arm
  - Back
  - Hand
  - Multiple locations, except fingers or toes alone
  - Other ill-defined locations
  - Unspecified location

840 Sprains and strains of shoulder and upper arm
- **840.4** Rotator cuff (capsule)

841 Sprains and strains of elbow and forearm

842 Sprains and strains of wrist and hand

843 Sprains and strains of hip and thigh

844 Sprains and strains of knee and leg

845 Sprains and strains of ankle and foot

846 Sprains and strains of sacroiliac region

847 Sprains and strains of other and unspecified parts of back

848 Other and ill-defined sprains and strains
- **848.1** Jaw
- **848.3** Ribs
- **848.4** Sternum
- **848.5** Pelvis
  Symphysis pubis

905 Late effects of musculoskeletal and connective tissue injuries
- **905.6** Late effect of dislocation
- **905.7** Late effect of sprain and strain without mention of tendon injury

941 Burn of face, head, and neck
- **941.0** Unspecified degree
- **941.1** Erythema [first degree]
- **941.2** Blisters, epidermal loss [second degree]
- **941.3** Full-thickness skin loss [third degree NOS]
- **941.4** Deep necrosis of underlying tissues [deep third degree] without mention of loss of a body part
- **941.5** Deep necrosis of underlying tissues [deep third degree] with loss of a body part

942 Burn of trunk
- **942.0** Unspecified degree
- **942.1** Erythema [first degree]
- **942.2** Blisters, epidermal loss [second degree]
- **942.3** Full-thickness skin loss [third degree NOS]
- **942.4** Deep necrosis of underlying tissues [deep third degree] without mention of loss of a body part
- **942.5** Deep necrosis of underlying tissues [deep third degree] with loss of a body part

943 Burn of upper limb, except wrist and hand
- **943.0** Unspecified degree
- **943.1** Erythema [first degree]
- **943.2** Blisters, epidermal loss [second degree]
- **943.3** Full-thickness skin loss [third degree NOS]
- **943.4** Deep necrosis of underlying tissues [deep third degree] without mention of loss of a body part
- **943.5** Deep necrosis of underlying tissues [deep third degree] with loss of a body part

944 Burn of wrist(s) and hand(s)
- **944.0** Unspecified degree
- **944.1** Erythema [first degree]
- **944.2** Blisters, epidermal loss [second degree]
- **944.3** Full-thickness skin loss [third degree NOS]
- **944.4** Deep necrosis of underlying tissues [deep third degree] without mention of loss of a body part
- **944.5** Deep necrosis of underlying tissues [deep third degree] with loss of a body part

945 Burn of lower limb(s)
- **945.0** Unspecified degree
- **945.1** Erythema [first degree]
- **945.2** Blisters, epidermal loss [second degree]
- **945.3** Full-thickness skin loss [third degree NOS]
- **945.4** Deep necrosis of underlying tissues [deep third degree] without mention of loss of a body part
- **945.5** Deep necrosis of underlying tissues [deep third degree] with loss of a body part

946 Burns of multiple specified sites
- **946.0** Unspecified degree
- **946.1** Erythema [first degree]
- **946.2** Blisters, epidermal loss [second degree]
- **946.3** Full-thickness skin loss [third degree NOS]
- **946.4** Deep necrosis of underlying tissues [deep third degree] without mention of loss of a body part
- **946.5** Deep necrosis of underlying tissues [deep third degree] with loss of a body part

947 Burn of internal organs
- **947.0** Mouth and pharynx
- **947.1** Larynx, trachea, and lung
- **947.2** Esophagus
- **947.3** Gastrointestinal tract
- **947.4** Vagina and uterus
- **947.8** Other unspecified parts
- **947.9** Unspecified site

948 Burns classified according to extent of body surface involved

949 Burn, unspecified
- **949.0** Unspecified degree
- **949.1** Erythema [first degree]
- **949.2** Blisters, epidermal loss [second degree]
- **949.3** Full-thickness skin loss [third degree NOS]
- **949.4** Deep necrosis of underlying tissues [deep third degree] without mention of loss of a body part
- **949.5** Deep necrosis of underlying tissues [deep third degree] with loss of a body part

Examination

Examination is a comprehensive screening and specific testing process that leads to a diagnostic classification or, when appropriate, to a referral to another practitioner. Examination is required prior to the initial intervention and is performed for all patients/clients. Through the examination, the physical therapist may identify impairments, functional limitations, disabilities, changes in physical function or overall health status, and needs related to restoration of health and to prevention, wellness, and fitness. The physical therapist synthesizes the examination findings to establish the diagnosis and the prognosis (including the plan of care). The patient/client, family, significant others, and caregivers may provide information during the examination process.

Examination has three components: the patient/client history, the systems review, and tests and measures. The *history* is a systematic gathering of past and current information (often from the patient/client) related to why the patient/client is seeking the services of the physical therapist. The *systems review* is a brief or limited examination of (1) the anatomical and physiological status of the cardiovascular/pulmonary, integumentary, musculoskeletal, and neuromuscular systems and (2) the communication ability, affect, cognition, language, and learning style of the patient/client. *Tests and measures* are the means of gathering data about the patient/client.

The selection of examination procedures and the depth of the examination vary based on patient/client age; severity of the problem; stage of recovery (acute, subacute, chronic); phase of rehabilitation (early, intermediate, late, return to activity); home, work (job/school/play), or community situation; and other relevant factors. *For clinical indications in selecting tests and measures and for listings of tests and measures, tools used to gather data, and the types of data generated by tests and measures, refer to Chapter 2.*

Patient/Client History

The history may include:

General Demographics

- Age
- Sex
- Race/ethnicity
- Primary language
- Education

Social History

- Cultural beliefs and behaviors
- Family and caregiver resources
- Social interactions, social activities, and support systems

Employment/Work (Job/School/Play)

- Current and prior work (job/school/play), community, and leisure actions, tasks, or activities

Growth and Development

- Developmental history
- Hand dominance

Living Environment

- Devices and equipment (eg, assistive, adaptive, orthotic, protective, supportive, prosthetic)
- Living environment and community characteristics
- Projected discharge destinations

General Health Status (Self-Report, Family Report, Caregiver Report)

- General health perception
- Physical function (eg, mobility, sleep patterns, restricted bed days)
- Psychological function (eg, memory, reasoning ability, depression, anxiety)
- Role function (eg, community, leisure, social, work)
- Social function (eg, social activity, social interaction, social support)

Social/Health Habits (Past and Current)

- Behavioral health risks (eg, smoking, drug abuse)
- Level of physical fitness

Family History

- Familial health risks

Medical/Surgical History

- Cardiovascular
- Endocrine/metabolic
- Gastrointestinal
- Genitourinary
- Gynecological
- Integumentary
- Musculoskeletal
- Neuromuscular
- Obstetrical
- Prior hospitalizations, surgeries, and preexisting medical and other health-related conditions
- Psychological
- Pulmonary

Current Condition(s)/Chief Complaint(s)

- Concerns that led patient/client to seek the services of a physical therapist
- Concerns or needs of patient/client who requires the services of a physical therapist
- Current therapeutic interventions
- Mechanisms of injury or disease, including date of onset and course of events
- Onset and pattern of symptoms
- Patient/client, family, significant other, and caregiver expectations and goals for the therapeutic intervention
- Patient/client, family, significant other, and caregiver perceptions of patient's/client's emotional response to the current clinical situation
- Previous occurrence of chief complaint(s)
- Prior therapeutic interventions

Functional Status and Activity Level

- Current and prior functional status in self-care and home management activities, including activities of daily living (ADL) and instrumental activities of daily living (IADL)
- Current and prior functional status in work (job/school/play), community, and leisure actions, tasks, or activities

Medications

- Medications for current condition
- Medications previously taken for current condition
- Medications for other conditions

Other Clinical Tests

- Laboratory and diagnostic tests
- Review of available records (eg, medical, education, surgical)
- Review of other clinical findings (eg, nutrition and hydration)

Systems Review

The systems review may include:

Anatomical and Physiological Status

- Cardiovascular/Pulmonary
  - Blood pressure
  - Edema
  - Heart rate
  - Respiratory rate
- Integumentary
  - Pliability (texture)
  - Presence of scar formation
  - Skin color
  - Skin integrity
- Musculoskeletal
  - Gross range of motion
  - Gross strength
  - Gross symmetry
  - Height
  - Weight
- Neuromuscular
  - Gross coordinated movements (eg, balance, gait, locomotion, transfers, transitions)
  - Motor function (motor control, motor learning)

Communication, Affect, Cognition, Language, and Learning Style

- Ability to make needs known
- Consciousness
- Expected emotional/behavioral responses
- Learning preferences (eg, education needs, learning barriers)
- Orientation (person, place, time)

Tests and Measures

Tests and measures for this pattern may include those that characterize or quantify:

Anthropometric Characteristics

- Edema (eg, girth measurement, palpation, scales, volume measurement)

Assistive and Adaptive Devices

- Assistive or adaptive devices and equipment use during functional activities (eg, activities of daily living [ADL] scales, functional scales, instrumental activities of daily living [IADL] scales, interviews, observations)
- Components, alignment, fit, and ability to care for the assistive or adaptive devices and equipment (eg, interviews, logs, observations, pressure-sensing maps, reports)
- Remediation of impairments, functional limitations, or disabilities with use of assistive or adaptive devices and equipment (eg, activity status indexes, ADL scales, aerobic capacity tests, functional performance inventories, health assessment questionnaires, IADL scales, pain scales, play scales, videographic assessments)
- Safety during use of assistive or adaptive devices and equipment (eg, diaries, fall scales, interviews, logs, observations, reports)

Cranial and Peripheral Nerve Integrity

- Motor distribution of the peripheral nerves (eg, dynamometry, muscle tests, observations, thoracic outlet tests)
- Response to neural provocation (eg, tension tests, vertebral artery compression tests)
- Sensory distribution of the peripheral nerves (eg, discrimination tests; tactile tests, including coarse and light touch, cold and heat, pain, pressure, and vibration; thoracic outlet tests)

Environmental, Home, and Work (Job/School/Play) Barriers

- Current and potential barriers (eg, checklists, interviews, observations, questionnaires)

Ergonomics and Body Mechanics

Ergonomics

- Dexterity and coordination during work (job/school/play) (eg, hand function tests, impairment rating scales, manipulative ability tests)
- Functional capacity and performance during work actions, tasks, or activities (eg, accelerometry, dynamometry, electroneuromyography, endurance tests, force platform tests, goniometry, interviews, observations, photographic assessments, physical capacity tests, postural loading analyses, technology-assisted assessments, videographic assessments, work analyses)
- Safety in work environments (eg, hazard identification checklists, job severity indexes, lifting standards, risk assessment scales, standards for exposure limits)
- Specific work conditions or activities (eg, handling checklists, job simulations, lifting models, preemployment screenings, task analysis checklists, workstation checklists)
- Tools, devices, equipment, and workstations related to work actions, tasks, or activities (eg, observations, tool analysis checklists, vibration assessments)

Body mechanics

- Body mechanics during self-care, home management, work, community, or leisure actions, tasks, or activities (eg, ADL scales, IADL scales, observations, photographic assessments, technology-assisted assessments, videographic assessments)

Gait, Locomotion, and Balance

- Balance during functional activities with or without the use of assistive, adaptive, orthotic, protective, supportive, or prosthetic devices or equipment (eg, ADL scales, IADL scales, observations, videographic assessments)
- Balance (dynamic and static) with or without the use of assistive, adaptive, orthotic, protective, supportive, or prosthetic devices or equipment (eg, balance scales, dizziness inventories, dynamic posturography, fall scales, motor impairment tests, observations, photographic assessments, postural control tests)
- Gait and locomotion during functional activities with or without the use of assistive, adaptive, orthotic, protective, supportive, or prosthetic devices or equipment (eg, ADL scales, gait indexes, IADL scales, mobility skill profiles, observations, videographic assessments)

- Gait and locomotion with or without the use of assistive, adaptive, orthotic, protective, supportive, or prosthetic devices or equipment (eg, dynamometry, electroneuromyography, footprint analyses, gait indexes, mobility skill profiles, observations, photographic assessments, technology-assisted assessments, videographic assessments, weight-bearing scales, wheelchair mobility tests)
- Safety during gait, locomotion, and balance (eg, confidence scales, diaries, fall scales, functional assessment profiles, logs, reports)

Joint Integrity and Mobility

- Joint integrity and mobility (eg, apprehension, compression and distraction, drawer, glide, impingement, shear, and valgus/varus stress tests; arthrometry; palpation)
- Joint play movements, including end feel (all joints of the axial and appendicular skeletal system) (eg, palpation)

Motor Function (Motor Control and Motor Learning)

- Dexterity, coordination, and agility (eg, coordination screens, motor impairment tests, motor proficiency tests, observations, videographic assessments)
- Hand function (eg, fine and gross motor control tests, finger dexterity tests, manipulative ability tests, observations)

Muscle Performance (Including Strength, Power, and Endurance)

- Electrophysiological integrity (eg, electroneuromyography)
- Muscle strength, power, and endurance (eg, dynamometry, manual muscle tests, muscle performance tests, physical capacity tests, technology-assisted assessments, timed activity tests)
- Muscle strength, power, and endurance during functional activities (eg, ADL scales, functional muscle tests, IADL scales, observations, videographic assessments)
- Muscle tension (eg, palpation)

Orthotic, Protective, and Supportive Devices

- Components, alignment, fit, and ability to care for orthotic, protective, and supportive devices and equipment (eg, interviews, logs, observations, pressure-sensing maps, reports)
- Orthotic, protective, and supportive devices and equipment use during functional activities (eg, ADL scales, functional scales, IADL scales, interviews, observations, profiles)
- Remediation of impairments, functional limitations, or disabilities with use of orthotic, protective, and supportive devices and equipment (eg, activity status indexes, ADL scales, aerobic capacity tests, functional performance inventories, health assessment questionnaires, IADL scales, pain scales, play scales, videographic assessments)
- Safety during use of orthotic, protective, and supportive devices and equipment (eg, diaries, fall scales, interviews, logs, observations, reports)

Pain

- Pain, soreness, and nociception (eg, analog scales, discrimination tests, pain drawings and maps, provocation tests, verbal and pictorial descriptor tests)
- Pain in specific body parts (eg, pain indexes, pain questionnaires, structural provocation tests)

Posture

- Postural alignment and position (dynamic and static), including symmetry and deviation from midline (eg, observations, grid measurements, technology-assisted assessments, photographic assessments, videographic assessments)
- Specific body parts (eg, angle assessments, forward-bending test, goniometry, observations, palpation, positional tests)

Range of Motion (ROM) (Including Muscle Length)

- Functional ROM (eg, observations, squat tests, toe touch tests)
- Joint active and passive movement (eg, goniometry, inclinometry, observations, photographic assessments, technology-assisted assessments, videographic assessments)
- Muscle length, soft tissue extensibility, and flexibility (eg, contracture tests, goniometry, inclinometry, ligamentous tests, linear measurement, multisegment flexibility tests, palpation)

Reflex Integrity

- Deep reflexes (eg, myotatic reflex scale, observations, reflex tests)
- Superficial reflexes and reactions (eg, observations, provocation tests)

Self-Care and Home Management (Including ADL and IADL)

- Ability to gain access to home environments (eg, barrier identification, observations, physical performance tests)
- Ability to perform self-care and home management activities with or without assistive, adaptive, orthotic, protective, supportive, or prosthetic devices and equipment (eg, ADL scales, aerobic capacity tests, IADL scales, interviews, observations, profiles)
- Safety in self-care and home management activities and environments (eg, diaries, fall scales, interviews, logs, observations, reports, videographic assessments)

Sensory Integrity

- Combined/cortical sensations (eg, stereognosis, tactile discrimination tests)
- Deep sensations (eg, kinesthesiometry, observations, photographic assessments, vibration tests)

Ventilation and Respiration/Gas Exchange

- Pulmonary signs of respiration/gas exchange, including breath sounds (eg, gas analyses, observations, oximetry)
- Pulmonary signs of ventilatory function, including airway protection; breath and voice sounds; respiratory rate, rhythm, and pattern; ventilatory flow, forces, and volumes (eg, airway clearance tests, observations, palpation, pulmonary function tests, ventilatory muscle force tests)
- Pulmonary symptoms (eg, dyspnea and perceived exertion indexes and scales)

Work (Job/School/Play), Community, and Leisure Integration or Reintegration (Including IADL)

- Ability to assume or resume work (job/school/play), community, and leisure activities with or without assistive, adaptive, orthotic, protective, supportive, or prosthetic devices and equipment (eg, activity profiles, disability indexes, functional status questionnaires, IADL scales, observations, physical capacity tests)
- Ability to gain access to work (job/school/play), community, and leisure environments (eg, barrier identification, interviews, observations, physical capacity tests, transportation assessments)
- Safety in work (job/school/play), community, and leisure activities and environments (eg, diaries, fall scales, interviews, logs, observations, videographic assessments)

Evaluation, Diagnosis, and Prognosis (Including Plan of Care)

Physical therapists perform *evaluations* (make clinical judgments) based on the data gathered from the history, systems review, and tests and measures. In the evaluation process, physical therapists synthesize the examination data to establish the diagnosis and prognosis (including the plan of care). Factors that influence the complexity of the evaluation include the clinical findings, extent of loss of function, chronicity or severity of the problem, possibility of multisite or multisystem involvement, preexisting condition(s), potential discharge destination, social considerations, physical function, and overall health status.

A *diagnosis* is a label encompassing a cluster of signs and symptoms, syndromes, or categories. It is the result of the systematic diagnostic process, which includes integrating and evaluating the data from the examination. The diagnostic label indicates the primary dysfunction(s) toward which the therapist will direct interventions. The *prognosis* is the determination of the predicted optimal level of improvement in function and the amount of time needed to reach that level and may also include a prediction of levels of improvement that may be reached at various intervals during the course of therapy. During the prognostic process, the physical therapist develops the plan of care. The *plan of care* identifies specific interventions, proposed frequency and duration of the interventions, anticipated goals, expected outcomes, and discharge plans. The plan of care identifies realistic anticipated goals and expected outcomes, taking into consideration the expectations of the patient/client and appropriate others. These anticipated goals and expected outcomes should be measureable and time limited.

The frequency of visits and duration of the episode of care may vary from a short episode with a high intensity of intervention to a longer episode with a diminishing intensity of intervention. Frequency and duration may vary greatly among patients/clients based on a variety of factors that the physical therapist considers throughout the evaluation process, such as anatomical and physiological changes related to growth and development; caregiver consistency or expertise; chronicity or severity of the current condition; living environment; multisite or multisystem involvement; social support; potential discharge destinations; probability of prolonged impairment, functional limitation, or disability; and stability of the condition.

Prognosis

Over the course of 2 weeks to 6 months, patient/client will demonstrate optimal joint mobility, muscle performance, and range of motion and the highest level of functioning in home, work (job/school/play), community, and leisure environments.

During the episode of care, patient/client will achieve (1) the anticipated goals and expected outcomes of the interventions that are described in the plan of care and (2) the global outcomes for patients/clients who are classified in this pattern.

Expected Range of Number of Visits Per Episode of Care

3 to 36

This range represents the lower and upper limits of the number of physical therapist visits required to achieve anticipated goals and expected outcomes. *It is anticipated that 80% of patients/clients who are classified into this pattern will achieve the anticipated goals and expected outcomes within 3 to 36 visits during a single continuous episode of care.* Frequency of visits and duration of the episode of care should be determined by the physical therapist to maximize effectiveness of care and efficiency of service delivery.

Factors That May Require New Episode of Care or That May Modify Frequency of Visits/Duration of Episode

- Accessibility and availability of resources
- Adherence to the intervention program
- Age
- Anatomical and physiological changes related to growth and development
- Caregiver consistency or expertise
- Chronicity or severity of the current condition
- Cognitive status
- Comorbitities, complications, or secondary impairments
- Concurrent medical, surgical, and therapeutic interventions
- Decline in functional independence
- Level of impairment
- Level of physical function
- Living environment
- Multisite or multisystem involvement
- Nutritional status
- Overall health status
- Potential discharge destinations
- Premorbid conditions
- Probability of prolonged impairment, functional limitation, or disability
- Psychological and socioeconomic factors
- Psychomotor abilities
- Social support
- Stability of the condition

Intervention

Intervention is the purposeful interaction of the physical therapist with the patient/client and, when appropriate, with other individuals involved in patient/client care, using various physical therapy procedures and techniques to produce changes in the condition consistent with the diagnosis and prognosis. Decisions about interventions are contingent on the timely monitoring of patient/client response and the progress made toward achieving the anticipated goals and expected outcomes.

Communication, coordination, and documentation and patient/client-related instruction are provided for all patients/clients across all settings. Procedural interventions are selected or modified based on the examination data and the evaluation, the diagnosis and the prognosis, and the anticipated goals and expected outcomes for a particular patient/client. *For clinical considerations in selecting interventions, listings of interventions, and listings of anticipated goals and expected outcomes, refer to Chapter 3.*

Coordination, Communication, and Documentation

Coordination, communication, and documentation may include:

Interventions

- Addressing required functions
  - advance directives
  - individualized family service plans (IFSPs) or individualized education plans (IEPs)
  - informed consent
  - mandatory communication and reporting (eg, patient advocacy and abuse reporting)
- Admission and discharge planning
- Case management
- Collaboration and coordination with agencies, including:
  - equipment suppliers
  - home care agencies
  - payer groups
  - schools
  - transportation agencies
- Communication across settings, including:
  - case conferences
  - documentation
  - education plans
- Cost-effective resource utilization
- Data collection, analysis, and reporting
  - outcome data
  - peer review findings
  - record reviews
- Documentation across settings, following APTA's *Guidelines for Physical Therapy Documentation* (Appendix 5), including:
  - changes in impairments, functional limitations, and disabilities
  - changes in interventions
  - elements of patient/client management (examination, evaluation, diagnosis, prognosis, intervention)
  - outcomes of intervention
- Interdisciplinary teamwork
  - case conferences
  - patient care rounds
  - patient/client family meetings
- Referrals to other professionals or resources

Anticipated Goals and Expected Outcomes

- Accountability for services is increased.
- Admission data and discharge planning are completed.
- Advance directives, individualized family service plans (IFSPs) or individualized education plans (IEPs), informed consent, and mandatory communication and reporting (eg, patient advocacy and abuse reporting) are obtained or completed.
- Available resources are maximally utilized.
- Care is coordinated with patient/client, family, significant others, caregivers, and other professionals.
- Case is managed throughout the episode of care.
- Collaboration and coordination occurs with agencies, including equipment suppliers, home care agencies, payer groups, schools, and transportation agencies.
- Communication enhances risk reduction and prevention.
- Communication occurs across settings through case conferences, education plans, and documentation.
- Data are collected, analyzed, and reported, including outcome data, peer review findings, and record reviews.
- Decision making is enhanced regarding health, wellness, and fitness needs.
- Decision making is enhanced regarding patient/client health and the use of health care resources by patient/client, family, significant others, and caregivers.
- Documentation occurs throughout patient/client management and across settings and follows APTA's *Guidelines for Physical Therapy Documentation* (Appendix 5).
- Interdisciplinary collaboration occurs through case conferences, patient care rounds, and patient/client family meetings.
- Patient/client, family, significant other, and caregiver understanding of anticipated goals and expected outcomes is increased.
- Placement needs are determined.
- Referrals are made to other professionals or resources whenever necessary and appropriate.
- Resources are utilized in a cost-effective way.

Patient/Client-Related Instruction

Patient/client-related instruction may include:

Interventions

- Instruction, education and training of patients/clients and caregivers regarding:
  - current condition (pathology/pathophysiology [disease, disorder, or condition], impairments, functional limitations, or disabilities)
  - enhancement of performance
  - health, wellness, and fitness programs
  - plan of care
  - risk factors for pathology/pathophysiology (disease, disorder, or condition), impairments, functional limitations, or disabilities
  - transitions across settings
  - transitions to new roles

Anticipated Goals and Expected Outcomes

- Ability to perform physical actions, tasks, or activities is improved.
- Awareness and use of community resources are improved.
- Behaviors that foster healthy habits, wellness, and prevention are acquired.
- Decision making is enhanced regarding patient/client health and the use of health care resources by patient/client, family, significant others, and caregivers.
- Disability associated with acute or chronic illnesses is reduced.
- Functional independence in activities of daily living (ADL) and instrumental activities of daily living (IADL) is increased.
- Health status is improved.
- Intensity of care is decreased.
- Level of supervision required for task performance is decreased.
- Patient/client, family, significant other, and caregiver knowledge and awareness of the diagnosis, prognosis, interventions, and anticipated goals and expected outcomes are increased.
- Patient/client knowledge of personal and environmental factors associated with the condition is increased.
- Performance levels in self-care, home management, work (job/school/play), community, or leisure actions, tasks, or activities are improved.
- Physical function is improved.
- Risk of recurrence of condition is reduced.
- Risk of secondary impairment is reduced.
- Safety of patient/client, family, significant others, and caregivers is improved.
- Self-management of symptoms is improved.
- Utilization and cost of health care services are decreased.

Procedural Interventions

Procedural interventions for this pattern may include:

Therapeutic Exercise

Interventions

- Aerobic capacity/endurance conditioning or reconditioning
  - aquatic programs
  - gait and locomotor training
  - increased workload over time
  - walking and wheelchair propulsion programs
- Balance, coordination, and agility training
  - developmental activities training
  - motor function (motor control and motor learning) training or retraining
  - neuromuscular education or reeducation
  - perceptual training
  - posture awareness training
  - standardized, programmatic, complementary exercise approaches
  - sensory training or retraining
  - task-specific performance training
- Body mechanics and postural stabilization
  - body mechanics training
  - posture awareness training
  - postural control training
  - postural stabilization activities
- Flexibility exercises
  - muscle lengthening
  - range of motion
  - stretching
- Gait and locomotion training
  - developmental activities training
  - gait training
  - implement and device training
  - perceptual training
  - standardized, programmatic, complementary exercise approaches
  - wheelchair training
- Relaxation
  - breathing strategies
  - movement strategies
  - relaxation techniques
  - standardized, programmatic, complementary exercise approaches
- Strength, power, and endurance training for head, neck, limb, pelvic-floor, trunk, and ventilatory muscles
  - active assistive, active, and resistive exercises (including concentric, dynamic/isotonic, eccentric, isokinetic, isometric, and plyometric)
  - aquatic programs
  - standardized, programmatic, complementary exercise approaches
  - task-specific performance training

Anticipated Goals and Expected Outcomes

- Impact on pathology/pathophysiology (disease, disorder, or condition)
  - Joint swelling, inflammation, or restriction is reduced.
  - Nutrient delivery to tissue is increased.
  - Osteogenic effects of exercise are maximized.
  - Pain is decreased.
  - Physiological response to increased oxygen demand is improved.
  - Soft tissue swelling, inflammation, or restriction is reduced.
  - Tissue perfusion and oxygenation are enhanced.
- Impact on impairments:
  - Aerobic capacity is increased.
  - Balance is improved.
  - Endurance is increased.
  - Energy expenditure per unit of work is decreased.
  - Gait, locomotion, and balance are improved.
  - Integumentary integrity is improved.
  - Joint integrity and mobility are improved.
  - Motor function (motor control and motor learning) is improved.
  - Muscle performance (strength, power, and endurance) is increased.
  - Postural control is improved.
  - Quality and quantity of movement between and across body segments are improved.
  - Range of motion is improved.
  - Relaxation is increased.
  - Weight-bearing status is improved.
  - Work of breathing is decreased.
- Impact on functional limitations
  - Ability to perform physical actions, tasks, or activities related to self-care, home management, work (job/school/play), community, and leisure is improved.
  - Level of supervision required for task performance is decreased.
  - Performance of and independence in activities of daily living (ADL) and instrumental activities of daily living (IADL) with or without devices and equipment are increased.
  - Tolerance of positions and activities is increased.
- Impact on disabilities
  - Ability to assume or resume required self-care, home management, work (job/school/play), community, and leisure roles is improved.
- Risk reduction/prevention
  - Preoperative and postoperative complications are reduced.
  - Risk factors are reduced.
  - Risk of recurrence of condition is reduced.
  - Risk of secondary impairments is reduced.
  - Safety is improved.
  - Self-management of symptoms is improved.
- Impact on health, wellness, and fitness
  - Fitness is improved.
  - Health status is improved.
  - Physical capacity is increased.
  - Physical function is improved.
- Impact on societal resources
  - Utilization of physical therapy services is optimized.
  - Utilization of physical therapy services results in efficient use of health care dollars.
- Patient/client satisfaction
  - Access, availability, and services provided are acceptable to patient/client.
  - Administrative management of practice is acceptable to patient/client.
  - Clinical proficiency of physical therapist is acceptable to patient/client.
  - Coordination of care is acceptable to patient/client.
  - Cost of health care services is decreased.
  - Intensity of care is decreased.
  - Interpersonal skills of physical therapist are acceptable to patient/client, family, and significant others.
  - Sense of well-being is improved.
  - Stressors are decreased.

Functional Training in Self-Care and Home Management [(Including Activities of Daily Living (ADL) and Instrumental Activities of Daily Living (IADL)]

Interventions

- ADL training
  - bathing
  - bed mobility and transfer training
  - developmental activities
  - dressing
  - eating
  - grooming
  - toileting
- Devices and equipment use and training
  - assistive and adaptive device or equipment training during ADL and IADL
  - orthotic, protective, or supportive device or equipment training during ADL and IADL
- Functional training programs
  - back schools
  - simulated environments and tasks
  - task adaptation
- IADL training
  - caring for dependents
  - home maintenance
  - household chores
  - shopping
  - structured play for infants and children
  - yard work
- Injury prevention or reduction
  - injury prevention education during self-care and home management
  - injury prevention or reduction with use of devices and equipment
  - safety awareness training during self-care and home management

Anticipated Goals and Expected Outcomes

- Impact on pathology/pathophysiology (disease, disorder, or condition)
  - Pain is decreased.
- Impact on impairments
  - Balance is improved.
  - Endurance is increased.
  - Energy expenditure per unit of work is decreased.
  - Motor function (motor control and motor learning) is improved.
  - Muscle performance (strength, power, and endurance) is increased.
  - Postural control is improved.
  - Sensory awareness is increased.
  - Weight-bearing status is improved.
  - Work of breathing is decreased.
- Impact on functional limitations
  - Ability to perform physical actions, tasks, or activities related to self-care and home management is improved.
  - Level of supervision required for task performance is decreased.
  - Performance of and independence in ADL and IADL with or without devices and equipment are increased.
  - Tolerance of positions and activities is increased.
- Impact on disabilities
  - Ability to assume or resume required self-care and home management roles is improved.
- Risk reduction/prevention
  - Risk factors are reduced.
  - Risk of secondary impairments is reduced.
  - Safety is improved.
  - Self-management of symptoms is improved.
- Impact on health, wellness, and fitness
  - Fitness is improved.
  - Health status is improved.
  - Physical capacity is increased.
  - Physical function is improved.
- Impact on societal resources
  - Utilization of physical therapy services is optimized.
  - Utilization of physical therapy services results in efficient use of health care dollars.
- Patient/client satisfaction
  - Access, availability, and services provided are acceptable to patient/client.
  - Administrative management of practice is acceptable to patient/client.
  - Clinical proficiency of physical therapist is acceptable to patient/client.
  - Coordination of care is acceptable to patient/client.
  - Cost of health care services is decreased.
  - Intensity of care is decreased.
  - Interpersonal skills of physical therapist are acceptable to patient/client, family, and significant others.
  - Sense of well-being is improved.
  - Stressors are decreased.

Functional Training in Work (Job/School/Play), Community, and Leisure Integration or Reintegration (Including Instrumental Activities of Daily Living [IADL], Work Hardening, and Work Conditioning)

Interventions

- Devices and equipment use and training
  - assistive and adaptive device or equipment training during IADL
  - orthotic, protective, or supportive device or equipment training during IADL
- Functional training programs
  - back schools
  - job coaching
  - simulated environments and tasks
  - task adaptation
  - task training
- IADL training
  - community service training involving instruments
  - school and play activities training including tools and instruments
  - work training with tools
- Injury prevention or reduction
  - injury prevention education during work (job/school/play), community, and leisure integration or reintegration
  - injury prevention or reduction with use of devices and equipment
  - safety awareness training during work (job/school/play), community, and leisure integration or reintegration
- Leisure and play activities and training

Anticipated Goals and Expected Outcomes

- Impact on pathology/pathophysiology (disease, disorder, or condition)
  - Pain is decreased.
- Impact on impairments
  - Balance is improved.
  - Endurance is increased.
  - Energy expenditure per unit of work is decreased.
  - Motor function (motor control and motor learning) is improved.
  - Muscle performance (strength, power, and endurance) is increased.
  - Postural control is improved.
  - Sensory awareness is increased.
  - Weight bearing status is improved.
  - Work of breathing is decreased.
- Impact on functional limitations
  - Ability to perform physical actions, tasks, or activities related to work (job/school/play), community, and leisure integration or reintegration is improved.
  - Level of supervision required for task performance is decreased.
  - Performance of and independence in IADL with or without devices and equipment are increased.
  - Tolerance of positions and activities is increased.
- Impact on disabilities
  - Ability to assume or resume required work (job/school/play), community, and leisure roles is improved.
- Risk reduction/prevention-
  - Risk factors are reduced.
  - Risk of secondary impairment is reduced.
  - Safety is improved.
  - Self-management of symptoms is improved.
- Impact on health, wellness, and fitness
  - Fitness is improved.
  - Health status is improved.
  - Physical capacity is increased.
  - Physical function is improved.
- Impact on societal resources
  - Costs of work-related injury or disability are reduced.
  - Utilization of physical therapy services is optimized.
  - Utilization of physical therapy services results in efficient use of health care dollars.
- Patient/client satisfaction
  - Access, availability, and services provided are acceptable to patient/client.
  - Administrative management of practice is acceptable to patient/client.
  - Clinical proficiency of physical therapist is acceptable to patient/client.
  - Coordination of care is acceptable to patient/client.
  - Cost of health care services is decreased.
  - Intensity of care is decreased.
  - Interpersonal skills of physical therapist are acceptable to patient/client, family, and significant others.
  - Sense of well-being is improved.
  - Stressors are decreased.

Manual Therapy Techniques (Including Mobilization/Manipulation)

Interventions

- Manual traction
- Massage
  - connective tissue massage
  - therapeutic massage
- Mobilization/manipulation
  - soft tissue
  - spinal and peripheral joints
- Passive range of motion

Anticipated Goals and Expected Outcomes

- Impact on pathology/pathophysiology (disease, disorder, or condition)
  - Edema, lymphedema, or effusion is reduced.
  - Joint swelling, inflammation, or restriction is reduced.
  - Neural compression is decreased.
  - Pain is decreased.
  - Soft tissue swelling, inflammation, or restriction is reduced.
- Impact on impairments
  - Balance is improved.
  - Energy expenditure per unit of work is decreased.
  - Gait, locomotion, and balance is improved.
  - Joint integrity and mobility are improved.
  - Muscle performance (strength, power, and endurance) is increased.
  - Postural control is improved.
  - Quality and quantity of movement between and across body segments are improved.
  - Range of motion is improved.
  - Relaxation is increased.
  - Sensory awareness is increased.
  - Weight-bearing status is improved.
  - Work of breathing is decreased.
- Impact on functional limitations
  - Ability to perform movement tasks is improved.
  - Ability to perform physical actions, tasks, or activities related to self-care, home management, work (job/school/play), community, and leisure is improved.
  - Tolerance of positions and activities is increased.
- Impact on disabilities
  - Ability to assume or resume required self-care, home management, work (job/school/play), community, and leisure roles is improved.
- Risk reduction/prevention
  - Risk factors are reduced.
  - Risk of recurrence of condition is reduced.
  - Risk of secondary impairment is reduced.
  - Self-management of symptoms is improved.
- Impact on health, wellness, and fitness
  - Fitness is improved.
  - Physical capacity is increased.
  - Physical function is improved.
- Impact on societal resources
  - Utilization of physical therapy services is optimized.
  - Utilization of physical therapy services results in efficient use of health care dollars.
- Patient/client satisfaction
  - Access, availability, and services provided are acceptable to patient/client.
  - Administrative management of practice is acceptable to patient/client.
  - Clinical proficiency of physical therapist is acceptable to patient/client.
  - Coordination of care is acceptable to patient/client.
  - Cost of health care services is decreased.
  - Intensity of care is decreased.
  - Interpersonal skills of physical therapist are acceptable to patient/client, family, and significant others.
  - Sense of well-being is improved.
  - Stressors are decreased.

Prescription, Application, and, as Appropriate, Fabrication of Devices and Equipment (Assistive, Adaptive, Orthotic, Protective, Supportive, and Prosthetic)

Interventions

- Adaptive devices
  - raised toilet seats
  - seating systems
- Assistive devices
  - canes
  - crutches
  - long-handled reachers
  - power devices
  - static and dynamic splints
  - walkers
  - wheelchairs
- Orthotic devices
  - braces
  - casts
  - shoe inserts
  - splints
- Protective devices
  - braces
  - cushions
  - protective taping
- Supportive devices
  - compression garments
  - corsets
  - elastic wraps
  - neck collars
  - serial casts
  - slings
  - supportive taping

Anticipated Goals and Expected Outcomes

- Impact on pathology/pathophysiology (disease, disorder, or condition)
  - Edema, lymphedema, or effusion is reduced.
  - Joint swelling, inflammation, or restriction is reduced.
  - Pain is decreased.
  - Soft tissue swelling, inflammation, or restriction is reduced.
- Impact on impairments
  - Balance is improved.
  - Endurance is increased.
  - Energy expenditure per unit of work is decreased.
  - Gait, locomotion, and balance are improved.
  - Joint stability is increased
  - Motor function (motor control and motor learning) is improved.
  - Muscle performance (strength, power, and endurance) is increased.
  - Optimal joint alignment is achieved.
  - Optimal loading on a body part is achieved.
  - Postural control is improved.
  - Quality and quantity of movement between and across body segments are improved.
  - Range of motion is improved.
  - Relaxation is increased.
  - Weight-bearing status is improved.
  - Work of breathing is decreased.
- Impact on functional limitations
  - Ability to perform physical actions, tasks, or activities related to self-care, home management, work (job/school/play), community, and leisure is improved.
  - Level of supervision required for task performance is decreased.
  - Performance of and independence in activities of daily living (ADL) and instrumental activities of daily living (IADL) with or without devices and equipment are increased.
  - Tolerance of positions and activities is improved.
- Impact on disabilities
  - Ability to assume or resume required self-care, home management, work (job/school/play), community, and leisure roles is improved.
- Risk reduction/prevention
  - Pressure on body tissues is reduced.
  - Protection of body parts is increased.
  - Risk factors are reduced.
  - Risk of secondary impairment is reduced.
  - Safety is improved.
  - Self-management of symptoms is improved.
  - Stresses precipitating injury are decreased.
- Impact on health, wellness, and fitness
  - Health status is improved.
  - Physical capacity is increased.
  - Physical function is improved.
- Impact on societal resources
  - Utilization of physical therapy services is optimized.
  - Utilization of physical therapy services results in efficient use of health care dollars.
- Patient/client satisfaction
  - Access, availability, and services provided are acceptable to patient/client.
  - Administrative management of practice is acceptable to patient/client.
  - Clinical proficiency of physical therapist is acceptable to patient/client.
  - Coordination of care is acceptable to patient/client.
  - Cost of health care services is decreased.
  - Intensity of care is decreased.
  - Interpersonal skills of physical therapist are acceptable to patient/client, family, and significant others.
  - Sense of well-being is improved.
  - Stressors are decreased.

Electrotherapeutic Modalities

Interventions

- Biofeedback
- Electrotherapeutic delivery of medications
  - iontophoresis
- Electrical stimulation
  - electrical muscle stimulation (EMS)
  - neuromuscular electrical stimulation (NMES)
  - transcutaneous electrical nerve stimulation (TENS)

Anticipated Goals and Expected Outcomes

- Impact on pathology/pathophysiology
  - Edema, lymphedema, or effusion is reduced.
  - Joint swelling, inflammation, or restriction is reduced.
  - Nutrient delivery to tissue is increased.
  - Osteogenic effects are enhanced.
  - Pain is decreased.
  - Soft tissue swelling, inflammation, or restriction is reduced.
  - Tissue perfusion and oxygenation are enhanced.
- Impact on impairments
  - Integumentary integrity is improved.
  - Motor function (motor control and motor learning) is improved.
  - Muscle performance (strength, power, and endurance) is increased.
  - Postural control is improved.
  - Quality and quantity of movement between and across body segments are improved.
  - Range of motion is improved.
  - Relaxation is increased.
  - Sensory awareness is increased.
- Impact on functional limitations
  - Ability to perform physical actions, tasks, or activities related to self-care, home management, community, work (job/ school/ play), and leisure is improved.
  - Level of supervision required for task performance is decreased.
  - Performance of and independence in activities of daily living (ADL) and instrumental activities of daily living (IADL) with or without devices and equipment are increased.
  - Tolerance of positions and activities is increased.
- Impact on disabilities
  - Ability to assume or resume required self-care, home management, work (job/school/play), community, and leisure roles is improved.
- Risk reduction/prevention
  - Complications of immobility are reduced.
  - Risk factors are reduced.
  - Risk of secondary impairment is reduced.
  - Self-management of symptoms is improved.
- Impact on health, wellness, and fitness
  - Physical capacity is increased.
  - Physical function is improved.
- Impact on societal resources
  - Utilization of physical therapy services is optimized.
  - Utilization of physical therapy services results in efficient use of health care dollars.
- Patient/client satisfaction
  - Access, availability, and services provided are acceptable to patient/client.
  - Administrative management of practice is acceptable to patient/client.
  - Clinical proficiency of physical therapist is acceptable to patient/client.
  - Coordination of care is acceptable to patient/client.
  - Interpersonal skills of physical therapist are acceptable to patient/client, family, and significant others.
  - Sense of well-being is improved.
  - Stressors are decreased.

Physical Agents and Mechanical Modalities

Interventions

Physical agents may include:

- Athermal agents
  - pulsed electromagnetic fields
- Cryotherapy
  - cold packs
  - ice massage
  - vapocoolant spray
- Hydrotherapy
  - whirlpool tanks
  - contrast bath
  - pools
- Light
  - infrared
  - laser
- Sound agents
  - phonophoresis
  - ultrasound
- Thermotherapy
  - dry heat
  - hot packs
  - paraffin baths

Mechanical modalities may include:

- Compression therapies
  - taping
  - vasopneumatic compression devices
- Mechanical motion devices
  - continuous passive motion (CPM)
- Traction devices
  - intermittent
  - positional
  - sustained

Anticipated Goals and Expected Outcomes

- Impact on pathology/pathophysiology (disease, disorder, or condition)
  - Edema, lymphedema, or effusion is reduced.
  - Joint swelling, inflammation, or restriction is reduced.
  - Neural compression is decreased.
  - Nutrient delivery to tissue is increased.
  - Pain is decreased.
  - Soft tissue swelling, inflammation, or restriction is reduced.
  - Tissue perfusion and oxygenation are enhanced.
- Impact on impairments:
  - Integumentary integrity is improved.
  - Muscle performance (strength, power, and endurance) is increased.
  - Range of motion is improved.
  - Weight-bearing status is improved.
- Impact on functional limitations
  - Ability to perform physical actions, tasks, or activities related to self-care, home management, work (job/school/play), community, and leisure is improved.
  - Performance of and independence in activities of daily living (ADL) and instrumental activities of daily living (IADL) with or without devices and equipment are increased.
  - Tolerance of positions and activities is increased.
- Impact on disabilities
  - Ability to assume or resume required self-care, home management, work (job/school/play), community, and leisure roles is improved.
- Risk reduction/prevention
  - Complications of soft tissue and circulation disorders.
  - Risk of secondary impairments is reduced.
  - Self-management of symptoms is improved.
  - Stresses precipitating injury are decreased.
- Impact on health, wellness, and fitness
  - Physical function is improved.
- Impact on societal resources
  - Utilization of physical therapy services is optimized.
- Patient/client satisfaction
  - Access, availability, and services provided are acceptable to patient/client.
  - Administrative management of practice is acceptable to patient/client.
  - Clinical proficiency of physical therapist is acceptable to patient/client.
  - Coordination of care is acceptable to patient/client.
  - Interpersonal skills of physical therapist are acceptable to patient/client, family, and significant others.
  - Sense of well-being is improved.
  - Stressors are decreased.

Reexamination

Reexamination is the process of performing selected tests and measures after the initial examination to evaluate progress and to modify or redirect interventions. Reexamination may be indicated more than once during a single episode of care. It also may be performed over the course of a disease, disorder, or condition, which for some patients/clients may be over the life span. Indications for reexamination include new clinical findings or failure to respond to physical therapy interventions.

Global Outcomes for Patients/Clients in This Pattern

Throughout the entire episode of care, the physical therapist determines the anticipated goals and expected outcomes for each intervention. These anticipated goals and expected outcomes are delineated in shaded boxes that accompany the lists of interventions in each preferred practice pattern. As the patient/client reaches the termination of physical therapy services and the end of the episode of care, the physical therapist measures the global outcomes of the physical therapy services by characterizing or quantifying the impact of the physical therapy interventions in the following domains:

- Pathology/pathophysiology (disease, disorder, or condition)
- Impairments
- Functional limitations
- Disabilities
- Risk reduction/prevention
- Health, wellness, and fitness
- Societal resources
- Patient/client satisfaction

In some instances, a particular anticipated goal or expected outcome is thoroughly achieved through implementation of a single form of intervention. More commonly, however, the anticipated goals and expected outcomes are achieved as a result of the combined effects of several forms of interventions, leading to enhancement of both health status and health-related quality of life.

Criteria for Termination of Physical Therapy Services

Discharge is the process of ending physical therapy services that have been provided during a single episode of care. It occurs when the anticipated goals and expected outcomes have been achieved. Discharge does *not* occur with a *transfer* (defined as the time when a patient is moved from one site to another site within the same setting or across settings during a single episode of care). Although there may be facility-specific or payer-specific requirements for documentation regarding the conclusion of physical therapy services, *discharge occurs based on the physical therapist's analysis of the achievement of anticipated goals and expected outcomes.*

Discontinuation is the process of ending physical therapy services that have been provided during a single episode of care when (1) the patient/client, caregiver, or legal guardian declines to continue intervention; (2) the patient/client is unable to continue to progress toward outcomes because of medical or psychosocial complications or because financial/insurance resources have been expended; or (3) the physical therapist determines that the patient/client will no longer benefit from physical therapy. When physical therapy services are terminated prior to achievement of anticipated goals and expected outcomes, patient/client status and the rationale for termination are documented.

For patients/clients who require multiple episodes of care, periodic follow-up is needed over the life span to ensure safety and effective adaptation following changes in physical status, caregivers, environment, or task demands. In consultation with appropriate individuals, and in consideration of the outcomes, the physical therapist plans for discharge or discontinuation and provides for appropriate follow-up or referral.

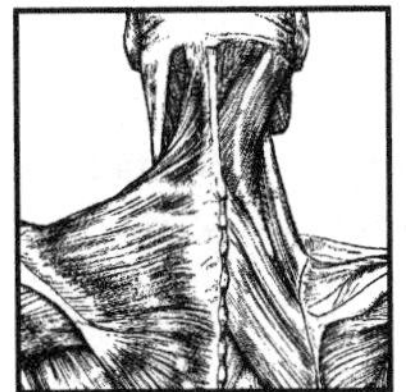

Impaired Joint Mobility, Motor Function, Muscle Performance, and Range of Motion Associated With Localized Inflammation

This preferred practice pattern describes the generally accepted elements of patient/client management that physical therapists provide for patients/clients who are classified in this pattern. The pattern title reflects the diagnosis made by the physical therapist. APTA emphasizes that preferred practice patterns are the boundaries within which a physical therapist may select any of a number of clinical alternatives, based on consideration of a wide variety of factors, such as individual patient/client needs; the profession's code of ethics and standards of practice; and patient/client age, culture, gender roles, race, sex, sexual orientation, and socioeconomic status.

Patient/Client Diagnostic Classification

Patients/clients will be classified into this pattern—for impaired joint mobility, motor function, muscle performance, and range of motion associated with localized inflammation—as a result of the physical therapist's evaluation of the examination data. The findings from the examination (history, systems review, and tests and measures) may indicate the presence or risk of pathology/pathophysiology (disease, disorder, or condition), impairments, functional limitations, or disabilities or the need for health, wellness, or fitness programs. The physical therapist integrates, synthesizes, and interprets the data to determine the diagnostic classification.

Inclusion

The following examples of examination findings may support the inclusion of patients/clients in this pattern:

Risk Factors or Consequences of Pathology/Pathophysiology (Disease, Disorder, or Condition)

- Abnormal response to provocation
- Ankylosing spondylitis
- Bursitis
- Capsulitis
- Epicondylitis
- Fasciitis
- Gout
- Osteoarthritis
- Prenatal and postnatal soft tissue inflammation
- Synovitis
- Tendinitis

Impairments, Functional Limitations, or Disabilities

- Edema
- Inability to perform self-care
- Inflammation of periarticular connective tissue
- Muscle strain
- Muscle weakness
- Pain
- Worker's inability to perform functional activities because of localized joint pain

Note:

Some risk factors or consequences of pathology/pathophysiology—such as *systemic disease processes*—may be severe and complex; *however, they do not necessarily exclude patients/ clients from this pattern.* Severe and complex risk factors or consequences may require modification of the frequency of visits and duration of care. (See "Evaluation, Diagnosis, and Prognosis," page 203.)

Exclusion or Multiple-Pattern Classification

The following examples of examination findings may support exclusion from this pattern or classification into additional patterns. Depending on the level of severity or complexity of the examination findings, the physical therapist may determine that the patient/client would be more appropriately managed through (1) classification in an entirely different pattern or (2) classification in both this and another pattern.

Findings That May Require Classification in a Different Pattern

- Deep vein thrombosis
- Fracture
- Impairments associated with dislocation
- Impairments associated with hemarthrosis
- Surgery

Findings That May Require Classification in Additional Patterns

- Open wound

ICD-9-CM Codes

The listing below contains the current (as of press time) and most typical 3- and 4-digit ICD-9-CM codes related to this preferred practice pattern. Because patient/client diagnostic classification is based on impairments, functional limitations, and disabilities—not on codes—patients/clients may be classified into the pattern even though the codes listed with the pattern may not apply to those clients.

This listing is intended for general information only and should not be used for coding purposes. The codes should be confirmed by referring to the World Health Organization's *International Classification of Diseases, 9th Revision, Clinical Modification (ICD-9-CM 2001)*, Volumes 1 and 3 (Chicago, Ill: American Medical Association; 2000) or subsequent revisions or by referring to other ICD-9-CM coding manuals that contain exclusion notes and instructions regarding fifth-digit requirements.

274 Gout
- **274.0** Gouty arthropathy

350 Trigeminal nerve disorders
- **350.1** Trigeminal neuralgia

353 Nerve root and plexus disorders
- **353.0** Brachial plexus lesions
- **353.4** Lumbosacral root lesions, not elsewhere classified

354 Mononeuritis of upper limb and mononeuritis multiplex
- **354.0** Carpal tunnel syndrome
- **354.2** Lesion of ulnar nerve
  Cubital tunnel syndrome

355 Mononeuritis of lower limb
- **355.5** Tarsal tunnel syndrome
- **355.6** Lesion of plantar nerve
  Morton's metarsalgia, neuralgia, or neuroma

524 Dentofacial anomalies, including malocclusion
- **524.6** Temporomandibular joint disorders

682 Other cellulitis and abscess

711 Arthropathy associated with infections

715 Osteoarthrosis and allied disorders

716 Other and unspecified arthropathies
- **716.6** Unspecified monoarthritis
- **716.9** Arthropathy, unspecified
  Inflammation of joint, not otherwise specified

717 Internal derangement of knee
- **717.7** Chondromalacia of patella

718 Other derangement of joint
- **718.8** Other joint derangement, not elsewhere classified
  Instability of joint

719 Other and unspecified disorders of joint
- **719.0** Effusion of joint
- **719.2** Villonodular synovitis

720 Ankylosing spondylitis and other inflammatory spondylopathies
- **720.2** Sacroiliitis, not elsewhere classified

722 Intervertebral disk disorders

724 Other and unspecified disorders of back
- **724.0** Spinal stenosis, other than cervical
- **724.2** Lumbago
  Low back pain
  Low back syndrome
  Lumbalgia

726 Peripheral enthesopathies and allied syndromes
- **726.0** Adhesive capsulitis of shoulder
- **726.1** Rotator cuff syndrome of shoulder and allied disorders
  - **726.10** Disorders of bursae and tendons in shoulder region, unspecified
- **726.2** Other affections of shoulder region, not elsewhere classified
- **726.3** Enthesopathy of elbow region
  - **726.31** Medial epicondylitis
  - **726.32** Lateral epicondylitis
- **726.5** Enthesopathy of hip region
  Bursitis of hip
- **726.6** Enthesopathy of knee
  - **726.60** Enthesopathy of knee, unspecified
- **726.9** Unspecified enthesopathy
  - **726.90** Enthesopathy of unspecified site

727 Other disorders of synovium, tendon, and bursa
- **727.0** Synovitis and tenosynovitis
  - **727.04** Radial styloid tenosynovitis
- **727.3** Other bursitis
- **727.6** Rupture of tendon, nontraumatic
  - **727.61** Complete rupture of rotator cuff
- **727.9** Unspecified disorder of synovium, tendon, and bursa

728 Disorders of muscle, ligament, and fascia
- **728.7** Other fibromatoses
  - **728.71** Plantar fascial fibromatosis
    Plantar fasciitis
- **728.9** Unspecified disorder of muscle, ligament, and fascia

729 Other disorders of soft tissues
- **729.1** Myalgia and myositis, unspecified
- **729.2** Neuralgia, neuritis, and radiculitis, unspecified
- **729.4** Fasciitis, unspecified
- **729.8** Other musculoskeletal symptoms referable to limbs
  - **729.81** Swelling of limb

732 Osteochondropathies
- **732.9** Unspecified osteochondropathy

840 Sprains and strains of shoulder and upper arm
- **840.4** Rotator cuff (capsule)

923 Contusion of upper limb

924 Contusion of lower limb and of other and unspecified sites

927 Crushing injury of upper limb

928 Crushing injury of lower limb

Examination

Examination is a comprehensive screening and specific testing process that leads to a diagnostic classification or, when appropriate, to a referral to another practitioner. Examination is required prior to the initial intervention and is performed for all patients/clients. Through the examination, the physical therapist may identify impairments, functional limitations, disabilities, changes in physical function or overall health status, and needs related to restoration of health and to prevention, wellness, and fitness. The physical therapist synthesizes the examination findings to establish the diagnosis and the prognosis (including the plan of care). The patient/client, family, significant others, and caregivers may provide information during the examination process.

Examination has three components: the patient/client history, the systems review, and tests and measures. The *history* is a systematic gathering of past and current information (often from the patient/client) related to why the patient/client is seeking the services of the physical therapist. The *systems review* is a brief or limited examination of (1) the anatomical and physiological status of the cardiovascular/pulmonary, integumentary, musculoskeletal, and neuromuscular systems and (2) the communication ability, affect, cognition, language, and learning style of the patient/client. *Tests and measures* are the means of gathering data about the patient/client.

The selection of examination procedures and the depth of the examination vary based on patient/client age; severity of the problem; stage of recovery (acute, subacute, chronic); phase of rehabilitation (early, intermediate, late, return to activity); home, work (job/school/play), or community situation; and other relevant factors. *For clinical indications in selecting tests and measures and for listings of tests and measures, tools used to gather data, and the types of data generated by tests and measures, refer to Chapter 2.*

Patient/Client History

The history may include:

General Demographics
- Age
- Sex
- Race/ethnicity
- Primary language
- Education

Social History
- Cultural beliefs and behaviors
- Family and caregiver resources
- Social interactions, social activities, and support systems

Employment/Work (Job/School/Play)
- Current and prior work (job/school/play), community, and leisure actions, tasks, or activities

Growth and Development
- Developmental history
- Hand dominance

Living Environment
- Devices and equipment (eg, assistive, adaptive, orthotic, protective, supportive, prosthetic)
- Living environment and community characteristics
- Projected discharge destinations

General Health Status (Self-Report, Family Report, Caregiver Report)
- General health perception
- Physical function (eg, mobility, sleep patterns, restricted bed days)
- Psychological function (eg, memory, reasoning ability, depression, anxiety)
- Role function (eg, community, leisure, social, work)
- Social function (eg, social activity, social interaction, social support)

Social/Health Habits (Past and Current)
- Behavioral health risks (eg, smoking, drug abuse)
- Level of physical fitness

Family History
- Familial health risks

Medical/Surgical History
- Cardiovascular
- Endocrine/metabolic
- Gastrointestinal
- Genitourinary
- Gynecological
- Integumentary
- Musculoskeletal
- Neuromuscular
- Obstetrical
- Prior hospitalizations, surgeries, and preexisting medical and other health-related conditions
- Psychological
- Pulmonary

Current Condition(s)/Chief Complaint(s)
- Concerns that led patient/client to seek the services of a physical therapist
- Concerns or needs of patient/client who requires the services of a physical therapist
- Current therapeutic interventions
- Mechanisms of injury or disease, including date of onset and course of events
- Onset and pattern of symptoms
- Patient/client, family, significant other, and caregiver expectations and goals for the therapeutic intervention
- Patient/client, family, significant other, and caregiver perceptions of patient's/client's emotional response to the current clinical situation
- Previous occurrence of chief complaint(s)
- Prior therapeutic interventions

Functional Status and Activity Level
- Current and prior functional status in self-care and home management activities, including activities of daily living (ADL) and instrumental activities of daily living (IADL)
- Current and prior functional status in work (job/school/play), community, and leisure actions, tasks, or activities

Medications
- Medications for current condition
- Medications previously taken for current condition
- Medications for other conditions

Other Clinical Tests
- Laboratory and diagnostic tests
- Review of available records (eg, medical, education, surgical)
- Review of other clinical findings (eg, nutrition and hydration)

Systems Review

The systems review may include:

Anatomical and Physiological Status

- Cardiovascular/Pulmonary
  - Blood pressure
  - Edema
  - Heart rate
  - Respiratory rate
- Integumentary
  - Pliability (texture)
  - Presence of scar formation
  - Skin color
  - Skin integrity
- Musculoskeletal
  - Gross range of motion
  - Gross strength
  - Gross symmetry
  - Height
  - Weight
- Neuromuscular
  - Gross coordinated movements (eg, balance, gait, locomotion, transfers, transitions)
  - Motor function (motor control, motor learning)

Communication, Affect, Cognition, Language, and Learning Style

- Ability to make needs known
- Consciousness
- Expected emotional/behavioral responses
- Learning preferences (eg, education needs, learning barriers)
- Orientation (person, place, time)

Tests and Measures

Tests and measures for this pattern may include those that characterize or quantify:

Aerobic Capacity and Endurance

- Aerobic capacity during functional activities (eg, activities of daily living [ADL] scales, indexes, instrumental activities of daily living [IADL] scales, observations)
- Aerobic capacity during standardized exercise test protocols (eg, ergometry, step tests, time/distance walk/run tests, treadmill tests, wheelchair tests)

Anthropometric Characteristics

- Edema (eg, girth measurement, palpation, scales, volume measurement)

Assistive and Adaptive Devices

- Assistive or adaptive devices and equipment use during functional activities (eg, ADL scales, functional scales, IADL scales, interviews, observations)
- Components, alignment, fit, and ability to care for the assistive or adaptive devices and equipment (eg, interviews, logs, observations, pressure-sensing maps, reports)
- Remediation of impairments, functional limitations, or disabilities with use of assistive or adaptive devices and equipment (eg, ADL scales, IADL scales, pain scales, play scales)
- Safety during use of assistive or adaptive devices and equipment (eg, diaries, fall scales, interviews, logs, observations, reports)

Cranial and Peripheral Nerve Integrity

- Electrophysiological integrity (eg, electroneuromyography)
- Motor distribution of the cranial nerves (eg, dynamometry, muscle tests, observations)
- Motor distribution of the peripheral nerves (eg, dynamometry, muscle tests, observations, thoracic outlet tests)
- Response to neural provocation (eg, tension tests, vertebral artery compression tests)
- Sensory distribution of the cranial nerves (eg, discrimination tests; tactile tests, including coarse and light touch, cold and heat, pain, pressure, and vibration)
- Sensory distribution of the peripheral nerves (eg, discrimination tests; tactile tests, including coarse and light touch, cold and heat, pain, pressure, and vibration; thoracic outlet tests)

Environmental, Home, and Work (Job/School/Play) Barriers

- Current and potential barriers (eg, checklists, interviews, observations, questionnaires)

Ergonomics and Body Mechanics

Ergonomics

- Dexterity and coordination during work (job/school/play) (eg, hand function tests, impairment rating scales, manipulative ability tests)
- Functional capacity and performance during work actions, tasks, or activities (eg, accelerometry, dynamometry, electroneuromyography, endurance tests, force platform tests, goniometry, interviews, observations, photographic assessments, physical capacity tests, postural loading analyses, technology-assisted assessments, videographic assessments, work analyses)
- Safety in work environments (eg, hazard identification checklists, job severity indexes, lifting standards, risk assessment scales, standards for exposure limits)
- Specific work conditions or activities (eg, handling checklists, job simulations, lifting models, preemployment screenings, task analysis checklists, workstation checklists)
- Tools, devices, equipment, and workstations related to work actions, tasks, or activities (eg, observations, tool analysis checklists, vibration assessments)

Body mechanics

- Body mechanics during self-care, home management, work, community, or leisure actions, tasks, or activities (eg, ADL scales, IADL scales, observations, photographic assessments, technology-assisted assessments, videographic assessments)

Gait, Locomotion, and Balance

- Balance during functional activities with or without the use of assistive, adaptive, orthotic, protective, supportive, or prosthetic devices or equipment (eg, ADL scales, IADL scales, observations, videographic assessments)
- Balance (dynamic and static) with or without the use of assistive, adaptive, orthotic, protective, supportive, or prosthetic devices or equipment (eg, balance scales, dizziness inventories, dynamic posturography, fall scales, motor impairment tests, observations, photographic assessments, postural control tests)
- Gait and locomotion during functional activities with or without the use of assistive, adaptive, orthotic, protective, supportive, or prosthetic devices or equipment (eg, ADL scales, gait indexes, IADL scales, mobility skill profiles, observations, videographic assessments)
- Gait and locomotion with or without the use of assistive, adaptive, orthotic, protective, supportive, or prosthetic devices or equipment (eg, dynamometry, electroneuromyography, footprint analyses, gait indexes, mobility skill profiles, observations, photographic assessments, technology-assisted assessments, videographic assessments, weight-bearing scales, wheelchair mobility tests)
- Safety during gait, locomotion, and balance (eg, confidence scales, diaries, fall scales, functional assessment profiles, logs, reports)

Integumentary Integrity

Associated skin

- Activities, positioning, and postures that produce or relieve trauma to the skin (eg, observations, pressure-sensing maps, scales)
- Skin characteristics, including blistering, continuity of skin color, dermatitis, hair growth, mobility, nail growth, sensation, temperature, texture, and turgor (eg, observations, palpation, photographic assessments, thermography)

Joint Integrity and Mobility

- Joint integrity and mobility (eg, apprehension, compression and distraction, drawer, glide, impingement, shear, and valgus/varus stress tests; arthrometry; palpation)
- Joint play movements, including end feel (all joints of the axial and appendicular skeletal system) (eg, palpation)

Motor Function (Motor Control and Motor Learning)

- Dexterity, coordination, and agility (eg, coordination screens, motor impairment tests, motor proficiency tests, observations, videographic assessments)
- Hand function (eg, fine and gross motor control tests, finger dexterity tests, manipulative ability tests, observations)

Muscle Performance (Including Strength, Power, and Endurance)

- Electrophysiological integrity (eg, electroneuromyography)
- Muscle strength, power, and endurance (eg, dynamometry, manual muscle tests, muscle performance tests, physical capacity tests, technology-assisted assessments, timed activity tests)
- Muscle strength, power, and endurance during functional activities (eg, ADL scales, functional muscle tests, IADL scales, observations, videographic assessments)
- Muscle tension (eg, palpation)

Orthotic, Protective, and Supportive Devices

- Components, alignment, fit, and ability to care for orthotic, protective, and supportive devices and equipment (eg, interviews, logs, observations, pressure-sensing maps, reports)
- Orthotic, protective, and supportive devices and equipment use during functional activities (eg, ADL scales, functional scales, IADL scales, interviews, observations, profiles)
- Remediation of impairments, functional limitations, or disabilities with use of orthotic, protective, and supportive devices and equipment (eg, activity status indexes, ADL scales, aerobic capacity tests, functional performance inventories, health assessment questionnaires, IADL scales, pain scales, play scales, videographic assessments)
- Safety during use of orthotic, protective, and supportive devices and equipment (eg, diaries, fall scales, interviews, logs, observations, reports)

Pain

- Pain, soreness, and nociception (eg, analog scales, discrimination tests, pain drawings and maps, provocation tests, verbal and pictorial descriptor tests)
- Pain in specific body parts (eg, pain indexes, pain questionnaires, structural provocation tests)

Posture

- Postural alignment and position (dynamic and static), including symmetry and deviation from midline (eg, observations, grid measurement, technology-assisted assessments, photographic assessments, videographic assessments)
- Specific body parts (eg, angle assessments, forward-bending test, goniometry, observations, palpation, positional tests)

Range of Motion (ROM) (Including Muscle Length)

- Functional ROM (eg, observations, squat tests, toe touch tests)
- Joint active and passive movement (eg, goniometry, inclinometry, observations, photographic assessments, videographic assessments)
- Muscle length, soft tissue extensibility, and flexibility (eg, contracture tests, goniometry, inclinometry, ligamentous tests, linear measurement, multisegment flexibility tests, palpation)

Reflex Integrity

- Deep reflexes (eg, myotatic reflex scale, observations, reflex tests)
- Superficial reflexes and reactions (eg, observations, provocation tests)

Self-Care and Home Management (Including ADL and IADL)

- Ability to gain access to home environments (eg, barrier identification, observations, physical performance tests)
- Ability to perform self-care and home management activities with or without assistive, adaptive, orthotic, protective, supportive, or prosthetic devices and equipment (eg, ADL scales, aerobic capacity tests, IADL scales, interviews, observations, profiles)
- Safety in self-care and home management activities and environments (eg, diaries, fall scales, interviews, logs, observations, reports, videographic assessments)

Sensory Integrity

- Deep sensations (eg, kinesthesiometry, observations, photographic assessments, vibration tests)
- Electrophysiological integrity (eg, electroneuromyography)

Work (Job/School/Play), Community, and Leisure Integration or Reintegration (Including IADL)

- Ability to assume or resume work (job/school/play), community, and leisure activities with or without assistive, adaptive, orthotic, protective, supportive, or prosthetic devices and equipment (eg, activity profiles, disability indexes, functional status questionnaires, IADL scales, observations, physical capacity tests)
- Ability to gain access to work (job/school/play), community, and leisure environments (eg, barrier identification, interviews, observations, physical capacity tests, transportation assessments)
- Safety in work (job/school/play), community, and leisure activities and environments (eg, diaries, fall scales, interviews, logs, observations, videographic assessments)

Ventilation and Respiration/Gas Exchange

- Pulmonary signs of respiration/gas exchange, including breath sounds (eg, gas analyses, observations, oximetry)
- Pulmonary signs of ventilatory function, including airway protection; breath and voice sounds; respiratory rate, rhythm, and pattern; ventilatory flow, forces, and volumes (eg, airway clearance tests, observations, palpation, pulmonary function tests, ventilatory muscle force tests)
- Pulmonary symptoms (eg, dyspnea and perceived exertion indexes and scales)

Evaluation, Diagnosis, and Prognosis (Including Plan of Care)

Physical therapists perform *evaluations* (make clinical judgments) based on the data gathered from the history, systems review, and tests and measures. In the evaluation process, physical therapists synthesize the examination data to establish the diagnosis and prognosis (including the plan of care). Factors that influence the complexity of the evaluation include the clinical findings, extent of loss of function, chronicity or severity of the problem, possibility of multisite or multisystem involvement, preexisting condition(s), potential discharge destination, social considerations, physical function, and overall health status.

A *diagnosis* is a label encompassing a cluster of signs and symptoms, syndromes, or categories. It is the result of the systematic diagnostic process, which includes integrating and evaluating the data from the examination. The diagnostic label indicates the primary dysfunction(s) toward which the therapist will direct interventions. The *prognosis* is the determination of the predicted optimal level of improvement in function and the amount of time needed to reach that level and may also include a prediction of levels of improvement that may be reached at various intervals during the course of therapy. During the prognostic process, the physical therapist develops the plan of care. The *plan of care* identifies specific interventions, proposed frequency and duration of the interventions, anticipated goals, expected outcomes, and discharge plans. The plan of care identifies realistic anticipated goals and expected outcomes, taking into consideration the expectations of the patient/client and appropriate others. These anticipated goals and expected outcomes should be measureable and time limited.

The frequency of visits and duration of the episode of care may vary from a short episode with a high intensity of intervention to a longer episode with a diminishing intensity of intervention. Frequency and duration may vary greatly among patients/clients based on a variety of factors that the physical therapist considers throughout the evaluation process, such as anatomical and physiological changes related to growth and development; caregiver consistency or expertise; chronicity or severity of the current condition; living environment; multisite or multisystem involvement; social support; potential discharge destinations; probability of prolonged impairment, functional limitation, or disability; and stability of the condition.

Prognosis

Over the course of 2 to 4 months, patient/client will demonstrate optimal joint mobility, motor function, muscle performance, and range of motion and the highest level of functioning in home, work (job/school/play), community, and leisure environments.

During the episode of care, patient/client will achieve (1) the anticipated goals and expected outcomes of the interventions that are described in the plan of care and (2) the global outcomes for patients/clients who are classified in this pattern.

Expected Range of Number of Visits Per Episode of Care

6 to 24

This range represents the lower and upper limits of the number of physical therapist visits required to achieve anticipated goals and expected outcomes. *It is anticipated that 80% of patients/clients who are classified into this pattern will achieve the anticipated goals and expected outcomes within 6 to 24 visits during a single continuous episode of care.* Frequency of visits and duration of the episode of care should be determined by the physical therapist to maximize effectiveness of care and efficiency of service delivery.

Factors That May Require New Episode of Care or That May Modify Frequency of Visits/Duration of Episode

- Accessibility and availability of resources
- Adherence to the intervention program
- Age
- Anatomical and physiological changes related to growth and development
- Caregiver consistency or expertise
- Chronicity or severity of the current condition
- Cognitive status
- Comorbitities, complications, or secondary impairments
- Concurrent medical, surgical, and therapeutic interventions
- Decline in functional independence
- Level of impairment
- Level of physical function
- Living environment
- Multisite or multisystem involvement
- Nutritional status
- Overall health status
- Potential discharge destinations
- Premorbid conditions
- Probability of prolonged impairment, functional limitation, or disability
- Psychological and socioeconomic factors
- Psychomotor abilities
- Social support
- Stability of the condition

Intervention

Intervention is the purposeful interaction of the physical therapist with the patient/client and, when appropriate, with other individuals involved in patient/client care, using various physical therapy procedures and techniques to produce changes in the condition consistent with the diagnosis and prognosis. Decisions about interventions are contingent on the timely monitoring of patient/client response and the progress made toward achieving the anticipated goals and expected outcomes.

Communication, coordination, and documentation and patient/client-related instruction are provided for all patients/clients across all settings. Procedural interventions are selected or modified based on the examination data and the evaluation, the diagnosis and the prognosis, and the anticipated goals and expected outcomes for a particular patient/client. *For clinical considerations in selecting interventions, listings of interventions, and listings of anticipated goals and expected outcomes, refer to Chapter 3.*

Coordination, Communication, and Documentation

Coordination, communication, and documentation may include:

Interventions

- Addressing required functions
  - advance directives
  - individualized family service plans (IFSPs) or individualized education plans (IEPs)
  - informed consent
  - mandatory communication and reporting (eg, patient advocacy and abuse reporting)
- Admission and discharge planning
- Case management
- Collaboration and coordination with agencies, including:
  - equipment suppliers
  - home care agencies
  - payer groups
  - schools
  - transportation agencies
- Communication across settings, including:
  - case conferences
  - documentation
  - education plans
- Cost-effective resource utilization
- Data collection, analysis, and reporting
  - outcome data
  - peer review findings
  - record reviews
- Documentation across settings, following APTA's *Guidelines for Physical Therapy Documentation* (Appendix 5), including:
  - changes in impairments, functional limitations, and disabilities
  - changes in interventions
  - elements of patient/client management (examination, evaluation, diagnosis, prognosis, intervention)
  - outcomes of intervention
- Interdisciplinary teamwork
  - case conferences
  - patient care rounds
  - patient/client family meetings
- Referrals to other professionals or resources

Anticipated Goals and Expected Outcomes

- Accountability for services is increased.
- Admission data and discharge planning are completed.
- Advance directives, individualized family service plans (IFSPs) or individualized education plans (IEPs), informed consent, and mandatory communication and reporting (eg, patient advocacy and abuse reporting) are obtained or completed.
- Available resources are maximally utilized.
- Care is coordinated with patient/client, family, significant others, caregivers, and other professionals.
- Case is managed throughout the episode of care.
- Collaboration and coordination occurs with agencies, including equipment suppliers, home care agencies, payer groups, schools, and transportation agencies.
- Communication enhances risk reduction and prevention.
- Communication occurs across settings through case conferences, education plans, and documentation.
- Data are collected, analyzed, and reported, including outcome data, peer review findings, and record reviews.
- Decision making is enhanced regarding health, wellness, and fitness needs.
- Decision making is enhanced regarding patient/client health and the use of health care resources by patient/client, family, significant others, and caregivers.
- Documentation occurs throughout patient/client management and across settings and follows APTA's *Guidelines for Physical Therapy Documentation* (Appendix 5).
- Interdisciplinary collaboration occurs through case conferences, patient care rounds, and patient/client family meetings.
- Patient/client, family, significant other, and caregiver understanding of anticipated goals and expected outcomes is increased.
- Placement needs are determined.
- Referrals are made to other professionals or resources whenever necessary and appropriate.
- Resources are utilized in a cost-effective way.

Patient/Client-Related Instruction

Patient/client-related instruction may include:

Interventions

- Instruction, education and training of patients/clients and caregivers regarding:
  - current condition (pathology/pathophysiology [disease, disorder, or condition], impairments, functional limitations, or disabilities)
  - enhancement of performance
  - health, wellness, and fitness
  - plan of care
  - risk factors for pathology/pathophysiology (disease, disorder, or condition), impairments, functional limitations, or disabilities
  - transitions across settings
  - transitions to new roles

Anticipated Goals and Expected Outcomes

- Ability to perform physical actions, tasks, or activities is improved.
- Awareness and use of community resources are improved.
- Behaviors that foster healthy habits, wellness, and prevention are acquired.
- Decision making is enhanced regarding patient/client health and the use of health care resources by patient/client, family, significant others, and caregivers.
- Disability associated with acute or chronic illnesses is reduced.
- Functional independence in activities of daily living (ADL) and instrumental activities of daily living (IADL) is increased.
- Health status is improved.
- Intensity of care is decreased.
- Level of supervision required for task performance is decreased.
- Patient/client, family, significant other, and caregiver knowledge and awareness of the diagnosis, prognosis, interventions, and anticipated goals and expected outcomes are increased.
- Patient/client knowledge of personal and environmental factors associated with the condition is increased.
- Performance levels in self-care, home management, work (job/school/play), community, or leisure actions, tasks, or activities are improved.
- Physical function is improved.
- Risk of recurrence of condition is reduced.
- Risk of secondary impairment is reduced.
- Safety of patient/client, family, significant others, and caregivers is improved.
- Self-management of symptoms is improved.
- Utilization and cost of health care services are decreased.

Procedural Interventions

Procedural interventions for this pattern may include:

Therapeutic Exercise

Interventions

- Aerobic capacity/endurance conditioning or reconditioning
  - aquatic programs
  - gait and locomotor training
  - increased workload over time
  - walking and wheelchair propulsion programs
- Balance, coordination, and agility training
  - developmental activities training
  - motor function (motor control and motor learning) training or retraining
  - neuromuscular education or reeducation
  - perceptual training
  - posture awareness training
  - standardized, programmatic, complementary exercise approaches
  - task-specific performance training
- Body mechanics and postural stabilization
  - body mechanics training
  - posture awareness training
  - postural control training
  - postural stabilization activities
- Flexibility exercises
  - muscle lengthening
  - range of motion
  - stretching
- Gait and locomotion training
  - developmental activities training
  - gait training
  - implement and device training
  - perceptual training
  - standardized, programmatic, complementary exercise approaches
  - wheelchair training
- Relaxation
  - breathing strategies
  - movement strategies
  - relaxation techniques
  - standardized, programmatic, complementary exercise approaches
- Strength, power, and endurance training for head, neck, limb, pelvic-floor, trunk, and ventilatory muscles
  - active assistive, active, and resistive exercises (including concentric, dynamic/isotonic, eccentric, isokinetic, isometric, and plyometric)
  - aquatic programs
  - standardized, programmatic, complementary exercise approaches
  - task-specific performance training

Anticipated Goals and Expected Outcomes

- Impact on pathology/pathophysiology (disease, disorder, or condition)
  - Joint swelling, inflammation, or restriction is reduced.
  - Nutrient delivery to tissue is increased.
  - Osteogenic effects of exercise are maximized.
  - Pain is decreased.
  - Physiological response to increased oxygen demand is improved.
  - Soft tissue swelling, inflammation, or restriction is reduced.
  - Tissue perfusion and oxygenation are enhanced.
- Impact on impairments
  - Aerobic capacity is increased.
  - Balance is improved.
  - Endurance is increased.
  - Energy expenditure per unit of work is decreased.
  - Gait, locomotion, and balance are improved.
  - Joint integrity and mobility are improved.
  - Motor function (motor control and motor learning) is improved.
  - Muscle performance (strength, power, and endurance) is increased.
  - Postural control is improved.
  - Quality and quantity of movement between and across body segments are improved.
  - Range of motion is improved.
  - Relaxation is increased.
  - Weight-bearing status is improved.
- Impact on functional limitations
  - Ability to perform physical actions, tasks, or activities related to self-care, home management, work (job/school/play), community, and leisure is improved.
  - Level of supervision required for task performance is decreased.
  - Performance of and independence in activities of daily living (ADL) and instrumental activities of daily living (IADL) with or without devices and equipment are increased.
  - Tolerance of positions and activities is increased.
- Impact on disabilities
  - Ability to assume or resume required self-care, home management, work (job/school/play), community, and leisure roles is improved.
- Risk reduction/prevention
  - Risk factors are reduced.
  - Risk of recurrence of condition is reduced.
  - Risk of secondary impairment is reduced.
  - Safety is improved.
  - Self-management of symptoms is improved.
- Impact on health, wellness, and fitness
  - Fitness is improved.
  - Health status is improved.
  - Physical capacity is increased.
  - Physical function is improved.
- Impact on societal resources
  - Utilization of physical therapy services is optimized.
  - Utilization of physical therapy services results in efficient use of health care dollars.
- Patient/client satisfaction
  - Access, availability, and services provided are acceptable to patient/client.
  - Administrative management of practice is acceptable to patient/client.
  - Clinical proficiency of physical therapist is acceptable to patient/client.
  - Coordination of care is acceptable to patient/client.
  - Cost of health care services is decreased.
  - Intensity of care is decreased.
  - Interpersonal skills of physical therapist are acceptable to patient/client, family, and significant others.
  - Sense of well-being is improved.
  - Stressors are decreased.

Functional Training in Self-Care and Home Management (Including Activities of Daily Living [ADL] and Instrumental Activities of Daily Living [IADL])

Interventions

- ADL training
  - bathing
  - bed mobility and transfer training
  - developmental activities
  - dressing
  - eating
  - grooming
  - toileting
- Devices and equipment use and training
  - assistive and adaptive device or equipment training during ADL and IADL
  - orthotic, protective, or supportive device or equipment training during ADL and IADL
- Functional training programs
  - back schools
  - simulated environments and tasks
  - task adaptation
- IADL training
  - caring for dependents
  - home maintenance
  - household chores
  - shopping
  - structured play for infants and children
  - yard work
- Injury prevention or reduction
  - injury prevention education during self-care and home management
  - injury prevention or reduction with use of devices and equipment
  - safety awareness training during self-care and home management

Anticipated Goals and Expected Outcomes

- Impact on pathology/pathophysiology (disease, disorder, or condition)
  - Pain is decreased.
- Impact on impairments
  - Balance is improved.
  - Endurance is increased.
  - Energy expenditure per unit of work is decreased.
  - Motor function (motor control and motor learning) is improved.
  - Muscle performance (strength, power, and endurance) is increased.
  - Postural control is improved.
  - Sensory awareness is increased.
  - Weight-bearing status is improved.
- Impact on functional limitations
  - Ability to perform physical actions, tasks, or activities related to self-care and home management is improved.
  - Level of supervision required for task performance is decreased.
  - Performance of and independence in ADL and IADL with or without devices and equipment are increased.
  - Tolerance of positions and activities is increased.
- Impact on disabilities
  - Ability to assume or resume required self-care and home management roles is improved.
- Risk reduction/prevention
  - Risk factors are reduced.
  - Risk of secondary impairments is reduced.
  - Safety is improved.
  - Self-management of symptoms is improved.
- Impact on health, wellness, and fitness
  - Fitness is improved.
  - Health status is improved.
  - Physical capacity is increased.
  - Physical function is improved.
- Impact on societal resources
  - Utilization of physical therapy services is optimized.
  - Utilization of physical therapy services results in efficient use of health care dollars.
- Patient/client satisfaction
  - Access, availability, and services provided are acceptable to patient/client.
  - Administrative management of practice is acceptable to patient/client.
  - Clinical proficiency of physical therapist is acceptable to patient/client.
  - Coordination of care is acceptable to patient/client.
  - Cost of health care services is decreased.
  - Intensity of care is decreased.
  - Interpersonal skills of physical therapist are acceptable to patient/client, family, and significant others.
  - Sense of well-being is improved.
  - Stressors are decreased.

Functional Training in Work (Job/School/Play), Community, and Leisure Integration or Reintegration (Including Instrumental Activities of Daily Living [IADL], Work Hardening, and Work Conditioning)

Interventions

- Devices and equipment use and training
  - assistive and adaptive device or equipment training during IADL
  - orthotic, protective, or supportive device or equipment training during IADL
- Functional training programs
  - back schools
  - job coaching
  - simulated environments and tasks
  - task adaptation
  - task training
- IADL training
  - community service training involving instruments
  - school and play activities training including tools and instruments
  - work training with tools
- Injury prevention or reduction
  - injury prevention education during work (job/school/play), community, and leisure integration or reintegration
  - injury prevention or reduction with use of devices and equipment
  - safety awareness training during work (job/school/play), community, and leisure integration or reintegration
- Leisure and play activities and training

Anticipated Goals and Expected Outcomes

- Impact on pathology/pathophysiology (disease, disorder, or condition)
  - Pain is decreased.
- Impact on impairments
  - Balance is improved.
  - Endurance is increased.
  - Energy expenditure per unit of work is decreased.
  - Motor function (motor control and motor learning) is improved.
  - Muscle performance (strength, power, and endurance) is increased.
  - Postural control is improved.
  - Sensory awareness is increased.
  - Weight-bearing status is improved.
  - Work of breathing is decreased.
- Impact on functional limitations
  - Ability to perform physical actions, tasks, or activities related to work (job/school/play), community, and leisure integration or reintegration is improved.
  - Level of supervision required for task performance is decreased.
  - Performance of and independence in IADL with or without devices and equipment are increased.
  - Tolerance of positions and activities is increased.
- Impact on disabilities
  - Ability to assume or resume required work (job/school/play), community, and leisure roles is improved.
- Risk reduction/prevention
  - Risk factors are reduced.
  - Risk of secondary impairment is reduced.
  - Safety is improved.
  - Self-management of symptoms is improved.
- Impact on health, wellness, and fitness
  - Fitness is improved.
  - Health status is improved.
  - Physical capacity is increased.
  - Physical function is improved.
- Impact on societal resources
  - Costs of work-related injury or disability are reduced.
  - Utilization of physical therapy services is optimized.
  - Utilization of physical therapy services results in efficient use of health care dollars.
- Patient/client satisfaction
  - Access, availability, and services provided are acceptable to patient/client.
  - Administrative management of practice is acceptable to patient/client.
  - Clinical proficiency of physical therapist is acceptable to patient/client.
  - Coordination of care is acceptable to patient/client.
  - Cost of health care services is decreased.
  - Intensity of care is decreased.
  - Interpersonal skills of physical therapist are acceptable to patient/client, family, and significant others.
  - Sense of well-being is improved.
  - Stressors are decreased.

Manual Therapy Techniques (Including Mobilization/Manipulation)

Interventions

- Manual traction
- Massage
  - connective tissue massage
  - therapeutic massage
- Mobilization/manipulation
  - soft tissue
  - spinal and peripheral joints
- Passive range of motion

Anticipated Goals and Expected Outcomes

- Impact on pathology/pathophysiology (disease, disorder, or condition)
  - Edema, lymphedema, or effusion is reduced.
  - Joint swelling, inflammation, or restriction is reduced.
  - Neural compression is decreased.
  - Pain is decreased.
  - Soft tissue swelling, inflammation, or restriction is reduced.
- Impact on impairments
  - Balance is improved.
  - Energy expenditure per unit of work is decreased.
  - Gait, locomotion, and balance are improved.
  - Joint integrity and mobility are improved.
  - Muscle performance (strength, power, and endurance) is increased.
  - Postural control is improved.
  - Quality and quantity of movement between and across body segments are improved.
  - Range of motion is improved.
  - Relaxation is increased.
  - Sensory awareness is increased.
  - Weight-bearing status is improved.
  - Work of breathing is decreased.
- Impact on functional limitations
  - Ability to perform movement tasks is improved.
  - Ability to perform physical actions, tasks, or activities related to self-care, home management, work (job/school/play), community, and leisure is improved.
  - Tolerance of positions and activities is increased.
- Impact on disabilities
  - Ability to assume or resume required self-care, home management, work (job/school/play), community, and leisure roles is improved.
- Risk reduction/prevention
  - Risk factors are reduced.
  - Risk of recurrence of condition is reduced.
  - Risk of secondary impairment is reduced.
  - Self-management of symptoms is improved.
- Impact on health, wellness, and fitness
  - Physical capacity is increased.
  - Physical function is improved.
- Impact on societal resources
  - Utilization of physical therapy services is optimized.
  - Utilization of physical therapy services results in efficient use of health care dollars.
- Patient/client satisfaction
  - Access, availability, and services provided are acceptable to patient/client.
  - Administrative management of practice is acceptable to patient/client.
  - Clinical proficiency of physical therapist is acceptable to patient/client.
  - Coordination of care is acceptable to patient/client.
  - Cost of health care services is decreased.
  - Intensity of care is decreased.
  - Interpersonal skills of physical therapist are acceptable to patient/client, family, and significant others.
  - Sense of well-being is improved.
  - Stressors are decreased.

Prescription, Application, and, as Appropriate, Fabrication of Devices and Equipment (Assistive, Adaptive, Orthotic, Protective, Supportive, and Prosthetic)

Interventions

- Adaptive devices
  - raised toilet seats
  - seating systems
- Assistive devices
  - canes
  - crutches
  - long-handled reachers
  - power devices
  - static and dynamic splints
  - walkers
  - wheelchairs
- Orthotic devices
  - braces
  - casts
  - shoe inserts
  - splints
- Protective devices
  - braces
  - cushions
  - protective taping
- Supportive devices
  - compression garments
  - corsets
  - elastic wraps
  - neck collars
  - serial casts
  - slings
  - supportive taping

Anticipated Goals and Expected Outcomes

- Impact on pathology/pathophysiology (disease, disorder, or condition)
  - Edema, lymphedema, or effusion is reduced.
  - Joint swelling, inflammation, or restriction is reduced.
  - Pain is decreased.
  - Soft tissue swelling, inflammation, or restriction is reduced.
- Impact on impairments
  - Balance is improved.
  - Endurance is increased.
  - Energy expenditure per unit of work is decreased.
  - Gait, locomotion, and balance are improved.
  - Joint stability is improved.
  - Motor function (motor control and motor learning) is improved.
  - Muscle performance (strength, power, and endurance) is increased.
  - Optimal joint alignment is achieved.
  - Optimal loading on a body part is achieved.
  - Postural control is improved.
  - Quality and quantity of movement between and across body segments are improved.
  - Range of motion is improved.
  - Relaxation is increased.
  - Weight-bearing status is improved.
- Impact on functional limitations
  - Ability to perform physical actions, tasks, or activities related to self-care, home management, work (job/school/play), community, and leisure is improved.
  - Level of supervision required for task performance is decreased.
  - Performance of and independence in activities of daily living (ADL) and instrumental activities of daily living (IADL) with or without devices and equipment are increased.
  - Tolerance of positions and activities is increased.
- Impact on disabilities
  - Ability to assume or resume required self-care, home management, work (job/school/play), community, and leisure roles is improved.
- Risk reduction/prevention
  - Pressure on body tissues is reduced.
  - Protection of body parts is increased.
  - Risk factors are reduced.
  - Risk of recurrence of condition is reduced.
  - Risk of secondary impairment is reduced.
  - Safety is improved.
  - Self-management of symptoms is improved.
  - Stresses precipitating injury are decreased.
- Impact on health, wellness, and fitness
  - Fitness is improved.
  - Health status is improved.
  - Physical capacity is increased.
  - Physical function is improved.
- Impact on societal resources
  - Utilization of physical therapy services is optimized.
  - Utilization of physical therapy services results in efficient use of health care dollars.
- Patient/client satisfaction
  - Access, availability, and services provided are acceptable to patient/client.
  - Administrative management of practice is acceptable to patient/client.
  - Clinical proficiency of physical therapist is acceptable to patient/client.
  - Coordination of care is acceptable to patient/client.
  - Cost of health care services is decreased.
  - Intensity of care is decreased.
  - Interpersonal skills of physical therapist are acceptable to patient/client, family, and significant others.
  - Sense of well-being is improved.
  - Stressors are decreased.

Electrotherapeutic Modalities

Interventions

- Electrotherapeutic delivery of medications
  - iontophoresis
- Electrical stimulation
  - electrical muscle stimulation (EMS)
  - functional electrical stimulation (FES)
  - high voltage pulsed current (HVPC)
  - neuromuscular electrical stimulation (NMES)
  - transcutaneous electrical nerve stimulation (TENS)

Anticipated Goals and Expected Outcomes

- Impact on pathology/pathophysiology (disease, disorder, or condition)
  - Edema, lymphedema, or effusion is reduced.
  - Joint swelling, inflammation, or restriction is reduced.
  - Nutrient delivery to tissue is increased.
  - Osteogenic effects are enhanced.
  - Pain is decreased.
  - Soft tissue swelling, inflammation, or restriction is reduced.
  - Tissue perfusion and oxygenation are enhanced.
- Impact on impairments
  - Motor function (motor control and motor learning) is improved.
  - Muscle performance (strength, power, and endurance) is increased.
  - Postural control is improved.
  - Quality and quantity of movement between and across body segments are improved.
  - Range of motion is improved.
  - Relaxation is increased.
  - Sensory awareness is increased.
- Impact on functional limitations
  - Ability to perform physical actions, tasks, or activities related to self-care, home management, work (job/school/play), community, and leisure is improved.
  - Level of supervision required for task performance is decreased.
  - Performance of and independence in activities of daily living (ADL) and instrumental activities of daily living (IADL) with or without devices and equipment are increased.
  - Tolerance of positions and activities is increased.
- Impact on disabilities
  - Ability to assume or resume required self-care, home management, work (job/school/play), community, and leisure roles is improved.
- Risk reduction/prevention
  - Complications of immobility are reduced.
  - Risk factors are reduced.
  - Risk of recurrence of condition is reduced.
  - Risk of secondary impairment is reduced.
  - Self-management of symptoms is improved.
- Impact on health, wellness, and fitness
  - Fitness is improved.
  - Physical capacity is increased.
  - Physical function is improved.
- Impact on societal resources
  - Utilization of physical therapy services is optimized.
  - Utilization of physical therapy services results in efficient use of health care dollars.
- Patient/client satisfaction
  - Access, availability, and services provided are acceptable to patient/client.
  - Administrative management of practice is acceptable to patient/client.
  - Clinical proficiency of physical therapist is acceptable to patient/client.
  - Coordination of care is acceptable to patient/client.
  - Interpersonal skills of physical therapist are acceptable to patient/client, family, and significant others.
  - Sense of well-being is improved.
  - Stressors are decreased.

Physical Agents and Mechanical Modalities

Interventions

Physical agents may include:

- Athermal agents
  - pulsed electromagnetic fields
- Cryotherapy
  - cold packs
  - ice massage
  - vapocoolant spray
- Hydrotherapy
  - whirlpool tanks
  - contrast bath
  - pools
- Light agents
  - infrared
  - laser
- Sound agents
  - phonophoresis
  - ultrasound
- Thermotherapy
  - diathermy
  - dry heat
  - hot packs
  - paraffin baths

Mechanical modalities may include:

- Compression therapies
  - taping
- Mechanical motion devices
  - continuous passive motion (CPM)

Anticipated Goals and Expected Outcomes

- Impact on pathology/pathophysiology (disease, disorder, or condition)
  - Edema, lymphedema, or effusion is reduced.
  - Joint swelling, inflammation, or restriction is reduced.
  - Nutrient delivery to tissue is increased.
  - Pain is decreased.
  - Soft tissue swelling, inflammation, or restriction is reduced.
  - Tissue perfusion and oxygenation are enhanced.
- Impact on impairments
  - Integumentary integrity is improved.
  - Muscle performance (strength, power, and endurance) is increased.
  - Range of motion is improved.
  - Weight-bearing status is improved.
- Impact on functional limitations
  - Ability to perform physical actions, tasks, or activities related to self-care, home management, work (job/school/play), community, and leisure is improved.
  - Performance of and independence in activities of daily living (ADL) and instrumental activities of daily living (IADL) with or without devices and equipment are increased.
  - Tolerance of positions and activities is increased.
- Impact on disabilities
  - Ability to assume or resume required self-care, home management, work (job/school/play), community, and leisure roles is improved.
- Risk reduction/prevention
  - Complications of soft tissue and circulatory disorders are decreased.
  - Risk of secondary impairment is reduced.
  - Self-management of symptoms is improved.
  - Stresses precipitating injury are decreased.
- Impact on health, wellness, and fitness
  - Physical function is improved.
- Impact on societal resources
  - Utilization of physical therapy services is optimized.
- Patient/client satisfaction
  - Access, availability, and services provided are acceptable to patient/client.
  - Administrative management of practice is acceptable to patient/client.
  - Clinical proficiency of physical therapist is acceptable to patient/client.
  - Coordination of care is acceptable to patient/client.
  - Interpersonal skills of physical therapist are acceptable to patient/client, family, and significant others.
  - Sense of well-being is improved.
  - Stressors are decreased.

Reexamination

Reexamination is the process of performing selected tests and measures after the initial examination to evaluate progress and to modify or redirect interventions. Reexamination may be indicated more than once during a single episode of care. It also may be performed over the course of a disease, disorder, or condition, which for some patients/clients may be over the life span. Indications for reexamination include new clinical findings or failure to respond to physical therapy interventions.

Global Outcomes for Patients/Clients in This Pattern

Throughout the entire episode of care, the physical therapist determines the anticipated goals and expected outcomes for each intervention. These anticipated goals and expected outcomes are delineated in shaded boxes that accompany the lists of interventions in each preferred practice pattern. As the patient/client reaches the termination of physical therapy services and the end of the episode of care, the physical therapist measures the global outcomes of the physical therapy services by characterizing or quantifying the impact of the physical therapy interventions in the following domains:

- Pathology/pathophysiology (disease, disorder, or condition)
- Impairments
- Functional limitations
- Disabilities
- Risk reduction/prevention
- Health, wellness, and fitness
- Societal resources
- Patient/client satisfaction

In some instances, a particular anticipated goal or expected outcome is thoroughly achieved through implementation of a single form of intervention. More commonly, however, the anticipated goals and expected outcomes are achieved as a result of the combined effects of several forms of interventions, leading to enhancement of both health status and health-related quality of life.

Criteria for Termination of Physical Therapy Services

Discharge is the process of ending physical therapy services that have been provided during a single episode of care. It occurs when the anticipated goals and expected outcomes have been achieved. Discharge does *not* occur with a *transfer* (defined as the time when a patient is moved from one site to another site within the same setting or across settings during a single episode of care). Although there may be facility-specific or payer-specific requirements for documentation regarding the conclusion of physical therapy services, *discharge occurs based on the physical therapist's analysis of the achievement of anticipated goals and expected outcomes.*

Discontinuation is the process of ending physical therapy services that have been provided during a single episode of care when (1) the patient/client, caregiver, or legal guardian declines to continue intervention; (2) the patient/client is unable to continue to progress toward outcomes because of medical or psychosocial complications or because financial/insurance resources have been expended; or (3) the physical therapist determines that the patient/client will no longer benefit from physical therapy. When physical therapy services are terminated prior to achievement of anticipated goals and expected outcomes, patient/client status and the rationale for termination are documented.

For patients/clients who require multiple episodes of care, periodic follow-up is needed over the life span to ensure safety and effective adaptation following changes in physical status, caregivers, environment, or task demands. In consultation with appropriate individuals, and in consideration of the outcomes, the physical therapist plans for discharge or discontinuation and provides for appropriate follow-up or referral.

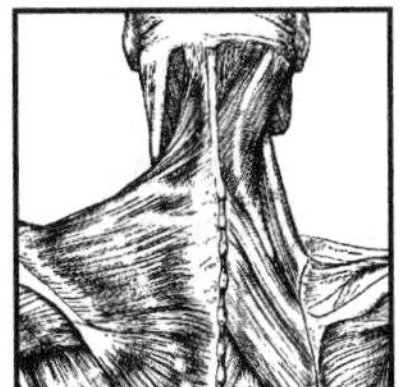

Impaired Joint Mobility, Motor Function, Muscle Performance, Range of Motion, and Reflex Integrity Associated With Spinal Disorders

This preferred practice pattern describes the generally accepted elements of patient/client management that physical therapists provide for patients/clients who are classified in this pattern. The pattern title reflects the diagnosis made by the physical therapist. APTA emphasizes that preferred practice patterns are the boundaries within which a physical therapist may select any of a number of clinical alternatives, based on consideration of a wide variety of factors, such as individual patient/client needs; the profession's code of ethics and standards of practice; and patient/client age, culture, gender roles, race, sex, sexual orientation, and socioeconomic status.

Patient/Client Diagnostic Classification

Patients/clients will be classified into this pattern—for impaired joint mobility, motor function, muscle performance, range of motion, and reflex integrity associated with spinal disorders—as a result of the physical therapist's evaluation of the examination data. The findings from the examination (history, systems review, and tests and measures) may indicate the presence or risk of pathology/pathophysiology (disease, disorder, or condition), impairments, functional limitations, or disabilities or the need for health, wellness, or fitness programs. The physical therapist integrates, synthesizes, and interprets the data to determine the diagnostic classification.

Inclusion

The following examples of examination findings may support the inclusion of patients/clients in this pattern:

Risk Factors or Consequences of Pathology/Pathophysiology (Disease, Disorder, or Condition)

- Degenerative disk disease
- Disk herniation
- History of spinal surgery
- Spinal stenosis
- Spondylolisthesis

Impairments, Functional Limitations, or Disabilities

- Abnormal neural tension
- Altered sensation
- Decreased deep tendon reflex
- Inability to perform lifting tasks
- Inability to perform self-care independently
- Inability to sit for prolonged periods
- Muscle weakness
- Pain with forward bending

Note:

Some risk factors or consequences of pathology/pathophysiology—such as *neoplasm*—may be severe and complex; *however, they do not necessarily exclude patients/clients from this pattern.* Severe and complex risk factors or consequences may require modification of the frequency of visits and duration of care. (See "Evaluation, Diagnosis, and Prognosis," page 221.)

Exclusion or Multiple-Pattern Classification

The following examples of examination findings may support exclusion from this pattern or classification into additional patterns. Depending on the level of severity or complexity of the examination findings, the physical therapist may determine that the patient/client would be more appropriately managed through (1) classification in an entirely different pattern or (2) classification in both this and another pattern.

Findings That May Require Classification in a Different Pattern

- Fracture
- Impairments associated with systemic conditions (eg, ankylosing spondylitis, Scheurermann disease, juvenile rheumatoid arthritis)
- Impairments associated with traumatic spinal cord injury

Findings That May Require Classification in Additional Patterns

- Neuromuscular disease

ICD-9-CM Codes

The listing below contains the current (as of press time) and most typical 3- and 4-digit ICD-9-CM codes related to this preferred practice pattern. Because patient/client diagnostic classification is based on impairments, functional limitations, and disabilities—not on codes—patients/clients may be classified into the pattern even though the codes listed with the pattern may not apply to those clients.

This listing is intended for general information only and should not be used for coding purposes. The codes should be confirmed by referring to the World Health Organization's *International Classification of Diseases, 9th Revision, Clinical Modification (ICD-9-CM 2001)*, Volumes 1 and 3 (Chicago, Ill: American Medical Association; 2000) or subsequent revisions or by referring to other ICD-9-CM coding manuals that contain exclusion notes and instructions regarding fifth-digit requirements.

353 Nerve root and plexus disorders
- **353.0** Brachial plexus lesions
- **353.1** Lumbosacral plexus lesions
- **353.2** Cervical root lesions, not elsewhere classified
- **353.4** Lumbosacral root lesions, not elsewhere classified

715 Osteoarthrosis and allied disorders

716 Other and unspecified arthropathies
- **716.9** Arthropathy, unspecified
  Inflammation of joint, not otherwise specified

718 Other derangement of joint
- **718.3** Recurrent dislocation of joint
- **718.9** Unspecified derangement of joint

719 Other and unspecified disorders of joint
- **719.8** Other specified disorders of joint
  Calcification of joint

720 Ankylosing spondylitis and other inflammatory spondylopathies

721 Spondylosis and allied disorders
- **721.1** Cervical spondylosis with myelopathy
- **721.4** Thoracic or lumbar spondylosis with myelopathy

722 Intervertebral disk disorders
- **722.4** Degeneration of cervical intervertebral disk
- **722.5** Degeneration of thoracic or lumbar intervertebral disk
- **722.6** Degeneration of intervertebral disk, site unspecified
- **722.7** Intervertebral disk disorder with myelopathy
- **722.8** Postlaminectomy syndrome

723 Other disorders of cervical region
- **723.0** Spinal stenosis in cervical region
- **723.1** Cervicalgia

724 Other and unspecified disorders of back
- **724.0** Spinal stenosis, other than cervical
- **724.2** Lumbago
  Low back pain
  Low back syndrome
  Lumbalgia
- **724.3** Sciatica
- **724.9** Other unspecified back disorders

727 Other disorders of synovium, tendon, and bursa
- **727.0** Synovitis and tenosynovitis

728 Disorders of muscle, ligament, and fascia
- **728.2** Muscular wasting and disuse atrophy, not elsewhere classified
- **728.8** Other disorders of muscle, ligament, and fascia
  - **728.85** Spasm of muscle
- **728.9** Unspecified disorder of muscle, ligament, and fascia

733 Other disorders of bone and cartilage
- **733.0** Osteoporosis

738 Other acquired deformity
- **738.4** Acquired spondylolisthesis
- **738.5** Other acquired deformity of back or spine

756 Other congenital musculoskeletal anomalies
- **756.1** Anomalies of spine
  - **756.11** Spondylolysis, lumbosacral region
  - **756.12** Spondylolisthesis

846 Sprains and strains of sacroiliac region
- **846.0** Lumbosacral (joint) (ligament)

847 Sprains and strains of other and unspecified parts of back

922 Contusion of trunk
- **922.3** Back

Examination

Examination is a comprehensive screening and specific testing process that leads to a diagnostic classification or, when appropriate, to a referral to another practitioner. Examination is required prior to the initial intervention and is performed for all patients/clients. Through the examination, the physical therapist may identify impairments, functional limitations, disabilities, changes in physical function or overall health status, and needs related to restoration of health and to prevention, wellness, and fitness. The physical therapist synthesizes the examination findings to establish the diagnosis and the prognosis (including the plan of care). The patient/client, family, significant others, and caregivers may provide information during the examination process.

Examination has three components: the patient/client history, the systems review, and tests and measures. The *history* is a systematic gathering of past and current information (often from the patient/client) related to why the patient/client is seeking the services of the physical therapist. The *systems review* is a brief or limited examination of (1) the anatomical and physiological status of the cardiovascular/pulmonary, integumentary, musculoskeletal, and neuromuscular systems and (2) the communication ability, affect, cognition, language, and learning style of the patient/client. *Tests and measures* are the means of gathering data about the patient/client.

The selection of examination procedures and the depth of the examination vary based on patient/client age; severity of the problem; stage of recovery (acute, subacute, chronic); phase of rehabilitation (early, intermediate, late, return to activity); home, work (job/school/play), or community situation; and other relevant factors. *For clinical indications in selecting tests and measures and for listings of tests and measures, tools used to gather data, and the types of data generated by tests and measures, refer to Chapter 2.*

Patient/Client History

The history may include:

General Demographics
- Age
- Sex
- Race/ethnicity
- Primary language
- Education

Social History
- Cultural beliefs and behaviors
- Family and caregiver resources
- Social interactions, social activities, and support systems

Employment/Work (Job/School/Play)
- Current and prior work (job/school/play), community, and leisure actions, tasks, or activities

Growth and Development
- Developmental history
- Hand dominance

Living Environment
- Devices and equipment (eg, assistive, adaptive, orthotic, protective, supportive, prosthetic)
- Living environment and community characteristics
- Projected discharge destinations

General Health Status (Self-Report, Family Report, Caregiver Report)
- General health perception
- Physical function (eg, mobility, sleep patterns, restricted bed days)
- Psychological function (eg, memory, reasoning ability, depression, anxiety)
- Role function (eg, community, leisure, social, work)
- Social function (eg, social activity, social interaction, social support)

Social/Health Habits (Past and Current)
- Behavioral health risks (eg, smoking, drug abuse)
- Level of physical fitness

Family History
- Familial health risks

Medical/Surgical History
- Cardiovascular
- Endocrine/metabolic
- Gastrointestinal
- Genitourinary
- Gynecological
- Integumentary
- Musculoskeletal
- Neuromuscular
- Obstetrical
- Prior hospitalizations, surgeries, and preexisting medical and other health-related conditions
- Psychological
- Pulmonary

Current Condition(s)/Chief Complaint(s)
- Concerns that led patient/client to seek the services of a physical therapist
- Concerns or needs of patient/client who requires the services of a physical therapist
- Current therapeutic interventions
- Mechanisms of injury or disease, including date of onset and course of events
- Onset and pattern of symptoms
- Patient/client, family, significant other, and caregiver expectations and goals for the therapeutic intervention
- Patient/client, family, significant other, and caregiver perceptions of patient's/client's emotional response to the current clinical situation
- Previous occurrence of chief complaint(s)
- Prior therapeutic interventions

Functional Status and Activity Level
- Current and prior functional status in self-care and home management activities, including activities of daily living (ADL) and instrumental activities of daily living (IADL)
- Current and prior functional status in work (job/school/play), community, and leisure actions, tasks, or activities

Medications
- Medications for current condition
- Medications previously taken for current condition
- Medications for other conditions

Other Clinical Tests
- Laboratory and diagnostic tests
- Review of available records (eg, medical, education, surgical)
- Review of other clinical findings (eg, nutrition and hydration)

Systems Review

The systems review may include:

Anatomical and Physiological Status

- Cardiovascular/Pulmonary
  - Blood pressure
  - Edema
  - Heart rate
  - Respiratory rate
- Integumentary
  - Pliability (texture)
  - Presence of scar formation
  - Skin color
  - Skin integrity
- Musculoskeletal
  - Gross range of motion
  - Gross strength
  - Gross symmetry
  - Height
  - Weight
- Neuromuscular
  - Gross coordinated movements (eg, balance, gait, locomotion, transfers, transitions)
  - Motor function (motor control, motor learning)

Communication, Affect, Cognition, Language, and Learning Style

- Ability to make needs known
- Consciousness
- Expected emotional/behavioral responses
- Learning preferences (eg, education needs, learning barriers)
- Orientation (person, place, time)

Tests and Measures

Tests and measures for this pattern may include those that characterize or quantify:

Aerobic Capacity and Endurance

- Aerobic capacity during functional activities (eg, activities of daily living [ADL] scales, indexes, instrumental activities of daily living [IADL] scales, observations)
- Aerobic capacity during standardized exercise test protocols (eg, ergometry, step tests, time/distance walk/run tests, treadmill tests, wheelchair tests)

Anthropometric Characteristics

- Body composition (eg, body mass index, impedance measurement, skinfold thickness measurement)
- Body dimensions (eg, girth measurement, length measurement)

Assistive and Adaptive Devices

- Assistive or adaptive devices and equipment use during functional activities (eg, ADL scales, functional scales, IADL scales, interviews, observations)
- Components, alignment, fit, and ability to care for the assistive or adaptive devices and equipment (eg, interviews, logs, observations, reports)
- Remediation of impairments, functional limitations, or disabilities with use of assistive or adaptive devices and equipment (eg, activity status indexes, ADL scales, aerobic capacity tests, functional performance inventories, health assessment questionnaires, IADL scales, pain scales, play scales, videographic assessments)
- Safety during use of assistive or adaptive devices and equipment (eg, diaries, fall scales, interviews, logs, observations, reports)

Cranial and Peripheral Nerve Integrity

- Electrophysiological integrity (eg, electroneuromyography)
- Motor distribution of the cranial nerves (eg, dynamometry, muscle tests, observations)
- Motor distribution of the peripheral nerves (eg, dynamometry, muscle tests, observations, thoracic outlet tests)
- Response to neural provocation (eg, tension tests, vertebral artery compression tests)
- Sensory distribution of the cranial nerves (eg, discrimination tests; tactile tests, including coarse and light touch, cold and heat, pain, pressure, and vibration)
- Sensory distribution of the peripheral nerves (eg, discrimination tests; tactile tests, including coarse and light touch, cold and heat, pain, pressure, and vibration; thoracic outlet tests)

Environmental, Home, and Work (Job/School/Play) Barriers

- Current and potential barriers (eg, checklists, interviews, observations, questionnaires)
- Physical space and environment (eg, compliance standards, observations, photographic assessments, questionnaires, structural specifications, videographic assessments)

Ergonomics and Body Mechanics

Ergonomics

- Dexterity and coordination during work (job/school/play) (eg, hand function tests, impairment rating scales, manipulative ability tests)
- Functional capacity and performance during work actions, tasks, or activities (eg, accelerometry, dynamometry, electroneuromyography, endurance tests, force platform tests, goniometry, interviews, observations, photographic assessments, physical capacity tests, postural loading analyses, technology-assisted assessments, videographic assessments, work analyses)
- Safety in work environments (eg, hazard identification checklists, job severity indexes, lifting standards, risk assessment scales, standards for exposure limits)
- Specific work conditions or activities (eg, handling checklists, job simulations, lifting models, preemployment screenings, task analysis checklists, workstation checklists)
- Tools, devices, equipment, and workstations related to work actions, tasks, or activities (eg, observations, tool analysis checklists, vibration assessments)

Body mechanics

- Body mechanics during self-care, home management, work, community, or leisure actions, tasks, or activities (eg, ADL scales, IADL scales, observations, photographic assessments, technology-assisted assessments, videographic assessments)

Gait, Locomotion, and Balance

- Balance during functional activities with or without the use of assistive, adaptive, orthotic, protective, supportive, or prosthetic devices or equipment (eg, ADL scales, IADL scales, observations, videographic assessments)
- Balance (dynamic and static) with or without the use of assistive, adaptive, orthotic, protective, supportive, or prosthetic devices or equipment (eg, balance scales, dizziness inventories, dynamic posturography, fall scales, motor impairment tests, observations, photographic assessments, postural control tests)
- Gait and locomotion during functional activities with or without the use of assistive, adaptive, orthotic, protective, supportive, or prosthetic devices or equipment (eg, ADL scales, gait indexes, IADL scales, mobility skill profiles, observations, videographic assessments)
- Gait and locomotion with or without the use of assistive, adaptive, orthotic, protective, supportive, or prosthetic devices or equipment (eg, dynamometry, electroneuromyography, footprint analyses, gait indexes, mobility skill profiles, observations, photographic assessments, technology-assisted assessments, videographic assessments, weight-bearing scales, wheelchair mobility tests)
- Safety during gait, locomotion, and balance (eg, confidence scales, diaries, fall scales, functional assessment profiles, logs, reports)

Joint Integrity and Mobility

- Joint integrity and mobility (eg, apprehension, compression and distraction, drawer, glide, impingement, shear, and valgus/varus stress tests; arthrometry; palpation)
- Joint play movements, including end feel (all joints of the axial and appendicular skeletal system) (eg, palpation)

Motor Function (Motor Control and Motor Learning)

- Dexterity, coordination, and agility (eg, coordination screens, motor impairment tests, motor proficiency tests, observations, videographic assessments)
- Hand function (eg, fine and gross motor control tests, finger dexterity tests, manipulative ability tests, observations)

Muscle Performance (Including Strength, Power, and Endurance)

- Electrophysiological integrity (eg, electroneuromyography)
- Muscle strength, power, and endurance (eg, dynamometry, manual muscle tests, muscle performance tests, physical capacity tests, technology-assisted assessments, timed activity tests)
- Muscle strength, power, and endurance during functional activities (eg, ADL scales, functional muscle tests, IADL scales, observations, videographic assessments)
- Muscle tension (eg, palpation)

Orthotic, Protective, and Supportive Devices

- Components, alignment, fit, and ability to care for orthotic, protective, and supportive devices and equipment (eg, interviews, logs, observations, pressure-sensing maps, reports)
- Orthotic, protective, and supportive devices and equipment use during functional activities (eg, ADL scales, functional scales, IADL scales, interviews, observations, profiles)
- Remediation of impairments, functional limitations, or disabilities with use of orthotic, protective, and supportive devices and equipment (eg, activity status indexes, ADL scales, aerobic capacity tests, functional performance inventories, health assessment questionnaires, IADL scales, pain scales, play scales, videographic assessments)
- Safety during use of orthotic, protective, and supportive devices and equipment (eg, diaries, fall scales, interviews, logs, observations, reports)

Pain

- Pain, soreness, and nociception (eg, analog scales, discrimination tests, pain drawings and maps, provocation tests, verbal and pictorial descriptor tests)
- Pain in specific body parts (eg, pain indexes, pain questionnaires, structural provocation tests)

Posture

- Postural alignment and position (static and dynamic), including symmetry and deviation from midline (eg, grid measurement, observations, photographic assessments, technology-assisted assessments, videographic assessments)
- Specific body parts (eg, angle assessments, forward-bending test, goniometry, observations, palpation, positional tests)

Range of Motion (ROM) (Including Muscle Length)

- Functional ROM (eg, observations, squat tests, toe touch tests)
- Joint active and passive movement (eg, goniometry, inclinometry, observations, photographic assessments, videographic assessments)
- Muscle length, soft tissue extensibility, and flexibility (eg, contracture tests, goniometry, inclinometry, ligamentous tests, linear measurement, multisegment flexibility tests, palpation)

Reflex Integrity

- Deep reflexes (eg, myotatic reflex scale, observations, reflex tests)
- Electrophysiological integrity (eg, electroneuromyography)
- Resistance to passive stretch (eg, tone scales)
- Superficial reflexes and reactions (eg, observations, provocation tests)

Self-Care and Home Management (Including ADL and IADL)

- Ability to gain access to home environments (eg, barrier identification, observations, physical performance tests)
- Ability to perform self-care and home management activities with or without assistive, adaptive, orthotic, protective, supportive, or prosthetic devices and equipment (eg, ADL scales, aerobic capacity tests, IADL scales, interviews, observations, profiles)
- Safety in self-care and home management activities and environments (eg, diaries, fall scales, interviews, logs, observations, reports, videographic assessments)

Sensory Integrity

- Combined/cortical sensations (eg, stereognosis tests, tactile discrimination tests)
- Deep sensations (eg, kinesthesiometry, observations, photographic assessments, vibration tests)
- Electrophysiological integrity (eg, electroneuromyography)

Work (Job/School/Play), Community, and Leisure Integration or Reintegration (Including IADL)

- Ability to assume or resume work (job/school/play), community, and leisure activities with or without assistive, adaptive, orthotic, protective, supportive, or prosthetic devices and equipment (eg, activity profiles, disability indexes, functional status questionnaires, IADL scales, observations, physical capacity tests)
- Ability to gain access to work (job/school/play), community, and leisure environments (eg, barrier identification, interviews, observations, physical capacity tests, transportation assessments)
- Safety in work (job/school/play), community, and leisure activities and environments (eg, diaries, fall scales, interviews, logs, observations, videographic assessments)

Evaluation, Diagnosis, and Prognosis (Including Plan of Care)

Physical therapists perform *evaluations* (make clinical judgments) based on the data gathered from the history, systems review, and tests and measures. In the evaluation process, physical therapists synthesize the examination data to establish the diagnosis and prognosis (including the plan of care). Factors that influence the complexity of the evaluation include the clinical findings, extent of loss of function, chronicity or severity of the problem, possibility of multisite or multisystem involvement, preexisting condition(s), potential discharge destination, social considerations, physical function, and overall health status.

A *diagnosis* is a label encompassing a cluster of signs and symptoms, syndromes, or categories. It is the result of the systematic diagnostic process, which includes integrating and evaluating the data from the examination. The diagnostic label indicates the primary dysfunction(s) toward which the therapist will direct interventions. The *prognosis* is the determination of the predicted optimal level of improvement in function and the amount of time needed to reach that level and may also include a prediction of levels of improvement that may be reached at various intervals during the course of therapy. During the prognostic process, the physical therapist develops the plan of care. The *plan of care* identifies specific interventions, proposed frequency and duration of the interventions, anticipated goals, expected outcomes, and discharge plans. The plan of care identifies realistic anticipated goals and expected outcomes, taking into consideration the expectations of the patient/client and appropriate others. These anticipated goals and expected outcomes should be measureable and time limited.

The frequency of visits and duration of the episode of care may vary from a short episode with a high intensity of intervention to a longer episode with a diminishing intensity of intervention. Frequency and duration may vary greatly among patients/clients based on a variety of factors that the physical therapist considers throughout the evaluation process, such as anatomical and physiological changes related to growth and development; caregiver consistency or expertise; chronicity or severity of the current condition; living environment; multisite or multisystem involvement; social support; potential discharge destinations; probability of prolonged impairment, functional limitation, or disability; and stability of the condition.

Prognosis

Over the course of 1 to 6 months, patient/client will demonstrate optimal joint mobility, motor function, muscle performance, range of motion, and reflex integrity and the highest level of functioning in home, work (job/school/play), community, and leisure environments.

During the episode of care, patient/client will achieve (1) the anticipated goals and expected outcomes of the interventions that are described in the plan of care and (2) the global outcomes for patients/clients who are classified in this pattern.

Expected Range of Number of Visits Per Episode of Care

8 to 24

This range represents the lower and upper limits of the number of physical therapist visits required to achieve anticipated goals and expected outcomes. *It is anticipated that 80% of patients/clients who are classified into this pattern will achieve the anticipated goals and expected outcomes within 8 to 24 visits during a single continuous episode of care.* Frequency of visits and duration of the episode of care should be determined by the physical therapist to maximize effectiveness of care and efficiency of service delivery.

Factors That May Require New Episode of Care or That May Modify Frequency of Visits/Duration of Episode

- Accessibility and availability of resources
- Adherence to the intervention program
- Age
- Anatomical and physiological changes related to growth and development
- Caregiver consistency or expertise
- Chronicity or severity of the current condition
- Cognitive status
- Comorbitities, complications, or secondary impairments
- Concurrent medical, surgical, and therapeutic interventions
- Decline in functional independence
- Level of impairment
- Level of physical function
- Living environment
- Multisite or multisystem involvement
- Nutritional status
- Overall health status
- Potential discharge destinations
- Premorbid conditions
- Probability of prolonged impairment, functional limitation, or disability
- Psychological and socioeconomic factors
- Psychomotor abilities
- Social support
- Stability of the condition

Intervention

Intervention is the purposeful interaction of the physical therapist with the patient/client and, when appropriate, with other individuals involved in patient/client care, using various physical therapy procedures and techniques to produce changes in the condition consistent with the diagnosis and prognosis. Decisions about interventions are contingent on the timely monitoring of patient/client response and the progress made toward achieving the anticipated goals and expected outcomes.

Communication, coordination, and documentation and patient/client-related instruction are provided for all patients/clients across all settings. Procedural interventions are selected or modified based on the examination data and the evaluation, the diagnosis and the prognosis, and the anticipated goals and expected outcomes for a particular patient/client. *For clinical considerations in selecting interventions, listings of interventions, and listings of anticipated goals and expected outcomes, refer to Chapter 3.*

Coordination, Communication, and Documentation

Coordination, communication, and documentation may include:

Interventions

- Addressing required functions
  - advance directives
  - individualized family service plans (IFSPs) or individualized education plans (IEPs)
  - informed consent
  - mandatory communication and reporting (eg, patient advocacy and abuse reporting)
- Admission and discharge planning
- Case management
- Collaboration and coordination with agencies, including:
  - equipment suppliers
  - home care agencies
  - payer groups
  - schools
  - transportation agencies
- Communication across settings, including:
  - case conferences
  - documentation
  - education plans
- Cost-effective resource utilization
- Data collection, analysis, and reporting
  - outcome data
  - peer review findings
  - record reviews
- Documentation across settings, following APTA's *Guidelines for Physical Therapy Documentation* (Appendix 5), including:
  - changes in impairments, functional limitations, and disabilities
  - changes in interventions
  - elements of patient/client management (examination, evaluation, diagnosis, prognosis, intervention)
  - outcomes of intervention
- Interdisciplinary teamwork
  - case conferences
  - patient care rounds
  - patient/client family meetings
- Referrals to other professionals or resources

Anticipated Goals and Expected Outcomes

- Accountability for services is increased.
- Admission data and discharge planning are completed.
- Advance directives, individualized family service plans (IFSPs) or individualized education plans (IEPs), informed consent, and mandatory communication and reporting (eg, patient advocacy and abuse reporting) are obtained or completed.
- Available resources are maximally utilized.
- Care is coordinated with patient/client, family, significant others, caregivers, and other professionals.
- Case is managed throughout the episode of care.
- Collaboration and coordination occurs with agencies, including equipment suppliers, home care agencies, payer groups, schools, and transportation agencies.
- Communication enhances risk reduction and prevention.
- Communication occurs across settings through case conferences, education plans, and documentation.
- Data are collected, analyzed, and reported, including outcome data, peer review findings, and record reviews.
- Decision making is enhanced regarding health, wellness, and fitness needs.
- Decision making is enhanced regarding patient/client health and the use of health care resources by patient/client, family, significant others, and caregivers.
- Documentation occurs throughout patient/client management and across settings and follows APTA's *Guidelines for Physical Therapy Documentation* (Appendix 5).
- Interdisciplinary collaboration occurs through case conferences, patient care rounds, and patient/client family meetings.
- Patient/client, family, significant other, and caregiver understanding of anticipated goals and expected outcomes is increased.
- Placement needs are determined.
- Referrals are made to other professionals or resources whenever necessary and appropriate.
- Resources are utilized in a cost-effective way.

Patient/Client-Related Instruction

Patient/client-related instruction may include:

Interventions

- Instruction, education and training of patients/clients and caregivers regarding:
  - current condition (pathology/pathophysiology [disease, disorder, or condition], impairments, functional limitations, or disabilities)
  - enhancement of performance
  - health, wellness, and fitness programs
  - plan of care
  - risk factors for pathology/pathophysiology (disease, disorder, or condition), impairments, functional limitations, or disabilities
  - transitions across settings
  - transitions to new roles

Anticipated Goals and Expected Outcomes

- Ability to perform physical actions, tasks, or activities is improved.
- Awareness and use of community resources are improved.
- Behaviors that foster healthy habits, wellness, and prevention are acquired.
- Decision making is enhanced regarding patient/client health and the use of health care resources by patient/client, family, significant others, and caregivers.
- Disability associated with acute or chronic illnesses is reduced.
- Functional independence in activities of daily living (ADL) and instrumental activities of daily living (IADL) is increased.
- Health status is improved.
- Intensity of care is decreased.
- Level of supervision required for task performance is decreased.
- Patient/client, family, significant other, and caregiver knowledge and awareness of the diagnosis, prognosis, interventions, and anticipated goals and expected outcomes are increased.
- Patient/client knowledge of personal and environmental factors associated with the condition is increased.
- Performance levels in self-care, home management, work (job/school/play), community, or leisure actions, tasks, or activities are improved.
- Physical functionis improved.
- Risk of recurrence of condition is reduced.
- Risk of secondary impairment is reduced.
- Safety of patient/client, family, significant others, and caregivers is improved.
- Self-management of symptoms is improved.
- Utilization and cost of health care services are decreased.

Procedural Interventions

Procedural interventions for this pattern may include:

Therapeutic Exercise

Interventions

- Aerobic capacity/endurance conditioning or reconditioning
  - aquatic programs
  - gait and locomotor training
  - increased workload over time
  - walking and wheelchair propulsion programs
- Balance, coordination, and agility training
  - developmental activities training
  - motor function (motor control and motor learning) training or retraining
  - neuromuscular education or reeducation
  - perceptual training
  - posture awareness training
  - standardized, programmatic, complementary exercise approaches
  - sensory training or retraining
  - task-specific performance training
- Body mechanics and postural stabilization
  - body mechanics training
  - posture awareness training
  - postural control training
  - postural stabilization activities
- Flexibility exercises
  - muscle lengthening
  - range of motion
  - stretching
- Gait and locomotion training
  - developmental activities training
  - gait training
  - implement and device training
  - perceptual training
  - standardized, programmatic, complementary exercise approaches
  - wheelchair training
- Relaxation
  - breathing strategies
  - movement strategies
  - relaxation techniques
  - standardized, programmatic, complementary exercise approaches
- Strength, power, and endurance training for head, neck, limb, pelvic-floor, trunk, and ventilatory muscles
  - active assistive, active, and resistive exercises (including concentric, dynamic/isotonic, eccentric, isokinetic, isometric, and plyometric)
  - aquatic programs
  - standardized, programmatic, complementary exercise approaches
  - task-specific performance training

Anticipated Goals and Expected Outcomes

- Impact on pathology/pathophysiology (disease, disorder, or condition)
  - Joint swelling, inflammation, or restriction is reduced.
  - Nutrient delivery to tissue is increased.
  - Osteogenic effects of exercise are maximized.
  - Pain is decreased.
  - Physiological response to increased oxygen demand is improved.
  - Soft tissue swelling, inflammation, or restriction is reduced.
  - Tissue perfusion and oxygenation are enhanced.
- Impact on impairments
  - Aerobic capacity is increased.
  - Balance is improved.
  - Endurance is increased.
  - Energy expenditure per unit of work is decreased.
  - Joint integrity and mobility are improved.
  - Motor function (motor control and motor learning) is improved.
  - Muscle performance (strength, power, and endurance) is increased.
  - Postural control is improved.
  - Quality and quantity of movement between and across body segments are improved.
  - Range of motion is improved.
  - Relaxation is increased.
  - Sensory awareness is increased.
  - Weight-bearing status is improved.
- Impact on functional limitations
  - Ability to perform physical actions, tasks, or activities related to self-care, home management, work (job/school/play), community, and leisure is improved.
  - Level of supervision required for task performance is decreased.
  - Performance of and independence in activities of daily living (ADL) and instrumental activities of daily living (IADL) with or without devices and equipment are increased.
  - Tolerance of positions and activities is increased.
- Impact on disabilities
  - Ability to assume or resume required self-care, home management, work (job/school/play), community, and leisure roles is improved.
- Risk reduction/prevention
  - Preoperative and postoperative complications are reduced.
  - Risk factors are reduced.
  - Risk of recurrence of condition is reduced.
  - Risk of secondary impairment is reduced.
  - Safety is improved.
  - Self-management of symptoms is improved.
- Impact on health, wellness, and fitness
  - Fitness is improved.
  - Health status is improved.
  - Physical capacity is increased.
  - Physical function is improved.
- Impact on societal resources
  - Utilization of physical therapy services is optimized.
  - Utilization of physical therapy services results in efficient use of health care dollars.
- Patient/client satisfaction
  - Access, availability, and services provided are acceptable to patient/client.
  - Administrative management of practice is acceptable to patient/client.
  - Clinical proficiency of physical therapist is acceptable to patient/client.
  - Coordination of care is acceptable to patient/client.
  - Cost of health care services is decreased.
  - Intensity of care is decreased.
  - Interpersonal skills of physical therapist are acceptable to patient/client, family, and significant others.
  - Sense of well-being is improved.
  - Stressors are decreased.

Functional Training in Self-Care and Home Management (Including Activities of Daily Living [ADL] and Instrumental Activities of Daily Living [IADL])

Interventions

- ADL training
  - bathing
  - bed mobility and transfer training
  - developmental activities
  - dressing
  - eating
  - grooming
  - toileting
- Devices and equipment use and training
  - assistive and adaptive device or equipment training during ADL and IADL
  - orthotic, protective, or supportive device or equipment training during ADL and IADL
- Functional training programs
  - back schools
  - simulated environments and tasks
  - task adaptation
- IADL training
  - caring for dependents
  - home maintenance
  - household chores
  - shopping
  - structured play for infants and children
  - yard work
- Injury prevention or reduction
  - injury prevention education during self-care and home management
  - injury prevention or reduction with use of devices and equipment
  - safety awareness training during self-care and home management

Anticipated Goals and Expected Outcomes

- Impact on pathology/pathophysiology (disease, disorder, or condition)
  - Pain is decreased.
  - Physiological response to increased oxygen demand is improved.
- Impact on impairments
  - Balance is improved.
  - Endurance is increased.
  - Energy expenditure per unit of work is decreased.
  - Motor function (motor control and motor learning) is improved.
  - Muscle performance (strength, power, and endurance) is increased.
  - Postural control is improved.
  - Sensory awareness is increased.
  - Weight-bearing status is improved.
- Impact on functional limitations
  - Ability to perform physical actions, tasks, or activities related to self-care and home management is improved.
  - Level of supervision required for task performance is decreased.
  - Performance of and independence in ADL and IADL with or without devices and equipment are increased.
  - Tolerance of positions and activities is increased.
- Impact on disabilities
  - Ability to assume or resume required self-care and home management roles is improved.
- Risk reduction/prevention
  - Risk factors are reduced.
  - Risk of secondary impairments is reduced.
  - Safety is improved.
  - Self-management of symptoms is improved.
- Impact on health, wellness, and fitness
  - Fitness is improved.
  - Health status is improved.
  - Physical capacity is increased.
  - Physical function is improved.
- Impact on societal resources
  - Utilization of physical therapy services is optimized.
  - Utilization of physical therapy services results in efficient use of health care dollars.
- Patient/client satisfaction
  - Access, availability, and services provided are acceptable to patient/client.
  - Administrative management of practice is acceptable to patient/client.
  - Clinical proficiency of physical therapist is acceptable to patient/client.
  - Coordination of care is acceptable to patient/client.
  - Cost of health care services is decreased.
  - Intensity of care is decreased.
  - Interpersonal skills of physical therapist are acceptable to patient/client, family, and significant others.
  - Sense of well-being is improved.
  - Stressors are decreased.

Functional Training in Work (Job/School/Play), Community, and Leisure Integration or Reintegration (Including Instrumental Activities of Daily Living [IADL], Work Hardening, and Work Conditioning)

Interventions

- Devices and equipment use and training
  - assistive and adaptive device or equipment training during IADL
  - orthotic, protective, or supportive device or equipment training during IADL
- Functional training programs
  - back schools
  - job coaching
  - simulated environments and tasks
  - task adaptation
  - task training
- IADL training
  - community service training involving instruments
  - school and play activities training including tools and instruments
  - work training with tools
- Injury prevention or reduction
  - injury prevention education during work (job/school/play), community, and leisure integration or reintegration
  - injury prevention or reduction with use of devices and equipment
  - safety awareness training during work (job/school/play), community, and leisure integration or reintegration
- Leisure and play activities and training

Anticipated Goals and Expected Outcomes

- Impact on pathology/pathophysiology (disease, disorder, or condition)
  - Pain is decreased.
  - Physiological response to increased oxygen demand is improved.
- Impact on impairments
  - Balance is improved.
  - Endurance is increased.
  - Energy expenditure per unit of work is decreased.
  - Motor function (motor control and motor learning) is improved.
  - Muscle performance (strength, power, and endurance) is increased.
  - Postural control is improved.
  - Sensory awareness is increased.
  - Weight-bearing status is improved.
- Impact on functional limitations
  - Ability to perform physical actions, tasks, or activities related to work (job/school/play), community, and leisure integration or reintegration is increased.
  - Level of supervision required for task performance is decreased.
  - Performance of and independence in IADL with or without devices and equipment are increased.
  - Tolerance of positions and activities is increased.
- Impact on disabilities
  - Ability to assume or resume required work (job/school/play), community, and leisure roles is improved.
- Risk reduction/prevention
  - Risk factors are reduced.
  - Risk of secondary impairment is reduced.
  - Safety is improved.
  - Self-management of symptoms is improved.
- Impact on health, wellness, and fitness
  - Fitness is improved.
  - Health status is improved.
  - Physical capacity is increased.
  - Physical function is improved.
- Impact on societal resources
  - Costs of work-related injury or disability are reduced.
  - Utilization of physical therapy services is optimized.
  - Utilization of physical therapy services results in efficient use of health care dollars.
- Patient/client satisfaction
  - Access, availability, and services provided are acceptable to patient/client.
  - Administrative management of practice is acceptable to patient/client.
  - Clinical proficiency of physical therapist is acceptable to patient/client.
  - Coordination of care is acceptable to patient/client.
  - Cost of health care services is decreased.
  - Intensity of care is decreased.
  - Interpersonal skills of physical therapist are acceptable to patient/client, family, and significant others.
  - Sense of well-being is improved.
  - Stressors are decreased.

Manual Therapy Techniques (Including Mobilization/Manipulation)

Interventions

- Manual traction
- Massage
  - connective tissue massage
  - therapeutic massage
- Mobilization/manipulation
  - soft tissue
  - spinal and peripheral joints
- Passive range of motion

Anticipated Goals and Expected Outcomes

- Impact on pathology/pathophysiology (disease, disorder, or condition)
  - Edema, lymphedema, or effusion is reduced.
  - Joint swelling, inflammation, or restriction is reduced.
  - Neural compression is decreased.
  - Pain is decreased.
  - Soft tissue swelling, inflammation, or restriction is reduced.
- Impact on impairments
  - Balance is improved.
  - Energy expenditure per unit of work is decreased.
  - Gait, locomotion, and balance are improved.
  - Joint integrity and mobility are improved.
  - Muscle performance (strength, power, and endurance) is increased.
  - Postural control is improved.
  - Quality and quantity of movement between and across body segments are improved.
  - Range of motion is improved.
  - Relaxation is increased.
  - Sensory awareness is increased.
  - Weight-bearing status is improved.
- Impact on functional limitations
  - Ability to perform movement tasks is improved.
  - Ability to perform physical actions, tasks, or activities related to self-care, home management, work (job/school/play), community, and leisure is improved.
  - Tolerance of positions and activities is increased.
- Impact on disabilities
  - Ability to assume or resume required self-care, home management, work (job/school/play), community, and leisure roles is improved.
- Risk reduction/prevention
  - Risk factors are reduced.
  - Risk of recurrence of condition is reduced.
  - Risk of secondary impairment is reduced.
  - Self-management of symptoms is improved.
- Impact on health, wellness, and fitness
  - Fitness is improved.
  - Physical capacity is increased.
  - Physical function is improved.
- Impact on societal resources
  - Utilization of physical therapy services is optimized.
  - Utilization of physical therapy services results in efficient use of health care dollars.
- Patient/client satisfaction
  - Access, availability, and services provided are acceptable to patient/client.
  - Administrative management of practice is acceptable to patient/client.
  - Clinical proficiency of physical therapist is acceptable to patient/client.
  - Coordination of care is acceptable to patient/client.
  - Cost of health care services is decreased.
  - Intensity of care is decreased.
  - Interpersonal skills of physical therapist are acceptable to patient/client, family, and significant others.
  - Sense of well-being is improved.
  - Stressors are decreased.

Prescription, Application, and, as Appropriate, Fabrication of Devices and Equipment (Assistive, Adaptive, Orthotic, Protective, Supportive, and Prosthetic)

Interventions

- Adaptive devices
  - hospital beds
  - raised toilet seats
  - seating systems
- Assistive devices
  - canes
  - crutches
  - long-handled reachers
  - power devices
  - static and dynamic splints
  - walkers
  - wheelchairs
- Orthotic devices
  - braces
  - casts
  - shoe inserts
  - splints
- Protective devices
  - braces
  - cushions
  - protective taping
- Supportive devices
  - compression garments
  - corsets
  - elastic wraps
  - neck collars
  - serial casts
  - slings
  - supportive taping

Anticipated Goals and Expected Outcomes

- Impact on pathology/pathophysiology (disease, disorder, or condition)
  - Edema, lymphedema, or effusion is reduced.
  - Joint swelling, inflammation, or restriction is reduced.
  - Pain is decreased.
  - Physiological response to increased oxygen demand is improved.
  - Soft tissue swelling, inflammation, or restriction is reduced.
- Impact on impairments
  - Balance is improved.
  - Endurance is increased.
  - Energy expenditure per unit of work is decreased.
  - Gait, locomotion, and balance are improved.
  - Joint stability is improved.
  - Muscle performance (strength, power, and endurance) is increased.
  - Optimal joint alignment is achieved.
  - Optimal loading on a body part is achieved.
  - Postural control is improved.
  - Quality and quantity of movement between and across body segments are improved.
  - Range of motion is improved.
  - Weight-bearing status is improved.
- Impact on functional limitations
  - Ability to perform physical actions, tasks, or activities related to self-care, home management, work (job/school/play), community, and leisure is improved.
  - Level of supervision required for task performance is decreased.
  - Performance of and independence in activities of daily living (ADL) and instrumental activities of daily living (IADL) with or without devices and equipment are increased.
  - Tolerance of positions and activities is increased.
- Impact on disabilities
  - Ability to assume or resume required self-care, home management, work (job/school/play), community, and leisure roles is improved.
- Risk reduction/prevention
  - Pressure on body tissues is reduced.
  - Protection of body parts is increased.
  - Risk factors are reduced.
  - Risk of recurrence of condition is reduced.
  - Risk of secondary impairment is reduced.
  - Safety is improved.
  - Self-management of symptoms is improved.
  - Stresses precipitating injury are decreased.
- Impact on health, wellness, and fitness
  - Fitness is improved.
  - Health status is improved.
  - Physical capacity is increased.
  - Physical function is improved.
- Impact on societal resources
  - Utilization of physical therapy services is optimized.
  - Utilization of physical therapy services results in efficient use of health care dollars.
- Patient/client satisfaction
  - Access, availability, and services provided are acceptable to patient/client.
  - Administrative management of practice is acceptable to patient/client.
  - Clinical proficiency of physical therapist is acceptable to patient/client.
  - Coordination of care is acceptable to patient/client.
  - Cost of health care services is decreased.
  - Intensity of care is decreased.
  - Interpersonal skills of physical therapist are acceptable to patient/client, family, and significant others.
  - Sense of well-being is improved.
  - Stressors are decreased.

Electrotherapeutic Modalities

Interventions

- Electrotherapeutic delivery of medications
  - iontophoresis
- Electrical stimulation
  - electrical muscle stimulation (EMS)
  - functional electrical stimulation (FES)
  - high voltage pulsed current (HVPC)
  - neuromuscular electrical stimulation (NMES)
  - transcutaneous electrical nerve stimulation (TENS)

Anticipated Goals and Expected Outcomes

- Impact on pathology/pathophysiology (disease, disorder, or condition)
  - Edema, lymphedema, or effusion is reduced.
  - Joint swelling, inflammation, or restriction is reduced.
  - Nutrient delivery to tissue is increased.
  - Osteogenic effects are enhanced.
  - Pain is decreased.
  - Soft tissue or wound healing is enhanced.
  - Soft tissue swelling, inflammation, or restriction is reduced.
  - Tissue perfusion and oxygenation are enhanced.
- Impact on impairments
  - Integumentary integrity is improved.
  - Motor function (motor control and motor learning) is improved.
  - Muscle performance (strength, power, and endurance) is increased.
  - Postural control is improved.
  - Quality and quantity of movement between and across body segments are improved.
  - Range of motion is improved.
  - Relaxation is increased.
  - Sensory awareness is increased.
- Impact on functional limitations
  - Ability to perform physical actions, tasks, or activities related to self-care, home management, work (job/school/play), community, and leisure is improved.
  - Level of supervision required for task performance is decreased.
  - Performance of and independence in activities of daily living (ADL) and instrumental activities of daily living (IADL) with or without devices and equipment are increased.
  - Tolerance of positions and activities is increased.
- Impact on disabilities
  - Ability to assume or resume required self-care, home management, work (job/school/play), community, and leisure roles is improved.
- Risk reduction/prevention
  - Preoperative and postoperative complications are reduced.
  - Risk factors are reduced.
  - Risk of recurrence of condition is reduced.
  - Risk of secondary impairment is reduced.
  - Self-management of symptoms is improved.
- Impact on health, wellness, and fitness
  - Fitness is improved.
  - Physical capacity is increased.
  - Physical function is improved.
- Impact on societal resources
  - Utilization of physical therapy services is optimized.
  - Utilization of physical therapy services results in efficient use of health care dollars.
- Patient/client satisfaction
  - Access, availability, and services provided are acceptable to patient/client.
  - Administrative management of practice is acceptable to patient/client.
  - Clinical proficiency of physical therapist is acceptable to patient/client.
  - Coordination of care is acceptable to patient/client.
  - Interpersonal skills of physical therapist are acceptable to patient/client, family, and significant others.
  - Sense of well-being is improved.
  - Stressors are decreased.

Physical Agents and Mechanical Modalities

Interventions

Physical agents may include:

- Athermal agents
  - pulsed electromagnetic fields
- Cryotherapy
  - cold packs
  - ice massage
  - vapocoolant spray
- Hydrotherapy
  - whirlpool tanks
  - contrast bath
  - pools
- Light agents
  - infrared
  - laser
- Sound agents
  - phonophoresis
  - ultrasound
- Thermotherapy
  - dry heat
  - hot packs
  - paraffin baths

Mechanical modalities may include:

- Compression therapies
  - taping
- Traction devices
  - intermittent
  - positional
  - sustained

Anticipated Goals and Expected Outcomes

- Impact on pathology/pathophysiology (disease, disorder, or condition)
  - Edema, lymphedema, or effusion is reduced.
  - Joint swelling, inflammation, or restriction is reduced.
  - Neural compression is decreased.
  - Nutrient delivery to tissue is increased.
  - Pain is decreased.
  - Soft tissue swelling, inflammation, or restriction is reduced.
  - Tissue perfusion and oxygenation are enhanced.
- Impact on impairments
  - Muscle performance (strength, power, and endurance) is increased.
  - Postural control is improved.
  - Range of motion is improved.
  - Weight-bearing status is improved.
- Impact on functional limitations
  - Ability to perform physical actions, tasks, or activities related to self-care, home management, work (job/school/play), community, and leisure is improved.
  - Performance of and independence in activities of daily living (ADL) and instrumental activities of daily living (IADL) with or without devices and equipment are increased.
  - Tolerance of positions and activities is increased.
- Impact on disabilities
  - Ability to assume or resume required self-care, home management, work (job/school/play), community, and leisure roles is improved.
- Risk reduction/prevention
  - Complications of soft tissue and circulatory disorders are decreased.
  - Risk of secondary impairment is reduced.
  - Self-management of symptoms is improved.
  - Stresses precipitating injury are decreased.
- Impact on health, wellness, and fitness
  - Fitness is improved.
  - Physical function is improved.
- Impact on societal resources
  - Utilization of physical therapy services is optimized.
- Patient/client satisfaction
  - Access, availability, and services provided are acceptable to patient/client.
  - Administrative management of practice is acceptable to patient/client.
  - Clinical proficiency of physical therapist is acceptable to patient/client.
  - Coordination of care is acceptable to patient/client.
  - Interpersonal skills of physical therapist are acceptable to patient/client, family, and significant others.
  - Sense of well-being is improved.
  - Stressors are decreased.

Reexamination

Reexamination is the process of performing selected tests and measures after the initial examination to evaluate progress and to modify or redirect interventions. Reexamination may be indicated more than once during a single episode of care. It also may be performed over the course of a disease, disorder, or condition, which for some patients/clients may be over the life span. Indications for reexamination include new clinical findings or failure to respond to physical therapy interventions.

Global Outcomes for Patients/Clients in This Pattern

Throughout the entire episode of care, the physical therapist determines the anticipated goals and expected outcomes for each intervention. These anticipated goals and expected outcomes are delineated in shaded boxes that accompany the lists of interventions in each preferred practice pattern. As the patient/client reaches the termination of physical therapy services and the end of the episode of care, the physical therapist measures the global outcomes of the physical therapy services by characterizing or quantifying the impact of the physical therapy interventions in the following domains:

- Pathology/pathophysiology (disease, disorder, or condition)
- Impairments
- Functional limitations
- Disabilities
- Risk reduction/prevention
- Health, wellness, and fitness
- Societal resources
- Patient/client satisfaction

In some instances, a particular anticipated goal or expected outcome is thoroughly achieved through implementation of a single form of intervention. More commonly, however, the anticipated goals and expected outcomes are achieved as a result of the combined effects of several forms of interventions, leading to enhancement of both health status and health-related quality of life.

Criteria for Termination of Physical Therapy Services

Discharge is the process of ending physical therapy services that have been provided during a single episode of care. It occurs when the anticipated goals and expected outcomes have been achieved. Discharge does *not* occur with a *transfer* (defined as the time when a patient is moved from one site to another site within the same setting or across settings during a single episode of care). Although there may be facility-specific or payer-specific requirements for documentation regarding the conclusion of physical therapy services, *discharge occurs based on the physical therapist's analysis of the achievement of anticipated goals and expected outcomes.*

Discontinuation is the process of ending physical therapy services that have been provided during a single episode of care when (1) the patient/client, caregiver, or legal guardian declines to continue intervention; (2) the patient/client is unable to continue to progress toward outcomes because of medical or psychosocial complications or because financial/insurance resources have been expended; or (3) the physical therapist determines that the patient/client will no longer benefit from physical therapy. When physical therapy services are terminated prior to achievement of anticipated goals and expected outcomes, patient/client status and the rationale for termination are documented.

For patients/clients who require multiple episodes of care, periodic follow-up is needed over the life span to ensure safety and effective adaptation following changes in physical status, caregivers, environment, or task demands. In consultation with appropriate individuals, and in consideration of the outcomes, the physical therapist plans for discharge or discontinuation and provides for appropriate follow-up or referral.

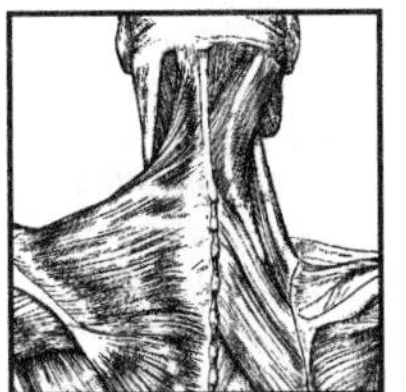

Impaired Joint Mobility, Muscle Performance, and Range of Motion Associated With Fracture

This preferred practice pattern describes the generally accepted elements of patient/client management that physical therapists provide for patients/clients who are classified in this pattern. The pattern title reflects the diagnosis made by the physical therapist. APTA emphasizes that preferred practice patterns are the boundaries within which a physical therapist may select any of a number of clinical alternatives, based on consideration of a wide variety of factors, such as individual patient/client needs; the profession's code of ethics and standards of practice; and patient/client age, culture, gender roles, race, sex, sexual orientation, and socioeconomic status.

Patient/Client Diagnostic Classification

Patients/clients will be classified into this pattern—for impaired joint mobility, muscle performance, and range of motion associated with fracture—as a result of the physical therapist's evaluation of the examination data. The findings from the examination (history, systems review, and tests and measures) may indicate the presence or risk of pathology/pathophysiology (disease, disorder, or condition), impairments, functional limitations, or disabilities or the need for health, wellness, or fitness programs. The physical therapist integrates, synthesizes, and interprets the data to determine the diagnostic classification.

Inclusion

The following examples of examination findings may support the inclusion of patients/clients in this pattern:

Risk Factors or Consequences of Pathology/Pathophysiology (Disease, Disorder, or Condition)

- Bone demineralization
- Fracture
- Hormonal changes
- Medications (eg, anti-epileptic medications, steroids, thyroid hormone)
- Menopause
- Nutritional deficiency
- Prolonged non-weight-bearing state
- Trauma

Impairments, Functional Limitations, or Disabilities

- Inability to access community
- Limited range of motion
- Muscle weakness from immobilization
- Pain with functional movements and activities

Note:

Some risk factors or consequences of pathology/pathophysiology—such as *neoplasm*—may be severe and complex; *however, they do not necessarily exclude patients/clients from this pattern.* Severe and complex risk factors or consequences may require modification of the frequency of visits and duration of care. (See "Evaluation, Diagnosis, and Prognosis," page 239.)

Exclusion or Multiple-Pattern Classification

The following examples of examination findings may support exclusion from this pattern or classification into additional patterns. Depending on the level of severity or complexity of the examination findings, the physical therapist may determine that the patient/client would be more appropriately managed through (1) classification in an entirely different pattern or (2) classification in both this and another pattern.

Findings That May Require Classification in a Different Pattern

- Flail chest

Findings That May Require Classification in Additional Patterns

- Osteogenesis imperfecta

ICD-9-CM Codes

The listing below contains the current (as of press time) and most typical 3- and 4-digit ICD-9-CM codes related to this preferred practice pattern. Because patient/client diagnostic classification is based on impairments, functional limitations, and disabilities—not on codes—patients/clients may be classified into the pattern even though the codes listed with the pattern may not apply to those clients.

This listing is intended for general information only and should not be used for coding purposes. The codes should be confirmed by referring to the World Health Organization's *International Classification of Diseases, 9th Revision, Clinical Modification (ICD-9-CM 2001)*, Volumes 1 and 3 (Chicago, Ill: American Medical Association; 2000) or subsequent revisions or by referring to other ICD-9-CM coding manuals that contain exclusion notes and instructions regarding fifth-digit requirements.

170 Malignant neoplasm of bone and articular cartilage
213 Benign neoplasm of bone and articular cartilage
262 Other severe, protein-calorie malnutrition
263 Other and unspecified protein-calorie malnutrition
268 Vitamin D deficiency
269 Other nutritional deficiencies
275 Disorders of mineral metabolism
627 Menopausal and postmenopausal disorders
715 Osteoarthrosis and allied disorders
719 Other and unspecified disorders of joint
- **719.5** Stiffness of joint, not elsewhere classified
- **719.8** Other specified disorders of joint
  - Calcification of joint

728 Disorders of muscle, ligament, and fascia
- **728.1** Muscular calcification and ossification

729 Other disorders of soft tissues
- **729.9** Other and unspecified disorders of soft tissue

730 Osteomyelitis, periostitis, and other infections involving bone
732 Osteochondropathies
- **732.4** Juvenile osteochondrosis of lower extremity, excluding foot

733 Other disorders of bone and cartilage
- **733.0** Osteoporosis
- **733.1** Pathologic fracture
- **733.2** Cyst of bone
- **733.4** Aseptic necrosis of bone
- **733.8** Malunion and nonunion of fracture
- **733.9** Other and unspecified disorders of bone and cartilage

736 Other acquired deformities of limbs
- **736.8** Acquired deformities of other parts of limbs

802 Fracture of face bones
805 Fracture of vertebral column without mention of spinal cord injury
- **805.6** Sacrum and coccyx, closed

808 Fracture of pelvis
810 Fracture of clavicle
811 Fracture of scapula
812 Fracture of humerus
813 Fracture of radius and ulna
- **813.4** Lower end, closed
- **813.5** Lower end, open

814 Fracture of carpal bone(s)
815 Fracture of metacarpal bone(s)
816 Fracture of one or more phalanges of hand
819 Multiple fractures involving both upper limbs, and upper limbs with ribs(s) and sternum
820 Fracture of neck of femur
821 Fracture of other and unspecified parts of femur
822 Fracture of patella
823 Fracture of tibia and fibula
824 Fracture of ankle
825 Fracture of one or more tarsal and metatarsal bones
826 Fracture of one or more phalanges of foot
827 Other, multiple, and ill-defined fractures of lower limb
828 Multiple fractures involving both lower limbs, lower with upper limb, and lower limb(s) with rib(s) and sternum
829 Fracture of unspecified bones

Examination

Examination is a comprehensive screening and specific testing process that leads to a diagnostic classification or, when appropriate, to a referral to another practitioner. Examination is required prior to the initial intervention and is performed for all patients/clients. Through the examination, the physical therapist may identify impairments, functional limitations, disabilities, changes in physical function or overall health status, and needs related to restoration of health and to prevention, wellness, and fitness. The physical therapist synthesizes the examination findings to establish the diagnosis and the prognosis (including the plan of care). The patient/client, family, significant others, and caregivers may provide information during the examination process.

Examination has three components: the patient/client history, the systems review, and tests and measures. The *history* is a systematic gathering of past and current information (often from the patient/client) related to why the patient/client is seeking the services of the physical therapist. The *systems review* is a brief or limited examination of (1) the anatomical and physiological status of the cardiovascular/pulmonary, integumentary, musculoskeletal, and neuromuscular systems and (2) the communication ability, affect, cognition, language, and learning style of the patient/client. *Tests and measures* are the means of gathering data about the patient/client.

The selection of examination procedures and the depth of the examination vary based on patient/client age; severity of the problem; stage of recovery (acute, subacute, chronic); phase of rehabilitation (early, intermediate, late, return to activity); home, work (job/school/play), or community situation; and other relevant factors. *For clinical indications in selecting tests and measures and for listings of tests and measures, tools used to gather data, and the types of data generated by tests and measures, refer to Chapter 2.*

Patient/Client History

The history may include:

General Demographics

- Age
- Sex
- Race/ethnicity
- Primary language
- Education

Social History

- Cultural beliefs and behaviors
- Family and caregiver resources
- Social interactions, social activities, and support systems

Employment/Work (Job/School/Play)

- Current and prior work (job/school/play), community, and leisure actions, tasks, or activities

Growth and Development

- Developmental history
- Hand dominance

Living Environment

- Devices and equipment (eg, assistive, adaptive, orthotic, protective, supportive, prosthetic)
- Living environment and community characteristics
- Projected discharge destinations

General Health Status (Self-Report, Family Report, Caregiver Report)

- General health perception
- Physical function (eg, mobility, sleep patterns, restricted bed days)
- Psychological function (eg, memory, reasoning ability, depression, anxiety)
- Role function (eg, community, leisure, social, work)
- Social function (eg, social activity, social interaction, social support)

Social/Health Habits (Past and Current)

- Behavioral health risks (eg, smoking, drug abuse)
- Level of physical fitness

Family History

- Familial health risks

Medical/Surgical History

- Cardiovascular
- Endocrine/metabolic
- Gastrointestinal
- Genitourinary
- Gynecological
- Integumentary
- Musculoskeletal
- Neuromuscular
- Obstetrical
- Prior hospitalizations, surgeries, and preexisting medical and other health-related conditions
- Psychological
- Pulmonary

Current Condition(s)/Chief Complaint(s)

- Concerns that led patient/client to seek the services of a physical therapist
- Concerns or needs of patient/client who requires the services of a physical therapist
- Current therapeutic interventions
- Mechanisms of injury or disease, including date of onset and course of events
- Onset and pattern of symptoms
- Patient/client, family, significant other, and caregiver expectations and goals for the therapeutic intervention
- Patient/client, family, significant other, and caregiver perceptions of patient's/client's emotional response to the current clinical situation
- Previous occurrence of chief complaint(s)
- Prior therapeutic interventions

Functional Status and Activity Level

- Current and prior functional status in self-care and home management activities, including activities of daily living (ADL) and instrumental activities of daily living (IADL)
- Current and prior functional status in work (job/school/play), community, and leisure actions, tasks, or activities

Medications

- Medications for current condition
- Medications previously taken for current condition
- Medications for other conditions

Other Clinical Tests

- Laboratory and diagnostic tests
- Review of available records (eg, medical, education, surgical)
- Review of other clinical findings (eg, nutrition and hydration)

Systems Review

The systems review may include:

Anatomical and Physiological Status

- Cardiovascular/Pulmonary
  - Blood pressure
  - Edema
  - Heart rate
  - Respiratory rate
- Integumentary
  - Pliability (texture)
  - Presence of scar formation
  - Skin color
  - Skin integrity
- Musculoskeletal
  - Gross range of motion
  - Gross strength
  - Gross symmetry
  - Height
  - Weight
- Neuromuscular
  - Gross coordinated movements (eg, balance, gait, locomotion, transfers, transitions)
  - Motor function (motor control, motor learning)

Communication, Affect, Cognition, Language, and Learning Style

- Ability to make needs known
- Consciousness
- Expected emotional/behavioral responses
- Learning preferences (eg, education needs, learning barriers)
- Orientation (person, place, time)

Tests and Measures

Tests and measures for this pattern may include those that characterize or quantify:

Aerobic Capacity and Endurance

- Aerobic capacity during functional activities (eg, activities of daily living [ADL] scales, indexes, instrumental activities of daily living [IADL] scales, observations)

Anthropometric Characteristics

- Body composition (eg, body mass index, impedance measurement, skinfold thickness measurement)
- Body dimensions (eg, girth measurement, length measurement)
- Edema (eg, girth measurement, palpation, scales, volume measurement)

Assistive and Adaptive Devices

- Assistive or adaptive devices and equipment use during functional activities (eg, activities of daily living [ADL] scales, functional scales, instrumental activities of daily living [IADL] scales, interviews, observations)
- Components, alignment, fit, and ability to care for the assistive or adaptive devices and equipment (eg, interviews, logs, observations, pressure-sensing maps, reports)
- Remediation of impairments, functional limitations, or disabilities with use of assistive or adaptive devices and equipment (eg, activity status indexes, ADL scales, aerobic capacity tests, functional performance inventories, health assessment questionnaires, IADL scales, pain scales, play scales, videographic assessments)
- Safety during use of assistive or adaptive devices and equipment (eg, diaries, fall scales, interviews, logs, observations, reports)

Cranial and Peripheral Nerve Integrity

- Electrophysiological integrity (eg, electroneuromyography)
- Motor distribution of the cranial nerves (eg, dynamometry, muscle tests, observations)
- Motor distribution of the peripheral nerves (eg, dynamometry, muscle tests, observations, thoracic outlet tests)
- Sensory distribution of the cranial nerves (eg, discrimination tests; tactile tests, including coarse and light touch, cold and heat, pain, pressure, and vibration)
- Sensory distribution of the peripheral nerves (eg, discrimination tests; tactile tests, including coarse and light touch, cold and heat, pain, pressure, and vibration; thoracic outlet tests)

Environmental, Home, and Work (Job/School/Play) Barriers

- Current and potential barriers (eg, checklists, interviews, observations, questionnaires)

Ergonomics and Body Mechanics

Ergonomics

- Dexterity and coordination during work (job/school/play) (eg, hand function tests, impairment rating scales, manipulative ability tests)
- Functional capacity and performance during work actions, tasks, or activities (eg, accelerometry, dynamometry, electroneuromyography, endurance tests, force platform tests, goniometry, interviews, observations, photographic assessments, physical capacity tests, postural loading analyses, technology-assisted assessments, videographic assessments, work analyses)
- Safety in work environments (eg, hazard identification checklists, job severity indexes, lifting standards, risk assessment scales, standards for exposure limits)
- Specific work conditions or activities (eg, handling checklists, job simulations, lifting models, preemployment screenings, task analysis checklists, workstation checklists)
- Tools, devices, equipment, and workstations related to work actions, tasks, or activities (eg, observations, tool analysis checklists, vibration assessments)

Body mechanics

- Body mechanics during self-care, home management, work, community, or leisure actions, tasks, or activities (eg, ADL scales, IADL scales, observations, photographic assessments, technology-assisted assessments, videographic assessments)

Gait, Locomotion, and Balance

- Balance during functional activities with or without the use of assistive, adaptive, orthotic, protective, supportive, or prosthetic devices or equipment (eg, ADL scales, IADL scales, observations, videographic assessments)
- Balance (dynamic and static) with or without the use of assistive, adaptive, orthotic, protective, supportive, or prosthetic devices or equipment (eg, balance scales, dizziness inventories, dynamic posturography, fall scales, motor impairment tests, observations, photographic assessments, postural control tests)
- Gait and locomotion during functional activities with or without the use of assistive, adaptive, orthotic, protective, supportive, or prosthetic devices or equipment (eg, ADL scales, gait indexes, IADL scales, mobility skill profiles, observations, videographic assessments)
- Gait and locomotion with or without the use of assistive, adaptive, orthotic, protective, supportive, or prosthetic devices or equipment (eg, dynamometry, electroneuromyography, footprint analyses, gait indexes, mobility skill profiles, observations, photographic assessments, technology-assisted assessments, videographic assessments, weight-bearing scales, wheelchair mobility tests)
- Safety during gait, locomotion, and balance (eg, confidence scales, diaries, fall scales, functional assessment profiles, logs, reports)

Integumentary Integrity

Associated skin

- Activities, positioning, and postures that produce or relieve trauma to the skin (eg, observations, pressure-sensing maps, scales)
- Assistive, adaptive, orthotic, protective, supportive or prosthetic devices and equipment that may produce or relieve trauma to the skin (eg, observations, pressure-sensing maps, risk assessment scales)
- Skin characteristics, including blistering, continuity of skin color, dermatitis, hair growth, mobility, nail growth, sensation, temperature, texture, and turgor (eg, observations, palpation, photographic assessments, thermography)

Joint Integrity and Mobility

- Joint integrity and mobility (eg, apprehension, compression and distraction, drawer, glide, impingement, shear, and valgus/varus stress tests; arthrometry; palpation)
- Joint play movements, including end feel (all joints of the axial and appendicular skeletal system) (eg, palpation)

Motor Function (Motor Control and Motor Learning)

- Dexterity, coordination, and agility (eg, coordination screens, motor impairment tests, motor proficiency tests, observations, videographic assessments)
- Hand function (eg, fine and gross motor control tests, finger dexterity tests, manipulative ability tests, observations)

Muscle Performance (Including Strength, Power, and Endurance)

- Electrophysiological integrity (eg, electroneuromyography)
- Muscle strength, power, and endurance (eg, dynamometry, manual muscle tests, muscle performance tests, physical capacity tests, technology-assisted assessments, timed activity tests)
- Muscle strength, power, and endurance during functional activities (eg, ADL scales, functional muscle tests, IADL scales, observations, videographic assessments)
- Muscle tension (eg, palpation)

Orthotic, Protective, and Supportive Devices

- Components, alignment, fit, and ability to care for orthotic, protective, and supportive devices and equipment (eg, interviews, logs, observations, pressure-sensing maps, reports)
- Orthotic, protective, and supportive devices and equipment use during functional activities (eg, ADL scales, functional scales, IADL scales, interviews, observations, profiles)
- Remediation of impairments, functional limitations, or disabilities with use of orthotic, protective, and supportive devices and equipment (eg, activity status indexes, ADL scales, aerobic capacity tests, functional performance inventories, health assessment questionnaires, IADL scales, pain scales, play scales, videographic assessments)
- Safety during use of orthotic, protective, and supportive devices and equipment (eg, diaries, fall scales, interviews, logs, observations, reports)

Pain

- Pain, soreness, and nociception (eg, analog scales, discrimination tests, pain drawings and maps, provocation tests, verbal and pictorial descriptor tests)
- Pain in specific body parts (eg, pain indexes, pain questionnaires, structural provocation tests)

Posture

- Postural alignment and position (static and dynamic), including symmetry and deviation from midline (eg, grid measurement, observations, photographic assessments, technology-assisted assessments, videographic assessments)
- Specific body parts (eg, angle assessments, forward-bending test, goniometry, observations, palpation, positional tests)

Range of Motion (ROM) (Including Muscle Length)

- Functional ROM (eg, observations, squat tests, toe touch tests)
- Joint active and passive movement (eg, goniometry, inclinometry, observations, photographic assessments, technology-assisted assessments, videographic assessments)
- Muscle length, soft tissue extensibility, and flexibility (eg, contracture tests, goniometry, inclinometry, ligamentous tests, linear measurement, multisegment flexibility tests, palpation)

Self-Care and Home Management (Including ADL and IADL)

- Ability to gain access to home environments (eg, barrier identification, observations, physical performance tests)
- Ability to perform self-care and home management activities with or without assistive, adaptive, orthotic, protective, supportive, or prosthetic devices and equipment (eg, ADL scales, aerobic capacity tests, IADL scales, interviews, observations, profiles)
- Safety in self-care and home management activities and environments (eg, diaries, fall scales, interviews, logs, observations, reports, videographic assessments)

Sensory Integrity

- Deep sensations (eg, kinesthesiometry, observations, photographic assessments, vibration tests)
- Electrophysiological integrity (eg, electroneuromyography)

Ventilation and Respiration/Gas Exchange

- Pulmonary signs of respiration/gas exchange, including breath sounds (eg, gas analyses, observations, oximetry)
- Pulmonary signs of ventilatory function, including airway protection; breath and voice sounds; respiratory rate, rhythm, and pattern; ventilatory flow, forces, and volumes (eg, airway clearance tests, observations, palpation, pulmonary function tests, ventilatory muscle force tests)
- Pulmonary symptoms (eg, dyspnea and perceived exertion indexes and scales)

Work (Job/School/Play), Community, and Leisure Integration or Reintegration (Including IADL)

- Ability to assume or resume work (job/school/play), community, and leisure activities with or without assistive, adaptive, orthotic, protective, supportive, or prosthetic devices and equipment (eg, activity profiles, disability indexes, functional status questionnaires, IADL scales, observations, physical capacity tests)
- Ability to gain access to work (job/school/play), community, and leisure environments (eg, barrier identification, interviews, observations, physical capacity tests, transportation assessments)
- Safety in work (job/school/play), community, and leisure activities and environments (eg, diaries, fall scales, interviews, logs, observations, videographic assessments)

Evaluation, Diagnosis, and Prognosis (Including Plan of Care)

Physical therapists perform *evaluations* (make clinical judgments) based on the data gathered from the history, systems review, and tests and measures. In the evaluation process, physical therapists synthesize the examination data to establish the diagnosis and prognosis (including the plan of care). Factors that influence the complexity of the evaluation include the clinical findings, extent of loss of function, chronicity or severity of the problem, possibility of multisite or multisystem involvement, preexisting condition(s), potential discharge destination, social considerations, physical function, and overall health status.

A *diagnosis* is a label encompassing a cluster of signs and symptoms, syndromes, or categories. It is the result of the systematic diagnostic process, which includes integrating and evaluating the data from the examination.The diagnostic label indicates the primary dysfunction(s) toward which the therapist will direct interventions. The *prognosis* is the determination of the predicted optimal level of improvement in function and the amount of time needed to reach that level and may also include a prediction of levels of improvement that may be reached at various intervals during the course of therapy. During the prognostic process, the physical therapist develops the plan of care. The *plan of care* identifies specific interventions, proposed frequency and duration of the interventions, anticipated goals, expected outcomes, and discharge plans. The plan of care identifies realistic anticipated goals and expected outcomes, taking into consideration the expectations of the patient/client and appropriate others.These anticipated goals and expected outcomes should be measureable and time limited.

The frequency of visits and duration of the episode of care may vary from a short episode with a high intensity of intervention to a longer episode with a diminishing intensity of intervention. Frequency and duration may vary greatly among patients/clients based on a variety of factors that the physical therapist considers throughout the evaluation process, such as anatomical and physiological changes related to growth and development; caregiver consistency or expertise; chronicity or severity of the current condition; living environment; multisite or multisystem involvement; social support; potential discharge destinations; probability of prolonged impairment, functional limitation, or disability; and stability of the condition.

Prognosis

Over the course of 3 to 6 months post-fracture, patient/client will demonstrate optimal joint mobility, muscle performance, and range of motion and the highest level of functioning in home, work (job/school/play), community, and leisure environments.

During the episode of care, patient/client will achieve (1) the anticipated goals and expected outcomes of the interventions that are described in the plan of care and (2) the global outcomes for patients/clients who are classified in this pattern.

Expected Range of Number of Visits Per Episode of Care

6 to 18

This range represents the lower and upper limits of the number of physical therapist visits required to achieve anticipated goals and expected outcomes. *It is anticipated that 80% of patients/clients who are classified into this pattern will achieve the anticipated goals and expected outcomes within 6 to 18 visits during a single continuous episode of care.* Frequency of visits and duration of the episode of care should be determined by the physical therapist to maximize effectiveness of care and efficiency of service delivery.

Factors That May Require New Episode of Care or That May Modify Frequency of Visits/ Duration of Episode

- Accessibility and availability of resources
- Adherence to the intervention program
- Age
- Anatomical and physiological changes related to growth and development
- Caregiver consistency or expertise
- Chronicity or severity of the current condition
- Cognitive status
- Comorbitities, complications, or secondary impairments
- Concurrent medical, surgical, and therapeutic interventions
- Decline in functional independence
- Level of impairment
- Level of physical function
- Living environment
- Multisite or multisystem involvement
- Nutritional status
- Overall health status
- Potential discharge destinations
- Premorbid conditions
- Probability of prolonged impairment, functional limitation, or disability
- Psychological and socioeconomic factors
- Psychomotor abilities
- Social support
- Stability of the condition

Intervention

Intervention is the purposeful interaction of the physical therapist with the patient/client and, when appropriate, with other individuals involved in patient/client care, using various physical therapy procedures and techniques to produce changes in the condition consistent with the diagnosis and prognosis. Decisions about interventions are contingent on the timely monitoring of patient/client response and the progress made toward achieving the anticipated goals and expected outcomes.

Communication, coordination, and documentation and patient/client-related instruction are provided for all patients/clients across all settings. Procedural interventions are selected or modified based on the examination data and the evaluation, the diagnosis and the prognosis, and the anticipated goals and expected outcomes for a particular patient/client. *For clinical considerations in selecting interventions, listings of interventions, and listings of anticipated goals and expected outcomes, refer to Chapter 3.*

Coordination, Communication, and Documentation

Coordination, communication, and documentation may include:

Interventions

- Addressing required functions
  - advance directives
  - individualized family service plans (IFSPs) or individualized education plans (IEPs)
  - informed consent
  - mandatory communication and reporting (eg, patient advocacy and abuse reporting)
- Admission and discharge planning
- Case management
- Collaboration and coordination with agencies, including:
  - equipment suppliers
  - home care agencies
  - payer groups
  - schools
  - transportation agencies
- Communication across settings, including:
  - case conferences
  - documentation
  - education plans
- Cost-effective resource utilization
- Data collection, analysis, and reporting
  - outcome data
  - peer review findings
  - record reviews
- Documentation across settings, following APTA's *Guidelines for Physical Therapy Documentation* (Appendix 5), including:
  - changes in impairments, functional limitations, and disabilities
  - changes in interventions
  - elements of patient/client management (examination, evaluation, diagnosis, prognosis, intervention)
  - outcomes of intervention
- Interdisciplinary teamwork
  - case conferences
  - patient care rounds
  - patient/client family meetings
- Referrals to other professionals or resources

Anticipated Goals and Expected Outcomes

- Accountability for services is increased.
- Admission data and discharge planning are completed.
- Advance directives, individualized family service plans (IFSPs) or individualized education plans (IEPs), informed consent, and mandatory communication and reporting (eg, patient advocacy and abuse reporting) are obtained or completed.
- Available resources are maximally utilized.
- Care is coordinated with patient/client, family, significant others, caregivers, and other professionals.
- Case is managed throughout the episode of care.
- Collaboration and coordination occurs with agencies, including equipment suppliers, home care agencies, payer groups, schools, and transportation agencies.
- Communication enhances risk reduction and prevention.
- Communication occurs across settings through case conferences, education plans, and documentation.
- Data are collected, analyzed, and reported, including outcome data, peer review findings, and record reviews.
- Decision making is enhanced regarding health, wellness, and fitness needs.
- Decision making is enhanced regarding patient/client health and the use of health care resources by patient/client, family, significant others, and caregivers.
- Documentation occurs throughout patient/client management and across settings and follows APTA's *Guidelines for Physical Therapy Documentation* (Appendix 5).
- Interdisciplinary collaboration occurs through case conferences, patient care rounds, and patient/client family meetings.
- Patient/client, family, significant other, and caregiver understanding of anticipated goals and expected outcomes is increased.
- Placement needs are determined.
- Referrals are made to other professionals or resources whenever necessary and appropriate.
- Resources are utilized in a cost-effective way.

Patient/Client-Related Instruction

Patient/client-related instruction may include:

Interventions

- Instruction, education and training of patients/clients and caregivers regarding:
  - current condition (pathology/pathophysiology [disease, disorder, or condition], impairments, functional limitations, or disabilities)
  - enhancement of performance
  - health, wellness, and fitness programs
  - plan of care
  - risk factors for pathology/pathophysiology (disease, disorder, or condition), impairments, functional limitations, or disabilities
  - transitions across settings
  - transitions to new roles

Anticipated Goals and Expected Outcomes

- Ability to perform physical actions, tasks, or activities is improved.
- Awareness and use of community resources are improved.
- Behaviors that foster healthy habits, wellness, and prevention are acquired.
- Decision making is enhanced regarding patient/client health and the use of health care resources by patient/client, family, significant others, and caregivers.
- Disability associated with acute or chronic illnesses is reduced.
- Functional independence in activities of daily living (ADL) and instrumental activities of daily living (IADL) is increased.
- Health status is improved.
- Intensity of care is decreased.
- Level of supervision required for task performance is decreased.
- Patient/client, family, significant other, and caregiver knowledge and awareness of the diagnosis, prognosis, interventions, and anticipated goals and expected outcomes are increased.
- Patient/client knowledge of personal and environmental factors associated with the condition is increased.
- Performance levels in self-care, home management, work (job/school/play), community, or leisure actions, tasks, or activities are improved.
- Physical function is improved.
- Risk of recurrence of condition is reduced.
- Risk of secondary impairment is reduced.
- Safety of patient/client, family, significant others, and caregivers is improved.
- Self-management of symptoms is improved.
- Utilization and cost of health care services are decreased.

Therapeutic Exercise

Interventions

- Aerobic capacity/endurance conditioning or reconditioning
  - aquatic programs
  - gait and locomotor training
  - increased workload over time
  - walking and wheelchair propulsion programs
- Balance, coordination, and agility training
  - developmental activities training
  - motor function (motor control and motor learning) training or retraining
  - neuromuscular education or reeducation
  - perceptual training
  - posture awareness training
  - standardized, programmatic, complementary exercise approaches
  - task-specific performance training
- Body mechanics and postural stabilization
  - body mechanics training
  - posture awareness training
  - postural control training
  - postural stabilization activities
- Flexibility exercises
  - muscle lengthening
  - range of motion
  - stretching
- Gait and locomotion training
  - developmental activities training
  - gait training
  - implement and device training
  - perceptual training
  - standardized, programmatic, complementary exercise approaches
  - wheelchair training
- Relaxation
  - breathing strategies
  - movement strategies
  - relaxation techniques
  - standardized, programmatic, complementary exercise approaches
- Strength, power, and endurance exercises for head, neck, limb, pelvic-floor, trunk, and ventilatory muscles
  - active assistive, active, and resistive exercises (including concentric, dynamic/isotonic, eccentric, isokinetic, isometric, and plyometric)
  - aquatic programs
  - standardized, programmatic, complementary exercise approaches
  - task-specific performance training

Anticipated Goals and Expected Outcomes

- Impact on pathology/pathophysiology (disease, disorder, or condition)
  - Joint swelling, inflammation, or restriction is reduced.
  - Nutrient delivery to tissue is increased.
  - Osteogenic effects of exercise are maximized.
  - Pain is decreased.
  - Physiological response to increased oxygen demand is improved.
  - Soft tissue swelling, inflammation, or restriction is reduced.
  - Tissue perfusion and oxygenation are enhanced.
- Impact on impairments
  - Aerobic capacity is increased.
  - Balance is improved.
  - Endurance is increased.
  - Energy expenditure per unit of work is decreased.
  - Gait, locomotion, and balance are improved.
  - Integumentary integrity is improved.
  - Joint integrity and mobility are improved.
  - Motor function (motor control and motor learning) is improved.
  - Muscle performance (strength, power, and endurance) is increased.
  - Postural control is improved.
  - Quality and quantity of movement between and across body segments are improved.
  - Range of motion is improved.
  - Relaxation is increased.
  - Sensory awareness is increased.
  - Weight-bearing status is improved.
- Impact on functional limitations
  - Ability to perform physical actions, tasks, or activities related to self-care, home management, work (job/school/play), community, and leisure is improved.
  - Level of supervision required for task performance is decreased.
  - Performance of and independence in activities of daily living (ADL) and instrumental activities of daily living (IADL) with or without devices and equipment are increased.
  - Tolerance of positions and activities is increased.
- Impact on disabilities
  - Ability to assume or resume required self-care, home management, work (job/school/play), community, and leisure roles is improved.
- Risk reduction/prevention
  - Risk factors are reduced.
  - Risk of secondary impairment is reduced.
  - Safety is improved.
  - Self-management of symptoms is improved.
- Impact on health, wellness, and fitness
  - Fitness is improved.
  - Health status is improved.
  - Physical capacity is increased.
  - Physical function is improved.
- Impact on societal resources
  - Utilization of physical therapy services is optimized.
  - Utilization of physical therapy services results in efficient use of health care dollars.
- Patient/client satisfaction
  - Access, availability, and services provided are acceptable to patient/client.
  - Administrative management of practice is acceptable to patient/client.
  - Clinical proficiency of physical therapist is acceptable to patient/client.
  - Coordination of care is acceptable to patient/client.
  - Cost of health care services is decreased.
  - Intensity of care is decreased.
  - Interpersonal skills of physical therapist are acceptable to patient/client, family, and significant others.
  - Sense of well-being is improved.
  - Stressors are decreased.

Functional Training in Self-Care and Home Management (Including Activities of Daily Living [ADL] and Instrumental Activities of Daily Living [IADL]

Interventions

- ADL training
  - bathing
  - bed mobility and transfer training
  - developmental activities
  - dressing
  - eating
  - grooming
  - toileting
- Devices and equipment use and training
  - assistive and adaptive device or equipment training during ADL and IADL
  - orthotic, protective, or supportive device or equipment training during ADL and IADL
  - prosthetic device or equipment training during ADL and IADL
- Functional training programs
  - back schools
  - simulated environments and tasks
  - task adaptation
- IADL training
  - caring for dependents
  - home maintenance
  - household chores
  - shopping
  - structured play for infants and children
  - yard work
- Injury prevention or reduction
  - injury prevention education during self-care and home management
  - injury prevention or reduction with use of devices and equipment
  - safety awareness training during self-care and home management

Anticipated Goals and Expected Outcomes

- Impact on pathology/pathophysiology (disease, disorder, or condition)
  - Pain is decreased.
  - Physiological response to increased oxygen demand is improved.
- Impact on impairments
  - Balance is improved.
  - Endurance is increased.
  - Energy expenditure per unit of work is decreased.
  - Motor function (motor control and motor learning) is improved.
  - Muscle performance (strength, power, and endurance) is increased.
  - Postural control is improved.
  - Sensory awareness is increased.
  - Weight-bearing status is improved.
- Impact on functional limitations
  - Ability to perform physical actions, tasks, or activities related to self-care and home management is increased.
  - Level of supervision required for task performance is decreased.
  - Performance of and independence in ADL and IADL with or without devices and equipment are increased.
  - Tolerance of positions and activities is increased.
- Impact on disabilities
  - Ability to assume or resume required self-care and home management roles are improved.
- Risk reduction/prevention
  - Risk factors are reduced.
  - Risk of secondary impairments is reduced.
  - Safety is improved.
  - Self-management of symptoms is improved.
- Impact on health, wellness, and fitness
  - Fitness is improved.
  - Health status is improved.
  - Physical capacity is increased.
  - Physical function is improved.
- Impact on societal resources
  - Utilization of physical therapy services is optimized.
  - Utilization of physical therapy services results in efficient use of health care dollars.
- Patient/client satisfaction
  - Access, availability, and services provided are acceptable to patient/client.
  - Administrative management of practice is acceptable to patient/client.
  - Clinical proficiency of physical therapist is acceptable to patient/client.
  - Coordination of care is acceptable to patient/client.
  - Cost of health care services is decreased.
  - Intensity of care is decreased.
  - Interpersonal skills of physical therapist are acceptable to patient/client, family, and significant others.
  - Sense of well-being is improved.
  - Stressors are decreased.

Functional Training in Work (Job/School/Play), Community, and Leisure Integration or Reintegration (Including Instrumental Activities of Daily Living [IADL], Work Hardening, and Work Conditioning)

Interventions

- Devices and equipment use and training
  - assistive and adaptive device or equipment training during IADL
  - orthotic, protective, or supportive device or equipment training during IADL
  - prosthetic device or equipment training during IADL
- Functional training programs
  - back schools
  - job coaching
  - simulated environments and tasks
  - task adaptation
  - task training
- IADL training
  - community service training involving instruments
  - school and play activities training including tools and instruments
  - work training with tools
- Injury prevention or reduction
  - injury prevention education during work (job/school/play), community, and leisure integration or reintegration
  - injury prevention or reduction with use of devices and equipment
  - safety awareness training during work (job/school/play), community, and leisure integration or reintegration
- Leisure and play activities and training

Anticipated Goals and Expected Outcomes

- Impact on pathology/pathophysiology (disease, disorder, or condition)
  - Pain is decreased.
  - Physiological response to increased oxygen demand is improved.
- Impact on impairments
  - Balance is improved.
  - Endurance is increased.
  - Energy expenditure per unit of work is decreased.
  - Motor function (motor control and motor learning) is improved.
  - Muscle performance (strength, power, and endurance) is increased.
  - Postural control is improved.
  - Sensory awareness is increased.
  - Weight-bearing status is improved.
- Impact on functional limitations
  - Ability to perform physical actions, tasks, or activities related to work (job/school/play), community, and leisure integration or reintegration is improved.
  - Level of supervision required for task performance is decreased.
  - Performance of and independence in IADL with or without devices and equipment are increased.
  - Tolerance of positions and activities is increased.
- Impact on disabilities
  - Ability to assume or resume required work (job/school/play), community, and leisure roles is improved.
- Risk reduction/prevention
  - Risk factors are reduced.
  - Risk of secondary impairment is reduced.
  - Safety is improved.
  - Self-management of symptoms is improved.
- Impact on health, wellness, and fitness
  - Fitness is improved.
  - Health status is improved.
  - Physical capacity is increased.
  - Physical function is improved.
- Impact on societal resources
  - Costs of work-related injury or disability are reduced.
  - Utilization of physical therapy services is optimized.
  - Utilization of physical therapy services results in efficient use of health care dollars.
- Patient/client satisfaction
  - Access, availability, and services provided are acceptable to patient/client.
  - Administrative management of practice is acceptable to patient/client.
  - Clinical proficiency of physical therapist is acceptable to patient/client.
  - Coordination of care is acceptable to patient/client.
  - Cost of health care services is decreased.
  - Intensity of care is decreased.
  - Interpersonal skills of physical therapist are acceptable to patient/client, family, and significant others.
  - Sense of well-being is improved.
  - Stressors are decreased.

Manual Therapy (Including Mobilization/Manipulation)

Interventions

- Massage
  - connective tissue massage
  - therapeutic massage
- Mobilization/manipulation
  - soft tissue
- Passive range of motion

Anticipated Goals and Expected Outcomes

- Impact on pathology/pathophysiology (disease, disorder, or condition)
  - Edema, lymphedema, or effusion is reduced.
  - Joint swelling, inflammation, or restriction is reduced.
  - Pain is decreased.
  - Soft tissue swelling, inflammation, or restriction is reduced.
- Impact on impairments
  - Gait, locomotion, and balance are improved.
  - Integumentary integrity is improved.
  - Joint integrity and mobility are improved.
  - Muscle performance (strength, power, and endurance) is increased.
  - Postural control is improved.
  - Quality and quantity of movement between and across body segments are improved.
  - Range of motion is improved.
  - Relaxation is increased.
  - Sensory awareness is increased.
  - Weight-bearing status is improved.
- Impact on functional limitations
  - Ability to perform movement tasks is improved.
  - Ability to perform physical actions, tasks, or activities related to self-care, home management, work (job/school/play), community, and leisure is improved.
  - Tolerance of positions and activities is increased.
- Impact on disabilities
  - Ability to assume or resume required self-care, home management, work (job/school/play), community, and leisure roles is improved.
- Risk reduction/prevention
  - Risk factors are reduced.
  - Risk of secondary impairment is reduced.
  - Self-management of symptoms is improved.
- Impact on health, wellness, and fitness
  - Fitness is improved.
  - Physical capacity is increased.
  - Physical function is improved.
- Impact on societal resources
  - Utilization of physical therapy services is optimized.
  - Utilization of physical therapy services results in efficient use of health care dollars.
- Patient/client satisfaction
  - Access, availability, and services provided are acceptable to patient/client.
  - Administrative management of practice is acceptable to patient/client.
  - Clinical proficiency of physical therapist is acceptable to patient/client.
  - Coordination of care is acceptable to patient/client.
  - Cost of health care services is decreased.
  - Intensity of care is decreased.
  - Interpersonal skills of physical therapist are acceptable to patient/client, family, and significant others.
  - Sense of well-being is improved.
  - Stressors are decreased.

Prescription, Application, and, as Appropriate, Fabrication of Devices and Equipment (Assistive, Adaptive, Orthotic, Protective, Supportive, and Prosthetic)

Interventions

- Adaptive devices
  - environmental controls
  - hospital beds
  - raised toilet seats
  - seating systems
- Assistive devices
  - canes
  - crutches
  - long-handled reachers
  - power devices
  - static and dynamic splints
  - walkers
  - wheelchairs
- Orthotic devices
  - braces
  - casts
  - shoe inserts
  - splints
- Protective devices
  - braces
  - cushions
  - helmets
  - protective taping
- Supportive devices
  - compression garments
  - corsets
  - elastic wraps
  - neck collars
  - serial casts
  - slings
  - supportive taping

Anticipated Goals and Expected Outcomes

- Impact on pathology/pathophysiology (disease, disorder, or condition)
  - Edema, lymphedema, or effusion is reduced.
  - Joint swelling, inflammation, or restriction is reduced.
  - Pain is decreased.
  - Soft tissue swelling, inflammation, or restriction is reduced.
- Impact on impairments
  - Balance is improved.
  - Endurance is increased.
  - Energy expenditure per unit of work is decreased.
  - Gait, locomotion, and balance are improved.
  - Integumentary integrity is improved.
  - Joint stability is improved.
  - Motor function (motor control and motor learning) is improved.
  - Muscle performance (strength, power, and endurance) is increased.
  - Optimal joint alignment is achieved.
  - Optimal loading on a body part is achieved.
  - Postural control is improved.
  - Quality and quantity of movement between and across body segments are improved.
  - Range of motion is improved.
  - Weight-bearing status is improved.
- Impact on functional limitations
  - Ability to perform physical actions, tasks, or activities related to self-care, home management, work (job/school/play), community, and leisure is improved.
  - Level of supervision required for task performance is decreased.
  - Performance of and independence in activities of daily living (ADL) and instrumental activities of daily living (IADL) with or without devices and equipment are increased.
  - Tolerance of positions and activities is increased.
- Impact on disabilities
  - Ability to assume or resume required self-care, home management, work (job/school/play), community, and leisure roles is improved.
- Risk reduction/prevention
  - Pressure on body tissues is reduced.
  - Protection of body parts is increased.
  - Risk factors are reduced.
  - Risk of recurrence of condition is reduced.
  - Risk of secondary impairment is reduced.
  - Safety is improved.
  - Self-management of symptoms is improved.
  - Stresses precipitating injury are decreased.
- Impact on health, wellness, and fitness
  - Fitness is improved.
  - Health status is improved.
  - Physical capacity is increased.
  - Physical function is improved.
- Impact on societal resources
  - Utilization of physical therapy services is optimized.
  - Utilization of physical therapy services results in efficient use of health care dollars.
- Patient/client satisfaction
  - Access, availability, and services provided are acceptable to patient/client.
  - Administrative management of practice is acceptable to patient/client.
  - Clinical proficiency of physical therapist is acceptable to patient/client.
  - Coordination of care is acceptable to patient/client.
  - Cost of health care services is decreased.
  - Intensity of care is decreased.
  - Interpersonal skills of physical therapist are acceptable to patient/client, family, and significant others.
  - Sense of well-being is improved.
  - Stressors are decreased.

Electrotherapeutic Modalities

Interventions

- Electrical stimulation
  - electrical muscle stimulation (EMS)
  - high voltage pulsed current (HVPC)
  - neuromuscular electrical stimulation (NMES)
  - transcutaneous electrical nerve stimulation (TENS)

Anticipated Goals and Expected Outcomes

- Impact on pathology/pathophysiology (disease, disorder, or condition)
  - Edema, lymphedema, or effusion is reduced.
  - Joint swelling, inflammation, or restriction is reduced.
  - Nutrient delivery to tissue is increased.
  - Osteogenic effects are enhanced.
  - Pain is decreased.
  - Soft tissue or wound healing is enhanced.
  - Soft tissue swelling, inflammation, or restriction is reduced.
  - Tissue perfusion and oxygenation are enhanced.
- Impact on impairments
  - Integumentary integrity is improved.
  - Motor function (motor control and motor learning) is improved.
  - Muscle performance (strength, power, and endurance) is increased.
  - Postural control is improved.
  - Quality and quantity of movement between and across body segments are improved.
  - Range of motion is improved.
  - Relaxation is increased.
  - Sensory awareness is increased.
- Impact on functional limitations
  - Ability to perform physical actions, tasks, or activities related to self-care, home management, work (job/school/play), community, and leisure is improved.
  - Level of supervision required for task performance is decreased.
  - Performance of and independence in activities of daily living (ADL) and instrumental activities of daily living (IADL) with or without devices and equipment are increased.
  - Tolerance of positions and activities is increased.
- Impact on disabilities
  - Ability to assume or resume required self-care, home management, work (job/school/play), community, and leisure roles is improved.
- Risk reduction/prevention
  - Complications of immobility are reduced.
  - Preoperative and postoperative complications are reduced.
  - Risk factors are reduced.
  - Risk of secondary impairment is reduced.
  - Self-management of symptoms is improved.
- Impact on health, wellness, and fitness
  - Fitness is improved.
  - Physical capacity is increased.
  - Physical function is improved.
- Impact on societal resources
  - Utilization of physical therapy services is optimized.
  - Utilization of physical therapy services results in efficient use of health care dollars.
- Patient/client satisfaction
  - Access, availability, and services provided are acceptable to patient/client.
  - Administrative management of practice is acceptable to patient/client.
  - Clinical proficiency of physical therapist is acceptable to patient/client.
  - Coordination of care is acceptable to patient/client.
  - Interpersonal skills of physical therapist are acceptable to patient/client, family, and significant others.
  - Sense of well-being is improved.
  - Stressors are decreased.

Physical Agents and Mechanical Modalities

Interventions

Physical agents may include:

- Athermal agents
  - pulsed electromagnetic fields
- Cryotherapy
  - cold packs
  - ice massage
  - vapocoolant spray
- Hydrotherapy
  - whirlpool tanks
  - contrast bath
  - pools
- Sound agents
  - phonophoresis
  - ultrasound
- Thermotherapy
  - dry heat
  - hot packs
  - paraffin baths

Mechanical modalities may include:

- Gravity-assisted compression devices
  - tilt table

Anticipated Goals and Expected Outcomes

- Impact on pathology/pathophysiology (disease, disorder, or condition)
  - Edema, lymphedema, or effusion is reduced.
  - Joint swelling, inflammation, or restriction is reduced.
  - Nutrient delivery to tissue is increased.
  - Osteogenic effects of exercise are maximized.
  - Pain is decreased.
  - Soft tissue swelling, inflammation, or restriction is reduced.
  - Tissue perfusion and oxygenation are enhanced.
- Impact on impairments
  - Integumentary integrity is improved.
  - Muscle performance (strength, power, and endurance) is increased.
  - Postural control is improved.
  - Range of motion is improved.
  - Weight-bearing status is improved.
- Impact on functional limitations
  - Ability to perform physical actions, tasks, or activities related to self-care, home management, work (job/school/play), community, and leisure is improved.
  - Performance of and independence in activities of daily living (ADL) and instrumental activities of daily living (IADL) with or without devices and equipment are increased.
  - Tolerance of positions and activities is increased.
- Impact on disabilities
  - Ability to assume or resume required self-care, home management, work (job/school/play), community, and leisure roles is improved.
- Risk reduction/prevention
  - Complications of soft tissue and circulatory disorders are decreased.
  - Risk factors are reduced.
  - Risk of secondary impairment is reduced.
  - Self-management of symptoms is improved.
- Impact on health, wellness, and fitness
  - Fitness is improved.
  - Physical capacity is increased.
  - Physical function is improved.
- Impact on societal resources
  - Utilization of physical therapy services is optimized.
- Patient/client satisfaction
  - Access, availability, and services provided are acceptable to patient/client.
  - Administrative management of practice is acceptable to patient/client.
  - Clinical proficiency of physical therapist is acceptable to patient/client.
  - Coordination of care is acceptable to patient/client.
  - Interpersonal skills of physical therapist are acceptable to patient/client, family, and significant others.
  - Sense of well-being is improved.
  - Stressors are decreased.

Reexamination

Reexamination is the process of performing selected tests and measures after the initial examination to evaluate progress and to modify or redirect interventions. Reexamination may be indicated more than once during a single episode of care. It also may be performed over the course of a disease, disorder, or condition, which for some patients/clients may be over the life span. Indications for reexamination include new clinical findings or failure to respond to physical therapy interventions.

Global Outcomes for Patients/Clients in This Pattern

Throughout the entire episode of care, the physical therapist determines the anticipated goals and expected outcomes for each intervention. These anticipated goals and expected outcomes are delineated in shaded boxes that accompany the lists of interventions in each preferred practice pattern. As the patient/client reaches the termination of physical therapy services and the end of the episode of care, the physical therapist measures the global outcomes of the physical therapy services by characterizing or quantifying the impact of the physical therapy interventions in the following domains:

- Pathology/pathophysiology (disease, disorder, or condition)
- Impairments
- Functional limitations
- Disabilities
- Risk reduction/prevention
- Health, wellness, and fitness
- Societal resources
- Patient/client satisfaction

In some instances, a particular anticipated goal or expected outcome is thoroughly achieved through implementation of a single form of intervention. More commonly, however, the anticipated goals and expected outcomes are achieved as a result of the combined effects of several forms of interventions, leading to enhancement of both health status and health-related quality of life.

Criteria for Termination of Physical Therapy Services

Discharge is the process of ending physical therapy services that have been provided during a single episode of care. It occurs when the anticipated goals and expected outcomes have been achieved. Discharge does *not* occur with a *transfer* (defined as the time when a patient is moved from one site to another site within the same setting or across settings during a single episode of care). Although there may be facility-specific or payer-specific requirements for documentation regarding the conclusion of physical therapy services, *discharge occurs based on the physical therapist's analysis of the achievement of anticipated goals and expected outcomes.*

Discontinuation is the process of ending physical therapy services that have been provided during a single episode of care when (1) the patient/client, caregiver, or legal guardian declines to continue intervention; (2) the patient/client is unable to continue to progress toward outcomes because of medical or psychosocial complications or because financial/insurance resources have been expended; or (3) the physical therapist determines that the patient/client will no longer benefit from physical therapy. When physical therapy services are terminated prior to achievement of anticipated goals and expected outcomes, patient/client status and the rationale for termination are documented.

For patients/clients who require multiple episodes of care, periodic follow-up is needed over the life span to ensure safety and effective adaptation following changes in physical status, caregivers, environment, or task demands. In consultation with appropriate individuals, and in consideration of the outcomes, the physical therapist plans for discharge or discontinuation and provides for appropriate follow-up or referral.

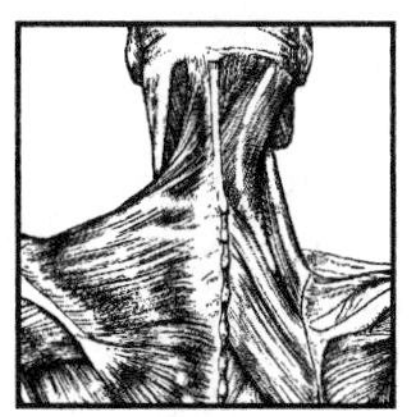

Impaired Joint Mobility, Motor Function, Muscle Performance, and Range of Motion Associated With Joint Arthroplasty

This preferred practice pattern describes the generally accepted elements of patient/client management that physical therapists provide for patients/clients who are classified in this pattern. The pattern title reflects the diagnosis made by the physical therapist. APTA emphasizes that preferred practice patterns are the boundaries within which a physical therapist may select any of a number of clinical alternatives, based on consideration of a wide variety of factors, such as individual patient/client needs; the profession's code of ethics and standards of practice; and patient/client age, culture, gender roles, race, sex, sexual orientation, and socioeconomic status.

Patient/Client Diagnostic Classification

Patients/clients will be classified into this pattern—for impaired joint mobility, motor function, muscle performance, and range of motion associated with joint arthroplasty—as a result of the physical therapist's evaluation of the examination data. The findings from the examination (history, systems review, and tests and measures) may indicate the presence or risk of pathology/pathophysiology (disease, disorder, or condition), impairments, functional limitations, or disabilities or the need for health, wellness, or fitness programs. The physical therapist integrates, synthesizes, and interprets the data to determine the diagnostic classification.

Inclusion

The following examples of examination findings may support the inclusion of patients/clients in this pattern:

Risk Factors or Consequences of Pathology/Pathophysiology (Disease, Disorder, or Condition)

- Ankylosing spondylitis
- Arthroplasties
- Avascular necrosis due to steroid use
- Juvenile rheumatoid arthritis
- Neoplasms of the bone
- Osteoarthritis
- Rheumatoid arthritis
- Trauma

Impairments, Functional Limitations, or Disabilities

- Decreased range of motion
- Inability to access transportation
- Inability to dress
- Muscle guarding
- Muscle weakness
- Pain

Note:

Some risk factors or consequences of pathology/pathophysiology—such as *multiple joint replacement, recurrent postoperative dislocation,* and *secondary postoperative infection*—may be severe and complex; *however, they do not necessarily exclude patients/clients from this pattern.* Severe and complex risk factors or consequences may require modification of the frequency of visits and duration of care. (See "Evaluation, Diagnosis, and Prognosis," page 257.)

Exclusion or Multiple-Pattern Classification

The following examples of examination findings may support exclusion from this pattern or classification into additional patterns. Depending on the level of severity or complexity of the examination findings, the physical therapist may determine that the patient/client would be more appropriately managed through (1) classification in an entirely different pattern or (2) classification in both this and another pattern.

Findings That May Require Classification in a Different Pattern

- Impairments associated with multisite trauma

Findings That May Require Classification in Additional Patterns

- Rheumatoid arthritis with deconditioning

ICD-9-CM Codes

The listing below contains the current (as of press time) and most typical 3- and 4-digit ICD-9-CM codes related to this preferred practice pattern. Because patient/client diagnostic classification is based on impairments, functional limitations, and disabilities—not on codes—patients/clients may be classified into the pattern even though the codes listed with the pattern may not apply to those clients.

This listing is intended for general information only and should not be used for coding purposes. The codes should be confirmed by referring to the World Health Organization's *International Classification of Diseases, 9th Revision, Clinical Modification (ICD-9-CM 2001)*, Volumes 1 and 3 (Chicago, Ill: American Medical Association; 2000) or subsequent revisions or by referring to other ICD-9-CM coding manuals that contain exclusion notes and instructions regarding fifth-digit requirements.

170 Malignant neoplasm of bone and articular cartilage

171 Malignant neoplasm of connective and other soft tissue

213 Benign neoplasm of bone and articular cartilage

215 Other benign neoplasm of connective and other soft tissue

524 Dentofacial anomalies, including malocclusion

- **524.6** Temporomandibular joint disorders

714 Rheumatoid arthritis and other inflammatory polyarthropathies

- **714.0** Rheumatoid arthritis
- **714.3** Juvenile chronic polyarthritis
  - **714.30** Polyarticular juvenile rheumatoid arthritis, chronic or unspecified

715 Osteoarthrosis and allied disorders

716 Other and unspecified arthropathies

- **716.8** Other specified arthropathy

717 Internal derangement of knee

- **717.9** Unspecified internal derangement of knee

718 Other derangement of joint

- **718.9** Unspecified derangement of joint

719 Other and unspecified disorders of joint

- **719.5** Stiffness of joint, not elsewhere classified
- **719.7** Difficulty in walking
- **719.8** Other specified disorders of joint
  Calcification of joint

729 Other disorders of soft tissues

- **729.8** Other musculoskeletal symptoms referable to limbs

730 Osteomyelitis, periostitis, and other infections involving bone

731 Osteitis deformans and osteopathies associated with other disorders classified elsewhere

- **731.0** Osteitis deformans without mention of bone tumor
  Paget's disease of bone

733 Other disorders of bone and cartilage

- **733.1** Pathologic fracture
- **733.8** Malunion and nonunion of fracture

808 Fracture of pelvis

- **808.0** Acetabulum, closed

812 Fracture of humerus

- **812.0** Upper end, closed

815 Fracture of metacarpal bone(s)

820 Fracture of neck of femur

- **820.8** Unspecified part of neck of femur, closed
- **820.9** Unspecified part of neck of femur, open

824 Fracture of ankle

835 Dislocation of hip

836 Dislocation of knee

- **836.5** Other dislocation of knee, closed

837 Dislocation of ankle

958 Certain early complications of trauma

- **958.3** Posttraumatic wound infection, not elsewhere classified

Supplemental Classification of Factors Influencing Health Status and Contact With Health Services

V43 Organ or tissue replaced by other means

- **V43.6** Joint
  - **V43.61** Shoulder
  - **V43.64** Hip
  - **V43.65** Knee
  - **V43.66** Ankle
  - **V43.70** Limb

Examination

Examination is a comprehensive screening and specific testing process that leads to a diagnostic classification or, when appropriate, to a referral to another practitioner. Examination is required prior to the initial intervention and is performed for all patients/clients. Through the examination, the physical therapist may identify impairments, functional limitations, disabilities, changes in physical function or overall health status, and needs related to restoration of health and to prevention, wellness, and fitness. The physical therapist synthesizes the examination findings to establish the diagnosis and the prognosis (including the plan of care). The patient/client, family, significant others, and caregivers may provide information during the examination process.

Examination has three components: the patient/client history, the systems review, and tests and measures. The *history* is a systematic gathering of past and current information (often from the patient/client) related to why the patient/client is seeking the services of the physical therapist. The *systems review* is a brief or limited examination of (1) the anatomical and physiological status of the cardiovascular/pulmonary, integumentary, musculoskeletal, and neuromuscular systems and (2) the communication ability, affect, cognition, language, and learning style of the patient/client. *Tests and measures* are the means of gathering data about the patient/client.

The selection of examination procedures and the depth of the examination vary based on patient/client age; severity of the problem; stage of recovery (acute, subacute, chronic); phase of rehabilitation (early, intermediate, late, return to activity); home, work (job/school/play), or community situation; and other relevant factors. *For clinical indications in selecting tests and measures and for listings of tests and measures, tools used to gather data, and the types of data generated by tests and measures, refer to Chapter 2.*

Patient/Client History

The history may include:

General Demographics

- Age
- Sex
- Race/ethnicity
- Primary language
- Education

Social History

- Cultural beliefs and behaviors
- Family and caregiver resources
- Social interactions, social activities, and support systems

Employment/Work (Job/School/Play)

- Current and prior work (job/school/play), community, and leisure actions, tasks, or activities

Growth and Development

- Developmental history
- Hand dominance

Living Environment

- Devices and equipment (eg, assistive, adaptive, orthotic, protective, supportive, prosthetic)
- Living environment and community characteristics
- Projected discharge destinations

General Health Status (Self-Report, Family Report, Caregiver Report)

- General health perception
- Physical function (eg, mobility, sleep patterns, restricted bed days)
- Psychological function (eg, memory, reasoning ability, depression, anxiety)
- Role function (eg, community, leisure, social, work)
- Social function (eg, social activity, social interaction, social support)

Social/Health Habits (Past and Current)

- Behavioral health risks (eg, smoking, drug abuse)
- Level of physical fitness

Family History

- Familial health risks

Medical/Surgical History

- Cardiovascular
- Endocrine/metabolic
- Gastrointestinal
- Genitourinary
- Gynecological
- Integumentary
- Musculoskeletal
- Neuromuscular
- Obstetrical
- Prior hospitalizations, surgeries, and preexisting medical and other health-related conditions
- Psychological
- Pulmonary

Current Condition(s)/Chief Complaint(s)

- Concerns that led patient/client to seek the services of a physical therapist
- Concerns or needs of patient/client who requires the services of a physical therapist
- Current therapeutic interventions
- Mechanisms of injury or disease, including date of onset and course of events
- Onset and pattern of symptoms
- Patient/client, family, significant other, and caregiver expectations and goals for the therapeutic intervention
- Patient/client, family, significant other, and caregiver perceptions of patient's/client's emotional response to the current clinical situation
- Previous occurrence of chief complaint(s)
- Prior therapeutic interventions

Functional Status and Activity Level

- Current and prior functional status in self-care and home management activities, including activities of daily living (ADL) and instrumental activities of daily living (IADL)
- Current and prior functional status in work (job/school/play), community, and leisure actions, tasks, or activities

Medications

- Medications for current condition
- Medications previously taken for current condition
- Medications for other conditions

Other Clinical Tests

- Laboratory and diagnostic tests
- Review of available records (eg, medical, education, surgical)
- Review of other clinical findings (eg, nutrition and hydration)

Systems Review

The systems review may include:

Anatomical and Physiological Status

- Cardiovascular/Pulmonary
  - Blood pressure
  - Edema
  - Heart rate
  - Respiratory rate
- Integumentary
  - Pliability (texture)
  - Presence of scar formation
  - Skin color
  - Skin integrity
- Musculoskeletal
  - Gross range of motion
  - Gross strength
  - Gross symmetry
  - Height
  - Weight
- Neuromuscular
  - Gross coordinated movements (eg, balance, gait, locomotion, transfers, transitions)
  - Motor function (motor control, motor learning)

Communication, Affect, Cognition, Language, and Learning Style

- Ability to make needs known
- Consciousness
- Expected emotional/behavioral responses
- Learning preferences (eg, education needs, learning barriers)
- Orientation (person, place, time)

Tests and Measures

Tests and measures for this pattern may include those that characterize or quantify:

Aerobic Capacity and Endurance

- Aerobic capacity during functional activities (eg, activities of daily living [ADL] scales, indexes, instrumental activities of daily living [IADL] scales, observations)

Anthropometric Characteristics

- Body dimensions (eg, girth measurement, length measurement)
- Edema (eg, girth measurement, palpation, scales, volume measurement)

Assistive and Adaptive Devices

- Assistive or adaptive devices and equipment use during functional activities (eg, ADL scales, functional scales, IADL scales, interviews, observations)
- Components, alignment, fit, and ability to care for the assistive or adaptive devices and equipment (eg, interviews, logs, observations, pressure-sensing maps, reports)
- Remediation of impairments, functional limitations, or disabilities with use of assistive or adaptive devices and equipment (eg, activity status indexes, ADL scales, aerobic capacity tests, functional performance inventories, health assessment questionnaires, IADL scales, pain scales, play scales, videographic assessments)
- Safety during use of assistive or adaptive devices and equipment (eg, diaries, fall scales, interviews, logs, observations, reports)

Cranial and Peripheral Nerve Integrity

- Electrophysiological integrity (eg, electroneuromyography)
- Motor distribution of the peripheral nerves (eg, dynamometry, muscle tests, observations, thoracic outlet tests)
- Sensory distribution of the peripheral nerves (eg, discrimination tests; tactile tests, including coarse and light touch, cold and heat, pain, pressure, and vibration; thoracic outlet tests)

Environmental, Home, and Work (Job/School/Play) Barriers

- Current and potential barriers (eg, checklists, interviews, observations, questionnaires
- Physical space and environment (eg, compliance standards, observations, photographic assessments, questionnaires, structural specifications, videographic assessments)

Ergonomics and Body Mechanics

Ergonomics :

- Dexterity and coordination during work (job/school/play) (eg, hand function tests, impairment rating scales, manipulative ability tests)
- Functional capacity and performance during work actions, tasks, or activities (eg, accelerometry, dynamometry, electroneuromyography, endurance tests, force platform tests, goniometry, interviews, observations, photographic assessments, physical capacity tests, postural loading analyses, technology-assisted assessments, videographic assessments, work analyses)
- Safety in work environments (eg, hazard identification checklists, job severity indexes, lifting standards, risk assessment scales, standards for exposure limits)
- Specific work conditions or activities (eg, handling checklists, job simulations, lifting models, preemployment screenings, task analysis checklists, workstation checklists)

Body mechanics

- Body mechanics during self-care, home management, work, community, or leisure actions, tasks, or activities (eg, ADL scales, IADL scales, observations, photographic assessments, technology-assisted assessments, videographic assessments)

Gait, Locomotion, and Balance

- Balance during functional activities with or without the use of assistive, adaptive, orthotic, protective, supportive, or prosthetic devices or equipment (eg, ADL scales, IADL scales, observations, videographic assessments)
- Balance (dynamic and static) with or without the use of assistive, adaptive, orthotic, protective, supportive, or prosthetic devices or equipment (eg, balance scales, dizziness inventories, dynamic posturography, fall scales, motor impairment tests, observations, photographic assessments, postural control tests)
- Gait and locomotion during functional activities with or without the use of assistive, adaptive, orthotic, protective, supportive, or prosthetic devices or equipment (eg, ADL scales, gait indexes, IADL scales, mobility skill profiles, observations, videographic assessments)
- Gait and locomotion with or without the use of assistive, adaptive, orthotic, protective, supportive, or prosthetic devices or equipment (eg, dynamometry, electroneuromyography, footprint analyses, gait indexes, mobility skill profiles, observations, photographic assessments, technology-assisted assessments, videographic assessments, weight-bearing scales, wheelchair mobility tests)
- Safety during gait, locomotion, and balance (eg, confidence scales, diaries, fall scales, functional assessment profiles, logs, reports)

Integumentary Integrity

Associated skin

- Activities, positioning, and postures that produce or relieve trauma to the skin (eg, observations, pressure-sensing maps, scales)
- Assistive, adaptive, orthotic, protective, supportive, or prosthetic devices and equipment that may produce or relieve trauma to the skin (eg, observations, risk assessment scales)
- Skin characteristics, including blistering, continuity of skin color, dermatitis, hair growth, mobility, nail growth, sensation, temperature, texture, and turgor (eg, observations, palpation, photographic assessments, thermography)

Motor Function (Motor Control and Motor Learning)

- Dexterity, coordination, and agility (eg, coordination screens, motor impairment tests, motor proficiency tests, observations, videographic assessments)
- Hand function (eg, fine and gross motor control tests, finger dexterity tests, manipulative ability tests, observations)

Muscle Performance (Including Strength, Power, and Endurance)

- Electrophysiological integrity (eg, electroneuromyography)
- Muscle strength, power, and endurance (eg, dynamometry, manual muscle tests, muscle performance tests, physical capacity tests, technology-assisted assessments, timed activity tests)
- Muscle strength, power, and endurance during functional activities (eg, ADL scales, functional muscle tests, IADL scales, observations, videographic assessments)
- Muscle tension (eg, palpation)

Orthotic, Protective, and Supportive Devices

- Components, alignment, fit, and ability to care for orthotic, protective, and supportive devices and equipment (eg, interviews, logs, observations, pressure-sensing maps, reports)
- Orthotic, protective, and supportive devices and equipment use during functional activities (eg, ADL scales, functional scales, IADL scales, interviews, observations, profiles)
- Remediation of impairments, functional limitations, or disabilities with use of orthotic, protective, and supportive devices and equipment (eg, activity status indexes, ADL scales, aerobic capacity tests, functional performance inventories, health assessment questionnaires, IADL scales, pain scales, play scales, videographic assessments)
- Safety during use of orthotic, protective, and supportive devices and equipment (eg, diaries, fall scales, interviews, logs, observations, reports)

Pain

- Pain, soreness, and nociception (eg, analog scales, discrimination tests, pain drawings and maps, provocation tests, verbal and pictorial descriptor tests)
- Pain in specific body parts (eg, pain indexes, pain questionnaires, structural provocation tests)

Posture

- Postural alignment and position (static and dynamic), including symmetry and deviation from midline (eg, observations, grid measurement, technology-assisted assessments, videographic assessments)
- Specific body parts (eg, angle assessments, forward-bending test, goniometry, observations, palpation, positional tests)

Range of Motion (ROM) (Including Muscle Length)

- Functional ROM (eg, observations, squat testing, toe touch tests)
- Joint active and passive movement (eg, goniometry, inclinometry, observations, photographic assessments, technology-assisted assessments, videographic assessments)
- Muscle length, soft tissue extensibility, and flexibility (eg, contracture tests, goniometry, inclinometry, ligamentous tests, linear measurement, multisegment flexibility tests, palpation)

Reflex Integrity

- Deep reflexes (eg, myotatic reflex scale, observations, reflex tests)
- Superficial reflexes and reactions (eg, observations, provocation tests)

Self-Care and Home Management (Including ADL and IADL)

- Ability to gain access to home environments (eg, barrier identification, observations, physical performance tests)
- Ability to perform self-care and home management activities with or without assistive, adaptive, orthotic, protective, supportive, or prosthetic devices and equipment (eg, ADL scales, aerobic capacity tests, IADL scales, interviews, observations, profiles)
- Safety in self-care and home management activities and environments (eg, diaries, fall scales, interviews, logs, observations, reports, videographic assessments)

Sensory Integrity

- Combined/cortical sensations (eg, stereognosis, tactile discrimination tests)
- Deep sensations (eg, kinesthesiometry, observations, photographic assessments, vibration tests)

Work (Job/School/Play), Community, and Leisure Integration or Reintegration (Including IADL)

- Ability to assume or resume work (job/school/play), community, and leisure activities with or without assistive, adaptive, orthotic, protective, supportive, or prosthetic devices and equipment (eg, activity profiles, disability indexes, functional status questionnaires, IADL scales, observations, physical capacity tests)
- Ability to gain access to work (job/school/play), community, and leisure environments (eg, barrier identification, interviews, observations, physical capacity tests, transportation assessments)
- Safety in work (job/school/play), community, and leisure activities and environments (eg, diaries, fall scales, interviews, logs, observations, videographic assessments)

Evaluation, Diagnosis, and Prognosis (Including Plan of Care)

Physical therapists perform *evaluations* (make clinical judgments) based on the data gathered from the history, systems review, and tests and measures. In the evaluation process, physical therapists synthesize the examination data to establish the diagnosis and prognosis (including the plan of care). Factors that influence the complexity of the evaluation include the clinical findings, extent of loss of function, chronicity or severity of the problem, possibility of multisite or multisystem involvement, preexisting condition(s), potential discharge destination, social considerations, physical function, and overall health status.

A *diagnosis* is a label encompassing a cluster of signs and symptoms, syndromes, or categories. It is the result of the systematic diagnostic process, which includes integrating and evaluating the data from the examination. The diagnostic label indicates the primary dysfunction(s) toward which the therapist will direct interventions. The *prognosis* is the determination of the predicted optimal level of improvement in function and the amount of time needed to reach that level and may also include a prediction of levels of improvement that may be reached at various intervals during the course of therapy. During the prognostic process, the physical therapist develops the plan of care. The *plan of care* identifies specific interventions, proposed frequency and duration of the interventions, anticipated goals, expected outcomes, and discharge plans. The plan of care identifies realistic anticipated goals and expected outcomes, taking into consideration the expectations of the patient/client and appropriate others. These anticipated goals and expected outcomes should be measureable and time limited.

The frequency of visits and duration of the episode of care may vary from a short episode with a high intensity of intervention to a longer episode with a diminishing intensity of intervention. Frequency and duration may vary greatly among patients/clients based on a variety of factors that the physical therapist considers throughout the evaluation process, such as anatomical and physiological changes related to growth and development; caregiver consistency or expertise; chronicity or severity of the current condition; living environment; multisite or multisystem involvement; social support; potential discharge destinations; probability of prolonged impairment, functional limitation, or disability; and stability of the condition.

Prognosis

Over the course of 6 months, patient/client will demonstrate optimal joint mobility, motor function, muscle performance, and range of motion and the highest level of functioning in home, work (job/school/play), community, and leisure environments.

During the episode of care, patient/client will achieve (1) the anticipated goals and expected outcomes of the interventions that are described in the plan of care and (2) the global outcomes for patients/clients who are classified in this pattern.

Expected Range of Number of Visits Per Episode of Care

12 to 60

This range represents the lower and upper limits of the number of physical therapist visits required to achieve anticipated goals and expected outcomes. *It is anticipated that 80% of patients/clients who are classified into this pattern will achieve the anticipated goals and expected outcomes within 12 to 60 visits during a single continuous episode of care.* Frequency of visits and duration of the episode of care should be determined by the physical therapist to maximize effectiveness of care and efficiency of service delivery.

Factors That May Require New Episode of Care or That May Modify Frequency of Visits/Duration of Episode

- Accessibility and availability of resources
- Adherence to the intervention program
- Age
- Anatomical and physiological changes related to growth and development
- Caregiver consistency or expertise
- Chronicity or severity of the current condition
- Cognitive status
- Comorbitities, complications, or secondary impairments
- Concurrent medical, surgical, and therapeutic interventions
- Decline in functional independence
- Level of impairment
- Level of physical function
- Living environment
- Multisite or multisystem involvement
- Nutritional status
- Overall health status
- Potential discharge destinations
- Premorbid conditions
- Probability of prolonged impairment, functional limitation, or disability
- Psychological and socioeconomic factors
- Psychomotor abilities
- Social support
- Stability of the condition

Intervention

Intervention is the purposeful interaction of the physical therapist with the patient/client and, when appropriate, with other individuals involved in patient/client care, using various physical therapy procedures and techniques to produce changes in the condition consistent with the diagnosis and prognosis. Decisions about interventions are contingent on the timely monitoring of patient/client response and the progress made toward achieving the anticipated goals and expected outcomes.

Communication, coordination, and documentation and patient/client-related instruction are provided for all patients/clients across all settings. Procedural interventions are selected or modified based on the examination data and the evaluation, the diagnosis and the prognosis, and the anticipated goals and expected outcomes for a particular patient/client. *For clinical considerations in selecting interventions, listings of interventions, and listings of anticipated goals and expected outcomes, refer to Chapter 3.*

Coordination, Communication, and Documentation

Coordination, communication, and documentation may include:

Interventions

- Addressing required functions
  - advance directives
  - individualized family service plans (IFSPs) or individualized education plans (IEPs)
  - informed consent
  - mandatory communication and reporting (eg, patient advocacy and abuse reporting)
- Admission and discharge planning
- Case management
- Collaboration and coordination with agencies, including:
  - equipment suppliers
  - home care agencies
  - payer groups
  - schools
  - transportation agencies
- Communication across settings, including:
  - case conferences
  - documentation
  - education plans
- Cost-effective resource utilization
- Data collection, analysis, and reporting
  - outcome data
  - peer review findings
  - record reviews
- Documentation across settings, following APTA's *Guidelines for Physical Therapy Documentation* (Appendix 5), including:
  - changes in impairments, functional limitations, and disabilities
  - changes in interventions
  - elements of patient/client management (examination, evaluation, diagnosis, prognosis, intervention)
  - outcomes of intervention
- Interdisciplinary teamwork
  - case conferences
  - patient care rounds
  - patient/client family meetings
- Referrals to other professionals or resources

Anticipated Goals and Expected Outcomes

- Accountability for services is increased.
- Admission data and discharge planning are completed.
- Advance directives, individualized family service plans (IFSPs) or individualized education plans (IEPs), informed consent, and mandatory communication and reporting (eg, patient advocacy and abuse reporting) are obtained or completed.
- Available resources are maximally utilized.
- Care is coordinated with patient/client, family, significant others, caregivers, and other professionals.
- Case is managed throughout the episode of care.
- Collaboration and coordination occurs with agencies, including equipment suppliers, home care agencies, payer groups, schools, and transportation agencies.
- Communication enhances risk reduction and prevention.
- Communication occurs across settings through case conferences, education plans, and documentation.
- Data are collected, analyzed, and reported, including outcome data, peer review findings, and record reviews.
- Decision making is enhanced regarding health, wellness, and fitness needs.
- Decision making is enhanced regarding patient/client health and the use of health care resources by patient/client, family, significant others, and caregivers.
- Documentation occurs throughout patient/client management and across settings and follows APTA's *Guidelines for Physical Therapy Documentation* (Appendix 5).
- Interdisciplinary collaboration occurs through case conferences, patient care rounds, and patient/client family meetings.
- Patient/client, family, significant other, and caregiver understanding of anticipated goals and expected outcomes is increased.
- Placement needs are determined.
- Referrals are made to other professionals or resources whenever necessary and appropriate.
- Resources are utilized in a cost-effective way.

Patient/Client-Related Instruction

Patient/client-related instruction may include:

Interventions

- Instruction, education and training of patients/clients and caregivers regarding:
  - current condition (pathology/pathophysiology [disease, disorder, or condition], impairments, functional limitations, or disabilities)
  - enhancement of performance
  - health, wellness, and fitness programs
  - plan of care
  - risk factors for pathology/pathophysiology (disease, disorder, or condition), impairments, functional limitations, or disabilities
  - transitions across settings
  - transitions to new roles

Anticipated Goals and Expected Outcomes

- Ability to perform physical actions, tasks, or activities is improved.
- Awareness and use of community resources are improved.
- Behaviors that foster healthy habits, wellness, and prevention are acquired.
- Decision making is enhanced regarding patient/client health and the use of health care resources by patient/client, family, significant others, and caregivers.
- Disability associated with acute or chronic illnesses is reduced.
- Functional independence in activities of daily living (ADL) and instrumental activities of daily living (IADL) is increased.
- Health status is improved.
- Intensity of care is decreased.
- Level of supervision required for task performance is decreased.
- Patient/client, family, significant other, and caregiver knowledge and awareness of the diagnosis, prognosis, interventions, and anticipated goals and expected outcomes are increased.
- Patient/client knowledge of personal and environmental factors associated with the condition is increased.
- Performance levels in self-care, home management, work (job/school/play), community, or leisure actions, tasks, or activities are improved.
- Physical function is improved.
- Risk of recurrence of condition is reduced.
- Risk of secondary impairment is reduced.
- Safety of patient/client, family, significant others, and caregivers is improved.
- Self-management of symptoms is improved.
- Utilization and cost of health care services are decreased.

Procedural Interventions

Procedural interventions for this pattern may include:

Therapeutic Exercise

Interventions

- Aerobic capacity/endurance conditioning or reconditioning
  - aquatic programs
  - gait and locomotor training
  - increased workload over time
  - walking and wheelchair propulsion programs
- Balance, coordination, and agility training
  - developmental activities training
  - motor function (motor control and motor learning) training or retraining
  - neuromuscular education or reeducation
  - perceptual training
  - posture awareness training
  - standardized, programmatic, complementary exercise approaches
  - task-specific performance training
- Body mechanics and postural stabilization
  - body mechanics training
  - posture awareness training
  - postural control training
  - postural stabilization activities
- Flexibility exercises
  - muscle lengthening
  - range of motion
  - stretching
- Gait and locomotion training
  - developmental activities training
  - gait training
  - implement and device training
  - perceptual training
  - standardized, programmatic, complementary exercise approaches
  - wheelchair training
- Relaxation
  - breathing strategies
  - movement strategies
  - relaxation techniques
  - standardized, programmatic, complementary exercise approaches
- Strength, power, and endurance training for head, neck, limb, pelvic-floor, trunk, and ventilatory muscles
  - active assistive, active, and resistive exercises (including concentric, dynamic/isotonic, eccentric, isokinetic, isometric, and plyometric)
  - aquatic programs
  - standardized, programmatic, complementary exercise approaches
  - task-specific performance training

Anticipated Goals and Expected Outcomes

- Impact on pathology/pathophysiology (disease, disorder, or condition)
  - Joint swelling, inflammation, or restriction is reduced.
  - Nutrient delivery to tissue is increased.
  - Osteogenic effects of exercise are maximized.
  - Pain is decreased.
  - Physiological response to increased oxygen demand is improved.
  - Soft tissue swelling, inflammation, or restriction is reduced.
  - Tissue perfusion and oxygenation are enhanced.
- Impact on impairments
  - Aerobic capacity is increased.
  - Airway clearance is improved.
  - Balance is improved.
  - Endurance is increased.
  - Energy expenditure per unit of work is decreased.
  - Gait, locomotion, and balance are improved.
  - Integumentary integrity is improved.
  - Joint integrity and mobility are improved.
  - Motor function (motor control and motor learning) is improved.
  - Muscle performance (strength, power, and endurance) is increased.
  - Postural control is improved.
  - Quality and quantity of movement between and across body segments are improved.
  - Range of motion is improved.
  - Relaxation is increased.
  - Sensory awareness is increased.
  - Weight-bearing status is improved.
- Impact on functional limitations
  - Ability to perform physical actions, tasks, or activities related to self-care, home management, work (job/school/play), community, and leisure is improved.
  - Level of supervision required for task performance is decreased.
  - Performance of and independence in activities of daily living (ADL) and instrumental activities of daily living (IADL) with or without devices and equipment are increased.
  - Tolerance of positions and activities is increased.
- Impact on disabilities
  - Ability to assume or resume required self-care, home management, work (job/school/play), community, and leisure roles is improved.
- Risk reduction/prevention
  - Preoperative and postoperative complications are reduced.
  - Risk factors are reduced.
  - Risk of secondary impairment is reduced.
  - Safety is improved.
  - Self-management of symptoms is improved.
- Impact on health, wellness, and fitness
  - Fitness is improved.
  - Health status is improved.
  - Physical capacity is increased.
  - Physical function is improved.
- Impact on societal resources
  - Utilization of physical therapy services is optimized.
  - Utilization of physical therapy services results in efficient use of health care dollars.
- Patient/client satisfaction
  - Access, availability, and services provided are acceptable to patient/client.
  - Administrative management of practice is acceptable to patient/client.
  - Clinical proficiency of physical therapist is acceptable to patient/client.
  - Coordination of care is acceptable to patient/client.
  - Cost of health care services is decreased.
  - Intensity of care is decreased.
  - Interpersonal skills of physical therapist are acceptable to patient/client, family, and significant others.
  - Sense of well-being is improved.
  - Stressors are decreased.

Functional Training in Self-Care and Home Management (Including Activities of Daily Living [ADL] and Instrumental Activities of Daily Living [IADL])

Interventions

- ADL training
  - bathing
  - bed mobility and transfer training
  - developmental activities
  - dressing
  - eating
  - grooming
  - toileting
- Devices and equipment use and training
  - assistive and adaptive device or equipment training during ADL and IADL
  - orthotic, protective, or supportive device or equipment training during ADL and IADL
  - prosthetic device or equipment training during ADL and IADL
- Functional training programs
  - back schools
  - simulated environments and tasks
  - task adaptation
- IADL training
  - caring for dependents
  - home maintenance
  - household chores
  - shopping
  - structured play for infants and children
  - yard work
- Injury prevention or reduction
  - injury prevention education during self-care and home management
  - injury prevention or reduction with use of devices and equipment
  - safety awareness training during self-care and home management

Anticipated Goals and Expected Outcomes

- Impact on pathology/pathophysiology (disease, disorder, or condition)
  - Pain is decreased.
  - Physiological response to increased oxygen demand is improved.
- Impact on impairments
  - Balance is improved.
  - Endurance is increased.
  - Energy expenditure per unit of work is decreased.
  - Motor function (motor control and motor learning) is improved.
  - Muscle performance (strength, power, and endurance) is increased.
  - Postural control is improved.
  - Sensory awareness is increased.
  - Weight-bearing status is improved.
- Impact on functional limitations
  - Ability to perform physical actions, tasks, or activities related to self-care and home management is increased.
  - Level of supervision required for task performance is decreased.
  - Performance of and independence in ADL and IADL with or without devices and equipment are increased.
  - Tolerance of positions and activities is increased.
- Impact on disabilities
  - Ability to assume or resume required self-care and home management roles is improved.
- Risk reduction/prevention
  - Risk factors are reduced.
  - Risk of secondary impairments is reduced.
  - Safety is improved.
  - Self-management of symptoms is improved.
- Impact on health, wellness, and fitness
  - Fitness is improved.
  - Health status is improved.
  - Physical capacity is increased.
  - Physical function is improved.
- Impact on societal resources
  - Utilization of physical therapy services is optimized.
  - Utilization of physical therapy services results in efficient use of health care dollars.
- Patient/client satisfaction
  - Access, availability, and services provided are acceptable to patient/client.
  - Administrative management of practice is acceptable to patient/client.
  - Clinical proficiency of physical therapist is acceptable to patient/client.
  - Coordination of care is acceptable to patient/client.
  - Cost of health care services is decreased.
  - Intensity of care is decreased.
  - Interpersonal skills of physical therapist are acceptable to patient/client, family, and significant others.
  - Sense of well-being is improved.
  - Stressors are decreased.

Functional Training in Work (Job/School/Play), Community, and Leisure Integration or Reintegration (Including Instrumental Activities of Daily Living [IADL], Work Hardening, and Work Conditioning)

Interventions

- Devices and equipment use and training
  - assistive and adaptive device or equipment training during IADL
  - orthotic, protective, or supportive device or equipment training during IADL
  - prosthetic device or equipment training during IADL
- Functional training programs
  - back schools
  - job coaching
  - simulated environments and tasks
  - task adaptation
  - task training
- IADL training
  - community service training involving instruments
  - school and play activities training including tools and instruments
  - work training with tools
- Injury prevention or reduction
  - injury prevention education during work (job/school/play), community, and leisure integration or reintegration
  - injury prevention or reduction with use of devices and equipment
  - safety awareness training during work (job/school/play), community, and leisure integration or reintegration
- Leisure and play activities and training

Anticipated Goals and Expected Outcomes

- Impact on pathology/pathophysiology (disease, disorder, or condition)
  - Pain is decreased.
  - Physiological response to increased oxygen demand is improved.
- Impact on impairments
  - Balance is improved.
  - Endurance is increased.
  - Energy expenditure per unit of work is decreased.
  - Motor function (motor control and motor learning) is improved.
  - Muscle performance (strength, power, and endurance) is increased.
  - Postural control is improved.
  - Sensory awareness is increased.
  - Weight-bearing status is improved.
- Impact on functional limitations
  - Ability to perform physical actions, tasks, or activities related to work (job/school/play), community, and leisure integration or reintegration is improved.
  - Level of supervision required for task performance is decreased.
  - Performance of and independence in IADL with or without devices and equipment are increased.
  - Tolerance of positions and activities is increased.
- Impact on disabilities
  - Ability to assume or resume required work (job/school/play), community, and leisure roles is improved.
- Risk reduction/prevention
  - Risk factors are reduced.
  - Risk of secondary impairment is reduced.
  - Safety is improved
  - Self-management of symptoms is improved.
- Impact on health, wellness, and fitness
  - Fitness is improved.
  - Health status is improved.
  - Physical capacity is increased.
  - Physical function is improved.
- Impact on societal resources
  - Costs of work-related injury or disability are reduced.
  - Utilization of physical therapy services is optimized.
  - Utilization of physical therapy services results in efficient use of health care dollars.
- Patient/client satisfaction
  - Access, availability, and services provided are acceptable to patient/client.
  - Administrative management of practice is acceptable to patient/client.
  - Clinical proficiency of physical therapist is acceptable to patient/client.
  - Coordination of care is acceptable to patient/client.
  - Cost of health care services is decreased.
  - Intensity of care is decreased.
  - Interpersonal skills of physical therapist are acceptable to patient/client, family, and significant others.
  - Sense of well-being is improved.
  - Stressors are decreased.

Manual Therapy Techniques (Including Mobilization/Manipulation)

Interventions

- Massage
  - connective tissue massage
  - therapeutic massage
- Mobilization/manipulation
  - soft tissue
- Passive range of motion

Anticipated Goals and Expected Outcomes

- Impact on pathology/pathophysiology (disease, disorder, or condition)
  - Edema, Lymphedema or effusion is reduced.
  - Joint swelling, inflammation, or restriction is reduced.
  - Pain is decreased.
  - Soft tissue swelling, inflammation, or restriction is reduced.
- Impact on impairments
  - Gait, locomotion, and balance are improved.
  - Integumentary integrity is improved.
  - Joint integrity and mobility are improved.
  - Muscle performance (strength, power, and endurance) is increased.
  - Postural control is improved.
  - Quality and quantity of movement between and across body segments are improved.
  - Range of motion is improved.
  - Relaxation is increased.
  - Sensory awareness is increased.
  - Weight-bearing status is improved.
- Impact on functional limitations
  - Ability to perform movement tasks is improved.
  - Ability to perform physical actions, tasks, or activities related to self-care, home management, work (job/school/play), community, and leisure is improved.
  - Tolerance of positions and activities is increased.
- Impact on disabilities
  - Ability to assume or resume required self-care, home management, work (job/school/play), community, and leisure roles is improved.
- Risk reduction/prevention
  - Risk factors are reduced.
  - Risk of secondary impairment is reduced.
  - Self-management of symptoms is improved.
- Impact on health, wellness, and fitness
  - Fitness is improved.
  - Physical capacity is increased.
  - Physical function is improved.
- Impact on societal resources
  - Utilization of physical therapy services is optimized.
  - Utilization of physical therapy services results in efficient use of health care dollars.
- Patient/client satisfaction
  - Access, availability, and services provided are acceptable to patient/client.
  - Administrative management of practice is acceptable to patient/client.
  - Clinical proficiency of physical therapist is acceptable to patient/client.
  - Coordination of care is acceptable to patient/client.
  - Cost of health care services is decreased.
  - Intensity of care is decreased.
  - Interpersonal skills of physical therapist are acceptable to patient/client, family, and significant others.
  - Sense of well-being is improved.
  - Stressors are decreased.

Prescription, Application, and, as Appropriate, Fabrication of Devices and Equipment (Assistive, Adaptive, Orthotic, Protective, Supportive, and Prosthetic)

Interventions

- Adaptive devices
  - environmental controls
  - hospital beds
  - raised toilet seats
  - seating systems
- Assistive devices
  - canes
  - crutches
  - long-handled reachers
  - power devices
  - static and dynamic splints
  - walkers
  - wheelchairs
- Orthotic devices
  - braces
  - casts
  - shoe inserts
  - splints
- Protective devices
  - braces
  - cushions
  - protective taping
- Supportive devices
  - compression garments
  - corsets
  - elastic wraps
  - neck collars
  - serial casts
  - slings
  - supportive taping

Anticipated Goals and Expected Outcomes

- Impact on pathology/pathophysiology (disease, disorder, or condition)
  - Edema, lymphedema, or effusion is reduced.
  - Joint swelling, inflammation, or restriction is reduced.
  - Soft tissue swelling, inflammation, or restriction is reduced.
  - Pain is decreased.
- Impact on impairments
  - Balance is improved.
  - Endurance is increased.
  - Energy expenditure per unit of work is decreased.
  - Gait, locomotion, and balance are improved.
  - Integumentary integrity is improved.
  - Joint stability is improved.
  - Motor function (motor control and motor learning) is improved.
  - Muscle performance (strength, power, and endurance) is increased.
  - Optimal joint alignment is achieved.
  - Optimal loading on a body part is achieved.
  - Postural control is improved.
  - Quality and quantity of movement between and across body segments are improved.
  - Range of motion is improved.
  - Weight-bearing status is improved.
- Impact on functional limitations
  - Ability to perform physical actions, tasks, or activities related to self-care, home management, work (job/school/play), community, and leisure is improved.
  - Level of supervision required for task performance is decreased.
  - Performance of and independence in activities of daily living (ADL) and instrumental activities of daily living (IADL) with or without devices and equipment are increased.
  - Tolerance of positions and activities is increased.
- Impact on disabilities
  - Ability to assume or resume required self-care, home management, work (job/school/play), community, and leisure roles is improved.
- Risk reduction/prevention
  - Pressure on body tissues is reduced.
  - Protection of body parts is increased.
  - Risk factors are reduced.
  - Risk of recurrence of condition is reduced.
  - Risk of secondary impairment is reduced.
  - Safety is improved.
  - Self-management of symptoms is improved.
  - Stresses precipitating injury are decreased.
- Impact on health, wellness, and fitness
  - Fitness is improved.
  - Health status is improved.
  - Physical capacity is increased.
  - Physical function is improved.
- Impact on societal resources
  - Utilization of physical therapy services is optimized.
  - Utilization of physical therapy services results in efficient use of health care dollars.
- Patient/client satisfaction
  - Access, availability, and services provided are acceptable to patient/client.
  - Administrative management of practice is acceptable to patient/client.
  - Clinical proficiency of physical therapist is acceptable to patient/client.
  - Coordination of care is acceptable to patient/client.
  - Cost of health care services is decreased.
  - Intensity of care is decreased.
  - Interpersonal skills of physical therapist are acceptable to patient/client, family, and significant others.
  - Sense of well-being is improved.
  - Stressors are decreased.

Electrotherapeutic Modalities

Interventions

- Biofeedback
- Electrical stimulation
  - electrical muscle stimulation (EMS)
  - functional electrical stimulation (FES)
  - high voltage pulsed current (HVPC)
  - neuromuscular electrical stimulation (NMES)
  - transcutaneous electrical nerve stimulation (TENS)

Anticipated Goals and Expected Outcomes

- Impact on pathology/pathophysiology (disease, disorder, or condition)
  - Edema, lymphedema, or effusion is reduced.
  - Joint swelling, inflammation, or restriction is reduced.
  - Nutrient delivery to tissue is increased.
  - Osteogenic effects are enhanced.
  - Pain is decreased.
  - Soft tissue or wound healing is enhanced.
  - Soft tissue swelling, inflammation, or restriction is reduced.
  - Tissue perfusion and oxygenation are enhanced.
- Impact on impairments
  - Integumentary integrity is improved.
  - Motor function (motor control and motor learning) is improved.
  - Muscle performance (strength, power, and endurance) is increased.
  - Postural control is improved.
  - Quality and quantity of movement between and across body segments are improved.
  - Range of motion is improved.
  - Relaxation is increased.
  - Sensory awareness is increased.
- Impact on functional limitations
  - Ability to perform physical actions, tasks, or activities related to self-care, home management, work (job/school/play), community, and leisure is improved.
  - Level of supervision required for task performance is decreased.
  - Performance of and independence in activities of daily living (ADL) and instrumental activities of daily living (IADL) with or without devices and equipment are increased.
  - Tolerance of positions and activities is increased.
- Impact on disabilities
  - Ability to assume or resume required self-care, home management, work (job/school/play), community, and leisure roles is improved.
- Risk reduction/prevention
  - Complications of immobility are reduced.
  - Preoperative and postoperative complications are reduced.
  - Risk factors are reduced.
  - Risk of secondary impairment is reduced.
  - Self-management of symptoms is improved.
- Impact on health, wellness, and fitness
  - Fitness is improved.
  - Physical capacity is increased.
  - Physical function is improved.
- Impact on societal resources
  - Utilization of physical therapy services is optimized.
  - Utilization of physical therapy services results in efficient use of health care dollars.
- Patient/client satisfaction
  - Access, availability, and services provided are acceptable to patient/client.
  - Administrative management of practice is acceptable to patient/client.
  - Clinical proficiency of physical therapist is acceptable to patient/client.
  - Coordination of care is acceptable to patient/client.
  - Interpersonal skills of physical therapist are acceptable to patient/client, family, and significant others.
  - Sense of well-being is improved.
  - Stressors are decreased.

Physical Agents and Mechanical Modalities

Interventions

Physical agents may include:

- Cryotherapy
  - cold packs
  - ice massage
  - vapocoolant spray
- Hydrotherapy
  - whirlpool tanks
  - contrast bath
  - pools
- Sound agents
  - phonophoresis
  - ultrasound
- Thermotherapy
  - dry heat
  - hot packs
  - paraffin baths

Mechanical modalities may include:

- Mechanical motion devices
  - continuous passive motion (CPM)

Anticipated Goals and Expected Outcomes

- Impact on pathology/pathophysiology (disease, disorder, or condition)
  - Edema, lymphedema, or effusion is reduced.
  - Joint swelling, inflammation, or restriction is reduced.
  - Nutrient delivery to tissue is increased.
  - Pain is decreased.
  - Soft tissue swelling, inflammation, or restriction is reduced.
  - Tissue perfusion and oxygenation are enhanced.
- Impact on impairments
  - Integumentary integrity is improved.
  - Muscle performance (strength, power, and endurance) is increased.
  - Range of motion is improved.
  - Weight-bearing status is improved.
- Impact on functional limitations
  - Ability to perform physical actions, tasks, or activities related to self-care, home management, work (job/school/play), community, and leisure is improved.
  - Performance of and independence in activities of daily living (ADL) and instrumental activities of daily living (IADL) with or without devices and equipment are increased.
  - Tolerance of positions and activities is increased.
- Impact on disabilities
  - Ability to assume or resume required self-care, home management, work (job/school/play), community, and leisure roles is improved.
- Risk reduction/prevention
  - Complications of soft tissue and circulatory disorders are decreased.
  - Risk factors are reduced.
  - Risk of secondary impairment is reduced.
  - Self-management of symptoms is improved.
- Impact on health, wellness, and fitness
  - Fitness is improved.
  - Physical capacity is improved.
  - Physical function is improved.
- Impact on societal resources
  - Utilization of physical therapy services is optimized.
- Patient/client satisfaction
  - Access, availability, and services provided are acceptable to patient/client.
  - Administrative management of practice is acceptable to patient/client.
  - Clinical proficiency of physical therapist is acceptable to patient/client.
  - Coordination of care is acceptable to patient/client.
  - Interpersonal skills of physical therapist are acceptable to patient/client, family, and significant others.
  - Sense of well-being is improved.
  - Stressors are decreased.

Reexamination

Reexamination is the process of performing selected tests and measures after the initial examination to evaluate progress and to modify or redirect interventions. Reexamination may be indicated more than once during a single episode of care. It also may be performed over the course of a disease, disorder, or condition, which for some patients/clients may be over the life span. Indications for reexamination include new clinical findings or failure to respond to physical therapy interventions.

Global Outcomes for Patients/Clients in This Pattern

Throughout the entire episode of care, the physical therapist determines the anticipated goals and expected outcomes for each intervention. These anticipated goals and expected outcomes are delineated in shaded boxes that accompany the lists of interventions in each preferred practice pattern. As the patient/client reaches the termination of physical therapy services and the end of the episode of care, the physical therapist measures the global outcomes of the physical therapy services by characterizing or quantifying the impact of the physical therapy interventions in the following domains:

- Pathology/pathophysiology (disease, disorder, or condition)
- Impairments
- Functional limitations
- Disabilities
- Risk reduction/prevention
- Health, wellness, and fitness
- Societal resources
- Patient/client satisfaction

In some instances, a particular anticipated goal or expected outcome is thoroughly achieved through implementation of a single form of intervention. More commonly, however, the anticipated goals and expected outcomes are achieved as a result of the combined effects of several forms of interventions, leading to enhancement of both health status and health-related quality of life.

Criteria for Termination of Physical Therapy Services

Discharge is the process of ending physical therapy services that have been provided during a single episode of care. It occurs when the anticipated goals and expected outcomes have been achieved. Discharge does *not* occur with a *transfer* (defined as the time when a patient is moved from one site to another site within the same setting or across settings during a single episode of care). Although there may be facility-specific or payer-specific requirements for documentation regarding the conclusion of physical therapy services, *discharge occurs based on the physical therapist's analysis of the achievement of anticipated goals and expected outcomes.*

Discontinuation is the process of ending physical therapy services that have been provided during a single episode of care when (1) the patient/client, caregiver, or legal guardian declines to continue intervention; (2) the patient/client is unable to continue to progress toward outcomes because of medical or psychosocial complications or because financial/insurance resources have been expended; or (3) the physical therapist determines that the patient/client will no longer benefit from physical therapy. When physical therapy services are terminated prior to achievement of anticipated goals and expected outcomes, patient/client status and the rationale for termination are documented.

For patients/clients who require multiple episodes of care, periodic follow-up is needed over the life span to ensure safety and effective adaptation following changes in physical status, caregivers, environment, or task demands. In consultation with appropriate individuals, and in consideration of the outcomes, the physical therapist plans for discharge or discontinuation and provides for appropriate follow-up or referral.

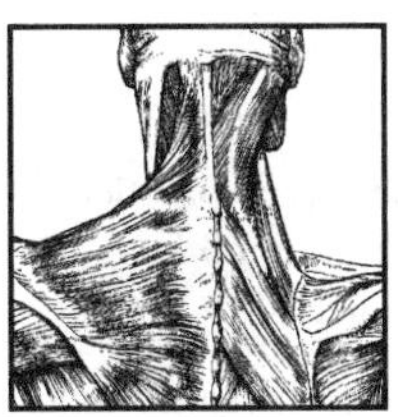

Impaired Joint Mobility, Motor Function, Muscle Performance, and Range of Motion Associated With Bony or Soft Tissue Surgery

This preferred practice pattern describes the generally accepted elements of patient/client management that physical therapists provide for patients/clients who are classified in this pattern. The pattern title reflects the diagnosis made by the physical therapist. APTA emphasizes that preferred practice patterns are the boundaries within which a physical therapist may select any of a number of clinical alternatives, based on consideration of a wide variety of factors, such as individual patient/client needs; the profession's code of ethics and standards of practice; and patient/client age, culture, gender roles, race, sex, sexual orientation, and socioeconomic status.

Patient/Client Diagnostic Classification

Patients/clients will be classified into this pattern—for impaired joint mobility, motor function, muscle performance, and range of motion associated with bony or soft tissue surgery—as a result of the physical therapist's evaluation of the examination data. The findings from the examination (history, systems review, and tests and measures) may indicate the presence or risk of pathology/pathophysiology (disease, disorder, or condition), impairments, functional limitations, or disabilities or the need for health, wellness, or fitness programs. The physical therapist integrates, synthesizes, and interprets the data to determine the diagnostic classification.

Inclusion

The following examples of examination findings may support the inclusion of patients/clients in this pattern:

Risk Factors or Consequences of Pathology/Pathophysiology (Disease, Disorder, or Condition)

- Ankylosis
- Bone graft and lengthening procedures
- Cesarean section
- Connective tissue repair or reconstruction
- Fascial releases
- Fusions
- Internal debridement
- Internal knee derangement
- Intervertebral disk disorder
- Laminectomies
- Muscle, tendon, ligament, capsule repair or reconstruction
- Multisite fractures
- Open reduction internal fixation
- Osteotomies
- Tibial tuberosity procedures

Impairments, Functional Limitations, or Disabilities

- Decreased range of motion
- Decreased strength and endurance due to inactivity
- Impaired joint mobility
- Limited independence in activities of daily living
- Pain
- Swelling

Note:

Some risk factors or consequences of pathology/pathophysiology—such as *failed surgeries*—may be severe and complex; *however, they do not necessarily exclude patients/clients from this pattern.* Severe and complex risk factors or consequences may require modification of the frequency of visits and duration of care. (See "Evaluation, Diagnosis, and Prognosis," page 276.)

Exclusion or Multiple-Pattern Classification

The following examples of examination findings may support exclusion from this pattern or classification into additional patterns. Depending on the level of severity or complexity of the examination findings, the physical therapist may determine that the patient/client would be more appropriately managed through (1) classification in an entirely different pattern or (2) classification in both this and another pattern.

Findings That May Require Classification in a Different Pattern

- Amputation
- Closed head trauma
- Non-union fractures
- Peripheral nerve lesions
- Total joint arthroplasties

Findings That May Require Classification in Additional Patterns

- Neurological sequelae
- Non-healing wound
- Vascular sequelae

ICD-9-CM Codes

The listing below contains the current (as of press time) and most typical 3- and 4-digit ICD-9-CM codes related to this preferred practice pattern. Because patient/client diagnostic classification is based on impairments, functional limitations, and disabilities—not on codes—patients/clients may be classified into the pattern even though the codes listed with the pattern may not apply to those clients.

This listing is intended for general information only and should not be used for coding purposes. The codes should be confirmed by referring to the World Health Organization's *International Classification of Diseases, 9th Revision, Clinical Modification (ICD-9-CM 2001)*, Volumes 1 and 3 (Chicago, Ill: American Medical Association; 2000) or subsequent revisions or by referring to other ICD-9-CM coding manuals that contain exclusion notes and instructions regarding fifth-digit requirements.

715 Osteoarthrosis and allied disorders

717 Internal derangement of knee
- **717.8** Other internal derangement of knee

718 Other derangement of joint
- **718.0** Articular cartilage disorder
- **718.2** Pathological dislocation
- **718.3** Recurrent dislocation of joint
- **718.4** Contracture of joint
- **718.5** Ankylosis of joint
- **718.9** Unspecified derangement of joint

719 Other and unspecified disorders of joint

721 Spondylosis and allied disorders

722 Intervertebral disk disorders
- **722.7** Intervertebral disk disorder with myelopathy

723 Other disorders of cervical region

724 Other and unspecified disorders of back
- **724.0** Spinal stenosis, other than cervical
- **724.3** Sciatica

726 Peripheral enthesopathies and allied syndromes
- **726.0** Adhesive capsulitis of shoulder
- **726.1** Rotator cuff syndrome of shoulder and allied disorders
- **726.2** Other affections of shoulder region, not elsewhere classified
  - Periarthritis of shoulder
  - Scapulohumeral fibrositis
- **726.9** Unspecified enthesopathy

727 Other disorders of synovium, tendon, and bursa
- **727.0** Synovitis and tenosynovitis
- **727.1** Bunion
- **727.4** Ganglion and cyst of synovium, tendon, and bursa
- **727.6** Rupture of tendon, nontraumatic

728 Disorders of muscle, ligament, and fascia
- **728.6** Contracture of palmar fascia
  - Dupuytren's contracture

731 Osteitis deformans and osteopathies associated with other disorders classified elsewhere
- **731.0** Osteitis deformans without mention of bone tumor
  - Paget's disease of bone

732 Osteochondropathies
- **732.4** Juvenile osteochondrosis of lower extremity, excluding foot
  - Tibial tubercle (of Osgood-Schlatter)
- **732.9** Unspecified osteochondropathy

733 Other disorders of bone and cartilage
- **733.1** Pathologic fracture
  - Spontaneous fracture
- **733.8** Malunion and nonunion of fracture
  - **733.82** Nonunion of fracture

736 Other acquired deformities of limbs
- **736.8** Acquired deformities of other parts of limbs

737 Curvature of spine

738 Other acquired deformity
- **738.4** Acquired spondylolisthesis

756 Other congenital musculoskeletal anomalies
- **756.1** Anomalies of spine

802 Fracture of face bones

805 Fracture of vertebral column without mention of spinal cord injury

808 Fracture of pelvis

810 Fracture of clavicle

811 Fracture of scapula

812 Fracture of humerus

813 Fracture of radius and ulna

814 Fracture of carpal bone(s)

815 Fracture of metacarpal bone(s)

816 Fracture of one or more phalanges of hand

820 Fracture of neck of femur

821 Fracture of other and unspecified parts of femur

822 Fracture of patella

823 Fracture of tibia and fibula

824 Fracture of ankle

825 Fracture of one or more tarsal and metatarsal bones

826 Fracture of one or more phalanges of foot

830 Dislocation of jaw

831 Dislocation of shoulder

832 Dislocation of elbow

833 Dislocation of wrist

834 Dislocation of finger

835 Dislocation of hip

836 Dislocation of knee

- **836.0** Tear of medial cartilage or meniscus of knee, current
- **836.1** Tear of lateral cartilage or meniscus of knee, current
- **836.2** Other tear of cartilage or meniscus of knee, current
- **836.5** Other dislocation of knee, closed

837 Dislocation of ankle

838 Dislocation of foot

839 Other, multiple, and ill-defined dislocations

- **839.0** Cervical vertebra, closed
- **839.3** Thoracic and lumbar vertebra, open
- **839.8** Multiple and ill-defined, closed
  - Arm
  - Back
  - Hand
  - Multiple locations, except for fingers or toes alone

840 Sprains and strains of shoulder and upper arm

- **840.4** Rotator cuff (capsule)

841 Sprains and strains of elbow and forearm

842 Sprains and strains of wrist and hand

843 Sprains and strains of hip and thigh

844 Sprains and strains of knee and leg

845 Sprains and strains of ankle and foot

846 Sprains and strains of sacroiliac region

847 Sprains and strains of other and unspecified parts of back

848 Other and ill-defined sprains and strains

959 Injury, other and unspecified

- **959.2** Shoulder and upper arm
- **959.9** Unspecified site

Examination

Examination is a comprehensive screening and specific testing process that leads to a diagnostic classification or, when appropriate, to a referral to another practitioner. Examination is required prior to the initial intervention and is performed for all patients/clients. Through the examination, the physical therapist may identify impairments, functional limitations, disabilities, changes in physical function or overall health status, and needs related to restoration of health and to prevention, wellness, and fitness. The physical therapist synthesizes the examination findings to establish the diagnosis and the prognosis (including the plan of care). The patient/client, family, significant others, and caregivers may provide information during the examination process.

Examination has three components: the patient/client history, the systems review, and tests and measures. The *history* is a systematic gathering of past and current information (often from the patient/client) related to why the patient/client is seeking the services of the physical therapist. The *systems review* is a brief or limited examination of (1) the anatomical and physiological status of the cardiovascular/pulmonary, integumentary, musculoskeletal, and neuromuscular systems and (2) the communication ability, affect, cognition, language, and learning style of the patient/client. *Tests and measures* are the means of gathering data about the patient/client.

The selection of examination procedures and the depth of the examination vary based on patient/client age; severity of the problem; stage of recovery (acute, subacute, chronic); phase of rehabilitation (early, intermediate, late, return to activity); home, work (job/school/play), or community situation; and other relevant factors. *For clinical indications in selecting tests and measures and for listings of tests and measures, tools used to gather data, and the types of data generated by tests and measures, refer to Chapter 2.*

Patient/Client History

The history may include:

General Demographics
- Age
- Sex
- Race/ethnicity
- Primary language
- Education

Social History
- Cultural beliefs and behaviors
- Family and caregiver resources
- Social interactions, social activities, and support systems

Employment/Work (Job/School/Play)
- Current and prior work (job/school/play), community, and leisure actions, tasks, or activities

Growth and Development
- Developmental history
- Hand dominance

Living Environment
- Devices and equipment (eg, assistive, adaptive, orthotic, protective, supportive, prosthetic)
- Living environment and community characteristics
- Projected discharge destinations

General Health Status (Self-Report, Family Report, Caregiver Report)
- General health perception
- Physical function (eg, mobility, sleep patterns, restricted bed days)
- Psychological function (eg, memory, reasoning ability, depression, anxiety)
- Role function (eg, community, leisure, social, work)
- Social function (eg, social activity, social interaction, social support)

Social/Health Habits (Past and Current)
- Behavioral health risks (eg, smoking, drug abuse)
- Level of physical fitness

Family History
- Familial health risks

Medical/Surgical History
- Cardiovascular
- Endocrine/metabolic
- Gastrointestinal
- Genitourinary
- Gynecological
- Integumentary
- Musculoskeletal
- Neuromuscular
- Obstetrical
- Prior hospitalizations, surgeries, and preexisting medical and other health-related conditions
- Psychological
- Pulmonary

Current Condition(s)/Chief Complaint(s)
- Concerns that led patient/client to seek the services of a physical therapist
- Concerns or needs of patient/client who requires the services of a physical therapist
- Current therapeutic interventions
- Mechanisms of injury or disease, including date of onset and course of events
- Onset and pattern of symptoms
- Patient/client, family, significant other, and caregiver expectations and goals for the therapeutic intervention
- Patient/client, family, significant other, and caregiver perceptions of patient's/client's emotional response to the current clinical situation
- Previous occurrence of chief complaint(s)
- Prior therapeutic interventions

Functional Status and Activity Level
- Current and prior functional status in self-care and home management activities, including activities of daily living (ADL) and instrumental activities of daily living (IADL)
- Current and prior functional status in work (job/school/play), community, and leisure actions, tasks, or activities

Medications
- Medications for current condition
- Medications previously taken for current condition
- Medications for other conditions

Other Clinical Tests
- Laboratory and diagnostic tests
- Review of available records (eg, medical, education, surgical)
- Review of other clinical findings (eg, nutrition and hydration)

Systems Review

The systems review may include:

Anatomical and Physiological Status

- Cardiovascular/Pulmonary
  - Blood pressure
  - Edema
  - Heart rate
  - Respiratory rate
- Integumentary
  - Pliability (texture)
  - Presence of scar formation
  - Skin color
  - Skin integrity
- Musculoskeletal
  - Gross range of motion
  - Gross strength
  - Gross symmetry
  - Height
  - Weight
- Neuromuscular
  - Gross coordinated movements (eg, balance, gait, locomotion, transfers, transitions)
  - Motor function (motor control, motor learning)

Communication, Affect, Cognition, Language, and Learning Style

- Ability to make needs known
- Consciousness
- Expected emotional/behavioral responses
- Learning preferences (eg, education needs, learning barriers)
- Orientation (person, place, time)

Tests and Measures

Tests and measures for this pattern may include those that characterize or quantify:

Aerobic Capacity and Endurance

- Aerobic capacity during functional activities (eg, activities of daily living [ADL] scales, indexes, instrumental activities of daily living [IADL] scales, observations)

Anthropometric Characteristics

- Body dimensions (eg, girth measurement, length measurement)
- Edema (eg, girth measurement, palpation, scales, volume measurement)

Assistive and Adaptive Devices

- Assistive or adaptive devices and equipment use during functional activities (eg, ADL scales, functional scales, IADL scales, interviews, observations)
- Components, alignment, fit, and ability to care for the assistive or adaptive devices and equipment (eg, interviews, logs, observations, pressure-sensing maps, reports)
- Remediation of impairments, functional limitations, or disabilities with use of assistive or adaptive devices and equipment (eg, activity status indexes, ADL scales, aerobic capacity tests, functional performance inventories, health assessment questionnaires, IADL scales, pain scales, play scales, videographic assessments)
- Safety during use of assistive or adaptive devices and equipment (eg, diaries, fall scales, interviews, logs, observations, reports)

Cranial and Peripheral Nerve Integrity

- Electrophysiological integrity (eg, electroneuromyography)
- Motor distribution of the cranial nerves (eg, dynamometry, muscle tests, observations)
- Motor distribution of the peripheral nerves (eg, dynamometry, muscle tests, observations, thoracic outlet tests)
- Sensory distribution of the cranial nerves (eg, discrimination tests; tactile tests, including coarse and light touch, cold and heat, pain, pressure, and vibration)
- Sensory distribution of the peripheral nerves (eg, discrimination tests; tactile tests, including coarse and light touch, cold and heat, pain, pressure, and vibration; thoracic outlet tests)

Environmental, Home, and Work (Job/School/Play) Barriers

- Current and potential barriers (eg, checklists, interviews, observations, questionnaires)
- Physical space and environment (eg, compliance standards, observations, photographic assessments, questionnaires, structural specifications, videographic assessments)

Ergonomics and Body Mechanics

Ergonomics

- Dexterity and coordination during work (job/school/play) (eg, hand function tests, impairment rating scales, manipulative ability tests)
- Functional capacity and performance during work actions, tasks, or activities (eg, accelerometry, dynamometry, electroneuromyography, endurance tests, force platform tests, goniometry, interviews, observations, photographic assessments, physical capacity tests, postural loading analyses, technology-assisted assessments, videographic assessments, work analyses)
- Safety in work environments (eg, hazard identification checklists, job severity indexes, lifting standards, risk assessment scales, standards for exposure limits)
- Specific work conditions or activities (eg, handling checklists, job simulations, lifting models, preemployment screenings, task analysis checklists, workstation checklists)
- Tools, devices, equipment, and workstations related to work actions, tasks, or activities (eg, observations, tool analysis checklists, vibration assessments)

Body mechanics

- Body mechanics during self-care, home management, work, community, or leisure actions, tasks, or activities (eg, ADL scales, IADL scales, observations, photographic assessments, technology-assisted assessments, videographic assessments)

Gait, Locomotion, and Balance

- Balance during functional activities with or without the use of assistive, adaptive, orthotic, protective, supportive, or prosthetic devices or equipment (eg, ADL scales, IADL scales, observations, videographic assessments)
- Balance (dynamic and static) with or without the use of assistive, adaptive, orthotic, protective, supportive, or prosthetic devices or equipment (eg, balance scales, dizziness inventories, dynamic posturography, fall scales, motor impairment tests, observations, photographic assessments, postural control tests)
- Gait and locomotion during functional activities with or without the use of assistive, adaptive, orthotic, protective, supportive, or prosthetic devices or equipment (eg, ADL scales, gait indexes, IADL scales, mobility skill profiles, observations, videographic assessments)
- Gait and locomotion with or without the use of assistive, adaptive, orthotic, protective, supportive, or prosthetic devices or equipment (eg, dynamometry, electroneuromyography, footprint analyses, gait indexes, mobility skill profiles, observations, photographic assessments, technology-assisted assessments, videographic assessments, weight-bearing scales, wheelchair mobility tests)
- Safety during gait, locomotion, and balance (eg, confidence scales, diaries, fall scales, functional assessment profiles, logs, reports)

Integumentary Integrity

Associated skin

- Activities, positioning, and postures that produce or relieve trauma to the skin (eg, observations, pressure-sensing maps, scales)
- Assistive, adaptive, orthotic, protective, supportive, or prosthetic devices and equipment that may produce or relieve trauma to the skin (eg, observations, pressure-sensing maps, risk assessment scales)
- Skin characteristics, including blistering, continuity of skin color, dermatitis, hair growth, mobility, nail growth, sensation, temperature, texture, and turgor (eg, observations, palpation, photographic assessments, thermography)

Wound

- Activities, positioning, and postures that aggravate the wound or scar or that produce or relieve trauma (eg, observations, pressure-sensing maps)
- Signs of infection (eg, cultures, observations, palpation)
- Wound scar tissue characteristics, including banding, pliability, sensation, and texture (eg, observations, scar-rating scales)

Joint Integrity and Mobility

- Joint integrity and mobility (eg, apprehension, compression and distraction, drawer, glide, impingement, shear, and valgus/varus stress tests; arthrometry; palpation)
- Joint play movements, including end feel (all joints of the axial and appendicular skeletal system) (eg, palpation)

Motor Function (Motor Control and Motor Learning)

- Dexterity, coordination, and agility (eg, coordination screens, motor impairment tests, motor proficiency tests, observations, videographic assessments)
- Hand function (eg, fine and gross motor control tests, finger dexterity tests, manipulative ability tests, observations)

Muscle Performance (Including Strength, Power, and Endurance)

- Electrophysiological integrity (eg, electroneuromyography)
- Muscle strength, power, and endurance (eg, dynamometry, manual muscle tests, muscle performance tests, physical capacity tests, technology-assisted assessments, timed activity tests)
- Muscle strength, power, and endurance during functional activities (eg, ADL scales, functional muscle tests, IADL scales, observations, videographic assessments)

Orthotic, Protective, and Supportive Devices

- Components, alignment, fit, and ability to care for orthotic, protective, and supportive devices and equipment (eg, interviews, logs, observations, pressure-sensing maps, reports)
- Orthotic, protective, and supportive devices and equipment use during functional activities (eg, ADL scales, functional scales, IADL scales, interviews, observations, profiles)
- Remediation of impairments, functional limitations, or disabilities with use of orthotic, protective, and supportive devices and equipment (eg, activity status indexes, ADL scales, aerobic capacity tests, functional performance inventories, health assessment questionnaires, IADL scales, pain scales, play scales, videographic assessments)
- Safety during use of orthotic, protective, and supportive devices and equipment (eg, diaries, fall scales, interviews, logs, observations, reports)

Pain

- Pain, soreness, and nociception (eg, analog scales, angina scales, discrimination tests, pain drawings and maps, provocation tests, verbal and pictorial descriptor tests)
- Pain in specific body parts (eg, pain indexes, pain questionnaires, structural provocation tests)

Posture

- Postural alignment and position (static and dynamic), including symmetry and deviation from midline (eg, grid measurement, observations, photographic assessment, technology-assisted assessments, videographic assessments)
- Specific body parts (eg, angle assessments, forward-bending test, goniometry, observations, palpation, positional tests)

Range of Motion (ROM) (Including Muscle Length)

- Functional ROM (eg, observations, squat testing, toe touch tests)
- Joint active and passive movement (eg, goniometry, inclinometry, observations, photographic assessments, technology-assisted assessments, videographic assessments)
- Muscle length, soft tissue extensibility, and flexibility (eg, contracture tests, goniometry, inclinometry, ligamentous tests, linear measurement, multisegment flexibility tests, palpation)

Reflex Integrity

- Deep reflexes (eg, myotatic reflex scale, observations, reflex tests)
- Superficial reflexes and reactions (eg, observations, provocation tests)

Self-Care and Home Management (Including ADL and IADL)

- Ability to gain access to home environments (eg, barrier identification, observations, physical performance tests)
- Ability to perform self-care and home management activities with or without assistive, adaptive, orthotic, protective, supportive, or prosthetic devices and equipment (eg, ADL scales, aerobic capacity tests, IADL scales, interviews, observations, profiles)
- Safety in self-care and home management activities and environments (eg, diaries, fall scales, interviews, logs, observations, reports, videographic assessments)

Sensory Integrity

- Combined/cortical sensations (eg, stereognosis tests, tactile discrimination tests)
- Deep sensations (eg, kinesthesiometry, observations, photographic assessments, vibration tests)
- Electrophysiological integrity (eg,electroneuromyography)

Work (Job/School/Play), Community, and Leisure Integration or Reintegration (Including IADL)

- Ability to assume or resume work (job/school/play), community, and leisure activities with or without assistive, adaptive, orthotic, protective, supportive, or prosthetic devices and equipment (eg, activity profiles, disability indexes, functional status questionnaires, IADL scales, observations, physical capacity tests)
- Ability to gain access to work (job/school/play), community, and leisure environments (eg, barrier identification, interviews, observations, physical capacity tests, transportation assessments)
- Safety in work (job/school/play), community, and leisure activities and environments (eg, diaries, fall scales, interviews, logs, observations, videographic assessments)

Evaluation, Diagnosis, and Prognosis (Including Plan of Care)

Physical therapists perform *evaluations* (make clinical judgments) based on the data gathered from the history, systems review, and tests and measures. In the evaluation process, physical therapists synthesize the examination data to establish the diagnosis and prognosis (including the plan of care). Factors that influence the complexity of the evaluation include the clinical findings, extent of loss of function, chronicity or severity of the problem, possibility of multisite or multisystem involvement, preexisting condition(s), potential discharge destination, social considerations, physical function, and overall health status.

A *diagnosis* is a label encompassing a cluster of signs and symptoms, syndromes, or categories. It is the result of the systematic diagnostic process, which includes integrating and evaluating the data from the examination.The diagnostic label indicates the primary dysfunction(s) toward which the therapist will direct interventions. The *prognosis* is the determination of the predicted optimal level of improvement in function and the amount of time needed to reach that level and may also include a prediction of levels of improvement that may be reached at various intervals during the course of therapy. During the prognostic process, the physical therapist develops the plan of care. The *plan of care* identifies specific interventions, proposed frequency and duration of the interventions, anticipated goals, expected outcomes, and discharge plans. The plan of care identifies realistic anticipated goals and expected outcomes, taking into consideration the expectations of the patient/client and appropriate others.These anticipated goals and expected outcomes should be measureable and time limited.

The frequency of visits and duration of the episode of care may vary from a short episode with a high intensity of intervention to a longer episode with a diminishing intensity of intervention. Frequency and duration may vary greatly among patients/clients based on a variety of factors that the physical therapist considers throughout the evaluation process, such as anatomical and physiological changes related to growth and development; caregiver consistency or expertise; chronicity or severity of the current condition; living environment; multisite or multisystem involvement; social support; potential discharge destinations; probability of prolonged impairment, functional limitation, or disability; and stability of the condition.

Prognosis

Over the course of 1 to 8 months, patient/client will demonstrate optimal joint mobility, motor function, muscle performance, and range of motion and the highest level of functioning in home, work (job/school/play), community, and leisure environments.

During the episode of care, patient/client will achieve (1) the anticipated goals and expected outcomes of the interventions that are described in the plan of care and (2) the global outcomes for patients/clients who are classified in this pattern.

Expected Range of Number of Visits Per Episode of Care

6 to 70

This range represents the lower and upper limits of the number of physical therapist visits required to achieve anticipated goals and expected outcomes. *It is anticipated that 80% of patients/clients who are classified into this pattern will achieve the anticipated goals and expected outcomes within 6 to 70 visits during a single continuous episode of care.* Frequency of visits and duration of the episode of care should be determined by the physical therapist to maximize effectiveness of care and efficiency of service delivery.

Factors That May Require New Episode of Care or That May Modify Frequency of Visits/ Duration of Episode

- Accessibility and availability of resources
- Adherence to the intervention program
- Age
- Anatomical and physiological changes related to growth and development
- Caregiver consistency or expertise
- Chronicity or severity of the current condition
- Cognitive status
- Comorbitities, complications, or secondary impairments
- Concurrent medical, surgical, and therapeutic interventions
- Decline in functional independence
- Level of impairment
- Level of physical function
- Living environment
- Multisite or multisystem involvement
- Nutritional status
- Overall health status
- Potential discharge destinations
- Premorbid conditions
- Probability of prolonged impairment, functional limitation, or disability
- Psychological and socioeconomic factors
- Psychomotor abilities
- Social support
- Stability of the condition

Intervention

Intervention is the purposeful interaction of the physical therapist with the patient/client and, when appropriate, with other individuals involved in patient/client care, using various physical therapy procedures and techniques to produce changes in the condition consistent with the diagnosis and prognosis. Decisions about interventions are contingent on the timely monitoring of patient/client response and the progress made toward achieving the anticipated goals and expected outcomes.

Communication, coordination, and documentation and patient/client-related instruction are provided for all patients/clients across all settings. Procedural interventions are selected or modified based on the examination data and the evaluation, the diagnosis and the prognosis, and the anticipated goals and expected outcomes for a particular patient/client. *For clinical considerations in selecting interventions, listings of interventions, and listings of anticipated goals and expected outcomes, refer to Chapter 3.*

Coordination, Communication, and Documentation

Coordination, communication, and documentation may include:

Interventions

- Addressing required functions
  - advance directives
  - individualized family service plans (IFSPs) or individualized education plans (IEPs)
  - informed consent
  - mandatory communication and reporting (eg, patient advocacy and abuse reporting)
- Admission and discharge planning
- Case management
- Collaboration and coordination with agencies, including:
  - equipment suppliers
  - home care agencies
  - payer groups
  - schools
  - transportation agencies
- Communication across settings, including:
  - case conferences
  - documentation
  - education plans
- Cost-effective resource utilization
- Data collection, analysis, and reporting
  - outcome data
  - peer review findings
  - record reviews
- Documentation across settings, following APTA's *Guidelines for Physical Therapy Documentation* (Appendix 5), including:
  - changes in impairments, functional limitations, and disabilities
  - changes in interventions
  - elements of patient/client management (examination, evaluation, diagnosis, prognosis, intervention)
  - outcomes of intervention
- Interdisciplinary teamwork
  - case conferences
  - patient care rounds
  - patient/client family meetings
- Referrals to other professionals or resources

Anticipated Goals and Expected Outcomes

- Accountability for services is increased.
- Admission data and discharge planning are completed.
- Advance directives, individualized family service plans (IFSPs) or individualized education plans (IEPs), informed consent, and mandatory communication and reporting (eg, patient advocacy and abuse reporting) are obtained or completed.
- Available resources are maximally utilized.
- Care is coordinated with patient/client, family, significant others, caregivers, and other professionals.
- Case is managed throughout the episode of care.
- Collaboration and coordination occurs with agencies, including equipment suppliers, home care agencies, payer groups, schools, and transportation agencies.
- Communication enhances risk reduction and prevention.
- Communication occurs across settings through case conferences, education plans, and documentation.
- Data are collected, analyzed, and reported, including outcome data, peer review findings, and record reviews.
- Decision making is enhanced regarding health, wellness, and fitness needs.
- Decision making is enhanced regarding patient/client health and the use of health care resources by patient/client, family, significant others, and caregivers.
- Documentation occurs throughout patient/client management and across settings and follows APTA's *Guidelines for Physical Therapy Documentation* (Appendix 5).
- Interdisciplinary collaboration occurs through case conferences, patient care rounds, and patient/client family meetings.
- Patient/client, family, significant other, and caregiver understanding of anticipated goals and expected outcomes is increased.
- Placement needs are determined.
- Referrals are made to other professionals or resources whenever necessary and appropriate.
- Resources are utilized in a cost-effective way.

Patient/Client-Related Instruction

Patient/client-related instruction may include:

Interventions

- Instruction, education and training of patients/clients and caregivers regarding:
    - current condition (pathology/pathophysiology [disease, disorder, or condition], impairments, functional limitations, or disabilities)
    - enhancement of performance
    - health, wellness, and fitness programs
    - plan of care
    - risk factors for pathology/pathophysiology (disease, disorder, or condition), impairments, functional limitations, or disabilities
    - transitions across settings
    - transitions to new roles

Anticipated Goals and Expected Outcomes

- Ability to perform physical actions, tasks, or activities is improved.
- Awareness and use of community resources are improved.
- Behaviors that foster healthy habits, wellness, and prevention are acquired.
- Decision making is enhanced regarding patient/client health and the use of health care resources by patient/client, family, significant others, and caregivers.
- Disability associated with acute or chronic illnesses is reduced.
- Functional independence in activities of daily living (ADL) and instrumental activities of daily living (IADL) is increased.
- Health status is improved.
- Intensity of care is decreased.
- Level of supervision required for task performance is decreased.
- Patient/client, family, significant other, and caregiver knowledge and awareness of the diagnosis, prognosis, interventions, and anticipated goals and expected outcomes are increased.
- Patient/client knowledge of personal and environmental factors associated with the condition is increased.
- Performance levels in self-care, home management, work (job/school/play), community, or leisure actions, tasks, or activities are improved.
- Physical function is improved.
- Risk of recurrence of condition is reduced.
- Risk of secondary impairment is reduced.
- Safety of patient/client, family, significant others, and caregivers is improved.
- Self-management of symptoms is improved.
- Utilization and cost of health care services are decreased.

Procedural Interventions

Procedural interventions for this pattern may include:

Therapeutic Exercise

Interventions

- Aerobic capacity/endurance conditioning or reconditioning
  - aquatic programs
  - gait and locomotor training
  - increased workload over time
  - walking and wheelchair propulsion programs
- Balance, coordination, and agility training
  - developmental activities training
  - motor function (motor control and motor learning) training or retraining
  - neuromuscular education or reeducation
  - perceptual training
  - posture awareness training
  - standardized, programmatic, complementary exercise approaches
  - sensory training or retraining
  - task-specific performance training
- Body mechanics and postural stabilization
  - body mechanics training
  - posture awareness training
  - postural control training
  - postural stabilization activities
- Flexibility exercises
  - muscle lengthening
  - range of motion
  - stretching
- Gait and locomotion training
  - developmental activities training
  - gait training
  - implement and device training
  - perceptual training
  - standardized, programmatic, complementary exercise approaches
  - wheelchair training
- Relaxation
  - breathing strategies
  - movement strategies
  - relaxation techniques
  - standardized, programmatic, complementary exercise approaches
- Strength, power, and endurance training for head, neck, limb, pelvic-floor, trunk, and ventilatory muscles
  - active assistive, active, and resistive exercises (including concentric, dynamic/isotonic, eccentric, isokinetic, isometric, and plyometric)
  - aquatic programs
  - standardized, programmatic, complementary exercise approaches
  - task-specific performance training

Anticipated Goals and Expected Outcomes

- Impact on pathology/pathophysiology (disease, disorder, or condition)
  - Joint swelling, inflammation, or restriction is reduced.
  - Nutrient delivery to tissue is increased.
  - Osteogenic effects of exercise are maximized.
  - Pain is decreased.
  - Physiological response to increased oxygen demand is improved.
  - Soft tissue swelling, inflammation, or restriction is reduced.
  - Tissue perfusion and oxygenation are enhanced.
- Impact on impairments
  - Aerobic capacity is increased.
  - Balance is improved.
  - Endurance is increased.
  - Energy expenditure per unit of work is decreased.
  - Gait, locomotion, and balance are improved.
  - Integumentary integrity is improved.
  - Joint integrity and mobility are improved.
  - Motor function (motor control and motor learning) is improved.
  - Muscle performance (strength, power, and endurance) is increased.
  - Postural control is improved.
  - Quality and quantity of movement between and across body segments are improved.
  - Range of motion is improved.
  - Relaxation is increased.
  - Sensory awareness is increased.
  - Weight-bearing status is improved.
- Impact on functional limitations
  - Ability to perform physical actions, tasks, or activities related to self-care, home management, work (job/school/play), community, and leisure is improved.
  - Level of supervision required for task performance is decreased.
  - Performance of and independence in activities of daily living (ADL) and instrumental activities of daily living (IADL) with or without devices and equipment are increased.
  - Tolerance of positions and activities is increased.
- Impact on disabilities
  - Ability to assume or resume required self-care, home management, work (job/school/play), community, and leisure roles is improved.
- Risk reduction/prevention
  - Preoperative and postoperative complications are reduced.
  - Risk factors are reduced.
  - Risk of secondary impairment is reduced.
  - Safety is improved.
  - Self-management of symptoms is improved.
- Impact on health, wellness, and fitness
  - Fitness is improved.
  - Health status is improved.
  - Physical capacity is increased.
  - Physical function is improved.
- Impact on societal resources
  - Utilization of physical therapy services is optimized.
  - Utilization of physical therapy services results in efficient use of health care dollars.
- Patient/client satisfaction
  - Access, availability, and services provided are acceptable to patient/client.
  - Administrative management of practice is acceptable to patient/client.
  - Clinical proficiency of physical therapist is acceptable to patient/client.
  - Coordination of care is acceptable to patient/client.
  - Cost of health care services is decreased.
  - Intensity of care is decreased.
  - Interpersonal skills of physical therapist are acceptable to patient/client, family, and significant others.
  - Sense of well-being is improved.
  - Stressors are decreased.

Functional Training in Self-Care and Home Management (Including Activities of Daily Living [ADL] and Instrumental Activities of Daily Living [IADL])

Interventions

- ADL training
  - bathing
  - bed mobility and transfer training
  - developmental activities
  - dressing
  - eating
  - grooming
  - toileting
- Devices and equipment use and training
  - assistive and adaptive device or equipment training during ADL and IADL
  - orthotic, protective, or supportive device or equipment training during ADL and IADL
  - prosthetic device or equipment training during ADL and IADL
- Functional training programs
  - back schools
  - simulated environments and tasks
  - task adaptation
- IADL training
  - caring for dependents
  - home maintenance
  - household chores
  - shopping
  - structured play for infants and children
  - yard work
- Injury prevention or reduction
  - injury prevention education during self-care and home management
  - injury prevention or reduction with use of devices and equipment
  - safety awareness training during self-care and home management

Anticipated Goals and Expected Outcomes

- Impact on pathology/pathophysiology (disease, disorder, or condition)
  - Pain is decreased.
  - Physiological response to increased oxygen demand is improved.
- Impact on impairments
  - Balance is improved.
  - Endurance is increased.
  - Energy expenditure per unit of work is decreased.
  - Motor function (motor control and motor learning) is improved.
  - Muscle performance (strength, power, and endurance) is increased.
  - Postural control is improved.
  - Sensory awareness is increased.
  - Weight-bearing status is improved.
- Impact on functional limitations
  - Ability to perform physical actions, tasks, or activities related to self-care and home management is improved.
  - Level of supervision required for task performance is decreased.
  - Performance of and independence in ADL and IADL with or without devices and equipment are increased.
  - Tolerance of positions and activities is increased.
- Impact on disabilities
  - Ability to assume or resume required self-care and home management roles is improved.
- Risk reduction/prevention
  - Risk factors are reduced.
  - Risk of secondary impairments is reduced.
  - Safety is improved.
  - Self-management of symptoms is improved.
- Impact on health, wellness, and fitness
  - Fitness is improved.
  - Health status is improved.
  - Physical capacity is increased.
  - Physical function is improved.
- Impact on societal resources
  - Utilization of physical therapy services is optimized.
  - Utilization of physical therapy services results in efficient use of health care dollars.
- Patient/client satisfaction
  - Access, availability, and services provided are acceptable to patient/client.
  - Administrative management of practice is acceptable to patient/client.
  - Clinical proficiency of physical therapist is acceptable to patient/client.
  - Coordination of care is acceptable to patient/client.
  - Cost of health care services is decreased.
  - Intensity of care is decreased.
  - Interpersonal skills of physical therapist are acceptable to patient/client, family, and significant others.
  - Sense of well-being is improved.
  - Stressors are decreased.

Functional Training in Work (Job/School/Play), Community, and Leisure Integration or Reintegration (Including Instrumental Activities of Daily Living [IADL], Work Hardening, and Work Conditioning)

Interventions

- Devices and equipment use and training
  - assistive and adaptive device or equipment training during IADL
  - orthotic, protective, or supportive device or equipment training during IADL
  - prosthetic device or equipment training during IADL
- Functional training programs
  - back schools
  - job coaching
  - simulated environments and tasks
  - task adaptation
  - task training
- IADL training
  - community service training involving instruments
  - school and play activities training including tools and instruments
  - work training with tools
- Injury prevention or reduction
  - injury prevention education during work (job/school/play), community, and leisure integration or reintegration
  - injury prevention or reduction with use of devices and equipment
  - safety awareness training during work (job/school/play), community, and leisure integration or reintegration
- Leisure and play activities and training

Anticipated Goals and Expected Outcomes

- Impact on pathology/pathophysiology (disease, disorder, or condition)
  - Pain is decreased.
  - Physiological response to increased oxygen demand is improved.
- Impact on impairments
  - Balance is improved.
  - Endurance is increased.
  - Energy expenditure per unit of work is decreased.
  - Motor function (motor control and motor learning) is improved.
  - Muscle performance (strength, power, and endurance) is increased.
  - Postural control is improved.
  - Sensory awareness is increased.
  - Weight-bearing status is improved.
- Impact on functional limitations
  - Ability to perform physical actions, tasks, or activities related to work (job/school/play), community, and leisure integration or reintegration is improved.
  - Level of supervision required for task performance is decreased.
  - Performance of and independence in IADL with or without devices and equipment are increased.
  - Tolerance of positions and activities is increased.
- Impact on disabilities
  - Ability to assume or resume required work (job/school/play), community, and leisure roles is improved.
- Risk reduction/prevention
  - Risk factors are reduced.
  - Risk of secondary impairment is reduced.
  - Safety is improved.
  - Self-management of symptoms is improved.
- Impact on health, wellness, and fitness
  - Fitness is improved.
  - Health status is improved.
  - Physical capacity is increased.
  - Physical function is improved.
- Impact on societal resources
  - Costs of work-related injury or disability are reduced.
  - Utilization of physical therapy services is optimized.
  - Utilization of physical therapy services results in efficient use of health care dollars.
- Patient/client satisfaction
  - Access, availability, and services provided are acceptable to patient/client.
  - Administrative management of practice is acceptable to patient/client.
  - Clinical proficiency of physical therapist is acceptable to patient/client.
  - Coordination of care is acceptable to patient/client.
  - Cost of health care services is decreased.
  - Intensity of care is decreased.
  - Interpersonal skills of physical therapist are acceptable to patient/client, family, and significant others.
  - Sense of well-being is improved.
  - Stressors are decreased.

Manual Therapy Techniques (Including Mobilization/Manipulation)

Interventions

- Manual lymphatic drainage
- Manual traction
- Massage
  - connective tissue massage
  - therapeutic massage
- Mobilization/manipulation
  - soft tissue
  - peripheral joints
- Passive range of motion

Anticipated Goals and Expected Outcomes

- Impact on pathology/pathophysiology (disease, disorder, or condition)
  - Edema, lymphedema, or effusion is reduced.
  - Joint swelling, inflammation, or restriction is reduced.
  - Neural compression is decreased.
  - Soft tissue swelling, inflammation, or restriction is reduced.
  - Pain is decreased.
- Impact on impairments
  - Gait, locomotion, and balance are improved.
  - Integumentary integrity is improved.
  - Joint integrity and mobility are improved.
  - Muscle performance (strength, power, and endurance) is increased.
  - Postural control is improved.
  - Quality and quantity of movement between and across body segments are improved.
  - Range of motion is improved.
  - Relaxation is increased.
  - Sensory awareness is increased.
  - Weight-bearing status is improved.
- Impact on functional limitations
  - Ability to perform movement tasks is improved.
  - Ability to perform physical actions, tasks, or activities related to self-care, home management, work (job/school/play), community, and leisure is improved.
  - Tolerance of positions and activities is increased.
- Impact on disabilities
  - Ability to assume or resume required self-care, home management, work (job/school/play), community, and leisure roles is improved.
- Risk reduction/prevention
  - Risk factors are reduced.
  - Risk of recurrence of condition is reduced.
  - Risk of secondary impairment is reduced.
  - Self-management of symptoms is improved.
- Impact on health, wellness, and fitness
  - Fitness is improved.
  - Physical capacity is increased.
  - Physical function is improved.
- Impact on societal resources
  - Utilization of physical therapy services is optimized.
  - Utilization of physical therapy services results in efficient use of health care dollars.
- Patient/client satisfaction
  - Access, availability, and services provided are acceptable to patient/client.
  - Administrative management of practice is acceptable to patient/client.
  - Clinical proficiency of physical therapist is acceptable to patient/client.
  - Coordination of care is acceptable to patient/client.
  - Cost of health care services is decreased.
  - Intensity of care is decreased.
  - Interpersonal skills of physical therapist are acceptable to patient/client, family, and significant others.
  - Sense of well-being is improved.
  - Stressors are decreased.

Prescription, Application, and, as Appropriate, Fabrication of Devices and Equipment (Assistive, Adaptive, Orthotic, Protective, Supportive, and Prosthetic)

Interventions

- Adaptive devices
  - environmental controls
  - hospital beds
  - raised toilet seats
  - seating systems
- Assistive devices
  - canes
  - crutches
  - long-handled reachers
  - power devices
  - static and dynamic splints
  - walkers
  - wheelchairs
- Orthotic devices
  - braces
  - casts
  - shoe inserts
  - splints
- Protective devices
  - braces
  - cushions
  - protective taping
- Supportive devices
  - compression garments
  - corsets
  - elastic wraps
  - neck collars
  - serial casts
  - slings
  - supportive taping

Anticipated Goals and Expected Outcomes

- Impact on pathology/pathophysiology (disease, disorder, or condition)
  - Edema, lymphedema, or effusion is reduced.
  - Joint swelling, inflammation, or restriction is reduced.
  - Pain is decreased.
  - Soft tissue swelling, inflammation, or restriction is reduced.
- Impact on impairments
  - Balance is improved.
  - Endurance is increased.
  - Energy expenditure per unit of work is decreased.
  - Gait, locomotion, and balance are improved.
  - Integumentary integrity is improved.
  - Joint integrity and mobility are improved.
  - Joint stability is improved.
  - Motor function (motor control and motor learning) is improved.
  - Muscle performance (strength, power, and endurance) is increased.
  - Optimal joint alignment is achieved.
  - Optimal loading on a body part is achieved.
  - Postural control is improved.
  - Quality and quantity of movement between and across body segments are improved.
  - Range of motion is improved.
  - Weight-bearing status is improved.
- Impact on functional limitations
  - Ability to perform physical actions, tasks, or activities related to self-care, home management, work (job/school/play), community, and leisure is improved.
  - Level of supervision required for task performance is decreased.
  - Performance of and independence in activities of daily living (ADL) and instrumental activities of daily living (IADL) with or without devices and equipment are increased.
  - Tolerance of positions and activities is increased.
- Impact on disabilities
  - Ability to assume or resume required self-care, home management, work (job/school/play), community, and leisure roles is improved.
- Risk reduction/prevention
  - Pressure on body tissues is reduced.
  - Protection of body parts is increased.
  - Risk factors are reduced.
  - Risk of recurrence of condition is reduced.
  - Risk of secondary impairment is reduced.
  - Safety is improved.
  - Self-management of symptoms is improved.
  - Stresses precipitating injury are decreased.
- Impact on health, wellness, and fitness
  - Health status is improved.
  - Physical capacity is increased.
  - Physical function is improved.
- Impact on societal resources
  - Utilization of physical therapy services is optimized.
  - Utilization of physical therapy services results in efficient use of health care dollars.
- Patient/client satisfaction
  - Access, availability, and services provided are acceptable to patient/client.
  - Administrative management of practice is acceptable to patient/client.
  - Clinical proficiency of physical therapist is acceptable to patient/client.
  - Coordination of care is acceptable to patient/client.
  - Cost of health care services is decreased.
  - Intensity of care is decreased.
  - Interpersonal skills of physical therapist are acceptable to patient/client, family, and significant others.
  - Sense of well-being is improved.
  - Stressors are decreased.

Electrotherapeutic Modalities

Interventions

- Biofeedback
- Electrotherapeutic delivery of medications
  - iontophoresis
- Electrical stimulation
  - electrical muscle stimulation (EMS)
  - functional electrical stimulation (FES)
  - high voltage pulsed current (HVPC)
  - neuromuscular electrical stimulation (NMES)
  - transcutaneous electrical nerve stimulation (TENS)

Anticipated Goals and Expected Outcomes

- Impact on pathology/pathophysiology (disease, disorder, or condition)
  - Edema, lymphedema, or effusion is reduced.
  - Joint swelling, inflammation, or restriction is reduced.
  - Nutrient delivery to tissue is increased.
  - Osteogenic effects are enhanced.
  - Pain is decreased.
  - Soft tissue or wound healing is enhanced.
  - Soft tissue swelling, inflammation, or restriction is reduced.
  - Tissue perfusion and oxygenation are enhanced.
- Impact on impairments
  - Integumentary integrity is improved.
  - Motor function (motor control and motor learning) is improved.
  - Muscle performance (strength, power, and endurance) is increased.
  - Postural control is improved.
  - Quality and quantity of movement between and across body segments are improved.
  - Range of motion is improved.
  - Relaxation is increased.
  - Sensory awareness is increased.
- Impact on functional limitations
  - Ability to perform physical actions, tasks, or activities related to self-care, home management, work (job/school/play), community, and leisure is improved.
  - Level of supervision required for task performance is decreased.
  - Performance of and independence in activities of daily living (ADL) and instrumental activities of daily living (IADL) with or without devices and equipment are increased.
  - Tolerance of positions and activities is increased.
- Impact on disabilities
  - Ability to assume or resume required self-care, home management, work (job/school/play), community, and leisure roles is improved.
- Risk reduction/prevention
  - Complications of immobility are reduced.
  - Preoperative and postoperative complications are reduced.
  - Risk factors are reduced.
  - Risk of secondary impairment is reduced.
  - Self-management of symptoms is improved.
- Impact on health, wellness, and fitness
  - Fitness is improved.
  - Physical capacity is increased.
  - Physical function is improved.
- Impact on societal resources
  - Utilization of physical therapy services is optimized.
  - Utilization of physical therapy services results in efficient use of health care dollars.
- Patient/client satisfaction
  - Access, availability, and services provided are acceptable to patient/client.
  - Administrative management of practice is acceptable to patient/client.
  - Clinical proficiency of physical therapist is acceptable to patient/client.
  - Coordination of care is acceptable to patient/client.
  - Interpersonal skills of physical therapist are acceptable to patient/client, family, and significant others.
  - Sense of well-being is improved.
  - Stressors are decreased.

Physical Agents and Mechanical Modalities

Interventions

Physical agents may include:

- Cryotherapy
  - cold packs
  - ice massage
  - vapocoolant spray
- Hydrotherapy
  - whirlpool tanks
  - contrast bath
  - pools
  - pulsatile lavage
- Sound agents
  - phonophoresis
  - ultrasound
- Thermotherapy
  - dry heat
  - hot packs
  - paraffin baths

Mechanical modalities may include:

- Compression therapies
  - compression bandaging
  - compression garments
  - taping
  - vasopneumatic compression devices
- Gravity-assisted compression devices
  - tilt table
- Mechanical motion devices
  - continuous passive motion (CPM)

Anticipated Goals and Expected Outcomes

- Impact on pathology/pathophysiology (disease, disorder, or condition)
  - Edema, lymphedema, or effusion is reduced.
  - Joint swelling, inflammation, or restriction is reduced.
  - Nutrient delivery to tissue is increased.
  - Osteogenic effects are enhanced.
  - Pain is decreased.
  - Soft tissue swelling, inflammation, or restriction is reduced.
  - Tissue perfusion and oxygenation are enhanced.
- Impact on impairments
  - Integumentary integrity is improved.
  - Muscle performance (strength, power, and endurance) is increased.
  - Range of motion is improved.
  - Weight-bearing status is improved.
- Impact on functional limitations
  - Ability to perform physical actions, tasks, or activities related to self-care, home management, work (job/school/play), community, and leisure is improved.
  - Performance of and independence in activities of daily living (ADL) and instrumental activities of daily living (IADL) with or without devices and equipment are increased.
  - Tolerance of positions and activities is increased.
- Impact on disabilities
  - Ability to assume or resume required self-care, home management, work (job/school/play), community, and leisure roles is improved.
- Risk reduction/prevention
  - Complications of soft tissue and circulatory disorders are decreased.
  - Risk factors are reduced.
  - Risk of secondary impairment is reduced.
  - Self-management of symptoms is improved.
- Impact on health, wellness, and fitness
  - Fitness is improved.
  - Physical capacity is increased.
  - Physical function is improved.
- Impact on societal resources
  - Utilization of physical therapy services is optimized.
- Patient/client satisfaction
  - Access, availability, and services provided are acceptable to patient/client.
  - Administrative management of practice is acceptable to patient/client.
  - Clinical proficiency of physical therapist is acceptable to patient/client.
  - Coordination of care is acceptable to patient/client.
  - Interpersonal skills of physical therapist are acceptable to patient/client, family, and significant others.
  - Sense of well-being is improved.
  - Stressors are decreased.

Reexamination

Reexamination is the process of performing selected tests and measures after the initial examination to evaluate progress and to modify or redirect interventions. Reexamination may be indicated more than once during a single episode of care. It also may be performed over the course of a disease, disorder, or condition, which for some patients/clients may be over the life span. Indications for reexamination include new clinical findings or failure to respond to physical therapy interventions.

Global Outcomes for Patients/Clients in This Pattern

Throughout the entire episode of care, the physical therapist determines the anticipated goals and expected outcomes for each intervention. These anticipated goals and expected outcomes are delineated in shaded boxes that accompany the lists of interventions in each preferred practice pattern. As the patient/client reaches the termination of physical therapy services and the end of the episode of care, the physical therapist measures the global outcomes of the physical therapy services by characterizing or quantifying the impact of the physical therapy interventions in the following domains:

- Pathology/pathophysiology (disease, disorder, or condition)
- Impairments
- Functional limitations
- Disabilities
- Risk reduction/prevention
- Health, wellness, and fitness
- Societal resources
- Patient/client satisfaction

In some instances, a particular anticipated goal or expected outcome is thoroughly achieved through implementation of a single form of intervention. More commonly, however, the anticipated goals and expected outcomes are achieved as a result of the combined effects of several forms of interventions, leading to enhancement of both health status and health-related quality of life.

Criteria for Termination of Physical Therapy Services

Discharge is the process of ending physical therapy services that have been provided during a single episode of care. It occurs when the anticipated goals and expected outcomes have been achieved. Discharge does *not* occur with a *transfer* (defined as the time when a patient is moved from one site to another site within the same setting or across settings during a single episode of care). Although there may be facility-specific or payer-specific requirements for documentation regarding the conclusion of physical therapy services, *discharge occurs based on the physical therapist's analysis of the achievement of anticipated goals and expected outcomes.*

Discontinuation is the process of ending physical therapy services that have been provided during a single episode of care when (1) the patient/client, caregiver, or legal guardian declines to continue intervention; (2) the patient/client is unable to continue to progress toward outcomes because of medical or psychosocial complications or because financial/insurance resources have been expended; or (3) the physical therapist determines that the patient/client will no longer benefit from physical therapy. When physical therapy services are terminated prior to achievement of anticipated goals and expected outcomes, patient/client status and the rationale for termination are documented.

For patients/clients who require multiple episodes of care, periodic follow-up is needed over the life span to ensure safety and effective adaptation following changes in physical status, caregivers, environment, or task demands. In consultation with appropriate individuals, and in consideration of the outcomes, the physical therapist plans for discharge or discontinuation and provides for appropriate follow-up or referral.

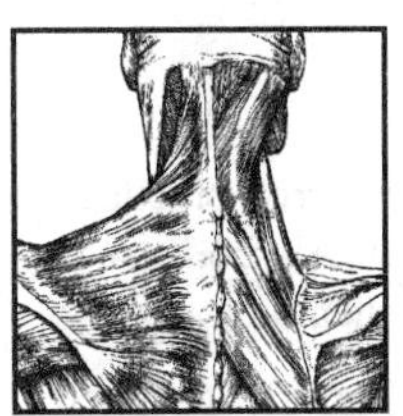

Impaired Motor Function, Muscle Performance, Range of Motion, Gait, Locomotion, and Balance Associated With Amputation

This preferred practice pattern describes the generally accepted elements of patient/client management that physical therapists provide for patients/clients who are classified in this pattern. The pattern title reflects the diagnosis made by the physical therapist. APTA emphasizes that preferred practice patterns are the boundaries within which a physical therapist may select any of a number of clinical alternatives, based on consideration of a wide variety of factors, such as individual patient/client needs; the profession's code of ethics and standards of practice; and patient/client age, culture, gender roles, race, sex, sexual orientation, and socioeconomic status.

Patient/Client Diagnostic Classification

Patients/clients will be classified into this pattern—for impaired motor function, muscle performance, range of motion, gait, locomotion, and balance associated with amputation—as a result of the physical therapist's evaluation of the examination data. The findings from the examination (history, systems review, and tests and measures) may indicate the presence or risk of pathology/pathophysiology (disease, disorder, or condition), impairments, functional limitations, or disabilities or the need for health, wellness, or fitness programs. The physical therapist integrates, synthesizes, and interprets the data to determine the diagnostic classification.

Inclusion

The following examples of examination findings may support the inclusion of patients/clients in this pattern:

Risk Factors or Consequences of Pathology/Pathophysiology (Disease, Disorder, or Condition)

- Amputation
- Diabetes
- Frostbite
- Peripheral vascular disease
- Trauma

Impairments, Functional Limitations, or Disabilities

- Decreased community access
- Difficulty with manipulation skills
- Edema
- Joint contracture
- Impaired aerobic capacity
- Impaired gait pattern
- Impaired integument and inadequate shape of residual limb
- Impaired performance during activities of daily living
- Residual limb pain

Note:

Some risk factors or consequences of pathology/pathophysiology—such as *multisystem involvement* and *traumatic amputation of multiple parts*—may be severe and complex; *however, they do not necessarily exclude patients/clients from this pattern.* Severe and complex risk factors or consequences may require modification of the frequency of visits and duration of care. (See "Evaluation, Diagnosis, and Prognosis," page 293.)

Exclusion or Multiple-Pattern Classification

The following examples of examination findings may support exclusion from this pattern or classification into additional patterns. Depending on the level of severity or complexity of the examination findings, the physical therapist may determine that the patient/client would be more appropriately managed through (1) classification in an entirely different pattern or (2) classification in both this and another pattern.

Findings That May Require Classification in a Different Pattern

- Amputation with respiratory failure

Findings That May Require Classification in Additional Patterns

- Open wound

ICD-9-CM Codes

The listing below contains the current (as of press time) and most typical 3- and 4-digit ICD-9-CM codes related to this preferred practice pattern. Because patient/client diagnostic classification is based on impairments, functional limitations, and disabilities—not on codes—patients/clients may be classified into the pattern even though the codes listed with the pattern may not apply to those clients.

This listing is intended for general information only and should not be used for coding purposes. The codes should be confirmed by referring to the World Health Organization's *International Classification of Diseases, 9th Revision, Clinical Modification (ICD-9-CM 2001)*, Volumes 1 and 3 (Chicago, Ill: American Medical Association; 2000) or subsequent revisions or by referring to other ICD-9-CM coding manuals that contain exclusion notes and instructions regarding fifth-digit requirements.

250 Diabetes mellitus

353 Nerve root and plexus disorders

- **353.6** Phantom limb (syndrome)

440 Atherosclerosis

- **440.2** Of native arteries of the extremities

442 Other aneurysm

- **442.3** Of artery of lower extremity

443 Other peripheral vascular disease

459 Other disorders of circulatory system

- **459.8** Other specified disorders of circulatory system

736 Other acquired deformities of limbs

747 Other congenital anomalies of circulatory system

- **747.6** Other anomalies of peripheral vascular system

755 Other congenital anomalies of limbs

- **755.0** Polydactyly
- **755.1** Syndactyly
- **755.2** Reduction deformities of upper limb
- **755.3** Reduction deformities of lower limb
- **755.4** Reduction deformities, unspecified limb
- **755.5** Other anomalies of upper limb, including shoulder girdle

781 Symptoms involving nervous and musculoskeletal systems

- **781.2** Abnormality of gait
- **781.5** Clubbing of fingers
- **781.9** Other symptoms involving nervous and musculoskeletal systems

885 Traumatic amputation of thumb (complete) (partial)

886 Traumatic amputation of other finger(s) (complete) (partial)

887 Traumatic amputation of arm and hand (complete) (partial)

895 Traumatic amputation of toe(s) (complete) (partial)

896 Traumatic amputation of foot (complete) (partial)

897 Traumatic amputation of leg(s) (complete) (partial)

905 Late effects of musculoskeletal and connective tissue injuries

- **905.9** Late effect of traumatic amputation

906 Late effects of injuries to skin and subcutaneous tissues

927 Crushing injury of upper limb

928 Crushing injury of lower limb

929 Crushing injury of multiple and unspecified sites

990 Effects of radiation, unspecified

991 Effects of reduced temperature

- **991.1** Frostbite of hand
- **991.2** Frostbite of foot

994 Effects of other external causes

- **994.0** Effects of lightning

997 Complications affecting specified body system, not elsewhere classified

- **997.6** Amputation stump complication

Examination

Examination is a comprehensive screening and specific testing process that leads to a diagnostic classification or, when appropriate, to a referral to another practitioner. Examination is required prior to the initial intervention and is performed for all patients/clients. Through the examination, the physical therapist may identify impairments, functional limitations, disabilities, changes in physical function or overall health status, and needs related to restoration of health and to prevention, wellness, and fitness. The physical therapist synthesizes the examination findings to establish the diagnosis and the prognosis (including the plan of care). The patient/client, family, significant others, and caregivers may provide information during the examination process.

Examination has three components: the patient/client history, the systems review, and tests and measures. The *history* is a systematic gathering of past and current information (often from the patient/client) related to why the patient/client is seeking the services of the physical therapist. The *systems review* is a brief or limited examination of (1) the anatomical and physiological status of the cardiovascular/pulmonary, integumentary, musculoskeletal, and neuromuscular systems and (2) the communication ability, affect, cognition, language, and learning style of the patient/client. *Tests and measures* are the means of gathering data about the patient/client.

The selection of examination procedures and the depth of the examination vary based on patient/client age; severity of the problem; stage of recovery (acute, subacute, chronic); phase of rehabilitation (early, intermediate, late, return to activity); home, work (job/school/play), or community situation; and other relevant factors. *For clinical indications in selecting tests and measures and for listings of tests and measures, tools used to gather data, and the types of data generated by tests and measures, refer to Chapter 2.*

Patient/Client History

The history may include:

General Demographics
- Age
- Sex
- Race/ethnicity
- Primary language
- Education

Social History
- Cultural beliefs and behaviors
- Family and caregiver resources
- Social interactions, social activities, and support systems

Employment/Work (Job/School/Play)
- Current and prior work (job/school/play), community, and leisure actions, tasks, or activities

Growth and Development
- Developmental history
- Hand dominance

Living Environment
- Devices and equipment (eg, assistive, adaptive, orthotic, protective, supportive, prosthetic)
- Living environment and community characteristics
- Projected discharge destinations

General Health Status (Self-Report, Family Report, Caregiver Report)
- General health perception
- Physical function (eg, mobility, sleep patterns, restricted bed days)
- Psychological function (eg, memory, reasoning ability, depression, anxiety)
- Role function (eg, community, leisure, social, work)
- Social function (eg, social activity, social interaction, social support)

Social/Health Habits (Past and Current)
- Behavioral health risks (eg, smoking, drug abuse)
- Level of physical fitness

Family History
- Familial health risks

Medical/Surgical History
- Cardiovascular
- Endocrine/metabolic
- Gastrointestinal
- Genitourinary
- Gynecological
- Integumentary
- Musculoskeletal
- Neuromuscular
- Obstetrical
- Prior hospitalizations, surgeries, and preexisting medical and other health-related conditions
- Psychological
- Pulmonary

Current Condition(s)/Chief Complaint(s)
- Concerns that led patient/client to seek the services of a physical therapist
- Concerns or needs of patient/client who requires the services of a physical therapist
- Current therapeutic interventions
- Mechanisms of injury or disease, including date of onset and course of events
- Onset and pattern of symptoms
- Patient/client, family, significant other, and caregiver expectations and goals for the therapeutic intervention
- Patient/client, family, significant other, and caregiver perceptions of patient's/client's emotional response to the current clinical situation
- Previous occurrence of chief complaint(s)
- Prior therapeutic interventions

Functional Status and Activity Level
- Current and prior functional status in self-care and home management activities, including activities of daily living (ADL) and instrumental activities of daily living (IADL)
- Current and prior functional status in work (job/school/play), community, and leisure actions, tasks, or activities

Medications
- Medications for current condition
- Medications previously taken for current condition
- Medications for other conditions

Other Clinical Tests
- Laboratory and diagnostic tests
- Review of available records (eg, medical, education, surgical)
- Review of other clinical findings (eg, nutrition and hydration)

Systems Review

The systems review may include:

Anatomical and Physiological Status

- Cardiovascular/Pulmonary
  - Blood pressure
  - Edema
  - Heart rate
  - Respiratory rate
- Integumentary
  - Pliability (texture)
  - Presence of scar formation
  - Skin color
  - Skin integrity
- Musculoskeletal
  - Gross range of motion
  - Gross strength
  - Gross symmetry
  - Height
  - Weight
- Neuromuscular
  - Gross coordinated movements (eg, balance, gait, locomotion, transfers, transitions)
  - Motor function (motor control, motor learning)

Communication, Affect, Cognition, Language, and Learning Style

- Ability to make needs known
- Consciousness
- Expected emotional/behavioral responses
- Learning preferences (eg, education needs, learning barriers)
- Orientation (person, place, time)

Tests and Measures

Tests and measures for this pattern may include those that characterize or quantify:

Aerobic Capacity and Endurance

- Aerobic capacity during functional activities (eg, activities of daily living [ADL] scales, indexes, instrumental activities of daily living [IADL] scales, observations)
- Aerobic capacity during standardized exercise test protocols (eg, ergometry, step tests, time/distance walk/run tests, treadmill tests, wheelchair tests)
- Cardiovascular signs and symptoms in response to increased oxygen demand with exercise or activity, including pressures and flow; heart rate, rhythm, and sounds; and superficial vascular responses (eg, electrocardiography, exertion scales, observations, palpation, sphygmomanometry)
- Pulmonary signs and symptoms in response to increased oxygen demand with exercise or activity, including breath and voice sounds; cyanosis; gas exchange; respiratory pattern, rate, and rhythm; and ventilatory flow, force, and volume (eg, auscultation, exertion scales, observations, oximetry, palpation)

Anthropometric Characteristics

- Body composition (eg, body mass index, impedance measurement, skinfold thickness measurement)
- Body dimensions (eg, girth measurement, length measurement)
- Edema (eg, girth measurement, palpation, scales, volume measurement)

Arousal, Attention, and Cognition

- Motivation (eg, adaptive behavior scales)

Assistive and Adaptive Devices

- Assistive or adaptive devices and equipment use during functional activities (eg, ADL scales, functional scales, IADL scales, interviews, observations)
- Components, alignment, fit, and ability to care for the assistive or adaptive devices and equipment (eg, interviews, logs, observations, pressure-sensing maps, reports)
- Remediation of impairments, functional limitations, or disabilities with use of assistive or adaptive devices and equipment (eg, activity status indexes, ADL scales, aerobic capacity tests, functional performance inventories, health assessment questionnaires, IADL scales, pain scales, play scales, videographic assessments)
- Safety during use of assistive or adaptive devices and equipment (eg, diaries, fall scales, interviews, logs, observations, reports)

Circulation (Arterial, Venous, and Lymphatic)

- Cardiovascular signs, including heart rate, rhythm, and sounds; pressures and flow; and superficial vascular responses (eg, auscultation, electrocardiography, girth measurement, observations, palpation, sphygmomanometry, thermography)
- Cardiovascular symptoms (eg, angina, claudication, and perceived exertion scales)
- Physiological responses to position change, including autonomic responses, central and peripheral pressures, heart rate and rhythm, respiratory rate and rhythm, ventilatory pattern (eg, auscultation, electrocardiography, observations, palpation, sphygmomanometry)

Cranial and Peripheral Nerve Integrity

- Electrophysiological integrity (eg, electroneuromyography)
- Motor distribution of the peripheral nerves (eg, dynamometry, muscle tests, observations, thoracic outlet tests)
- Sensory distribution of the peripheral nerves (eg, discrimination tests; tactile tests, including coarse and light touch, cold and heat, pain, pressure, and vibration; thoracic outlet tests)

Environmental, Home, and Work (Job/School/Play) Barriers

- Current and potential barriers (eg, checklists, interviews, observations, questionnaires)
- Physical space and environment (eg, compliance standards, observations, photographic assessments, questionnaires, structural specifications, videographic assessments)

Ergonomics and Body Mechanics

Ergonomics

- Dexterity and coordination during work (job/school/play) (eg, hand function tests, impairment rating scales, manipulative ability tests)
- Functional capacity and performance during work actions, tasks, or activities (eg, accelerometry, dynamometry, electroneuromyography, endurance tests, force platform tests, goniometry, interviews, observations, photographic assessments, physical capacity tests, postural loading analyses, technology-assisted assessments, videographic assessments, work analyses)
- Safety in work environments (eg, hazard identification checklists, job severity indexes, lifting standards, risk assessment scales, standards for exposure limits)
- Specific work conditions or activities (eg, handling checklists, job simulations, lifting models, preemployment screenings, task analysis checklists, workstation checklists)
- Tools, devices, equipment, and workstations related to work actions, tasks, or activities (eg, observations, tool analysis checklists, vibration assessments)

Body mechanics

- Body mechanics during self-care, home management, work, community, or leisure actions, tasks, or activities (eg, ADL scales, IADL scales, observations, photographic assessments, technology-assisted assessments, videographic assessments)

Gait, Locomotion, and Balance

- Balance during functional activities with or without the use of assistive, adaptive, orthotic, protective, supportive, or prosthetic devices or equipment (eg, ADL scales, IADL scales, observations, videographic assessments)
- Balance (dynamic and static) with or without the use of assistive, adaptive, orthotic, protective, supportive, or prosthetic devices or equipment (eg, balance scales, dizziness inventories, dynamic posturography, fall scales, motor impairment tests, observations, photographic assessments, postural control tests)
- Gait and locomotion during functional activities with or without the use of assistive, adaptive, orthotic, protective, supportive, or prosthetic devices or equipment (eg, ADL scales, gait indexes, IADL scales, mobility skill profiles, observations, videographic assessments)
- Gait and locomotion with or without the use of assistive, adaptive, orthotic, protective, supportive, or prosthetic devices or equipment (eg, dynamometry, electroneuromyography, footprint analyses, gait indexes, mobility skill profiles, observations, photographic assessments, technology-assisted assessments, videographic assessments, weight-bearing scales, wheelchair mobility tests)
- Safety during gait, locomotion, and balance (eg, confidence scales, diaries, fall scales, functional assessment profiles, logs, reports)

Integumentary Integrity

Associated skin

- Activities, positioning, and postures that produce or relieve trauma to the skin (eg, observations, pressure-sensing maps, scales)
- Assistive, adaptive, orthotic, protective, supportive, or prosthetic devices and equipment that may produce or relieve trauma to the skin (eg, observations, pressure-sensing maps, risk assessment scales)
- Skin characteristics, including blistering, continuity of skin color, dermatitis, hair growth, mobility, nail growth, sensation, temperature, texture, and turgor (eg, observations, palpation, photographic assessments, thermography)

Wound

- Activities, positioning, and postures that aggravate the wound or scar or that produce or relieve trauma (eg, observations, pressure-sensing maps)
- Signs of infection (eg, cultures, observations, palpation)
- Wound scar tissue characteristics, including banding, pliability, sensation, and texture (eg, observations, scar-rating scales)

Joint Integrity and Mobility

- Joint integrity and mobility (eg, apprehension, compression and distraction, drawer, glide, impingement, shear, and valgus/varus stress tests; arthrometry; palpation)
- Joint play movements, including end feel (all joints of the axial and appendicular skeletal system) (eg, palpation)

Motor Function (Motor Control and Motor Learning)

- Dexterity, coordination, and agility (eg, coordination screens, motor impairment tests, motor proficiency tests, observations, videographic assessments)
- Hand function (eg, fine and gross motor control tests, finger dexterity tests, manipulative ability tests, observations)

Muscle Performance (Including Strength, Power, and Endurance)

- Muscle strength, power, and endurance (eg, dynamometry, manual muscle tests, muscle performance tests, physical capacity tests, technology-assisted assessments, timed activity tests)
- Muscle strength, power, and endurance during functional activities (eg, ADL scales, functional muscle tests, IADL scales, observations, videographic assessments)
- Muscle tension (eg, palpation)

Orthotic, Protective, and Supportive Devices

- Components, alignment, fit, and ability to care for orthotic, protective, and supportive devices and equipment (eg, interviews, logs, observations, pressure-sensing maps, reports)
- Orthotic, protective, and supportive devices and equipment use during functional activities (eg, ADL scales, functional scales, IADL scales, interviews, observations, profiles)
- Remediation of impairments, functional limitations, or disabilities with use of orthotic, protective, and supportive devices and equipment (eg, activity status indexes, ADL scales, aerobic capacity tests, functional performance inventories, health assessment questionnaires, IADL scales, pain scales, play scales, videographic assessments)
- Safety during use of orthotic, protective, and supportive devices and equipment (eg, diaries, fall scales, interviews, logs, observations, reports)

Pain

- Pain, soreness, and nociception (eg, analog scales, angina scales, discrimination tests, pain drawings and maps, provocation tests, verbal and pictorial descriptor tests)
- Pain in specific body parts (eg, pain indexes, pain questionnaires, structural provocation tests)

Posture

- Postural alignment and position (static and dynamic), including symmetry and deviation from midline (eg, grid measurement, observations, photographic assessments, technology-assisted assessments, videographic assessments)
- Specific body parts (eg, angle assessments, forward-bending test, goniometry, observations, palpation, positional tests)

Prosthetic Requirements

- Components, alignment, fit, and ability to care for the prosthetic device (eg, interviews, logs, observations, pressure-sensing maps, reports)
- Prosthetic device use during functional activities (eg, ADL scales, functional scales, IADL scales, interviews, observations)
- Remediation of impairments, functional limitations, or disabilities with use of the prosthetic device (eg, aerobic capacity tests, activity status indexes, ADL scales, functional performance inventories, health assessment questionnaires, IADL scales, pain scales, play scales, videographic assessments)
- Residual limb or adjacent segment, including edema, range of motion, skin integrity, and strength (eg, goniometry, muscle tests, observations, palpation, photographic assessments, skin integrity tests, videographic assessments, volume measurement)
- Safety during use of the prosthetic device (eg, diaries, fall scales, interviews, logs, observations, reports)

Range of Motion (ROM) (Including Muscle Length)

- Functional ROM (eg, observations, squat testing, toe touch tests)
- Joint active and passive movement (eg, goniometry, inclinometry, observations, photographic assessments, videographic assessments)
- Muscle length, soft tissue extensibility, and flexibility (eg, contracture tests, goniometry, inclinometry, ligamentous tests, linear measurement, multisegment flexibility tests, palpation)

Self-Care and Home Management (Including ADL and IADL)

- Ability to gain access to home environments (eg, barrier identification, observations, physical performance tests)
- Ability to perform self-care and home management activities with or without assistive, adaptive, orthotic, protective, supportive, or prosthetic devices and equipment (eg, ADL scales, aerobic capacity tests, IADL scales, interviews, observations, profiles)
- Safety in self-care and home management activities and environments (eg, diaries, fall scales, interviews, logs, observations, reports, videographic assessments)

Sensory Integrity

- Combined/cortical sensations (eg, stereognosis, tactile discrimination tests)
- Deep sensations (eg, kinesthesiometry, observations, photographic assessments, vibration tests)

Work (Job/School/Play), Community, and Leisure Integration or Reintegration (Including IADL)

- Ability to assume or resume work (job/school/play), community, and leisure activities with or without assistive, adaptive, orthotic, protective, supportive, or prosthetic devices and equipment (eg, activity profiles, disability indexes, functional status questionnaires, IADL scales, observations, physical capacity tests)
- Ability to gain access to work (job/school/play), community, and leisure environments (eg, barrier identification, interviews, observations, physical capacity tests, transportation assessments)
- Safety in work (job/school/play), community, and leisure activities and environments (eg, diaries, fall scales, interviews, logs, observations, videographic assessments)

Evaluation, Diagnosis, and Prognosis (Including Plan of Care)

Physical therapists perform *evaluations* (make clinical judgments) based on the data gathered from the history, systems review, and tests and measures. In the evaluation process, physical therapists synthesize the examination data to establish the diagnosis and prognosis (including the plan of care). Factors that influence the complexity of the evaluation include the clinical findings, extent of loss of function, chronicity or severity of the problem, possibility of multisite or multisystem involvement, preexisting condition(s), potential discharge destination, social considerations, physical function, and overall health status.

A *diagnosis* is a label encompassing a cluster of signs and symptoms, syndromes, or categories. It is the result of the systematic diagnostic process, which includes integrating and evaluating the data from the examination. The diagnostic label indicates the primary dysfunction(s) toward which the therapist will direct interventions. The *prognosis* is the determination of the predicted optimal level of improvement in function and the amount of time needed to reach that level and may also include a prediction of levels of improvement that may be reached at various intervals during the course of therapy. During the prognostic process, the physical therapist develops the plan of care. The *plan of care* identifies specific interventions, proposed frequency and duration of the interventions, anticipated goals, expected outcomes, and discharge plans. The plan of care identifies realistic anticipated goals and expected outcomes, taking into consideration the expectations of the patient/client and appropriate others. These anticipated goals and expected outcomes should be measureable and time limited.

The frequency of visits and duration of the episode of care may vary from a short episode with a high intensity of intervention to a longer episode with a diminishing intensity of intervention. Frequency and duration may vary greatly among patients/clients based on a variety of factors that the physical therapist considers throughout the evaluation process, such as anatomical and physiological changes related to growth and development; caregiver consistency or expertise; chronicity or severity of the current condition; living environment; multisite or multisystem involvement; social support; potential discharge destinations; probability of prolonged impairment, functional limitation, or disability; and stability of the condition.

Prognosis

Over the course of 6 months, patient/client will demonstrate optimal motor function; muscle performance; range of motion; and gait, locomotion, and balance; and the highest level of functioning in home, work (job/school/play), community, and leisure environments.

During the episode of care, patient/client will achieve (1) the anticipated goals and expected outcomes of the interventions that are described in the plan of care and (2) the global outcomes for patients/clients who are classified in this pattern.

Expected Range of Number of Visits Per Episode of Care

15 to 45

This range represents the lower and upper limits of the number of physical therapist visits required to achieve anticipated goals and expected outcomes. *It is anticipated that 80% of patients/clients who are classified into this pattern will achieve the anticipated goals and expected outcomes within 15 to 45 visits during a single continuous episode of care.* Frequency of visits and duration of the episode of care should be determined by the physical therapist to maximize effectiveness of care and efficiency of service delivery.

Factors That May Require New Episode of Care or That May Modify Frequency of Visits/Duration of Episode

- Accessibility and availability of resources
- Adherence to the intervention program
- Age
- Anatomical and physiological changes related to growth and development
- Caregiver consistency or expertise
- Chronicity or severity of the current condition
- Cognitive status
- Comorbitities, complications, or secondary impairments
- Concurrent medical, surgical, and therapeutic interventions
- Decline in functional independence
- Level of impairment
- Level of physical function
- Living environment
- Multisite or multisystem involvement
- Nutritional status
- Overall health status
- Potential discharge destinations
- Premorbid conditions
- Probability of prolonged impairment, functional limitation, or disability
- Psychological and socioeconomic factors
- Psychomotor abilities
- Social support
- Stability of the condition

Intervention

Intervention is the purposeful interaction of the physical therapist with the patient/client and, when appropriate, with other individuals involved in patient/client care, using various physical therapy procedures and techniques to produce changes in the condition consistent with the diagnosis and prognosis. Decisions about interventions are contingent on the timely monitoring of patient/client response and the progress made toward achieving the anticipated goals and expected outcomes.

Communication, coordination, and documentation and patient/client-related instruction are provided for all patients/clients across all settings. Procedural interventions are selected or modified based on the examination data and the evaluation, the diagnosis and the prognosis, and the anticipated goals and expected outcomes for a particular patient/client. *For clinical considerations in selecting interventions, listings of interventions, and listings of anticipated goals and expected outcomes, refer to Chapter 3.*

Coordination, Communication, and Documentation

Coordination, communication, and documentation may include:

Interventions

- Addressing required functions
  - advance directives
  - individualized family service plans (IFSPs) or individualized education plans (IEPs)
  - informed consent
  - mandatory communication and reporting (eg, patient advocacy and abuse reporting)
- Admission and discharge planning
- Case management
- Collaboration and coordination with agencies, including:
  - equipment suppliers
  - home care agencies
  - payer groups
  - schools
  - transportation agencies
- Communication across settings, including:
  - case conferences
  - documentation
  - education plans
- Cost-effective resource utilization
- Data collection, analysis, and reporting
  - outcome data
  - peer review findings
  - record reviews
- Documentation across settings, following APTA's *Guidelines for Physical Therapy Documentation* (Appendix 5), including:
  - changes in impairments, functional limitations, and disabilities
  - changes in interventions
  - elements of patient/client management (examination, evaluation, diagnosis, prognosis, intervention)
  - outcomes of intervention
- Interdisciplinary teamwork
  - case conferences
  - patient care rounds
  - patient/client family meetings
- Referrals to other professionals or resources

Anticipated Goals and Expected Outcomes

- Accountability for services is increased.
- Admission data and discharge planning are completed.
- Advance directives, individualized family service plans (IFSPs) or individualized education plans (IEPs), informed consent, and mandatory communication and reporting (eg, patient advocacy and abuse reporting) are obtained or completed.
- Available resources are maximally utilized.
- Care is coordinated with patient/client, family, significant others, caregivers, and other professionals.
- Case is managed throughout the episode of care.
- Collaboration and coordination occurs with agencies, including equipment suppliers, home care agencies, payer groups, schools, and transportation agencies.
- Communication enhances risk reduction and prevention.
- Communication occurs across settings through case conferences, education plans, and documentation.
- Data are collected, analyzed, and reported, including outcome data, peer review findings, and record reviews.
- Decision making is enhanced regarding health, wellness, and fitness needs.
- Decision making is enhanced regarding patient/client health and the use of health care resources by patient/client, family, significant others, and caregivers.
- Documentation occurs throughout patient/client management and across settings and follows APTA's *Guidelines for Physical Therapy Documentation* (Appendix 5).
- Interdisciplinary collaboration occurs through case conferences, patient care rounds, and patient/client family meetings.
- Patient/client, family, significant other, and caregiver understanding of anticipated goals and expected outcomes is increased.
- Placement needs are determined.
- Referrals are made to other professionals or resources whenever necessary and appropriate.
- Resources are utilized in a cost-effective way.

Patient/Client-Related Instruction

Patient/client-related instruction may include:

Interventions

- Instruction, education and training of patients/clients and caregivers regarding:
  - current condition (pathology/pathophysiology [disease, disorder, or condition], impairments, functional limitations, or disabilities)
  - enhancement of performance
  - health, wellness, and fitness programs
  - plan of care
  - risk factors for pathology/pathophysiology (disease, disorder, or condition), impairments, functional limitations, or disabilities
  - transitions across settings
  - transitions to new roles

Anticipated Goals and Expected Outcomes

- Ability to perform physical actions, tasks, or activities is improved.
- Awareness and use of community resources are improved.
- Behaviors that foster healthy habits, wellness, and prevention are acquired.
- Decision making is enhanced regarding patient/client health and the use of health care resources by patient/client, family, significant others, and caregivers.
- Disability associated with acute or chronic illnesses is reduced.
- Functional independence in activities of daily living (ADL) and instrumental activities of daily living (IADL) is increased.
- Health status is improved.
- Intensity of care is decreased.
- Level of supervision required for task performance is decreased.
- Patient/client, family, significant other, and caregiver knowledge and awareness of the diagnosis, prognosis, interventions, and anticipated goals and expected outcomes are increased.
- Patient/client knowledge of personal and environmental factors associated with the condition is increased.
- Performance levels in self-care, home management, work (job/school/play), community, or leisure actions, tasks, or activities are improved.
- Physical function is improved.
- Risk of recurrence of condition is reduced.
- Risk of secondary impairment is reduced.
- Safety of patient/client, family, significant others, and caregivers is improved.
- Self-management of symptoms is improved.
- Utilization and cost of health care services are decreased.

Procedural Interventions

Procedural interventions for this pattern may include:

Therapeutic Exercise

Interventions

- Aerobic capacity/endurance conditioning or reconditioning
  - aquatic programs
  - gait and locomotor training
  - increased workload over time
  - walking and wheelchair propulsion programs
- Balance, coordination, and agility training
  - motor function (motor control and motor learning) training or retraining
  - neuromuscular education or reeducation
  - perceptual training
  - posture awareness training
  - standardized, programmatic, complementary exercise approaches
  - sensory training or retraining
  - task-specific performance training
- Body mechanics and postural stabilization
  - body mechanics training
  - developmental activities training
  - posture awareness training
  - postural control training
  - postural stabilization activities
- Flexibility exercises
  - muscle lengthening
  - range of motion
  - stretching
- Gait and locomotion training
  - developmental activities training
  - gait training
  - implement and device training
  - perceptual training
  - standardized, programmatic, complementary exercise approaches
  - wheelchair training
- Relaxation
  - breathing strategies
  - movement strategies
  - relaxation techniques
  - standardized, programmatic, complementary exercise approaches
- Strength, power, and endurance training for head, neck, limb, pelvic-floor, trunk, and ventilatory muscles
  - active assistive, active, and resistive exercises (including concentric, dynamic/isotonic, eccentric, isokinetic, isometric, and plyometric)
  - aquatic programs
  - standardized, programmatic, complementary exercise approaches
  - task-specific performance training

Anticipated Goals and Expected Outcomes

- Impact on pathology/pathophysiology (disease, disorder, or condition)
  - Joint swelling, inflammation, or restriction is reduced.
  - Nutrient delivery to tissue is increased.
  - Osteogenic effects of exercise are maximized.
  - Pain is decreased.
  - Physiological response to increased oxygen demand is improved.
  - Soft tissue swelling, inflammation, or restriction is reduced.
  - Tissue perfusion and oxygenation are enhanced.
- Impact on impairments
  - Aerobic capacity is increased.
  - Balance is improved.
  - Endurance is increased.
  - Energy expenditure per unit of work is decreased.
  - Gait, locomotion, and balance are improved.
  - Integumentary integrity is improved.
  - Joint integrity and mobility are improved.
  - Motor function (motor control and motor learning) is improved.
  - Muscle performance (strength, power, and endurance) is increased.
  - Postural control is improved.
  - Quality and quantity of movement between and across body segments are improved.
  - Range of motion is improved.
  - Relaxation is increased.
  - Sensory awareness is increased.
  - Weight-bearing status is improved.
- Impact on functional limitations
  - Ability to perform physical actions, tasks, or activities related to self-care, home management, work (job/school/play), community, and leisure is improved.
  - Level of supervision required for task performance is decreased.
  - Performance of and independence in activities of daily living (ADL) and instrumental activities of daily living (IADL) with or without devices and equipment are increased.
  - Tolerance of positions and activities is increased.
- Impact on disabilities
  - Ability to assume or resume required self-care, home management, work (job/school/play), community, and leisure roles is improved.
- Risk reduction/prevention
  - Preoperative and postoperative complications are reduced.
  - Risk factors are reduced.
  - Risk of secondary impairment is reduced.
  - Safety is improved.
  - Self-management of symptoms is improved.
- Impact on health, wellness, and fitness
  - Fitness is improved.
  - Health status is improved.
  - Physical capacity is increased.
  - Physical function is improved.
- Impact on societal resources
  - Utilization of physical therapy services is optimized.
  - Utilization of physical therapy services results in efficient use of health care dollars.
- Patient/client satisfaction
  - Access, availability, and services provided are acceptable to patient/client.
  - Administrative management of practice is acceptable to patient/client.
  - Clinical proficiency of physical therapist is acceptable to patient/client.
  - Coordination of care is acceptable to patient/client.
  - Cost of health care services is decreased.
  - Intensity of care is decreased.
  - Interpersonal skills of physical therapist are acceptable to patient/client, family, and significant others.
  - Sense of well-being is improved.
  - Stressors are decreased.

Functional Training in Self-Care and Home Management (Including Activities of Daily Living [ADL] and Instrumental Activities of Daily Living [IADL])

Interventions

- ADL training
  - bathing
  - bed mobility and transfer training
  - developmental activities
  - dressing
  - eating
  - grooming
  - toileting
- Devices and equipment use and training
  - assistive and adaptive device or equipment training during ADL and IADL
  - orthotic, protective, or supportive device or equipment training during ADL and IADL
  - prosthetic device or equipment training during ADL and IADL
- Functional training programs
  - back schools
  - simulated environments and tasks
  - task adaptation
- IADL training
  - caring for dependents
  - home maintenance
  - household chores
  - shopping
  - structured play for infants and children
  - yard work
- Injury prevention or reduction
  - injury prevention education during self-care and home management
  - injury prevention or reduction with use of devices and equipment
  - safety awareness training during self-care and home management

Anticipated Goals and Expected Outcomes

- Impact on pathology/pathophysiology (disease, disorder, or condition)
  - Pain is decreased.
  - Physiological response to increased oxygen demand is improved.
- Impact on impairments
  - Balance is improved.
  - Endurance is increased.
  - Energy expenditure per unit of work is decreased.
  - Motor function (motor control and motor learning) is improved.
  - Muscle performance (strength, power, and endurance) is increased.
  - Postural control is improved.
  - Sensory awareness is increased.
  - Weight-bearing status is improved.
- Impact on functional limitations
  - Ability to perform physical actions, tasks, or activities related to self-care and home management is improved.
  - Level of supervision required for task performance is decreased.
  - Performance of and independence in ADL and IADL with or without devices and equipment are increased.
  - Tolerance of positions and activities is increased.
- Impact on disabilities
  - Ability to assume or resume required self-care and home management roles is improved.
- Risk reduction/prevention
  - Risk factors are reduced.
  - Risk of secondary impairments is reduced.
  - Safety is improved.
  - Self-management of symptoms is improved.
- Impact on health, wellness, and fitness
  - Fitness is improved.
  - Health status is improved.
  - Physical capacity is increased.
  - Physical function is improved.
- Impact on societal resources
  - Utilization of physical therapy services is optimized.
  - Utilization of physical therapy services results in efficient use of health care dollars.
- Patient/client satisfaction
  - Access, availability, and services provided are acceptable to patient/client.
  - Administrative management of practice is acceptable to patient/client.
  - Clinical proficiency of physical therapist is acceptable to patient/client.
  - Coordination of care is acceptable to patient/client.
  - Cost of health care services is decreased.
  - Intensity of care is decreased.
  - Interpersonal skills of physical therapist are acceptable to patient/client, family, and significant others.
  - Sense of well-being is improved.
  - Stressors are decreased.

Functional Training in Work (Job/School/Play), Community, and Leisure Integration or Reintegration (Including Instrumental Activities of Daily Living [IADL], Work Hardening, and Work Conditioning)

Interventions

- Devices and equipment use and training
  - assistive and adaptive device or equipment training during IADL
  - orthotic, protective, or supportive device or equipment training during IADL
  - prosthetic device or equipment training during IADL
- Functional training programs
  - back schools
  - job coaching
  - simulated environments and tasks
  - task adaptation
  - task training
- IADL training
  - community service training involving instruments
  - school and play activities training including tools and instruments
  - work training with tools
- Injury prevention or reduction
  - injury prevention education during work (job/school/play), community, and leisure integration or reintegration
  - injury prevention or reduction with use of devices and equipment
  - safety awareness training during work (job/school/play), community, and leisure integration or reintegration
- Leisure and play activities and training

Anticipated Goals and Outcomes

- Impact on pathology/pathophysiology (disease, disorder, or condition)
  - Pain is decreased.
  - Physiological response to increased oxygen demand is improved.
- Impact on impairments
  - Balance is improved.
  - Endurance is increased.
  - Energy expenditure per unit of work is decreased.
  - Motor function (motor control and motor learning) is improved.
  - Muscle performance (strength, power, and endurance) is increased.
  - Postural control is improved.
  - Sensory awareness is increased.
  - Weight-bearing status is improved.
- Impact on functional limitations
  - Ability to perform physical actions, tasks, or activities related to work (job/school/play), community, and leisure integration or reintegration is improved.
  - Level of supervision required for task performance is decreased.
  - Performance of and independence in IADL with or without devices and equipment are increased.
  - Tolerance of positions and activities is increased.
- Impact on disabilities
  - Ability to assume or resume required work (job/school/play), community, and leisure roles is improved.
- Risk reduction/prevention
  - Risk factors are reduced.
  - Risk of secondary impairment is reduced.
  - Safety is improved.
  - Self-management of symptoms is improved.
- Impact on health, wellness, and fitness
  - Fitness is improved.
  - Health status is improved.
  - Physical capacity is increased.
  - Physical function is improved.
- Impact on societal resources
  - Costs of work-related injury or disability are reduced.
  - Utilization of physical therapy services is optimized.
  - Utilization of physical therapy services results in efficient use of health care dollars.
- Patient/client satisfaction
  - Access, availability, and services provided are acceptable to patient/client.
  - Administrative management of practice is acceptable to patient/client.
  - Clinical proficiency of physical therapist is acceptable to patient/client.
  - Coordination of care is acceptable to patient/client.
  - Cost of health care services is decreased.
  - Intensity of care is decreased.
  - Interpersonal skills of physical therapist are acceptable to patient/client, family, and significant others.
  - Sense of well-being is improved.
  - Stressors are decreased.

Manual Therapy Techniques (Including Mobilization/Manipulation)

Interventions

- Manual lymphatic drainage
- Massage
  - connective tissue massage
  - therapeutic massage
- Mobilization/manipulation
  - soft tissue
- Passive range of motion

Anticipated Goals and Expected Outcomes

- Impact on pathology/pathophysiology (disease, disorder, or condition)
  - Edema, lymphedema, or effusion is reduced.
  - Joint swelling, inflammation, or restriction is reduced.
  - Pain is decreased.
  - Soft tissue swelling, inflammation, or restriction is reduced.
- Impact on impairments
  - Balance is improved.
  - Energy expenditure per unit of work is decreased.
  - Gait, locomotion, and balance are improved.
  - Integumentary integrity is improved.
  - Muscle performance (strength, power, and endurance) is increased.
  - Postural control is improved.
  - Quality and quantity of movement between and across body segments are improved.
  - Range of motion is improved.
  - Relaxation is increased.
  - Sensory awareness is increased.
  - Weight-bearing status is improved.
- Impact on functional limitations
  - Ability to perform movement tasks is improved.
  - Ability to perform physical actions, tasks, or activities related to self-care, home management, work (job/school/play), community, and leisure is improved.
  - Tolerance of positions and activities is increased.
- Impact on disabilities
  - Ability to assume or resume required self-care, home management, work (job/school/play), community, and leisure roles is improved.
- Risk reduction/prevention
  - Risk factors are reduced.
  - Risk of secondary impairment is reduced.
  - Self-management of symptoms is improved.
- Impact on health, wellness, and fitness
  - Fitness is improved.
  - Physical capacity is increased.
  - Physical function is improved.
- Impact on societal resources
  - Utilization of physical therapy services is optimized.
  - Utilization of physical therapy services results in efficient use of health care dollars.
- Patient/client satisfaction
  - Access, availability, and services provided are acceptable to patient/client.
  - Administrative management of practice is acceptable to patient/client.
  - Clinical proficiency of physical therapist is acceptable to patient/client.
  - Coordination of care is acceptable to patient/client.
  - Cost of health care services is decreased.
  - Intensity of care is decreased.
  - Interpersonal skills of physical therapist are acceptable to patient/client, family, and significant others.
  - Sense of well-being is improved.
  - Stressors are decreased.

Prescription, Application, and, as Appropriate, Fabrication of Devices and Equipment (Assistive, Adaptive, Orthotic, Protective, Supportive, and Prosthetic)

Interventions

- Adaptive devices
  - environmental controls
  - hospital beds
  - raised toilet seats
  - seating systems
  - assistive devices
  - canes
  - crutches
  - long-handled reachers
  - power devices
  - static and dynamic splints
  - walkers
  - wheelchairs
- Orthotic devices
  - braces
  - casts
  - shoe inserts
  - splints
- Prosthetic devices (lower-extremity and upper-extremity)
- Protective devices
  - braces
  - cushions
  - helmets
  - protective taping
- Supportive devices
  - compression garments
  - corsets
  - elastic wraps
  - neck collars
  - serial casts
  - slings
  - supportive taping

Anticipated Goals and Outcomes

- Impact on pathology/pathophysiology (disease, disorder, or condition)
  - Edema, lymphedema, or effusion is reduced.
  - Joint swelling, inflammation, or restriction is reduced.
  - Pain is decreased.
  - Physiological response to increased oxygen demand is improved.
  - Soft tissue swelling, inflammation, or restriction is reduced.
- Impact on impairments
  - Balance is improved.
  - Energy expenditure per unit of work is decreased.
  - Gait, locomotion, and balance are improved.
  - Integumentary integrity is improved.
  - Joint stability is improved.
  - Motor function (motor control and motor learning) is improved.
  - Muscle performance (strength, power, and endurance) is increased.
  - Optimal joint alignment is achieved.
  - Optimal loading on a body part is achieved.
  - Postural control is improved.
  - Prosthetic fit is achieved.
  - Quality and quantity of movement between and across body segments are improved.
  - Range of motion is improved.
  - Weight-bearing status is improved.
- Impact on functional limitations
  - Ability to perform physical actions, tasks, or activities related to self-care, home management, work (job/school/play), community, and leisure is improved.
  - Level of supervision required for task performance is decreased.
  - Performance of and independence in activities of daily living (ADL) and instrumental activities of daily living (IADL) with or without devices and equipment are increased.
  - Tolerance of positions and activities is increased.
- Impact on disabilities
  - Ability to assume or resume required self-care, home management, work (job/school/play), community, and leisure roles is improved.
- Risk reduction/prevention
  - Pressure on body tissues is reduced.
  - Protection of body parts is increased.
  - Risk factors are reduced.
  - Risk of secondary impairment is reduced.
  - Safety is improved.
  - Self-management of symptoms is improved.
- Impact on health, wellness, and fitness
  - Fitness is improved.
  - Health status is improved.
  - Physical capacity is increased.
  - Physical function is improved.
- Impact on societal resources
  - Utilization of physical therapy services is optimized.
  - Utilization of physical therapy services results in efficient use of health care dollars.
- Patient/client satisfaction
  - Access, availability, and services provided are acceptable to patient/client.
  - Administrative management of practice is acceptable to patient/client.
  - Clinical proficiency of physical therapist is acceptable to patient/client.
  - Coordination of care is acceptable to patient/client.
  - Cost of health care services is decreased.
  - Intensity of care is decreased.
  - Interpersonal skills of physical therapist are acceptable to patient/client, family, and significant others.
  - Sense of well-being is improved.
  - Stressors are decreased.

Electrotherapeutic Modalities

Interventions

- Electrical stimulation
  - high voltage pulsed current (HVPC)
  - neuromuscular electrical stimulation (NMES)
  - transcutaneous electrical nerve stimulation (TENS)

Anticipated Goals and Expected Outcomes

- Impact on pathology/pathophysiology (disease, disorder, or condition)
  - Edema, lymphedema, or effusion is reduced.
  - Joint swelling, inflammation, or restriction is reduced.
  - Nutrient delivery to tissue is increased.
  - Osteogenic effects are enhanced.
  - Pain is decreased.
  - Soft tissue or wound healing is enhanced.
  - Soft tissue swelling, inflammation, or restriction is reduced.
  - Tissue perfusion and oxygenation are enhanced.
- Impact on impairments
  - Integumentary integrity is improved.
  - Motor function (motor control and motor learning) is improved.
  - Muscle performance (strength, power, and endurance) is increased.
  - Postural control is improved.
  - Quality and quantity of movement between and across body segments are improved.
  - Range of motion is improved.
  - Relaxation is increased.
  - Sensory awareness is increased.
- Impact on functional limitations
  - Ability to perform physical actions, tasks, or activities related to self-care, home management, work (job/school/play), community, and leisure is improved.
  - Level of supervision required for task performance is decreased.
  - Performance of and independence in activities of daily living (ADL) and instrumental activities of daily living (IADL) with or without devices and equipment are increased.
  - Tolerance of positions and activities is increased.
- Impact on disabilities
  - Ability to assume or resume required self-care, home management, work (job/school/play), community, and leisure roles is improved.
- Risk reduction/prevention
  - Preoperative and postoperative complications are reduced.
  - Risk factors are reduced.
  - Risk of recurrence of condition is reduced.
  - Risk of secondary impairment is reduced.
  - Self-management of symptoms is improved.
- Impact on health, wellness, and fitness
  - Fitness is improved.
  - Physical capacity is increased.
  - Physical function is improved.
- Impact on societal resources
  - Utilization of physical therapy services is optimized.
  - Utilization of physical therapy services results in efficient use of health care dollars.
- Patient/client satisfaction
  - Access, availability, and services provided are acceptable to patient/client.
  - Administrative management of practice is acceptable to patient/client.
  - Clinical proficiency of physical therapist is acceptable to patient/client.
  - Coordination of care is acceptable to patient/client.
  - Interpersonal skills of physical therapist are acceptable to patient/client, family, and significant others.
  - Sense of well-being is improved.
  - Stressors are decreased.

Physical Agents and Mechanical Modalities

Interventions

Physical agents may include:

- Cryotherapy
  - cold packs
  - ice massage
- Hydrotherapy
  - contrast bath
  - pools
- Thermotherapy
  - dry heat

Mechanical modalities may include:

- Compression therapies
  - compression bandaging
  - compression garments
  - taping
  - total contact casting
  - vasopneumatic compression devices

Anticipated Goals and Expected Outcomes

- Impact on pathology/pathophysiology (disease, disorder, or condition)
  - Edema, lymphedema, or effusion is reduced.
  - Joint swelling, inflammation, or restriction is reduced.
  - Nutrient delivery to tissue is increased.
  - Pain is decreased.
  - Soft tissue swelling, inflammation, or restriction is reduced.
  - Tissue perfusion and oxygenation are enhanced.
- Impact on impairments
  - Muscle performance (strength, power, and endurance) is increased.
  - Range of motion is improved.
- Impact on functional limitations
  - Ability to perform physical actions, tasks, or activities related to self-care, home management, work (job/school/play), community, and leisure is improved.
  - Performance of and independence in activities of daily living (ADL) and instrumental activities of daily living (IADL) with or without devices and equipment are increased.
  - Tolerance of positions and activities is increased.
- Impact on disabilities
  - Ability to assume or resume required self-care, home management, work (job/school/play), community, and leisure roles is improved.
- Risk reduction/prevention
  - Complications of soft tissue and circulatory disorders are decreased.
  - Risk of secondary impairment is reduced.
  - Self-management of symptoms is improved.
- Impact on health, wellness, and fitness
  - Fitness is improved.
  - Physical capacity is increased.
  - Physical function is improved.
- Impact on societal resources
  - Utilization of physical therapy services is optimized.
- Patient/client satisfaction
  - Access, availability, and services provided are acceptable to patient/client.
  - Administrative management of practice is acceptable to patient/client.
  - Clinical proficiency of physical therapist is acceptable to patient/client.
  - Coordination of care is acceptable to patient/client.
  - Interpersonal skills of physical therapist are acceptable to patient/client, family, and significant others.
  - Sense of well-being is improved.
  - Stressors are decreased.

Reexamination

Reexamination is the process of performing selected tests and measures after the initial examination to evaluate progress and to modify or redirect interventions. Reexamination may be indicated more than once during a single episode of care. It also may be performed over the course of a disease, disorder, or condition, which for some patients/clients may be over the life span. Indications for reexamination include new clinical findings or failure to respond to physical therapy interventions.

Global Outcomes for Patients/Clients in This Pattern

Throughout the entire episode of care, the physical therapist determines the anticipated goals and expected outcomes for each intervention. These anticipated goals and expected outcomes are delineated in shaded boxes that accompany the lists of interventions in each preferred practice pattern. As the patient/client reaches the termination of physical therapy services and the end of the episode of care, the physical therapist measures the global outcomes of the physical therapy services by characterizing or quantifying the impact of the physical therapy interventions in the following domains:

- Pathology/pathophysiology (disease, disorder, or condition)
- Impairments
- Functional limitations
- Disabilities
- Risk reduction/prevention
- Health, wellness, and fitness
- Societal resources
- Patient/client satisfaction

In some instances, a particular anticipated goal or expected outcome is thoroughly achieved through implementation of a single form of intervention. More commonly, however, the anticipated goals and expected outcomes are achieved as a result of the combined effects of several forms of interventions, leading to enhancement of both health status and health-related quality of life.

Criteria for Termination of Physical Therapy Services

Discharge is the process of ending physical therapy services that have been provided during a single episode of care. It occurs when the anticipated goals and expected outcomes have been achieved. Discharge does *not* occur with a *transfer* (defined as the time when a patient is moved from one site to another site within the same setting or across settings during a single episode of care). Although there may be facility-specific or payer-specific requirements for documentation regarding the conclusion of physical therapy services, *discharge occurs based on the physical therapist's analysis of the achievement of anticipated goals and expected outcomes.*

Discontinuation is the process of ending physical therapy services that have been provided during a single episode of care when (1) the patient/client, caregiver, or legal guardian declines to continue intervention; (2) the patient/client is unable to continue to progress toward outcomes because of medical or psychosocial complications or because financial/insurance resources have been expended; or (3) the physical therapist determines that the patient/client will no longer benefit from physical therapy. When physical therapy services are terminated prior to achievement of anticipated goals and expected outcomes, patient/client status and the rationale for termination are documented.

For patients/clients who require multiple episodes of care, periodic follow-up is needed over the life span to ensure safety and effective adaptation following changes in physical status, caregivers, environment, or task demands. In consultation with appropriate individuals, and in consideration of the outcomes, the physical therapist plans for discharge or discontinuation and provides for appropriate follow-up or referral.

CHAPTER 5

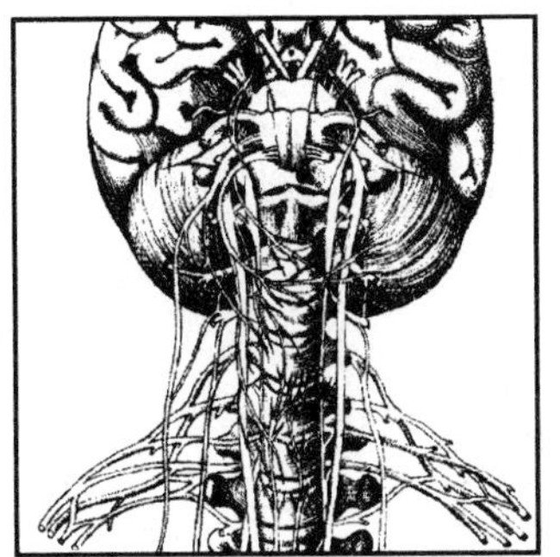

Preferred Physical Therapist Practice Patterns: Neuromuscular

Preferred Physical Therapist Practice Patterns describe the five elements of patient/client management that are provided by physical therapists: examination (history, systems review, and tests and measures), evaluation, diagnosis, prognosis (including plan of care), and intervention (with anticipated goals and expected outcomes). Each pattern also addresses reexamination, global outcomes, and criteria for termination of physical therapy services. Examples of ICD-9-CM codes are included.

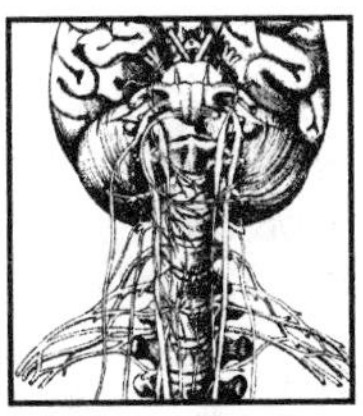

Primary Prevention/Risk Reduction for Loss of Balance and Falling

This preferred practice pattern describes the generally accepted elements of patient/client management that physical therapists provide for patients/clients who are classified in this pattern. The pattern title reflects the diagnosis made by the physical therapist. APTA emphasizes that preferred practice patterns are the boundaries within which a physical therapist may select any of a number of clinical alternatives, based on consideration of a wide variety of factors, such as individual patient/client needs; the profession's code of ethics and standards of practice; and patient/client age, culture, gender roles, race, sex, sexual orientation, and socioeconomic status.

Patient/Client Diagnostic Classification

Patients/clients will be classified into this primary prevention/risk reduction pattern as a result of the physical therapist's evaluation of the examination data. The findings from the examination (history, systems review, and tests and measures) may indicate the need for a prevention/risk reduction program. The physical therapist integrates, synthesizes, and interprets the data to determine inclusion in this diagnostic category.

Inclusion

The following examples of examination findings may support the inclusion of patients/clients in this pattern:

Risk Factors or Consequences of Pathology/Pathophysiology (Disease, Disorder, or Condition)

- Advanced age
- Alteration in senses (auditory, visual, somatosensory)
- Dementia
- Depression
- Dizziness
- Fear of falling
- History of falls
- Medications
- Musculoskeletal diseases
- Neuromuscular diseases
- Prolonged inactivity
- Vestibular pathology

Impairments, Functional Limitations, or Disabilities

- Deconditioning
- Difficulty negotiating in community environment
- Difficulty negotiating terrains
- Disequilibrium
- Generalized weakness
- Impaired gait pattern
- Impaired position sense

Note:

Prevention and risk reduction are inherent in all practice patterns. Patients/clients included in this pattern are in need of primary prevention/risk reduction only.

ICD-9-CM Codes

The listing below contains the current (as of press time) and most typical 3- and 4-digit ICD-9-CM codes related to this preferred practice pattern. Because patient/client diagnostic classification is based on impairments, functional limitations, and disabilities—not on codes—patients/clients may be classified into the pattern even though the codes listed with the pattern may not apply to those patients/clients.

This listing is intended for general information only and should not be used for coding purposes. The codes should be confirmed by referring to the World Health Organization's *International Classification of Diseases, 9th Revision, Clinical Modification (ICD-9-CM 2001)*, Volumes 1 and 3 (Chicago, Ill: American Medical Association; 2000) or subsequent revisions or by referring to other ICD-9-CM coding manuals that contain exclusion notes and instructions regarding fifth-digit requirements.

331 Other cerebral degenerations
- **331.0** Alzheimer's disease

332 Parkinson's disease

333 Other extrapyramidal disease and abnormal movement disorders

334 Spinocerebellar disease

335 Anterior horn cell disease

336 Other diseases of spinal cord

340 Multiple sclerosis

342 Hemiplegia and hemiparesis

345 Epilepsy

359 Muscular dystrophies and other myopathies

386 Vertiginous syndromes and other disorders of vestibular system
- **386.0** Ménière's disease
- **386.1** Other and unspecified peripheral vertigo
- **386.2** Vertigo of central origin
- **386.3** Labyrinthitis

780 General symptoms
- **780.0** Alteration of consciousness
- **780.2** Syncope and collapse
- **780.4** Dizziness and giddiness
- **780.7** Malaise and fatigue

781 Symptoms involving nervous and musculoskeletal systems
- **781.0** Abnormal involuntary movements
- **781.2** Abnormality of gait
- **781.3** Lack of coordination

797 Senility without mention of psychosis

Examination

Examination is a comprehensive screening and specific testing process that leads to a diagnostic classification or, when appropriate, to a referral to another practitioner. Examination is required prior to the initial intervention and is performed for all patients/clients. Through the examination, the physical therapist may identify impairments, functional limitations, disabilities, changes in physical function or overall health status, and needs related to restoration of health and to prevention, wellness, and fitness. The physical therapist synthesizes the examination findings to establish the diagnosis and the prognosis (including the plan of care). The patient/client, family, significant others, and caregivers may provide information during the examination process.

Examination has three components: the patient/client history, the systems review, and tests and measures. The *history* is a systematic gathering of past and current information (often from the patient/client) related to why the patient/client is seeking the services of the physical therapist. The *systems review* is a brief or limited examination of (1) the anatomical and physiological status of the cardiovascular/pulmonary, integumentary, musculoskeletal, and neuromuscular systems and (2) the communication ability, affect, cognition, language, and learning style of the patient/client. *Tests and measures* are the means of gathering data about the patient/client.

The selection of examination procedures and the depth of the examination vary based on patient/client age; severity of the problem; stage of recovery (acute, subacute, chronic); phase of rehabilitation (early, intermediate, late, return to activity); home, work (job/school/play), or community situation; and other relevant factors. *For clinical indications in selecting tests and measures and for listings of tests and measures, tools used to gather data, and the types of data generated by tests and measures, refer to Chapter 2.*

Patient/Client History

The history may include:

General Demographics
- Age
- Sex
- Race/ethnicity
- Primary language
- Education

Social History
- Cultural beliefs and behaviors
- Family and caregiver resources
- Social interactions, social activities, and support systems

Employment/Work (Job/School/Play)
- Current and prior work (job/school/play), community, and leisure actions, tasks, or activities

Growth and Development
- Developmental history
- Hand dominance

Living Environment
- Devices and equipment (eg, assistive, adaptive, orthotic, protective, supportive, prosthetic)
- Living environment and community characteristics
- Projected discharge destinations

General Health Status (Self-Report, Family Report, Caregiver Report)
- General health perception
- Physical function (eg, mobility, sleep patterns, restricted bed days)
- Psychological function (eg, memory, reasoning ability, depression, anxiety)
- Role function (eg, community, leisure, social, work)
- Social function (eg, social activity, social interaction, social support)

Social/Health Habits (Past and Current)
- Behavioral health risks (eg, smoking, drug abuse)
- Level of physical fitness

Family History
- Familial health risks

Medical/Surgical History
- Cardiovascular
- Endocrine/metabolic
- Gastrointestinal
- Genitourinary
- Gynecological
- Integumentary
- Musculoskeletal
- Neuromuscular
- Obstetrical
- Prior hospitalizations, surgeries, and preexisting medical and other health-related conditions
- Psychological
- Pulmonary

Current Condition(s)/Chief Complaint(s)
- Concerns that led patient/client to seek the services of a physical therapist
- Concerns or needs of patient/client who requires the services of a physical therapist
- Current therapeutic interventions
- Mechanisms of injury or disease, including date of onset and course of events
- Onset and pattern of symptoms
- Patient/client, family, significant other, and caregiver expectations and goals for the therapeutic intervention
- Patient/client, family, significant other, and caregiver perceptions of patient's/client's emotional response to the current clinical situation
- Previous occurrence of chief complaint(s)
- Prior therapeutic interventions

Functional Status and Activity Level
- Current and prior functional status in self-care and home management activities, including activities of daily living (ADL) and instrumental activities of daily living (IADL)
- Current and prior functional status in work (job/school/play), community, and leisure actions, tasks, or activities

Medications
- Medications for current condition
- Medications previously taken for current condition
- Medications for other conditions

Other Clinical Tests
- Laboratory and diagnostic tests
- Review of available records (eg, medical, education, surgical)
- Review of other clinical findings (eg, nutrition and hydration)

Systems Review

The systems review may include:

Anatomical and Physiological Status

- Cardiovascular/Pulmonary
  - Blood pressure
  - Edema
  - Heart rate
  - Respiratory rate
- Integumentary
  - Pliability (texture)
  - Presence of scar formation
  - Skin color
  - Skin integrity
- Musculoskeletal
  - Gross range of motion
  - Gross strength
  - Gross symmetry
  - Height
  - Weight
- Neuromuscular
  - Gross coordinated movements (eg, balance, gait, locomotion, transfers, transitions)
  - Motor function (motor control, motor learning)

Communication, Affect, Cognition, Language, and Learning Style

- Ability to make needs known
- Consciousness
- Expected emotional/behavioral responses
- Learning preferences (eg, education needs, learning barriers)
- Orientation (person, place, time)

Tests and Measures

Test and measures for this pattern may include those that characterize or quantify:

Aerobic Capacity and Endurance

- Aerobic capacity during functional activities (eg, activities of daily living [ADL] scales, indexes, instrumental activities of daily living [IADL] scales, observations)
- Aerobic capacity during standardized exercise test protocols (eg, ergometry, step tests, time/distance walk/run tests, treadmill tests, wheelchair tests)

Arousal, Attention, and Cognition

- Arousal and attention (eg, adaptability tests, arousal and awareness scales, indexes, profiles, questionnaires)
- Cognition, including ability to process commands (eg, indexes, interviews, mental state scales, observations, questionnaires, safety checklists)
- Motivation (eg, adaptive behavior scales)
- Orientation to time, person, place, and situation (eg, attention tests, learning profiles, mental state scales)
- Recall, including memory and retention (eg, assessment scales, interviews, questionnaires)

Assistive and Adaptive Devices

- Assistive or adaptive devices and equipment use during functional activities (eg, ADL scales, functional scales, IADL scales, interviews, observations)
- Components, alignment, fit, and ability to care for the assistive or adaptive devices and equipment (eg, interviews, observations, reports)
- Remediation of impairments, functional limitations, or disabilities with use of assistive or adaptive devices and equipment (eg, activity status indexes, ADL scales, aerobic capacity tests, functional performance inventories, health assessment questionnaires, IADL scales, pain scales, play scales, videographic assessments)
- Safety during use of assistive or adaptive devices and equipment (eg, fall scales, reports, interviews, observations)

Cranial and Peripheral Nerve Integrity

- Motor distribution of the peripheral nerves (eg, dynamometry, muscle tests, observations)
- Response to stimuli, including auditory, gustatory, olfactory, pharyngeal, vestibular, and visual (eg, observations, provocation tests)
- Sensory distribution of the cranial nerves (eg, discrimination tests; tactile tests, including coarse and light touch, cold and heat, pain, pressure, and vibration)
- Sensory distribution of the peripheral nerves (eg, discrimination tests; tactile tests, including coarse and light touch, cold and heat, pain, pressure, and vibration; thoracic outlet tests)

Environmental, Home, and Work (Job/School/Play) Barriers

- Current and potential barriers (eg, checklists, interviews, observations, questionnaires)

Ergonomics and Body Mechanics

Body mechanics

- Body mechanics during self-care, home management, work, community, or leisure actions, tasks, or activities (eg, ADL scales, IADL scales, observations, photographic assessments, technology-assisted assessments, videographic assessments)

Gait, Locomotion, and Balance

- Balance during functional activities with or without the use of assistive, adaptive, orthotic, protective, supportive, or prosthetic devices or equipment (eg, ADL scales, IADL scales, observations, videographic assessments)
- Balance (dynamic and static) with or without the use of assistive, adaptive, orthotic, protective, supportive, or prosthetic devices or equipment (eg, balance scales, dizziness inventories, dynamic posturography, fall scales, motor impairment tests, observations, photographic assessments, postural control tests)
- Gait and locomotion during functional activities with or without the use of assistive, adaptive, orthotic, protective, supportive, or prosthetic devices or equipment (eg, ADL scales, gait indexes, IADL scales, mobility skill profiles, observations)
- Gait and locomotion with or without the use of assistive, adaptive, orthotic, protective, supportive, or prosthetic devices or equipment (eg, dynamometry, electroneuromyography, footprint analyses, gait indexes, mobility skill profiles, observations, photographic assessments, technology-assisted assessments, videographic assessments, weight-bearing scales, wheelchair mobility tests)
- Safety during gait, locomotion, and balance (eg, confidence scales, fall scales, functional assessment profiles, reports)

Motor Function (Motor Control and Motor Learning)

- Dexterity, coordination, and agility (eg, coordination screens, motor impairment tests, motor proficiency tests, observations, videographic assessments)
- Initiation, modification, and control of movement patterns and voluntary postures (eg, activity indexes, developmental scales, gross motor function profiles, motor scales, movement assessment batteries, neuromotor tests, observations, physical performance tests, postural challenge tests, videographic assessments)

Muscle Performance (Including Strength, Power, and Endurance)

- Muscle strength, power, and endurance (eg, dynamometry, manual muscle tests, muscle performance tests, physical capacity tests,technology-assisted assessments, timed activity tests)
- Muscle strength, power, and endurance during functional activities (eg, ADL scales, functional muscle tests, IADL scales, observations, videographic assessments)

Orthotic, Protective, and Supportive Devices

- Components, alignment, fit, and ability to care for orthotic, protective, and supportive devices and equipment (eg, interviews, observations, reports)
- Orthotic, protective, and supportive devices and equipment use during functional activities (eg, ADL scales, functional scales, IADL scales, interviews, observations, profiles)
- Safety during use of orthotic, protective, and supportive devices and equipment (eg, fall scales, reports, interviews, observations)

Posture

- Postural alignment and position (static and dynamic), including symmetry and deviation from midline (eg, grid measurement, photographic assessments, observations, technology-assisted assessments, videographic assessments)
- Specific body parts (eg, angle assessments, forward-bending test, goniometry, observations, palpation, positional tests)

Range of Motion (Including Muscle Length)

- Functional ROM (eg, observations, squat testing, toe touch tests)
- Joint active and passive movement (eg, goniometry, inclinometry, observations, photographic assessments, technology-assisted assessments, videographic assessments)
- Muscle length, soft tissue extensibility, and flexibility (eg, contracture tests, goniometry, inclinometry, ligamentous tests, linear measurement, multisegment flexibility tests, palpation)

Reflex Integrity

- Deep reflexes (eg, myotatic reflex scale, observations, reflex tests)
- Postural reflexes and reactions, including righting, equilibrium, and protective reactions (eg, observations, postural challenge tests, reflex profiles, videographic assessments)
- Resistance to passive stretch (eg, tone scales)

Self-Care and Home Management (Including Activities of Daily Living and Instrumental Activities of Daily Living)

- Ability to gain access to home environments (eg, barrier identification, observations, physical performance tests)
- Safety in self-care and home management activities and environments (eg, diaries, fall scales, interviews, logs, observations, reports, videographic assessments)

Sensory Integrity

- Combined/cortical sensations (eg, stereognosis, tactile discrimination tests)
- Deep sensations (eg, kinesthesiometry, observations, photographic assessments, vibration tests)

Work (Job/School/Play), Community, and Leisure Integration or Reintegration (Including IADL)

- Ability to gain access to work (job/school/play), community, and leisure environments (eg, barrier identification, interviews, observations, physical capacity, transportation assessments)
- Safety in work (job/school/play), community, and leisure activities and environments (eg, fall scales, interviews, observations)

Evaluation, Diagnosis, and Prognosis (Including Plan of Care)

Physical therapists perform *evaluations* (make clinical judgments) based on the data gathered from the history, systems review, and tests and measures. In the evaluation process, physical therapists synthesize the examination data to establish the diagnosis and prognosis (including the plan of care). Factors that influence the complexity of the evaluation include the clinical findings, extent of loss of function, chronicity or severity of the problem, possibility of multisite or multisystem involvement, preexisting condition(s), potential discharge destination, social considerations, physical function, and overall health status.

A *diagnosis* is a label encompassing a cluster of signs and symptoms, syndromes, or categories. It is the result of the systematic diagnostic process, which includes integrating and evaluating the data from the examination. The diagnostic label indicates the primary dysfunction(s) toward which the therapist will direct interventions. The *prognosis* is the determination of the predicted optimal level of improvement in function and the amount of time needed to reach that level and may also include a prediction of levels of improvement that may be reached at various intervals during the course of therapy. During the prognostic process, the physical therapist develops the plan of care. The *plan of care* identifies specific interventions, proposed frequency and duration of the interventions, anticipated goals, expected outcomes, and discharge plans. The plan of care identifies realistic anticipated goals and expected outcomes, taking into consideration the expectations of the patient/client and appropriate others. These anticipated goals and expected outcomes should be measureable and time limited.

The frequency of visits and duration of the episode of care may vary from a short episode with a high intensity of intervention to a longer episode with a diminishing intensity of intervention. Frequency and duration may vary greatly among patients/clients based on a variety of factors that the physical therapist considers throughout the evaluation process, such as anatomical and physiological changes related to growth and development; caregiver consistency or expertise; chronicity or severity of the current condition; living environment; multisite or multisystem involvement; social support; potential discharge destinations; probability of prolonged impairment, functional limitation, or disability; and stability of the condition.

Prognosis

Patient/client will reduce the risk of falling through therapeutic exercise, balance training, and lifestyle modification.

Expected Range of Number of Visits Per Episode of Care

2 to 18

This range represents the lower and upper limits of the number of physical therapist visits required to achieve anticipated goals and expected outcomes. *It is anticipated that 80% of patients/clients who are classified into this pattern will achieve the anticipated goals and expected outcomes within 2 to 18 visits during a single continuous episode of care.*

Frequency of visits and duration of the episode of care should be determined by the physical therapist to maximize effectiveness of care and efficiency of service delivery.

Factors That May Require New Episode of Care or That May Modify Frequency of Visits/Duration of Care

- Accessibility and availability of resources
- Adherence to the intervention program
- Age
- Anatomical and physiological changes related to growth and development
- Caregiver consistency or expertise
- Chronicity or severity of the current condition
- Cognitive status
- Comorbitities, complications, or secondary impairments
- Concurrent medical, surgical, and therapeutic interventions
- Decline in functional independence
- Level of impairment
- Level of physical function
- Living environment
- Multisite or multisystem involvement
- Nutritional status
- Overall health status
- Potential discharge destinations
- Premorbid conditions
- Probability of prolonged impairment, functional limitation, or disability
- Psychological and socioeconomic factors
- Psychomotor abilities
- Social support
- Stability of the condition

Intervention

Intervention is the purposeful interaction of the physical therapist with the patient/client and, when appropriate, with other individuals involved with the patient/client, using various physical therapy procedures and techniques to produce changes in the condition consistent with the diagnosis and prognosis. Decisions about interventions are contingent on the timely monitoring of patient/client response and the progress made toward achieving the anticipated goals and expected outcomes.

Communication, coordination, and documentation and patient/client-related instruction are provided for all patients/clients across all settings. Procedural interventions are selected or modified based on the examination data and the evaluation, the diagnosis and the prognosis, and the anticipated goals and expected outcomes for a particular patient/client. *For clinical considerations in selecting interventions, listings of interventions, and listings of anticipated goals and expected outcomes, refer to Chapter 3.*

Coordination, Communication, and Documentation

Coordination, communication, and documentation for primary prevention/risk reduction may include:

Interventions

- Addressing required functions
  - individualized family service plans (IFSPs) or individualized education plans (IEPs)
  - informed consent
  - mandatory communication and reporting (eg, patient/client advocacy and abuse reporting)
- Collaboration and coordination with agencies, including:
  - equipment suppliers
  - home care agencies
  - payer groups
  - schools
  - transportation agencies
- Communication, including:
  - education plans
  - documentation
- Data collection, analysis and reporting
  - outcome data
  - peer review findings
  - record reviews
- Documentation
  - elements of patient/client management (examination, evaluation, diagnosis, prognosis, intervention)
  - outcomes of intervention
- Referrals to other professionals or resources

Anticipated Goals and Expected Outcomes

- Accountability for services is increased.
- Individualized family service plans (IFSPs) or individualized education plans (IEPs), informed consent, and mandatory communication and reporting (eg, patient/client advocacy and abuse reporting) are obtained or completed.
- Available resources are maximally utilized.
- Collaboration and coordination occurs with agencies, including equipment suppliers, home care agencies, payer groups, schools, and transportation agencies.
- Communication occurs through education plans and documentation.
- Data are collected, analyzed, and reported, including outcome data, peer review findings, and record reviews.
- Decision making is enhanced regarding patient/client health and the use of health care resources by patient/client, family, significant others, and caregivers.
- Documentation occurs throughout client management and follows APTA's *Guidelines for Physical Therapy Documentation* (Appendix 5).
- Patient/client, family, significant other, and caregiver understanding of anticipated goals and expected outcomes is increased.
- Referrals are made to other professionals or resources whenever necessary and appropriate.
- Resources are utilized in a cost-effective way.

Patient/Client-Related Instruction

Patient/client-related instruction may include:

Interventions

- Instruction, education, and training of patients/clients and caregivers regarding:
  - enhancement of performance
  - health, wellness, and fitness programs
  - plan for intervention
  - risk factors for pathology/pathophysiology (disease, disorder, or condition), impairments, functional limitations, or disabilities

Anticipated Goals and Expected Outcomes

- Ability to perform physical actions, tasks, or activities is improved.
- Awareness and use of community resources are improved.
- Behaviors that foster healthy habits, wellness, and prevention are acquired.
- Decision making is enhanced regarding patient/client health and the use of health care resources by patient/client, family, significant others, and caregivers.
- Health status is improved.
- Patient/client, family, significant other, and caregiver knowledge and awareness of the diagnosis, prognosis, interventions, and anticipated goals and expected outcomes are increased.
- Patient/client knowledge of personal and environmental factors associated with the condition is increased.
- Performance levels in self-care, home management, work (job/school/play), community, or leisure actions, tasks, or activities are improved.
- Physical function is improved.
- Risk of recurrence of condition is reduced.
- Safety of patient/client, family, significant others, and caregivers is improved.
- Utilization and cost of health care services are decreased.

Procedural Interventions

Procedural interventions for this pattern may include:

Therapeutic Exercise

Interventions

- Aerobic capacity/endurance conditioning or reconditioning
  - aquatic programs
  - gait and locomotor training
  - increased workload over time
  - walking and wheelchair propulsion programs
- Balance, coordination, and agility training
  - motor function (motor control and motor learning) training or retraining
  - neuromuscular education or reeducation
  - perceptual training
  - posture awareness training
  - standardized, programmatic, complementary exercise approaches
  - sensory training or retraining
  - task-specific performance training
  - vestibular training
- Body mechanics and postural stabilization
  - body mechanics training
  - posture awareness training
  - postural control training
  - postural stabilization activities
- Flexibility exercises
  - muscle lengthening
  - range of motion
  - stretching
- Gait and locomotion training
  - gait training
  - implement and device training
  - perceptual training
  - standardized, programmatic, complementary exercise approaches
  - wheelchair training
- Relaxation
  - breathing strategies
  - movement strategies
  - relaxation techniques
  - standardized, programmatic, complementary exercise approaches
- Strength, power, and endurance training for head, neck, limb, pelvic-floor, trunk, and ventilatory muscles
  - active assistive, active, and resistive exercises (including concentric, dynamic/isotonic, eccentric, isokinetic, isometric, and plyometric)
  - aquatic programs
  - standardized, programmatic, complementary exercise approaches
  - task-specific performance training

Anticipated Goals and Expected Outcomes

- Impact on pathology/pathophysiology (disease, disorder, or condition)
  - Nutrient delivery to tissue is increased.
  - Osteogenic effects of exercise are maximized.
  - Physiological response to increased oxygen demand is improved.
  - Tissue perfusion and oxygenation are enhanced.
- Impact on impairments
  - Aerobic capacity is increased.
  - Balance is improved.
  - Endurance is increased.
  - Energy expenditure per unit of work is decreased.
  - Gait, locomotion, and balance are improved.
  - Joint integrity and mobility are improved.
  - Integumentary integrity is improved.
  - Motor function (motor control and motor learning) is improved.
  - Muscle performance (strength, power, and endurance) is increased.
  - Postural control is improved.
  - Quality and quantity of movement between and across body segments are improved.
  - Range of motion is improved.
  - Relaxation is increased.
  - Sensory awareness is increased.
  - Weight-bearing status is improved.
- Impact on functional limitations
  - Ability to perform physical actions, tasks, or activities related to self-care, home management, work (job/school/play), community, and leisure is improved.
  - Level of supervision required for task performance is decreased.
  - Performance of and independence in activities of daily living (ADL) and instrumental activities of daily living (IADL) with or without devices and equipment are increased.
  - Tolerance of positions and activities is increased.
- Impact on disabilities
  - Ability to assume or resume required self-care, home management, work (job/school/play), community, and leisure roles is improved.
- Risk reduction/prevention
  - Risk factors are reduced.
  - Risk of secondary impairment is reduced.
  - Safety is improved.
  - Self-management of symptoms is improved.
- Impact on health, wellness, and fitness
  - Fitness is improved.
  - Health status is improved.
  - Physical capacity is increased.
  - Physical function is improved.
- Impact on societal resources
  - Utilization of physical therapy services is optimized.
  - Utilization of physical therapy services results in efficient use of health care dollars.
- Patient/client satisfaction
  - Access, availability, and services provided are acceptable to patient/client.
  - Administrative management of practice is acceptable to patient/client.
  - Clinical proficiency of physical therapist is acceptable to patient/client.
  - Coordination of care is acceptable to patient/client.
  - Cost of health care services is decreased.
  - Interpersonal skills of physical therapist are acceptable to patient/client, family, and significant others.
  - Sense of well-being is improved.
  - Stressors are decreased.

Functional Training in Self-Care and Home Management (Including Activities of Daily Living [ADL] and Instrumental Activities of Daily Living [IADL])

Interventions

- Injury prevention or reduction
  - injury prevention education during self-care and home management
  - injury prevention or reduction with use of devices and equipment
  - safety awareness training during self-care and home management
- Functional training programs
  - simulated environments and tasks
  - task adaptation

Anticipated Goals and Expected Outcomes

- Impact on pathology/pathophysiology (disease, disorder, or condition)
  - Physiological response to increased oxygen demand is improved.
- Impact on impairments
  - Postural control is improved.
  - Weight-bearing status is improved.
- Impact on functional limitations
  - Ability to perform physical actions, tasks, or activities related to self-care and home management is improved.
  - Level of supervision required for task performance is decreased.
  - Performance of and independence in ADL and IADL with or without devices and equipment are increased.
  - Tolerance of positions and activities is increased.
- Impact on disabilities
  - Ability to assume or resume required self-care and home management roles is improved.
- Risk reduction/prevention
  - Risk factors are reduced.
  - Risk of secondary impairments is reduced.
  - Safety is improved.
  - Self-management of symptoms is improved.
- Impact on health, wellness, and fitness
  - Health status is improved.
  - Physical function is improved.
- Impact on societal resources
  - Utilization of physical therapy services is optimized.
  - Utilization of physical therapy services results in efficient use of health care dollars.
- Patient/client satisfaction
  - Access, availability, and services provided are acceptable to patient/client.
  - Administrative management of practice is acceptable to patient/client.
  - Clinical proficiency of physical therapist is acceptable to patient/client.
  - Coordination of care is acceptable to patient/client.
  - Cost of health care services is decreased.
  - Interpersonal skills of physical therapist are acceptable to patient/client, family, and significant others.
  - Sense of well-being is improved.
  - Stressors are decreased.

Functional Training in Work (Job/School/Play), Community, and Leisure Integration or Reintegration (Including Instrumental Activities of Daily Living [IADL], Work Hardening, and Work Conditioning)

Interventions

- Injury prevention or reduction
  - injury prevention education during work (job/school/play), community, and leisure integration or reintegration
  - injury prevention or reduction with use of devices and equipment
  - safety awareness training during work (job/school/play), community, and leisure integration or reintegration
- Functional training programs
  - simulated environments and tasks
  - task adaptation
  - task training
  - travel training

Anticipated Goals and Expected Outcomes

- Impact on pathology/pathophysiology (disease, disorder, or condition)
  - Physiological response to increased oxygen demand is improved.
- Impact on impairments
  - Postural control is improved.
  - Weight-bearing status is improved.
- Impact on functional limitations
  - Ability to perform physical actions, tasks, or activities related to work (job/school/play), community, and leisure integration or reintegration is improved.
  - Level of supervision required for task performance is decreased.
  - Performance of and independence in IADL with or without devices and equipment are increased.
  - Tolerance of positions and activities is increased.
- Impact on disabilities
  - Ability to assume or resume required work (job/school/play), community, and leisure roles is improved.
- Risk reduction/prevention
  - Risk factors are reduced.
  - Risk of secondary impairment is reduced.
  - Safety is improved.
  - Self-management of symptoms is improved.
- Impact on health, wellness, and fitness
  - Health status is improved.
  - Physical function is improved.
- Impact on societal resources
  - Costs of work-related injury or disability are reduced.
  - Utilization of physical therapy services is optimized.
  - Utilization of physical therapy services results in efficient use of health care dollars.
- Patient/client satisfaction
  - Access, availability, and services provided are acceptable to patient/client.
  - Administrative management of practice is acceptable to patient/client.
  - Clinical proficiency of physical therapist is acceptable to patient/client.
  - Coordination of care is acceptable to patient/client.
  - Cost of health care services is decreased.
  - Interpersonal skills of physical therapist are acceptable to patient/client, family, and significant others.
  - Sense of well-being is improved.
  - Stressors are decreased.

Prescription, Application, and, as Appropriate, Fabrication of Devices and Equipment (Assistive, Adaptive, Orthotic, Protective, Supportive, and Prosthetic)

Interventions

- Assistive devices
  - canes
  - crutches
  - long-handled reachers
  - walkers
- Protective devices
  - braces
  - helmets
- Orthotic devices
  - braces
  - shoe inserts

Anticipated Goals and Expected Outcomes

- Impact on pathology/pathophysiology (disease, disorder, or condition)
  - Pain is decreased.
  - Physiological response to increased oxygen demand is improved.
- Impact on impairments
  - Balance is improved.
  - Energy expenditure per unit of work is decreased.
  - Gait, locomotion, and balance are improved.
  - Joint stability is improved.
  - Motor function (motor control and motor learning) is improved.
  - Muscle performance (strength, power, and endurance) is increased.
  - Optimal joint alignment is achieved.
  - Optimal loading on a body part is achieved.
  - Postural control is improved.
  - Quality and quantity of movement between and across body segments are improved.
  - Weight-bearing status is improved.
- Impact on functional limitations
  - Ability to perform physical actions, tasks, or activities related to self-care, home management, work (job/school/play), community, and leisure is improved.
  - Level of supervision required for task performance is decreased.
  - Performance of and independence in activities of daily living (ADL) and instrumental activities of daily living (IADL) with or without devices and equipment are increased.
  - Tolerance of positions and activities is increased.
- Impact on disabilities
  - Ability to assume or resume required self-care, home management, work (job/school/play), community, and leisure roles is improved.
- Risk reduction/prevention
  - Pressure on body tissues is reduced.
  - Protection of body parts is increased.
  - Risk factors are reduced.
  - Risk of recurrence of condition is reduced.
  - Risk of secondary impairment is reduced.
  - Safety is improved.
  - Self-management of symptoms is improved.
  - Stresses precipitating injury are decreased.
- Impact on health, wellness, and fitness
  - Health status is improved.
  - Physical capacity is increased.
  - Physical function is improved.
- Impact on societal resources
  - Utilization of physical therapy services is optimized.
  - Utilization of physical therapy services results in efficient use of health care dollars.
- Patient/client satisfaction
  - Access, availability, and services provided are acceptable to patient/client.
  - Administrative management of practice is acceptable to patient/client.
  - Clinical proficiency of physical therapist is acceptable to patient/client.
  - Coordination of care is acceptable to patient/client.
  - Cost of health care services is decreased.
  - Interpersonal skills of physical therapist are acceptable to patient/client, family, and significant others.
  - Sense of well-being is improved.
  - Stressors are decreased.

Reexamination

Reexamination is the process of performing selected tests and measures after the initial examination to evaluate progress and to modify or redirect interventions. Reexamination may be indicated more than once during a single episode of care. It also may be performed over the course of a disease, disorder, or condition, which for some patients/clients may be over the life span. Indications for reexamination include new clinical findings or failure to respond to physical therapy interventions.

Global Outcomes for Patients/Clients in This Pattern

Throughout the entire episode of care, the physical therapist determines the anticipated goals and expected outcomes for each intervention. These anticipated goals and expected outcomes are delineated in shaded boxes that accompany the lists of interventions in each preferred practice pattern. As the patient/client reaches the termination of physical therapy services and the end of the episode of care, the physical therapist measures the global outcomes of the physical therapy services by characterizing or quantifying the impact of the physical therapy interventions in the following domains:

- Pathology/pathophysiology (disease, disorder, or condition)
- Impairments
- Functional limitations
- Disabilities
- Risk reduction/prevention
- Health, wellness, and fitness
- Societal resources
- Patient/client satisfaction

In some instances, a particular anticipated goal or expected outcome is thoroughly achieved through implementation of a single form of intervention. More commonly, however, the anticipated goals and expected outcomes are achieved as a result of the combined effects of several forms of interventions, leading to enhancement of both health status and health-related quality of life.

Criteria for Termination of Physical Therapy Services

Discharge is the process of ending physical therapy services that have been provided during a single episode of care. It occurs when the anticipated goals and expected outcomes have been achieved. Discharge does *not* occur with a *transfer* (defined as the time when a patient is moved from one site to another site within the same setting or across settings during a single episode of care). Although there may be facility-specific or payer-specific requirements for documentation regarding the conclusion of physical therapy services, *discharge occurs based on the physical therapist's analysis of the achievement of anticipated goals and expected outcomes.*

Discontinuation is the process of ending physical therapy services that have been provided during a single episode of care when (1) the patient/client, caregiver, or legal guardian declines to continue intervention; (2) the patient/client is unable to continue to progress toward outcomes because of medical or psychosocial complications or because financial/insurance resources have been expended; or (3) the physical therapist determines that the patient/client will no longer benefit from physical therapy. When physical therapy services are terminated prior to achievement of anticipated goals and expected outcomes, patient/client status and the rationale for termination are documented.

For patients/clients who require multiple episodes of care, periodic follow-up is needed over the life span to ensure safety and effective adaptation following changes in physical status, caregivers, environment, or task demands. In consultation with appropriate individuals, and in consideration of the outcomes, the physical therapist plans for discharge or discontinuation and provides for appropriate follow-up or referral.

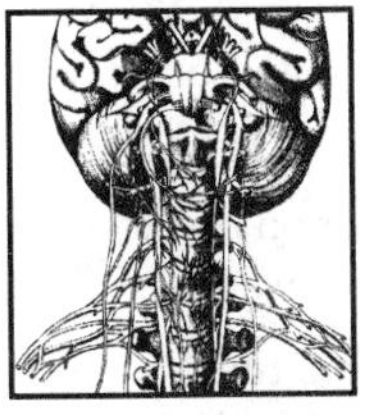

Impaired Neuromotor Development

This preferred practice pattern describes the generally accepted elements of patient/client management that physical therapists provide for patients/clients who are classified in this pattern. The pattern title reflects the diagnosis made by the physical therapist. APTA emphasizes that preferred practice patterns are the boundaries within which a physical therapist may select any of a number of clinical alternatives, based on consideration of a wide variety of factors, such as individual patient/client needs; the profession's code of ethics and standards of practice; and patient/client age, culture, gender roles, race, sex, sexual orientation, and socioeconomic status.

Patient/Client Diagnostic Classification

Patients/clients will be classified into this pattern for impaired neuromotor development as a result of the physical therapist's evaluation of the examination data. The findings from the examination (history, systems review, and tests and measures) may indicate the presence or risk of pathology/pathophysiology (disease, disorder, or condition), impairments, functional limitations, or disabilities or the need for health, wellness, or fitness programs. The physical therapist integrates, synthesizes, and interprets the data to determine the diagnostic classification.

Inclusion

The following examples of examination findings may support the inclusion of patients/clients in this pattern:

Risk Factors or Consequences of Pathology/Pathophysiology (Disease, Disorder, or Condition)

- Alteration in senses (auditory, visual)
- Birth trauma
- Cognitive delay
- Developmental coordination disorder
- Developmental delay
- Dyspraxia
- Fetal alcohol syndrome
- Genetic syndromes
- Prematurity

Impairments, Functional Limitations, or Disabilities

- Clumsiness during play
- Delayed motor skills
- Delayed oral motor development
- Impaired arousal, attention, and cognition
- Impaired locomotion
- Impaired sensory integration

Note:

Some risk factors or consequences of pathology/pathophysiology—such as *neoplasm*—may be severe and complex; *however, they do not necessarily exclude patients/clients from this pattern.* Severe and complex risk factors or consequences may require modification of the frequency of visits and duration of care. (See "Evaluation, Diagnosis, and Prognosis," page 326.)

Exclusion or Multiple-Pattern Classification

The following examples of examination findings may support exclusion from this pattern or classification into additional patterns. Depending on the level of severity or complexity of the examination findings, the physical therapist may determine that the patient/client would be more appropriately managed through (1) classification in an entirely different pattern or (2) classification in both this and another pattern.

Findings That May Require Classification in a Different Pattern

- Spinal cord injury

Findings That May Require Classification in Additional Patterns

- Arthritis
- Congenital heart defect

ICD-9-CM Codes

The listing below contains the current (as of press time) and most typical 3- and 4-digit ICD-9-CM codes related to this preferred practice pattern. Because patient/client diagnostic classification is based on impairments, functional limitations, and disabilities—not on codes—patients/clients may be classified into the pattern even though the codes listed with the pattern may not apply to those clients.

This listing is intended for general information only and should not be used for coding purposes. The codes should be confirmed by referring to the World Health Organization's *International Classification of Diseases, 9th Revision, Clinical Modification (ICD-9-CM 2001)*, Volumes 1 and 3 (Chicago, Ill: American Medical Association; 2000) or subsequent revisions or by referring to other ICD-9-CM coding manuals that contain exclusion notes and instructions regarding fifth-digit requirements.

191 Malignant neoplasm of brain
192 Malignant neoplasm of other and unspecified parts of nervous system
225 Benign neoplasm of brain and other parts of nervous system
252 Disorders of parathyroid gland
- **252.0** Hyperparathyroidism

253 Disorders of the pituitary gland and its hypothalamic control
- **253.3** Pituitary dwarfism

262 Other severe, protein-calorie malnutrition
299 Psychoses with origin specific to childhood
- **299.0** Infantile autism

315 Specific delays in development
- **315.4** Coordination disorder
- **315.9** Unspecified delay in development

333 Other extrapyramidal disease and abnormal movement disorders
- **333.7** Symptomatic torsion dystonia

345 Epilepsy
- **345.1** Generalized convulsive epilepsy
- **345.2** Petit mal status
- **345.3** Grand mal status
- **345.9** Epilepsy, unspecified

348 Other conditions of brain
- **348.1** Anoxic brain damage
- **348.3** Encephalopathy, unspecified

358 Myoneural disorders
359 Muscular dystrophies and other myopathies
389 Hearing loss
714 Rheumatoid arthritis and other inflammatory polyarthropathies
- **714.3** Juvenile chronic polyarthritis

728 Disorders of muscle, ligament, and fascia
- **728.3** Other specific muscle disorders
  Arthrogryposis

741 Spina bifida
742 Other congenital anomalies of nervous system
- **742.3** Congenital hydrocephalus
- **742.5** Other specified anomalies of spinal cord

745 Bulbus cordis anomalies and anomalies of cardiac septal closure
- **745.1** Transposition of great vessels
- **745.2** Tetralogy of Fallot
- **745.4** Ventricular septal defect
- **745.5** Ostium secundum type atrial septal defect

746 Other congenital anomalies of heart
- **746.0** Anomalies of pulmonary valve

747 Other congenital anomalies of circulatory system
- **747.1** Coarctation of aorta

748 Congenital anomalies of respiratory system
754 Certain congenital musculoskeletal deformities
- **754.2** Of spine
- **754.3** Congenital dislocation of hip

755 Other congenital anomalies of limbs
756 Other congenital musculoskeletal anomalies
- **756.5** Osteodystrophies
  - **756.51** Osteogenesis imperfecta

758 Chromosomal anomalies
Includes: syndromes associated with anomalies in the number and form of chromosomes
759 Other and unspecified congenital anomalies
760 Fetus or newborn affected by maternal conditions which may be unrelated to present pregnancy
- **760.7** Noxious influences affecting fetus via placenta or breast milk

762 Fetus or newborn affected by complications of placenta, cord, and membranes
- **762.5** Other compression of umbilical cord

763 Fetus or newborn affected by other complications of labor and delivery
764 Slow fetal growth and fetal malnutrition
765 Disorders relating to short gestation and unspecified low birth weight
767 Birth trauma
- **767.0** Subdural and cerebral hemorrhage
- **767.9** Birth trauma, unspecified

768 Intrauterine hypoxia and birth asphyxia
- **768.5** Severe birth asphyxia
- **768.6** Mild or moderate birth asphyxia
- **768.9** Unspecified birth asphyxia in liveborn infant

770 Other respiratory conditions of fetus and newborn
- **770.1** Meconium aspiration syndrome
- **770.7** Chronic respiratory disease arising in the perinatal period

771 Infections specific to the perinatal period
- **771.2** Other congenital infections
  Congenital toxoplasmosis

779 Other and ill-defined conditions originating in the perinatal period
780 General symptoms
- **780.3** Convulsions

783 Symptoms concerning nutrition, metabolism, and development

799 Other ill-defined and unknown causes of morbidity and mortality

- **799.0** Asphyxia

800 Fracture of vault of skull

801 Fracture of base of skull

803 Other and unqualified skull fractures

804 Multiple fractures involving skull or face with other bones

850 Concussion

851 Cerebral laceration and contusion

852 Subarachnoid, subdural, and extradural hemorrhage, following injury

853 Other and unspecified intracranial hemorrhage following injury

854 Intracranial injury of other and unspecified nature

994 Effects of other external causes

- **994.1** Drowning and nonfatal submersion

995 Certain adverse effects not elsewhere classified

- **995.5** Child maltreatment syndrome

Examination

Examination is a comprehensive screening and specific testing process that leads to a diagnostic classification or, when appropriate, to a referral to another practitioner. Examination is required prior to the initial intervention and is performed for all patients/clients. Through the examination, the physical therapist may identify impairments, functional limitations, disabilities, changes in physical function or overall health status, and needs related to restoration of health and to prevention, wellness, and fitness. The physical therapist synthesizes the examination findings to establish the diagnosis and the prognosis (including the plan of care). The patient/client, family, significant others, and caregivers may provide information during the examination process.

Examination has three components: the patient/client history, the systems review, and tests and measures. The *history* is a systematic gathering of past and current information (often from the patient/client) related to why the patient/client is seeking the services of the physical therapist. The *systems review* is a brief or limited examination of (1) the anatomical and physiological status of the cardiovascular/pulmonary, integumentary, musculoskeletal, and neuromuscular systems and (2) the communication ability, affect, cognition, language, and learning style of the patient/client. *Tests and measures* are the means of gathering data about the patient/client.

The selection of examination procedures and the depth of the examination vary based on patient/client age; severity of the problem; stage of recovery (acute, subacute, chronic); phase of rehabilitation (early, intermediate, late, return to activity); home, work (job/school/play), or community situation; and other relevant factors. *For clinical indications in selecting tests and measures and for listings of tests and measures, tools used to gather data, and the types of data generated by tests and measures, refer to Chapter 2.*

Patient/Client History

The history may include:

General Demographics

- Age
- Sex
- Race/ethnicity
- Primary language
- Education

Social History

- Cultural beliefs and behaviors
- Family and caregiver resources
- Social interactions, social activities, and support systems

Employment/Work (Job/School/Play)

- Current and prior work (job/school/play), community, and leisure actions, tasks, and activities

Growth and Development

- Developmental history
- Hand dominance

Living Environment

- Devices and equipment (eg, assistive, adaptive, orthotic, protective, supportive, prosthetic)
- Living environment and community characteristics
- Projected discharge destinations

General Health Status (Self-Report, Family Report, Caregiver Report)

- General health perception
- Physical function (eg, mobility, sleep patterns, restricted bed days)
- Psychological function (eg, memory, reasoning ability, depression, anxiety)
- Role function (eg, community, leisure, social, work)
- Social function (eg, social activity, social interaction, social support)

Social/Health Habits (Past and Current)

- Behavioral health risks (eg, smoking, drug abuse)
- Level of physical fitness

Family History

- Familial health risks

Medical/Surgical History

- Cardiovascular
- Endocrine/metabolic
- Gastrointestinal
- Genitourinary
- Gynecological
- Integumentary
- Musculoskeletal
- Neuromuscular
- Obstetrical
- Prior hospitalizations, surgeries, and preexisting medical and other health-related conditions
- Psychological
- Pulmonary

Current Condition(s)/Chief Complaint(s)

- Concerns that led patient/client to seek the services of a physical therapist
- Concerns or needs of patient/client who requires the services of a physical therapist
- Current therapeutic interventions
- Mechanisms of injury or disease, including date of onset and course of events
- Onset and pattern of symptoms
- Patient/client, family, significant other, and caregiver expectations and goals for the therapeutic intervention
- Patient/client, family, significant other, and caregiver perceptions of patient's/client's emotional response to the current clinical situation
- Previous occurrence of chief complaint(s)
- Prior therapeutic interventions

Functional Status and Activity Level

- Current and prior functional status in self-care and home management activities, including activities of daily living (ADL) and instrumental activities of daily living (IADL)
- Current and prior functional status in work (job/school/play), community, and leisure actions, tasks, or activities

Medications

- Medications for current condition
- Medications previously taken for current condition
- Medications for other conditions

Other Clinical Tests

- Laboratory and diagnostic tests
- Review of available records (eg, medical, education, surgical)
- Review of other clinical findings (eg, nutrition and hydration)

Systems Review

The systems review may include:

Anatomical and Physiological Status

- Cardiovascular/Pulmonary
  - Blood pressure
  - Edema
  - Heart rate
  - Respiratory rate
- Integumentary
  - Pliability (texture)
  - Presence of scar formation
  - Skin color
  - Skin integrity
- Musculoskeletal
  - Gross range of motion
  - Gross strength
  - Gross symmetry
  - Height
  - Weight
- Neuromuscular
  - Gross coordinated movements (eg, balance, gait, locomotion, transfers, transitions)
  - Motor function (motor control, motor learning)

Communication, Affect, Cognition, Language, and Learning Style

- Ability to make needs known
- Consciousness
- Expected emotional/behavioral responses
- Learning preferences (eg, education needs, learning barriers)
- Orientation (person, place, time)

Tests and Measures

Test and measures for this pattern may include those that characterize or quantify:

Aerobic Capacity and Endurance

- Aerobic capacity during functional activities (eg, activities of daily living [ADL] scales, indexes, instrumental activities of daily living [IADL] scales, observations)
- Aerobic capacity during standardized exercise test protocols (eg, ergometry, step tests, time/distance walk/run tests, treadmill tests, wheelchair tests)
- Cardiovascular signs and symptoms in response to increased oxygen demand with exercise or activity, including pressures and flow; heart rate, rhythm, and sounds; and superficial vascular responses (eg, angina, claudication, and exertion scales; electrocardiography; observations; palpation; sphygmomanometry)
- Pulmonary signs and symptoms in response to increased oxygen demand with exercise or activity, including breath and voice sounds; cyanosis; gas exchange; respiratory pattern, rate, and rhythm; and ventilatory flow, force, and volume (eg, auscultation, dyspnea and exertion scales, gas analyses, observations, oximetry, palpation, pulmonary function tests)

Anthropometric Characteristics

- Body composition (eg, impedance measurement, skinfold thickness measurement)
- Body dimensions (eg, girth measurement, length measurement)

Arousal, Attention, and Cognition

- Arousal and attention (eg, adaptability tests, arousal and awareness scales, indexes, profiles, questionnaires)
- Cognition, including ability to process commands (eg, developmental inventories, indexes, interviews, mental state scales, observations, questionnaires, safety checklists)
- Communication (eg, functional communication profiles, interviews, inventories, observations, questionnaires)
- Motivation (eg, adaptive behavior scales)
- Orientation to time, person, place, and situation (eg, attention tests, learning profiles, mental state scales)
- Recall, including memory and retention (eg, assessment scales, interviews, questionnaires)

Assistive and Adaptive Devices

- Assistive or adaptive devices and equipment use during functional activities (eg, ADL scales, functional scales, IADL scales, interviews, observations)
- Components, alignment, fit, and ability to care for the assistive or adaptive devices and equipment (eg, interviews, logs, observations, pressure-sensing maps, reports)
- Remediation of impairments, functional limitations, or disabilities with use of assistive or adaptive devices and equipment (eg, activity status indexes, ADL scales, aerobic capacity tests, functional performance inventories, health assessment questionnaires, IADL scales, pain scales, play scales, videographic assessments)
- Safety during use of assistive or adaptive devices and equipment (eg, diaries, fall scales, interviews, logs, observations, reports)

Circulation (Arterial, Venous, Lymphatic)

- Cardiovascular signs, including heart rate, rhythm, and sounds; pressures and flow; and superficial vascular responses (eg, auscultation, electrocardiography, girth measurement, observations, palpation, sphygmomanometry, thermography)
- Cardiovascular symptoms (eg, angina, claudication, and perceived exertion scales)
- Physiological responses to position change, including autonomic responses, central and peripheral pressures, heart rate and rhythm, respiratory rate and rhythm, ventilatory pattern (eg, auscultation, electrocardiography, observations, palpation, sphygmomanometry)

Cranial and Peripheral Nerve Integrity

- Electrophysiological integrity (eg, electroneuromyography)
- Motor distribution of the cranial nerves (eg, dynamometry, muscle tests, observations)
- Motor distribution of the peripheral nerves (eg, dynamometry, muscle tests, observations, thoracic outlet tests)
- Response to stimuli, including auditory, gustatory, olfactory, pharyngeal, vestibular, and visual (eg, observations, provocation tests)
- Sensory distribution of the cranial nerves (eg, discrimination tests; tactile tests, including coarse and light touch, cold and heat, pain, pressure, and vibration)
- Sensory distribution of the peripheral nerves (eg, discrimination tests; tactile tests, including coarse and light touch, cold and heat, pain, pressure, and vibration; thoracic outlet tests)

Environmental, Home, and Work (Job/School/Play) Barriers

- Current and potential barriers (eg, checklists, interviews, observations, questionnaires)
- Physical space and environment (eg, compliance standards, observations, photographic assessments, questionnaires, structural specifications, videographic assessments)

Ergonomics and Body Mechanics

Ergonomics

- Dexterity and coordination during work (job/school/play) (eg, hand function tests, impairment rating scales, manipulative ability tests)
- Functional capacity and performance during work actions, tasks, or activities (eg, accelerometry, dynamometry, electroneuromyography, endurance tests, force platform tests, goniometry, interviews, observations, photographic assessments, physical capacity tests, postural loading analyses, technology-assisted assessments, videographic assessments, work analyses)
- Safety in work environments (eg, hazard identification checklists, job severity indexes, lifting standards, risk assessment scales, standards for exposure limits)
- Specific work conditions or activities (eg, handling checklists, job simulations, lifting models, preemployment screenings, task analysis checklists, workstation checklists)
- Tools, devices, equipment, and workstations related to work actions, tasks, or activities (eg, observations, tool analysis checklists, vibration assessments, tool analysis checklists, vibration assessments)

Body mechanics

- Body mechanics during self-care, home management, work, community, or leisure actions, tasks, or activities (eg, ADL scales, IADL scales, observations, photographic assessments, technology-assisted assessments, videographic assessments)

Gait, Locomotion, and Balance

- Balance during functional activities with or without the use of assistive, adaptive, orthotic, protective, supportive, or prosthetic devices or equipment (eg, ADL scales, IADL scales, observations, videographic assessments)
- Balance (dynamic and static) with or without the use of assistive, adaptive, orthotic, protective, supportive, or prosthetic devices or equipment (eg, balance scales, dizziness inventories, dynamic posturography, fall scales, motor impairment tests, observations, photographic assessments, postural control tests)
- Gait and locomotion during functional activities with or without the use of assistive, adaptive, orthotic, protective, supportive, or prosthetic devices or equipment (eg, ADL scales, gait indexes, IADL scales, mobility skill profiles, observations, videographic assessments)
- Gait and locomotion with or without the use of assistive, adaptive, orthotic, protective, supportive, or prosthetic devices or equipment (eg, dynamometry, electroneuromyography, footprint analyses, gait indexes, mobility skill profiles, observations, photographic assessments, technology-assisted assessments, videographic assessments, weight-bearing scales, wheelchair mobility tests)
- Safety during gait, locomotion, and balance (eg, confidence scales, diaries, fall scales, functional assessment profiles, logs, reports)

Integumentary Integrity

Associated skin

- Activities, positioning, and postures that produce or relieve trauma to the skin (eg, observations, pressure-sensing maps, scales)
- Assistive, adaptive, orthotic, protective, supportive, or prosthetic devices and equipment that may produce or relieve trauma to the skin (eg, observations, pressure-sensing maps, risk assessment scales)
- Skin characteristics, including blistering, continuity of skin color, dermatitis, hair growth, mobility, nail growth, sensation, temperature, texture, and turgor (eg, observations, palpation, photographic assessments, thermography)

Joint Integrity and Mobility

- Joint integrity and mobility (eg, apprehension, compression and distraction, drawer, glide, impingement, shear, and valgus/varus stress tests; arthrometry; palpation)
- Joint play movements, including end feel (all joints of the axial and appendicular skeletal system) (eg, palpation)

Motor Function (Motor Control and Motor Learning)

- Dexterity, coordination, and agility (eg, coordination screens, motor impairment tests, motor proficiency tests, observations, videographic assessments)
- Electrophysiological integrity (eg, electroneuromyography)
- Hand function (eg, fine and gross motor control tests, finger dexterity tests, manipulative ability tests, observations)
- Initiation, modification, and control of movement patterns and voluntary postures (eg, activity indexes, developmental scales, gross motor function profiles, motor scales, movement assessment batteries, neuromotor tests, observations, physical performance tests, postural challenge tests, videographic assessments)

Muscle Performance (Including Strength, Power, and Endurance)

- Electrophysiological integrity (eg, electroneuromyography)
- Muscle strength, power, and endurance (eg, dynamometry, manual muscle tests, muscle performance tests, physical capacity tests, technology-assisted assessments, timed activity tests)
- Muscle strength, power, and endurance during functional activities (eg, ADL scales, functional muscle tests, IADL scales, observations, videographic assessments)
- Muscle tension (eg, palpation)

Neuromotor Development and Sensory Integration

- Acquisition and evolution of motor skills, including age-appropriate development (eg, activity indexes, developmental inventories and questionnaires, infant and toddler motor assessments, learning profiles, motor function tests, motor proficiency assessments, neuromotor assessments, reflex tests, screens, videographic assessments)
- Oral motor function, phonation, and speech production (eg, interviews, observations)
- Sensorimotor integration, including postural, equilibrium, and righting reactions (eg, behavioral assessment scales, motor and processing skill tests, observations, postural challenge tests, reflex tests, sensory profiles, visual perceptual skill tests)

Orthotic, Protective, and Supportive Devices

- Components, alignment, fit, and ability to care for orthotic, protective, and supportive devices and equipment (eg, interviews, logs, observations, pressure-sensing maps, reports)
- Orthotic, protective, and supportive devices and equipment use during functional activities (eg, ADL scales, functional scales, IADL scales, interviews, observations, profiles)
- Remediation of impairments, functional limitations, or disabilities with use of orthotic, protective, and supportive devices and equipment (eg, activity status indexes, ADL scales, aerobic capacity tests, functional performance inventories, health assessment questionnaires, IADL scales, pain scales, play scales, videographic assessments)
- Safety during use of orthotic, protective, and supportive devices and equipment (eg, diaries, fall scales, interviews, logs, observations, reports)

Pain

- Pain, soreness, and nociception (eg, analog scales, discrimination tests, pain drawings and maps, provocation tests, verbal and pictorial descriptor tests)
- Pain in specific body parts (eg, pain indexes, pain questionnaires, structural provocation tests)

Posture

- Postural alignment and position (static and dynamic), including symmetry and deviation from midline (eg, grid measurement, observations, photographic assessments, technology-assisted assessments, videographic assessments)
- Specific body parts (eg, angle assessments, forward-bending test, goniometry, observations, palpation, positional tests)

Prosthetic Requirements

- Components, alignment, fit, and ability to care for the prosthetic device (eg, interviews, logs, observations, pressure-sensing maps, reports)
- Prosthetic device use during functional activities (eg, ADL scales, functional scales, IADL scales, interviews, observations)
- Safety during use of the prosthetic device (eg, diaries, fall scales, interviews, logs, observations, reports)

Range of Motion (Including Muscle Length)

- Functional ROM (eg, observations, squat testing, toe touch tests)
- Joint active and passive movement (eg, goniometry, inclinometry, observations, photographic assessments, technology-assisted assessments, videographic assessments)
- Muscle length, soft tissue extensibility, and flexibility (eg, contracture tests, goniometry, inclinometry, ligamentous tests, linear measurement, multisegment flexibility tests, palpation)

Reflex Integrity

- Deep reflexes (eg, myotatic reflex scale, observations, reflex tests)
- Electrophysiological integrity (eg, electroneuromyography)
- Postural reflexes and reactions, including righting, equilibrium, and protective reactions (eg, observations, postural challenge tests, reflex profiles, videographic assessments)
- Primitive reflexes and reactions, including developmental (eg, reflex profiles, screening tests)
- Resistance to passive stretch (eg, tone scales)
- Superficial reflexes and reactions (eg, observations, provocation tests)

Self-Care and Home Management (Including ADL and IADL)

- Ability to gain access to home environments (eg, barrier identification, observations, physical performance tests)
- Ability to perform self-care and home management activities with or without assistive, adaptive, orthotic, protective, supportive, or prosthetic devices and equipment (eg, ADL scales, aerobic capacity tests, IADL scales, interviews, observations, profiles)
- Safety in self-care and home management activities and environments (eg, diaries, fall scales, interviews, logs, observations, reports, videographic assessments)

Sensory Integrity

- Combined/cortical sensations (eg, stereognosis tests, tactile discrimination tests)
- Deep sensations (eg, kinesthesiometry, observations, photographic assessments, vibration tests)

Ventilation and Respiration/Gas Exchange

- Pulmonary signs of respiration/gas exchange, including breath sounds (eg, gas analyses, observations, oximetry)
- Pulmonary signs of ventilatory function, including airway protection; breath and voice sounds; respiratory rate, rhythm, and pattern; ventilatory flow, forces, and volumes (eg, airway clearance tests, observations, palpation, pulmonary function tests, ventilatory muscle force tests)
- Pulmonary symptoms (eg, dyspnea and perceived exertion indexes and scales)

Work (Job/School/Play), Community, and Leisure Integration or Reintegration (Including IADL)

- Ability to assume or resume work (job/school/play), community, and leisure activities with or without assistive, adaptive, orthotic, protective, supportive, or prosthetic devices and equipment (eg, activity profiles, disability indexes, functional status questionnaires, IADL scales, observations, physical capacity tests)
- Ability to gain access to work (job/school/play), community, and leisure environments (eg, barrier identification, interviews, observations, physical capacity, transportation assessments)
- Safety in work (job/school/play), community, and leisure activities and environments (eg, diaries, fall scales, interviews, logs, observations, videographic assessments)

Evaluation, Diagnosis, and Prognosis (Including Plan of Care)

Physical therapists perform *evaluations* (make clinical judgments) based on the data gathered from the history, systems review, and tests and measures. In the evaluation process, physical therapists synthesize the examination data to establish the diagnosis and prognosis (including the plan of care). Factors that influence the complexity of the evaluation include the clinical findings, extent of loss of function, chronicity or severity of the problem, possibility of multisite or multisystem involvement, preexisting condition(s), potential discharge destination, social considerations, physical function, and overall health status.

A *diagnosis* is a label encompassing a cluster of signs and symptoms, syndromes, or categories. It is the result of the systematic diagnostic process, which includes integrating and evaluating the data from the examination. The diagnostic label indicates the primary dysfunction(s) toward which the therapist will direct interventions. The *prognosis* is the determination of the predicted optimal level of improvement in function and the amount of time needed to reach that level and may also include a prediction of levels of improvement that may be reached at various intervals during the course of therapy. During the prognostic process, the physical therapist develops the plan of care. The *plan of care* identifies specific interventions, proposed frequency and duration of the interventions, anticipated goals, expected outcomes, and discharge plans. The plan of care identifies realistic anticipated goals and expected outcomes, taking into consideration the expectations of the patient/client and appropriate others. These anticipated goals and expected outcomes should be measureable and time limited.

The frequency of visits and duration of the episode of care may vary from a short episode with a high intensity of intervention to a longer episode with a diminishing intensity of intervention. Frequency and duration may vary greatly among patients/clients based on a variety of factors that the physical therapist considers throughout the evaluation process, such as anatomical and physiological changes related to growth and development; caregiver consistency or expertise; chronicity or severity of the current condition; living environment; multisite or multisystem involvement; social support; potential discharge destinations; probability of prolonged impairment, functional limitation, or disability; and stability of the condition.

Prognosis

Over the course of 12 months, patient/client will demonstrate optimal neuromotor development and the highest level of functioning in home, work (job/school/play), community, and leisure environments, within the context of the impairments, functional limitations, and disabilities.

During the episode of care, patient/client will achieve (1) the anticipated goals and expected outcomes of the interventions that are described in the plan of care and (2) the global outcomes for patients/clients who are classified in this pattern.

Expected Range of Number of Visits Per Episode of Care

6 to 90

This range represents the lower and upper limits of the number of physical therapist visits required to achieve anticipated goals and expected outcomes. *It is anticipated that 80% of patients/clients who are classified into this pattern will achieve the anticipated goals and expected outcomes within 6 to 90 visits during a single continuous episode of care.* Frequency of visits and duration of the episode of care should be determined by the physical therapist to maximize effectiveness of care and efficiency of service delivery.

Note:

These patients/clients may require multiple episodes of care over the lifetime to ensure safety and effective adaptation following changes in physical status, caregivers, environment, or task demands. Factors that may lead to these additional episodes of care include:

- Cognitive maturation
- Periods of rapid growth

Factors That May Require New Episode of Care or That May Modify Frequency of Visits/Duration of Episode

- Accessibility and availability of resources
- Adherence to the intervention program
- Age
- Anatomical and physiological changes related to growth and development
- Caregiver consistency or expertise
- Chronicity or severity of the current condition
- Cognitive status
- Comorbitities, complications, or secondary impairments
- Concurrent medical, surgical, and therapeutic interventions
- Decline in functional independence
- Level of impairment
- Level of physical function
- Living environment
- Multisite or multisystem involvement
- Nutritional status
- Overall health status
- Potential discharge destinations
- Premorbid conditions
- Probability of prolonged impairment, functional limitation, or disability
- Psychological and socioeconomic factors
- Psychomotor abilities
- Social support
- Stability of the condition

Intervention

Intervention is the purposeful interaction of the physical therapist with the patient/client and, when appropriate, with other individuals involved in patient/client care, using various physical therapy procedures and techniques to produce changes in the condition consistent with the diagnosis and prognosis. Decisions about interventions are contingent on the timely monitoring of patient/client response and the progress made toward achieving the anticipated goals and expected outcomes.

Communication, coordination, and documentation and patient/client-related instruction are provided for all patients/clients across all settings. Procedural interventions are selected or modified based on the examination data and the evaluation, the diagnosis and the prognosis, and the anticipated goals and expected outcomes for a particular patient/client. *For clinical considerations in selecting interventions, listings of interventions, and listings of anticipated goals and expected outcomes, refer to Chapter 3.*

Coordination, Communication, and Documentation

Coordination, communication, and documentation may include:

Interventions

- Addressing required functions
  - advance directives
  - individualized family service plans (IFSPs) or individualized education plans (IEPs)
  - informed consent
  - mandatory communication and reporting (eg, patient advocacy and abuse reporting)
- Admission and discharge planning
- Case management
- Collaboration and coordination with agencies, including:
  - equipment suppliers
  - home care agencies
  - payer groups
  - schools
  - transportation agencies
- Communication across settings, including:
  - case conferences
  - documentation
  - education plans
- Cost-effective resource utilization
- Data collection, analysis, and reporting
  - outcome data
  - peer review findings
  - record reviews
- Documentation across settings, following APTA's *Guidelines for Physical Therapy Documentation* (Appendix 5), including:
  - changes in impairments, functional limitations, and disabilities
  - changes in interventions
  - elements of patient/client management (examination, evaluation, diagnosis, prognosis, intervention)
  - outcomes of intervention
- Interdisciplinary teamwork
  - case conferences
  - patient care rounds
  - patient/client family meetings
- Referrals to other professionals or resources

Anticipated Goals and Expected Outcomes

- Accountability for services is increased.
- Admission data and discharge planning are completed.
- Advance directives, individualized family service plans (IFSPs) or individualized education plans (IEPs), informed consent, and mandatory communication and reporting (eg, patient advocacy and abuse reporting) are obtained or completed.
- Available resources are maximally utilized.
- Care is coordinated with patient/client, family, significant others, caregivers, and other professionals.
- Case is managed throughout the episode of care.
- Collaboration and coordination occurs with agencies, including equipment suppliers, home care agencies, payer groups, schools, and transportation agencies.
- Communication enhances risk reduction and prevention.
- Communication occurs across settings through case conferences, education plans, and documentation.
- Data are collected, analyzed, and reported, including outcome data, peer review findings, and record reviews.
- Decision making is enhanced regarding health, wellness, and fitness needs.
- Decision making is enhanced regarding patient/client health and the use of health care resources by patient/client, family, significant others, and caregivers.
- Documentation occurs throughout patient/client management and across settings and follows APTA's *Guidelines for Physical Therapy Documentation* (Appendix 5).
- Interdisciplinary collaboration occurs through case conferences, patient care rounds, and patient/client family meetings.
- Patient/client, family, significant other, and caregiver understanding of anticipated goals and expected outcomes is increased.
- Placement needs are determined.
- Referrals are made to other professionals or resources whenever necessary and appropriate.
- Resources are utilized in a cost-effective way.

Patient/Client-Related Instruction

Patient/client-related instruction may include:

Interventions

- Instruction, education and training of patients/clients and caregivers regarding:
  - current condition (pathology/pathophysiology [disease, disorder, or condition], impairments, functional limitations, or disabilities)
  - enhancement of performance
  - health, wellness, and fitness programs
  - plan of care
  - risk factors for pathology/pathophysiology (disease, disorder, or condition), impairments, functional limitations, or disabilities
  - transitions across settings
  - transitions to new roles

Anticipated Goals and Expected Outcomes

- Ability to perform physical actions, tasks, or activities is improved.
- Awareness and use of community resources are improved.
- Behaviors that foster healthy habits, wellness, and prevention are acquired.
- Decision making is enhanced regarding patient/client health and the use of health care resources by patient/client, family, significant others, and caregivers.
- Disability associated with acute or chronic illnesses is reduced.
- Functional independence in activities of daily living (ADL) and instrumental activities of daily living (IADL) is increased.
- Health status is improved.
- Intensity of care is decreased.
- Level of supervision required for task performance is decreased.
- Patient/client, family, significant other, and caregiver knowledge and awareness of the diagnosis, prognosis, interventions, and anticipated goals and expected outcomes are increased.
- Patient/client knowledge of personal and environmental factors associated with the condition is increased.
- Performance levels in self-care, home management, work (job/school/play), community, or leisure actions, tasks, or activities are improved.
- Physical function is improved.
- Risk of recurrence of condition is reduced.
- Risk of secondary impairment is reduced.
- Safety of patient/client, family, significant others, and caregivers is improved.
- Self-management of symptoms is improved.
- Utilization and cost of health care services are decreased.

Procedural Interventions

Procedural interventions for this pattern may include:

Therapeutic Exercise

Interventions

- Aerobic capacity/endurance conditioning or reconditioning
  - aquatic programs
  - gait and locomotor training
  - increased workload over time
  - walking and wheelchair propulsion programs
- Balance, coordination, and agility training
  - developmental activities training
  - motor function (motor control and motor learning) training or retraining
  - neuromuscular education or reeducation
  - perceptual training
  - posture awareness training
  - standardized, programmatic, complementary exercise approaches
  - sensory training or retraining
  - task-specific performance training
- Body mechanics and postural stabilization
  - body mechanics training
  - posture awareness training
  - postural control training
  - postural stabilization activities
- Neuromotor development training
  - developmental activities training
  - motor training
  - movement pattern training
  - neuromuscular education or reeducation
- Flexibility exercises
  - muscle lengthening
  - range of motion
  - stretching
- Gait and locomotion training
  - developmental activities training
  - gait training
  - implement and device training
  - perceptual training
  - wheelchair training
- Relaxation
  - breathing strategies
  - movement strategies
  - relaxation techniques
- Strength, power, and endurance training for head, neck, limb, pelvic-floor, trunk, and ventilatory muscles
  - active assistive, active, and resistive exercises (including concentric, dynamic/isotonic, eccentric, isokinetic, isometric, and plyometric)
  - aquatic programs
  - standardized, programmatic, complementary exercise approaches
  - task-specific performance training

Anticipated Goals and Expected Outcomes

- Impact on pathology/pathophysiology (disease, disorder, or condition)
  - Nutrient delivery to tissue is increased.
  - Osteogenic effects of exercise are maximized.
  - Pain is decreased.
  - Physiological response to increased oxygen demand is improved.
- Impact on impairments:
  - Aerobic capacity is increased.
  - Balance is improved.
  - Endurance is increased.
  - Energy expenditure per unit of work is decreased.
  - Gait, locomotion, and balance are improved.
  - Joint integrity and mobility are improved.
  - Motor function (motor control and motor learning) is improved.
  - Muscle performance (strength, power, and endurance) is increased.
  - Postural control is improved.
  - Quality and quantity of movement between and across body segments are improved.
  - Range of motion is improved.
  - Relaxation is increased.
  - Sensory awareness is increased.
  - Weight-bearing status is improved.
  - Work of breathing is decreased.
- Impact on functional limitations
  - Ability to perform physical actions, tasks, or activities related to self-care, home management, work (job/school/play), community, and leisure is improved.
  - Level of supervision required for task performance is decreased.
  - Performance of and independence in ADL and IADL with or without devices and equipment are increased.
  - Tolerance of positions and activities is increased.
- Impact on disabilities
  - Ability to assume or resume required self-care, home management, work (job/school/play), community, and leisure roles is improved.
- Risk reduction/prevention
  - Risk factors are reduced.
  - Risk of secondary impairments is reduced.
  - Safety is improved.
  - Self-management of symptoms is improved.
- Impact on health, wellness, and fitness
  - Fitness is improved.
  - Health status is improved.
  - Physical capacity is increased.
  - Physical function is improved.
- Impact on societal resources
  - Utilization of physical therapy services is optimized.
  - Utilization of physical therapy services results in efficient use of health care dollars.
- Patient/client satisfaction
  - Access, availability, and services provided are acceptable to patient/client.
  - Administrative management of practice is acceptable to patient/client.
  - Clinical proficiency of physical therapist is acceptable to patient/client.
  - Coordination of care is acceptable to patient/client.
  - Cost of health care services is decreased.
  - Intensity of care is decreased.
  - Interpersonal skills of physical therapist are acceptable to patient/client, family, and significant others.
  - Sense of well-being is improved.
  - Stressors are decreased.

Functional Training in Self-Care and Home Management (Including Activities of Daily Living [ADL] and Instrumental Activities of Daily Living [IADL])

Interventions

- ADL training
  - bathing
  - bed mobility and transfer training
  - developmental activities
  - dressing
  - eating
  - grooming
  - toileting
- Functional training programs
  - simulated environments and tasks
  - task adaptation
  - travel training
- IADL training
  - home maintenance
  - household chores
  - shopping
  - structured play for infants and children
  - travel training
  - yard work
- Devices and equipment use and training
  - assistive and adaptive device or equipment training during ADL and IADL
  - orthotic, protective, or supportive device or equipment training during ADL and IADL
  - prosthetic device or equipment training during ADL and IADL
- Injury prevention or reduction
  - injury prevention education during self-care and home management
  - injury prevention or reduction with use of devices and equipment
  - safety awareness training during self-care and home management

Anticipated Goals and Expected Outcomes

- Impact on pathology/pathophysiology (disease, disorder, or condition)
  - Pain is decreased.
  - Physiological response to increased oxygen demand is improved.
- Impact on impairments
  - Balance is improved.
  - Endurance is increased.
  - Energy expenditure per unit of work is decreased
  - Motor function (motor control and motor learning) is improved.
  - Muscle performance (strength, power, and endurance) is increased.
  - Postural control is improved.
  - Sensory awareness is increased.
  - Weight-bearing status is improved.
  - Work of breathing is decreased.
- Impact on functional limitations
  - Ability to perform physical actions, tasks, or activities related to self-care and home management is improved.
  - Level of supervision required for task performance is decreased.
  - Performance of and independence in ADL and IADL with or without devices and equipment are increased.
  - Tolerance of positions and activities is increased.
- Impact on disabilities
  - Ability to assume or resume required self-care and home management roles is improved.
- Risk reduction/prevention
  - Risk factors are reduced.
  - Risk of secondary impairments is reduced.
  - Safety is improved.
  - Self-management of symptoms is improved.
- Impact on health, wellness, and fitness
  - Health status is improved.
  - Physical capacity is increased.
  - Physical function is improved.
- Impact on societal resources
  - Utilization of physical therapy services is optimized.
  - Utilization of physical therapy services results in efficient use of health care dollars.
- Patient/client satisfaction
  - Access, availability, and services provided are acceptable to patient/client.
  - Administrative management of practice is acceptable to patient/client.
  - Clinical proficiency of physical therapist is acceptable to patient/client.
  - Coordination of care is acceptable to patient/client.
  - Cost of health care services is decreased.
  - Intensity of care is decreased.
  - Interpersonal skills of physical therapist are acceptable to patient/client, family, and significant others.
  - Sense of well-being is improved.
  - Stressors are decreased.

Functional Training in Work (Job/School/Play), Community, and Leisure Integration or Reintegration (Including Instrumental Activities of Daily Living [IADL], Work Hardening, and Work Conditioning)

Interventions

- Devices and equipment use and training
  - assistive and adaptive device or equipment training during IADL
  - orthotic, protective, or supportive device or equipment training during IADL
  - prosthetic device or equipment training during IADL
- Functional training programs
  - job coaching
  - simulated environments and tasks
  - task adaptation
  - task training
  - travel training
- IADL training
  - community service training involving instruments
  - school and play activities training including tools and instruments
  - work training with tools
- Injury prevention or reduction
  - injury prevention education during work (job/school/play), community, and leisure integration or reintegration
  - injury prevention or reduction with use of devices and equipment
  - safety awareness training during work (job/school/play), community, and leisure integration or reintegration
- Leisure and play activities training

Anticipated Goals and Expected Outcomes

- Impact on pathology/pathophysiology (disease, disorder, or condition)
  - Pain is decreased.
  - Physiological response to increased oxygen demand is improved.
- Impact on impairments
  - Balance is improved.
  - Endurance is increased.
  - Energy expenditure per unit of work is decreased.
  - Motor function (motor control and motor learning) is improved.
  - Muscle performance (strength, power, and endurance) is increased.
  - Postural control is improved.
  - Sensory awareness is increased.
  - Weight-bearing status is improved.
  - Work of breathing is decreased.
- Impact on functional limitations
  - Ability to perform physical actions, tasks, or activities related to work (job/school/play), community, and leisure integration or reintegration is improved.
  - Level of supervision required for task performance is decreased.
  - Performance of and independence in IADL with or without devices and equipment are increased.
  - Tolerance of positions and activities is increased.
- Impact on disabilities
  - Ability to assume or resume required work (job/school/play), community, and leisure roles is improved.
- Risk reduction/prevention
  - Risk factors are reduced.
  - Risk of secondary impairment is reduced.
  - Safety is improved.
  - Self-management of symptoms is improved.
- Impact on health, wellness, and fitness
  - Fitness is improved.
  - Health status is improved.
  - Physical capacity is increased.
  - Physical function is improved.
- Impact on societal resources
  - Costs of work-related injury or disability are reduced.
  - Utilization of physical therapy services is optimized.
  - Utilization of physical therapy services results in efficient use of health care dollars.
- Patient/client satisfaction
  - Access, availability, and services provided are acceptable to patient/client.
  - Administrative management of practice is acceptable to patient/client.
  - Clinical proficiency of physical therapist is acceptable to patient/client.
  - Coordination of care is acceptable to patient/client.
  - Cost of health care services is decreased.
  - Intensity of care is decreased.
  - Interpersonal skills of physical therapist are acceptable to patient/client, family, and significant others.
  - Sense of well-being is improved.
  - Stressors are decreased.

Manual Therapy Techniques (Including Mobilization/Manipulation)

Interventions

- Manual traction
- Massage
  - connective tissue massage
  - therapeutic massage
- Mobilization/manipulation
  - Soft tissue mobilization
- Passive range of motion

Anticipated Goals and Expected Outcomes

- Impact on pathology/pathophysiology (disease, disorder, or condition)
  - Edema, lymphedema, or effusion is reduced.
  - Joint swelling, inflammation, or restriction is reduced.
  - Soft tissue swelling, inflammation, or restriction is reduced.
  - Pain is decreased.
- Impact on impairments
  - Balance is improved.
  - Energy expenditure per unit of work is decreased.
  - Gait, locomotion, and balance are improved.
  - Joint integrity and mobility are improved.
  - Muscle performance (strength, power, and endurance) is increased.
  - Postural control is improved.
  - Quality and quantity of movement between and across body segments are improved.
  - Range of motion is improved.
  - Relaxation is increased.
  - Sensory awareness is increased.
  - Work of breathing is decreased.
- Impact on functional limitations
  - Ability to perform movement tasks is improved.
  - Ability to perform physical actions, tasks, or activities related to self-care, home management, work (job/school/play), community, and leisure is improved.
  - Tolerance of positions and activities is increased.
- Impact on disabilities
  - Ability to assume or resume required self-care, home management, work (job/school/play), community, and leisure roles is improved.
- Risk reduction/prevention
  - Risk factors are reduced.
  - Risk of secondary impairment is reduced.
  - Self-management of symptoms is improved.
- Impact on health, wellness, and fitness
  - Physical capacity is increased.
  - Physical function is improved.
- Impact on societal resources
  - Utilization of physical therapy services is optimized.
  - Utilization of physical therapy services results in efficient use of health care dollars.
- Patient/client satisfaction
  - Access, availability, and services provided are acceptable to patient/client.
  - Administrative management of practice is acceptable to patient/client.
  - Clinical proficiency of physical therapist is acceptable to patient/client.
  - Coordination of care is acceptable to patient/client.
  - Cost of health care services is decreased.
  - Intensity of care is decreased.
  - Interpersonal skills of physical therapist are acceptable to patient/client, family, and significant others.
  - Sense of well-being is improved.
  - Stressors are decreased.

Procedural Interventions continued

Prescription, Application, and, as Appropriate, Fabrication of Devices and Equipment (Assistive, Adaptive, Orthotic, Protective, Supportive, and Prosthetic)

Interventions

- Adaptive devices
  - environmental controls
  - hospital beds
  - raised toilet seats
  - seating systems
- Assistive devices
  - canes
  - crutches
  - long-handled reachers
  - power devices
  - static and dynamic splints
  - walkers
  - wheelchairs
- Orthotic devices
  - braces
  - casts
  - shoe inserts
  - splints
- Prosthetic devices (lower-extremity and upper-extremity)
- Protective devices
  - braces
  - cushions
  - helmets
  - protective taping
- Supportive devices
  - compression garments
  - corsets
  - elastic wraps
  - neck collars
  - supplemental oxygen

Anticipated Goals and Expected Outcomes

- Impact on pathology/pathophysiology (disease, disorder, or condition)
  - Edema, lymphedema, or effusion is reduced.
  - Joint swelling, inflammation, or restriction is reduced.
  - Pain is decreased.
  - Physiological response to increased oxygen demand is improved.
  - Soft tissue swelling, inflammation, or restriction is reduced.
- Impact on impairments
  - Balance is improved.
  - Endurance is increased.
  - Energy expenditure per unit of work is decreased.
  - Gait, locomotion, and balance are improved.
  - Integumentary integrity is improved.
  - Joint stability is improved.
  - Motor function (motor control and motor learning) is improved.
  - Muscle performance (strength, power, and endurance) is increased.
  - Optimal joint alignment is achieved.
  - Optimal loading on a body part is achieved.
  - Postural control is improved.
  - Quality and quantity of movement between and across body segments are improved.
  - Range of motion is improved.
  - Weight-bearing status is improved.
- Impact on functional limitations
  - Ability to perform physical actions, tasks, or activities related to self-care, home management, work (job/school/play), community, and leisure is improved.
  - Level of supervision required for task performance is decreased.
  - Performance of and independence in activities of daily living (ADL) and instrumental activities of daily living (IADL) with or without devices and equipment are increased.
  - Tolerance of positions and activities is improved.
- Impact on disabilities
  - Ability to assume or resume required self-care, home management, work (job/school/play), community, and leisure roles is improved.
- Risk reduction/prevention
  - Pressure on body tissues is reduced.
  - Protection of body parts is increased.
  - Risk factors are reduced.
  - Risk of secondary impairment is reduced.
  - Safety is improved.
  - Self-management of symptoms is improved.
- Impact on health, wellness, and fitness
  - Health status is improved.
  - Physical capacity is increased.
  - Physical function is improved.
- Impact on societal resources
  - Utilization of physical therapy services is optimized.
  - Utilization of physical therapy services results in efficient use of health care dollars.
- Patient/client satisfaction
  - Access, availability, and services provided are acceptable to patient/client.
  - Administrative management of practice is acceptable to patient/client.
  - Clinical proficiency of physical therapist is acceptable to patient/client.
  - Coordination of care is acceptable to patient/client.
  - Cost of health care services is decreased.
  - Intensity of care is decreased.
  - Interpersonal skills of physical therapist are acceptable to patient/client, family, and significant others.
  - Sense of well-being is improved.
  - Stressors are decreased.

Airway Clearance Techniques

Interventions

- Breathing strategies
  - active cycle of breathing or forced expiratory techniques
  - assisted cough/huff techniques
  - autogenic drainage
  - paced breathing
  - pursed lip breathing
  - techniques to maximize ventilation (eg, maximum inspiratory hold, staircase breathing, manual hyperinflation)
- Positioning
  - positioning to alter work of breathing
  - positioning to maximize ventilation and perfusion
  - pulmonary postural drainage

Anticipated Goals and Expected Outcomes

- Impact on pathology/pathophysiology(disease, disorder, or condition)
  - Nutrient delivery to tissue is increased.
  - Physiological response to increased oxygen demand is improved.
  - Symptoms associated with increased oxygen demand are decreased.
  - Tissue perfusion and oxygenation are enhanced.
- Impact on impairments
  - Airway clearance is improved.
  - Cough is improved.
  - Endurance is increased.
  - Energy expenditure per unit of work is decreased.
  - Muscle performance (strength, power, and endurance) is increased.
  - Ventilation and respiration/gas exchange are improved.
  - Work of breathing is decreased.
- Impact on functional limitations
  - Ability to perform physical actions, tasks, or activities related to self-care, home management, community, work (job/ school/ play), and leisure is improved.
  - Performance of and independence in activities of daily living (ADL) and instrumental activities of daily living (IADL) with or without devices and equipment are increased.
  - Tolerance of positions and activities is increased.
- Impact on disabilities
  - Ability to assume or resume required self-care, home management, work (job/school/play), community, and leisure roles is improved.
- Risk reduction/prevention
  - Risk factors are reduced.
  - Risk of secondary impairment is reduced.
  - Safety is improved.
  - Self-management of symptoms is improved.
- Impact on health, wellness, and fitness
  - Health status is improved.
  - Physical capacity is increased.
  - Physical function is improved.
- Impact on societal resources
  - Utilization of physical therapy services is optimized.
  - Utilization of physical therapy services results in efficient use of health care dollars.
- Patient/client satisfaction
  - Access, availability, and services provided are acceptable to patient/client.
  - Administrative management of practice is acceptable to patient/client.
  - Clinical proficiency of physical therapist is acceptable to patient/client.
  - Coordination of care is acceptable to patient/client.
  - Cost of health care services is decreased.
  - Intensity of care is decreased.
  - Interpersonal skills of physical therapist are acceptable to patient/client, family, and significant others.
  - Sense of well-being is improved.
  - Stressors are decreased.

Electrotherapeutic Modalities

Interventions

- Biofeedback
- Electrical muscle stimulation
  - electrical muscle stimulation (EMS)
  - neuromuscular electrical stimulation (NMES)
  - transcutaneous electrical nerve stimulation (TENS)

Anticipated Goals and Expected Outcomes

- Impact on pathology/pathophysiology
  - Edema, lymphedema, or effusion is reduced.
  - Joint swelling, inflammation, or restriction is reduced.
  - Nutrient delivery to tissue is increased.
  - Osteogenic effects are enhanced.
  - Pain is decreased.
  - Soft tissue swelling, inflammation, or restriction is reduced.
  - Tissue perfusion and oxygenation are enhanced.
- Impact on impairments
  - Motor function (motor control and motor learning) is improved.
  - Muscle performance (strength, power, and endurance) is increased.
  - Postural control is improved.
  - Quality and quantity of movement between and across body segments are improved.
  - Range of motion is improved.
  - Sensory awareness is increased.
- Impact on functional limitations
  - Ability to perform physical actions, tasks, or activities related to self-care, home management, community, work (job/ school/ play), and leisure is improved.
  - Level of supervision required for task performance is decreased.
  - Performance of and independence in activities of daily living (ADL) and instrumental activities of daily living (IADL) with or without devices and equipment are increased.
  - Tolerance of positions and activities is increased.
- Impact on disabilities
  - Ability to assume or resume required self-care, home management, work (job/school/play), community, and leisure roles is improved.
- Risk reduction/prevention
  - Complications of immobility are reduced.
  - Risk factors are reduced.
  - Risk of secondary impairment is reduced.
  - Self-management of symptoms is improved.
- Impact on health, wellness, and fitness
  - Physical function is improved.
- Impact on societal resources
  - Utilization of physical therapy services is optimized.
  - Utilization of physical therapy services results in efficient use of health care dollars.
- Patient/client satisfaction
  - Access, availability, and services provided are acceptable to patient/client.
  - Administrative management of practice is acceptable to patient/client.
  - Clinical proficiency of physical therapist is acceptable to patient/client.
  - Coordination of care is acceptable to patient/client.
  - Interpersonal skills of physical therapist are acceptable to patient/client, family, and significant others.
  - Sense of well-being is improved.
  - Stressors are decreased.

Physical Agents and Mechanical Modalities

Interventions

Mechanical modalities may include:

- Compression therapies
  - compression bandaging
  - compression garments
  - taping
  - total contact casting
  - vasopneumatic compression devices
- Gravity-assisted compression devices
  - standing frame
  - tilt table

Anticipated Goals and Expected Outcomes

- Impact on pathology/pathophysiology (disease, disorder, or condition)
  - Edema, lymphedema, or effusion is reduced.
  - Joint swelling, inflammation, or restriction is reduced.
  - Nutrient delivery to tissue is increased.
  - Osteogenic effects are enhanced..
  - Pain is decreased.
  - Soft tissue swelling, inflammation, or restriction is reduced.
  - Tissue perfusion and oxygenation are enhanced.
- Impact on impairments:
  - Integumentary integrity is improved.
  - Muscle performance (strength, power, and endurance) is increased.
  - Range of motion is improved.
  - Weight-bearing status is improved.
- Impact on functional limitations
  - Ability to perform physical actions, tasks, or activities related to self-care, home management, work (job/school/play), community, and leisure is improved.
  - Performance of and independence in activities of daily living (ADL) and instrumental activities of daily living (IADL) with or without devices and equipment are increased.
  - Tolerance of positions and activities is increased.
- Impact on disabilities
  - Ability to assume or resume required self-care, home management, work (job/school/play), community, and leisure roles is improved.
- Risk reduction/prevention
  - Complications of soft tissue and circulatory disorders are decreased.
  - Risk of secondary impairments is reduced.
  - Self-management of symptoms is improved.
- Impact on health, wellness, and fitness
  - Physical function is improved.
- Impact on societal resources
  - Utilization of physical therapy services is optimized.
- Patient/client satisfaction
  - Access, availability, and services provided are acceptable to patient/client.
  - Administrative management of practice is acceptable to patient/client.
  - Clinical proficiency of physical therapist is acceptable to patient/client.
  - Coordination of care is acceptable to patient/client.
  - Interpersonal skills of physical therapist are acceptable to patient/client, family, and significant others.
  - Sense of well-being is improved.
  - Stressors are decreased.

Reexamination

Reexamination is the process of performing selected tests and measures after the initial examination to evaluate progress and to modify or redirect interventions. Reexamination may be indicated more than once during a single episode of care. It also may be performed over the course of a disease, disorder, or condition, which for some patients/clients may be over the life span. Indications for reexamination include new clinical findings or failure to respond to physical therapy interventions.

Global Outcomes for Patients/Clients in This Pattern

Throughout the entire episode of care, the physical therapist determines the anticipated goals and expected outcomes for each intervention. These anticipated goals and expected outcomes are delineated in shaded boxes that accompany the lists of interventions in each preferred practice pattern. As the patient/client reaches the termination of physical therapy services and the end of the episode of care, the physical therapist measures the global outcomes of the physical therapy services by characterizing or quantifying the impact of the physical therapy interventions in the following domains:

- Pathology/pathophysiology (disease, disorder, or condition)
- Impairments
- Functional limitations
- Disabilities
- Risk reduction/prevention
- Health, wellness, and fitness
- Societal resources
- Patient/client satisfaction

In some instances, a particular anticipated goal or expected outcome is thoroughly achieved through implementation of a single form of intervention. More commonly, however, the anticipated goals and expected outcomes are achieved as a result of the combined effects of several forms of interventions, leading to enhancement of both health status and health-related quality of life.

Criteria for Termination of Physical Therapy Services

Discharge is the process of ending physical therapy services that have been provided during a single episode of care. It occurs when the anticipated goals and expected outcomes have been achieved. Discharge does *not* occur with a *transfer* (defined as the time when a patient is moved from one site to another site within the same setting or across settings during a single episode of care). Although there may be facility-specific or payer-specific requirements for documentation regarding the conclusion of physical therapy services, *discharge occurs based on the physical therapist's analysis of the achievement of anticipated goals and expected outcomes.*

Discontinuation is the process of ending physical therapy services that have been provided during a single episode of care when (1) the patient/client, caregiver, or legal guardian declines to continue intervention; (2) the patient/client is unable to continue to progress toward outcomes because of medical or psychosocial complications or because financial/insurance resources have been expended; or (3) the physical therapist determines that the patient/client will no longer benefit from physical therapy. When physical therapy services are terminated prior to achievement of anticipated goals and expected outcomes, patient/client status and the rationale for termination are documented.

For patients/clients who require multiple episodes of care, periodic follow-up is needed over the life span to ensure safety and effective adaptation following changes in physical status, caregivers, environment, or task demands. In consultation with appropriate individuals, and in consideration of the outcomes, the physical therapist plans for discharge or discontinuation and provides for appropriate follow-up or referral.

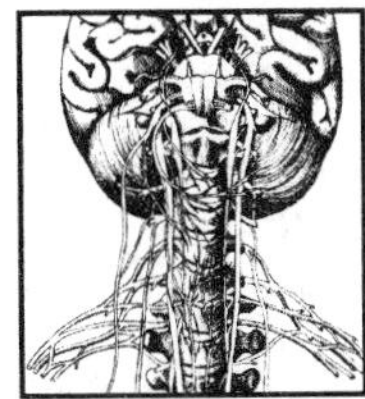

Impaired Motor Function and Sensory Integrity Associated With Nonprogressive Disorders of the Central Nervous System—Congenital Origin or Acquired in Infancy or Childhood

This preferred practice pattern describes the generally accepted elements of patient/client management that physical therapists provide for patients/clients who are classified in this pattern. The pattern title reflects the diagnosis made by the physical therapist. APTA emphasizes that preferred practice patterns are the boundaries within which a physical therapist may select any of a number of clinical alternatives, based on consideration of a wide variety of factors, such as individual patient/client needs; the profession's code of ethics and standards of practice; and patient/client age, culture, gender roles, race, sex, sexual orientation, and socioeconomic status.

Patient/Client Diagnostic Classification

Patients/clients will be classified into this pattern—for impaired motor function and sensory integrity associated with nonprogressive disorders of the central nervous system (congenital origin or acquired in infancy or childhood)—as a result of the physical therapist's evaluation of the examination data. The findings from the examination (history, systems review, and tests and measures) may indicate the presence or risk of pathology/pathophysiology (disease, disorder, or condition), impairments, functional limitations, or disabilities or the need for health, wellness, or fitness programs. The physical therapist integrates, synthesizes, and interprets the data to determine the diagnostic classification.

Inclusion

The following examples of examination findings may support the inclusion of patients/clients in this pattern:

Risk Factors or Consequences of Pathology/Pathophysiology (Disease, Disorder, or Condition)

- Anoxia or hypoxia
- Birth trauma
- Brain anomalies
- Cerebral palsy
- Encephalitis
- Genetic syndromes affecting central nervous system (CNS)
- Hydrocephalus
- Infectious disease affecting CNS
- Meningocele
- Neoplasm
- Prematurity
- Tethered cord
- Traumatic brain injury

Impairments, Functional Limitations, or Disabilities

- Difficulty negotiating terrains
- Difficulty planning movements
- Difficulty with manipulation skills
- Difficulty with positioning
- Frequent falls
- Impaired affect
- Impaired arousal, attention, and cognition
- Impaired expressive or receptive communication
- Impaired motor function
- Loss of balance during daily activities
- Inability to keep up with peers
- Inability to perform work (job/school/play) activities

Note:

Some risk factors or consequences of pathology/pathophysiology—such as *neoplasm*—may be severe and complex; *however, they do not necessarily exclude patients/clients from this pattern.* Severe and complex risk factors or consequences may require modification of the frequency of visits and duration of care. (See "Evaluation, Diagnosis, and Prognosis," page 345.)

Exclusion or Multiple-Pattern Classification

The following examples of examination findings may support exclusion from this pattern or classification into additional patterns. Depending on the level of severity or complexity of the examination findings, the physical therapist may determine that the patient/client would be more appropriately managed through (1) classification in an entirely different pattern or (2) classification in both this and another pattern.

Findings That May Require Classification in a Different Pattern

- Amputation
- Coma
- Spinal cord injury

Findings That May Require Classification in Additional Patterns

- Congenital Heart Defect
- Fracture

ICD-9-CM Codes

The listing below contains the current (as of press time) and most typical 3- and 4-digit ICD-9-CM codes related to this preferred practice pattern. Because patient/client diagnostic classification is based on impairments, functional limitations, and disabilities—not on codes—patients/clients may be classified into the pattern even though the codes listed with the pattern may not apply to those clients.

This listing is intended for general information only and should not be used for coding purposes. The codes should be confirmed by referring to the World Health Organization's *International Classification of Diseases, 9th Revision, Clinical Modification (ICD-9-CM 2001)*, Volumes 1 and 3 (Chicago, Ill: American Medical Association; 2000) or subsequent revisions or by referring to other ICD-9-CM coding manuals that contain exclusion notes and instructions regarding fifth-digit requirements.

036 Meningococcal infection
- **036.1** Meningococcal encephalitis

052 Chickenpox
- **052.0** Postvaricella encephalitis

055 Measles
- **055.0** Postmeasles encephalitis

056 Rubella
- **056.0** With neurological complications

072 Mumps
- **072.2** Mumps encephalitis

090 Congenital syphilis
- **090.4** Juvenile neurosyphilis

225 Benign neoplasm of brain and other parts of nervous system

320 Bacterial meningitis
- **320.9** Meningitis due to unspecified bacterium

321 Meningitis due to other organisms
- **321.8** Meningitis due to other nonbacterial organisms classified elsewhere*

322 Meningitis of unspecified cause
- **322.9** Meningitis, unspecified

323 Encephalitis, myelitis, and encephalomyelitis
- **323.4** Other encephalitis due to infection classified elsewhere*
- **323.5** Encephalitis following immunization procedures
- **323.6** Postinfectious encephalitis*
- **323.8** Other causes of encephalitis
- **323.9** Unspecified cause of encephalitis

333 Other extrapyramidal disease and abnormal movement disorders
- **333.7** Symptomatic torsion dystonia
  Athetoid cerebral palsy [Vogt's disease]; double athetosis (syndrome)

343 Infantile cerebral palsy

345 Epilepsy
- **345.1** Generalized convulsive epilepsy
- **345.2** Petit mal status
- **345.3** Grand mal status
- **345.9** Epilepsy, unspecified

348 Other conditions of brain
- **348.1** Anoxic brain damage
- **348.3** Encephalopathy, unspecified

741 Spina bifida

742 Other congenital anomalies of nervous system
- **742.3** Congenital hydrocephalus

756 Other congenital musculoskeletal anomalies
- **756.1** Anomalies of spine

758 Chromosomal anomalies
Includes: syndromes associated with anomalies in the number and form of chromosomes

759 Other and unspecified congenital anomalies

765 Disorders relating to short gestation and unspecified low birth weight

767 Birth trauma
- **767.0** Subdural and cerebral hemorrhage
- **767.9** Birth trauma, unspecified

768 Intrauterine hypoxia and birth asphyxia
- **768.5** Severe birth asphyxia
- **768.6** Mild or moderate birth asphyxia
- **768.9** Unspecified birth asphyxia in liveborn infant

771 Infections specific to the perinatal period
- **771.2** Other congenital infections
  Congenital toxoplasmosis

780 General symptoms
- **780.3** Convulsions

799 Other ill-defined and unknown causes of morbidity. and mortality
- **799.0** Asphyxia

800 Fracture of vault of skull

801 Fracture of base of skull

803 Other and unqualified skull fractures

804 Multiple fractures involving skull or face with other bones

850 Concussion

851 Cerebral laceration and contusion

852 Subarachnoid, subdural, and extradural hemorrhage, following injury

853 Other and unspecified intracranial hemorrhage following injury

854 Intracranial injury of other and unspecified nature

984 Toxic effect of lead and its compounds (including fumes)

985 Toxic effect of other metals

994 Effects of other external causes
- **994.1** Drowning and nonfatal submersion

* Not a primary diagnosis

Examination

Examination is a comprehensive screening and specific testing process that leads to a diagnostic classification or, when appropriate, to a referral to another practitioner. Examination is required prior to the initial intervention and is performed for all patients/clients. Through the examination, the physical therapist may identify impairments, functional limitations, disabilities, changes in physical function or overall health status, and needs related to restoration of health and to prevention, wellness, and fitness. The physical therapist synthesizes the examination findings to establish the diagnosis and the prognosis (including the plan of care). The patient/client, family, significant others, and caregivers may provide information during the examination process.

Examination has three components: the patient/client history, the systems review, and tests and measures. The *history* is a systematic gathering of past and current information (often from the patient/client) related to why the patient/client is seeking the services of the physical therapist. The *systems review* is a brief or limited examination of (1) the anatomical and physiological status of the cardiovascular/pulmonary, integumentary, musculoskeletal, and neuromuscular systems and (2) the communication ability, affect, cognition, language, and learning style of the patient/client. *Tests and measures* are the means of gathering data about the patient/client.

The selection of examination procedures and the depth of the examination vary based on patient/client age; severity of the problem; stage of recovery (acute, subacute, chronic); phase of rehabilitation (early, intermediate, late, return to activity); home, work (job/school/play), or community situation; and other relevant factors. *For clinical indications in selecting tests and measures and for listings of tests and measures, tools used to gather data, and the types of data generated by tests and measures, refer to Chapter 2.*

Patient/Client History

The history may include:

General Demographics

- Age
- Sex
- Race/ethnicity
- Primary language
- Education

Social History

- Cultural beliefs and behaviors
- Family and caregiver resources
- Social interactions, social activities, and support systems

Employment/Work (Job/School/Play)

- Current and prior work (job/school/play), community, and leisure actions, tasks, or activities

Growth and Development

- Developmental history
- Hand dominance

Living Environment

- Devices and equipment (eg, assistive, adaptive, orthotic, protective, supportive, prosthetic)
- Living environment and community characteristics
- Projected discharge destinations

General Health Status (Self-Report, Family Report, Caregiver Report)

- General health perception
- Physical function (eg, mobility, sleep patterns, restricted bed days)
- Psychological function (eg, memory, reasoning ability, depression, anxiety)
- Role function (eg, community, leisure, social, work)
- Social function (eg, social activity, social interaction, social support)

Social/Health Habits (Past and Current)

- Behavioral health risks (eg, smoking, drug abuse)
- Level of physical fitness

Family History

- Familial health risks

Medical/Surgical History

- Cardiovascular
- Endocrine/metabolic
- Gastrointestinal
- Genitourinary
- Gynecological
- Integumentary
- Musculoskeletal
- Neuromuscular
- Obstetrical
- Prior hospitalizations, surgeries, and preexisting medical and other health-related conditions
- Psychological
- Pulmonary

Current Condition(s)/Chief Complaint(s)

- Concerns that led patient/client to seek the services of a physical therapist
- Concerns or needs of patient/client who requires the services of a physical therapist
- Current therapeutic interventions
- Mechanisms of injury or disease, including date of onset and course of events
- Onset and pattern of symptoms
- Patient/client, family, significant other, and caregiver expectations and goals for the therapeutic intervention
- Patient/client, family, significant other, and caregiver perceptions of patient's/client's emotional response to the current clinical situation
- Previous occurrence of chief complaint(s)
- Prior therapeutic interventions

Functional Status and Activity Level

- Current and prior functional status in self-care and home management activities, including activities of daily living (ADL) and instrumental activities of daily living (IADL)
- Current and prior functional status in work (job/school/play), community, and leisure actions, tasks, or activities

Medications

- Medications for current condition
- Medications previously taken for current condition
- Medications for other conditions

Other Clinical Tests

- Laboratory and diagnostic tests
- Review of available records (eg, medical, education, surgical)
- Review of other clinical findings (eg, nutrition and hydration)

Systems Review

The systems review may include:

Anatomical and Physiological Status

- Cardiovascular/Pulmonary
  - Blood pressure
  - Edema
  - Heart rate
  - Respiratory rate
- Integumentary
  - Pliability (texture)
  - Presence of scar formation
  - Skin color
  - Skin integrity
- Musculoskeletal
  - Gross range of motion
  - Gross strength
  - Gross symmetry
  - Height
  - Weight
- Neuromuscular
  - Gross coordinated movements (eg, balance, gait, locomotion, transfers, transitions)
  - Motor function (motor control, motor learning)

Communication, Affect, Cognition, Language, and Learning Style

- Ability to make needs known
- Consciousness
- Expected emotional/behavioral responses
- Learning preferences (eg, education needs, learning barriers)
- Orientation (person, place, time)

Tests and Measures

Test and measures for this pattern may include those that characterize or quantify:

Aerobic Capacity and Endurance

- Aerobic capacity during functional activities (eg, activities of daily living [ADL] scales, indexes, instrumental activities of daily living [IADL] scales, observations)
- Aerobic capacity during standardized exercise test protocols (eg, ergometry, step tests, time/distance walk/run tests, treadmill tests, wheelchair tests)

Anthropometric Characteristics

- Body composition (eg, body mass index, impedance measurement, skinfold thickness measurement)
- Body dimensions (eg, girth measurement, length measurement)

Arousal, Attention, and Cognition

- Arousal and attention (eg, adaptability tests, arousal and awareness scales, indexes, profiles, questionnaires)
- Cognition, including ability to process commands (eg, developmental inventories, indexes, interviews, mental state scales, observations, questionnaires, safety checklists)
- Communication (eg, functional communication profiles, interviews, inventories, observations, questionnaires)
- Motivation (eg, adaptive behavior scales)
- Orientation to time, person, place, and situation (eg, attention tests, learning profiles, mental state scales)
- Recall, including memory and retention (eg, assessment scales, interviews, questionnaires)

Assistive and Adaptive Devices

- Assistive or adaptive devices and equipment use during functional activities (eg, ADL scales, functional scales, IADL scales, interviews, observations)
- Components, alignment, fit, and ability to care for the assistive or adaptive devices and equipment (eg, interviews, logs, observations, pressure-sensing maps, reports)
- Remediation of impairments, functional limitations, or disabilities with use of assistive or adaptive devices and equipment (eg, activity status indexes, ADL scales, aerobic capacity tests, functional performance inventories, health assessment questionnaires, IADL scales, pain scales, play scales, videographic assessments)
- Safety during use of assistive or adaptive devices and equipment (eg, diaries, fall scales, interviews, logs, observations, reports)

Circulation (Arterial, Venous, and Lymphatic)

- Cardiovascular signs, including heart rate, rhythm, and sounds; pressures and flow; and superficial vascular responses (eg, auscultation, electrocardiography, girth measurement, observations, palpation, sphygmomanometry, thermography)
- Cardiovascular symptoms (eg, angina, claudication, and perceived exertion scales)
- Physiological responses to position change, including autonomic responses, central and peripheral pressures, heart rate and rhythm, respiratory rate and rhythm, ventilatory pattern (eg, auscultation, electrocardiography, observations, palpation, sphygmomanometry)

Cranial and Peripheral Nerve Integrity

- Electrophysiological integrity (eg, electroneuromyography)
- Motor distribution of the cranial nerves (eg, dynamometry, muscle tests, observations)
- Motor distribution of the peripheral nerves (eg, dynamometry, muscle tests, observations, thoracic outlet tests)
- Response to stimuli, including auditory, gustatory, olfactory, pharyngeal, vestibular, and visual (eg, observations, provocation tests)
- Sensory distribution of the cranial nerves (eg, discrimination tests; tactile tests, including coarse and light touch, cold and heat, pain, pressure, and vibration)
- Sensory distribution of the peripheral nerves (eg, discrimination tests; tactile tests, including coarse and light touch, cold and heat, pain, pressure, and vibration; thoracic outlet tests)

Environmental, Home, and Work (Job/School/Play) Barriers

- Current and potential barriers (eg, checklists, interviews, observations, questionnaires)
- Physical space and environment (eg, compliance standards, observations, photographic assessments, questionnaires, structural specifications, videographic assessments)

Ergonomics and Body Mechanics

Ergonomics

- Dexterity and coordination during work (job/school/play) (eg, hand function tests, impairment rating scales, manipulative ability tests)
- Functional capacity and performance during work actions, tasks, or activities (eg, accelerometry, dynamometry, electroneuromyography, endurance tests, force platform tests, goniometry, interviews, observations, photographic assessments, physical capacity tests, postural loading analyses, technology-assisted assessments, videographic assessments, work analyses)
- Safety in work environments (eg, hazard identification checklists, job severity indexes, lifting standards, risk assessment scales, standards for exposure limits)
- Specific work conditions or activities (eg, handling checklists, job simulations, lifting models, preemployment screenings, task analysis checklists, workstation checklists)
- Tools, devices, equipment, and workstations related to work actions, tasks, or activities (eg, observations, tool analysis checklists, vibration assessments)

Body mechanics

- Body mechanics during self-care, home management, work, community, or leisure actions, tasks, or activities (eg, ADL scales, IADL scales, observations, photographic assessments, technology-assisted assessments, videographic assessments)

Gait, Locomotion, and Balance

- Balance during functional activities with or without the use of assistive, adaptive, orthotic, protective, supportive, or prosthetic devices or equipment (eg, ADL scales, IADL scales, observations, videographic assessments)
- Balance (dynamic and static) with or without the use of assistive, adaptive, orthotic, protective, supportive, or prosthetic devices or equipment (eg, balance scales, dizziness inventories, dynamic posturography, fall scales, motor impairment tests, observations, photographic assessments, postural control tests)
- Gait and locomotion during functional activities with or without the use of assistive, adaptive, orthotic, protective, supportive, or prosthetic devices or equipment (eg, ADL scales, gait indexes, IADL scales, mobility skill profiles, observations, videographic assessments)
- Gait and locomotion with or without the use of assistive, adaptive, orthotic, protective, supportive, or prosthetic devices or equipment (eg, dynamometry, electroneuromyography, footprint analyses, gait indexes, mobility skill profiles, observations, photographic assessments, technology-assisted assessments, videographic assessments, weight-bearing scales, wheelchair mobility tests)
- Safety during gait, locomotion, and balance (eg, confidence scales, diaries, fall scales, functional assessment profiles, logs, reports)

Integumentary Integrity

Associated skin

- Activities, positioning, and postures that produce or relieve trauma to the skin (eg, observations, pressure-sensing maps, scales)
- Assistive, adaptive, orthotic, protective, supportive, or prosthetic devices and equipment that may produce or relieve trauma to the skin (eg, observations, pressure-sensing maps, risk assessment scales)
- Skin characteristics, including blistering, continuity of skin color, dermatitis, hair growth, mobility, nail growth, sensation, temperature, texture, and turgor (eg, observations, palpation, photographic assessments, thermography)

Joint Integrity and Mobility

- Joint integrity and mobility (eg, apprehension, compression and distraction, drawer, glide, impingement, shear, and valgus/varus stress tests; arthrometry; palpation)

Motor Function (Motor Control and Motor Learning)

- Dexterity, coordination, and agility (eg, coordination screens, motor impairment tests, motor proficiency tests, observations, videographic assessments)
- Electrophysiological integrity (eg, electroneuromyography)
- Hand function (eg, fine and gross motor control tests, finger dexterity tests, manipulative ability tests, observations)
- Initiation, modification, and control of movement patterns and voluntary postures (eg, activity indexes, developmental scales, gross motor function profiles, motor scales, movement assessment batteries, neuromotor tests, observations, physical performance tests, postural challenge tests, videographic assessments)

Muscle Performance (Including Strength, Power, and Endurance)

- Electrophysiological integrity (eg, electroneuromyography)
- Muscle strength, power, and endurance (eg, dynamometry, manual muscle tests, muscle performance tests, physical capacity tests, technology-assisted assessments, timed activity tests)
- Muscle strength, power, and endurance during functional activities (eg, ADL scales, functional muscle tests, IADL scales, observations, videographic assessments)
- Muscle tension (eg, palpation)

Neuromotor Development and Sensory Integration

- Acquisition and evolution of motor skills, including age-appropriate development (eg, activity indexes, developmental inventories and questionnaires, infant and toddler motor assessments, learning profiles, motor function tests, motor proficiency assessments, neuromotor assessments, reflex tests, screens, videographic assessments)
- Oral motor function, phonation, and speech production (eg, interviews, observations)
- Sensorimotor integration, including postural, equilibrium, and righting reactions (eg, behavioral assessment scales, motor and processing skill tests, observations, postural challenge tests, reflex tests, sensory profiles, visual perceptual skill tests)

Orthotic, Protective, and Supportive Devices

- Components, alignment, fit, and ability to care for orthotic, protective, and supportive devices and equipment (eg, interviews, logs, observations, pressure-sensing maps, reports)
- Orthotic, protective, and supportive devices and equipment use during functional activities (eg, ADL scales, functional scales, IADL scales, interviews, observations, profiles)
- Remediation of impairments, functional limitations, or disabilities with use of orthotic, protective, and supportive devices and equipment (eg, activity status indexes, ADL scales, aerobic capacity tests, functional performance inventories, health assessment questionnaires, IADL scales, pain scales, play scales, videographic assessments)
- Safety during use of orthotic, protective, and supportive devices and equipment (eg, diaries, fall scales, interviews, logs, observations, reports)

Pain

- Pain, soreness, and nociception (eg, analog scales, discrimination tests, pain drawings and maps, provocation tests, verbal and pictorial descriptor tests)
- Pain in specific body parts (eg, pain indexes, pain questionnaires, structural provocation tests)

Posture

- Postural alignment and position (static and dynamic), including symmetry and deviation from midline (eg, grid measurement, observations, photographic assessments, technology-assisted assessments, videographic assessments)
- Specific body parts (eg, angle assessments, forward-bending test, goniometry, observations, palpation, positional tests)

Range of Motion (ROM) (Including Muscle Length)

- Functional ROM (eg, observations, squat testing, toe touch tests)
- Joint active and passive movement (eg, goniometry, inclinometry, observations, photographic assessments, technology-assisted assessments, videographic assessments)
- Muscle length, soft tissue extensibility, and flexibility (eg, contracture tests, goniometry, inclinometry, ligamentous tests, linear measurement, multisegment flexibility tests, palpation)

Reflex Integrity

- Deep reflexes (eg, myotatic reflex scale, observations, reflex tests)
- Electrophysiological integrity (eg, electroneuromyography)
- Postural reflexes and reactions, including righting, equilibrium, and protective reactions (eg, observations, postural challenge tests, reflex profiles, videographic assessments)
- Primitive reflexes and reactions, including developmental (eg, reflex profiles)
- Resistance to passive stretch (eg, tone scales)
- Superficial reflexes and reactions (eg, observations, provocation tests)

Self-Care and Home Management (Including ADL and IADL)

- Ability to gain access to home environments (eg, barrier identification, observations, physical performance tests)
- Ability to perform self-care and home management activities with or without assistive, adaptive, orthotic, protective, supportive, or prosthetic devices and equipment (eg, ADL scales, aerobic capacity tests, IADL scales, interviews, observations, profiles)
- Safety in self-care and home management activities and environments (eg, diaries, fall scales, interviews, logs, observations, reports, videographic assessments)

Sensory Integrity

- Combined/cortical sensations (eg, stereognosis, tactile discrimination tests)
- Deep sensations (eg, kinesthesiometry, observations, photographic assessments, vibration tests)
- Electrophysiological integrity (eg,electroneuromyography)

Ventilation and Respiration/Gas Exchange

- Pulmonary signs of respiration/gas exchange, including breath sounds (eg, gas analyses, observations, oximetry)
- Pulmonary signs of ventilatory function, including airway protection; breath and voice sounds; respiratory rate, rhythm, and pattern; ventilatory flow, forces, and volumes (eg, airway clearance tests, observations, palpation, pulmonary function tests, ventilatory muscle force tests)
- Pulmonary symptoms (eg, dyspnea and perceived exertion indexes and scales)

Work (Job/School/Play), Community, and Leisure Integration or Reintegration (Including IADL)

- Ability to assume or resume work (job/school/play), community, and leisure activities with or without assistive, adaptive, orthotic, protective, supportive, or prosthetic devices and equipment (eg, activity profiles, disability indexes, functional status questionnaires, IADL scales, observations, physical capacity tests)
- Ability to gain access to work (job/school/play), community, and leisure environments (eg, barrier identification, interviews, observations, physical capacity tests, transportation assessments)
- Safety in work (job/school/play), community, and leisure activities and environments (eg, diaries, fall scales, interviews, logs, observations, videographic assessments)

Evaluation, Diagnosis, and Prognosis (Including Plan of Care)

Physical therapists perform *evaluations* (make clinical judgments) based on the data gathered from the history, systems review, and tests and measures. In the evaluation process, physical therapists synthesize the examination data to establish the diagnosis and prognosis (including the plan of care). Factors that influence the complexity of the evaluation include the clinical findings, extent of loss of function, chronicity or severity of the problem, possibility of multisite or multisystem involvement, preexisting condition(s), potential discharge destination, social considerations, physical function, and overall health status.

A *diagnosis* is a label encompassing a cluster of signs and symptoms, syndromes, or categories. It is the result of the systematic diagnostic process, which includes integrating and evaluating the data from the examination. The diagnostic label indicates the primary dysfunction(s) toward which the therapist will direct interventions. The *prognosis* is the determination of the predicted optimal level of improvement in function and the amount of time needed to reach that level and may also include a prediction of levels of improvement that may be reached at various intervals during the course of therapy. During the prognostic process, the physical therapist develops the plan of care. The *plan of care* identifies specific interventions, proposed frequency and duration of the interventions, anticipated goals, expected outcomes, and discharge plans. The plan of care identifies realistic anticipated goals and expected outcomes, taking into consideration the expectations of the patient/client and appropriate others. These anticipated goals and expected outcomes should be measureable and time limited.

The frequency of visits and duration of the episode of care may vary from a short episode with a high intensity of intervention to a longer episode with a diminishing intensity of intervention. Frequency and duration may vary greatly among patients/clients based on a variety of factors that the physical therapist considers throughout the evaluation process, such as anatomical and physiological changes related to growth and development; caregiver consistency or expertise; chronicity or severity of the current condition; living environment; multisite or multisystem involvement; social support; potential discharge destinations; probability of prolonged impairment, functional limitation, or disability; and stability of the condition.

Prognosis

Patient/client will demonstrate optimal motor function and sensory integrity and the highest level of functioning in home, work (job/school/play), community, and leisure environments, within the context of the impairments, functional limitations, and disabilities.

During the episode of care, patient/client will achieve (1) the anticipated goals and expected outcomes of the interventions that are described in the plan of care and (2) the global outcomes for patients/clients who are classified in this pattern.

Expected Range of Number of Visits Per Episode of Care

6 to 90

This range represents the lower and upper limits of the number of physical therapist visits required to achieve anticipated goals and expected outcomes. *It is anticipated that 80% of patients/clients who are classified into this pattern will achieve the anticipated goals and expected outcomes within 6 to 90 visits during a single continuous episode of care.* Frequency of visits and duration of the episode of care should be determined by the physical therapist to maximize effectiveness of care and efficiency of service delivery.

Note:

These patients/clients may require multiple episodes of care over the lifetime to ensure safety and effective adaptation following changes in physical status, caregivers, environment, or task demands. Factors that may lead to these additional episodes of care include:

- Cognitive maturation
- Periods of rapid growth

Factors That May Require New Episode of Care or That May Modify Frequency of Visits/Duration of Care

- Accessibility and availability of resources
- Adherence to the intervention program
- Age
- Anatomical and physiological changes related to growth and development
- Caregiver consistency or expertise
- Chronicity or severity of the current condition
- Cognitive status
- Comorbitities, complications, or secondary impairments
- Concurrent medical, surgical, and therapeutic interventions
- Decline in functional independence
- Level of impairment
- Level of physical function
- Living environment
- Multisite or multisystem involvement
- Nutritional status
- Overall health status
- Potential discharge destinations
- Premorbid conditions
- Probability of prolonged impairment, functional limitation, or disability
- Psychological and socioeconomic factors
- Psychomotor abilities
- Social support
- Stability of the condition

Intervention

Intervention is the purposeful interaction of the physical therapist with the patient/client and, when appropriate, with other individuals involved in patient/client care, using various physical therapy procedures and techniques to produce changes in the condition consistent with the diagnosis and prognosis. Decisions about interventions are contingent on the timely monitoring of patient/client response and the progress made toward achieving the anticipated goals and expected outcomes.

Communication, coordination, and documentation and patient/client-related instruction are provided for all patients/clients across all settings. Procedural interventions are selected or modified based on the examination data and the evaluation, the diagnosis and the prognosis, and the anticipated goals and expected outcomes for a particular patient/client. *For clinical considerations in selecting interventions, listings of interventions, and listings of anticipated goals and expected outcomes, refer to Chapter 3.*

Coordination, Communication, and Documentation

Coordination, communication, and documentation may include:

Interventions

- Addressing required functions
  - advance directives
  - individualized family service plans (IFSPs) or individualized education plans (IEPs)
  - informed consent
  - mandatory communication and reporting (eg, patient advocacy and abuse reporting)
- Admission and discharge planning
- Case management
- Collaboration and coordination with agencies, including:
  - equipment suppliers
  - home care agencies
  - payer groups
  - schools
  - transportation agencies
- Communication across settings, including:
  - case conferences
  - documentation
  - education plans
- Cost-effective resource utilization
- Data collection, analysis, and reporting
  - outcome data
  - peer review findings
  - record reviews
- Documentation across settings, following APTA's *Guidelines for Physical Therapy Documentation* (Appendix 5), including:
  - changes in impairments, functional limitations, and disabilities
  - changes in interventions
  - elements of patient/client management (examination, evaluation, diagnosis, prognosis, intervention)
  - outcomes of intervention
- Interdisciplinary teamwork
  - case conferences
  - patient care rounds
  - patient/client family meetings
- Referrals to other professionals or resources

Anticipated Goals and Expected Outcomes

- Accountability for services is increased.
- Admission data and discharge planning are completed.
- Advance directives, individualized family service plans (IFSPs) or individualized education plans (IEPs), informed consent, and mandatory communication and reporting (eg, patient advocacy and abuse reporting) are obtained or completed.
- Available resources are maximally utilized.
- Care is coordinated with patient/client, family, significant others, caregivers, and other professionals.
- Case is managed throughout the episode of care.
- Collaboration and coordination occurs with agencies, including equipment suppliers, home care agencies, payer groups, schools, and transportation agencies.
- Communication enhances risk reduction and prevention.
- Communication occurs across settings through case conferences, education plans, and documentation.
- Data are collected, analyzed, and reported, including outcome data, peer review findings, and record reviews.
- Decision making is enhanced regarding health, wellness, and fitness needs.
- Decision making is enhanced regarding patient/client health and the use of health care resources by patient/client, family, significant others, and caregivers.
- Documentation occurs throughout patient/client management and across settings and follows APTA's *Guidelines for Physical Therapy Documentation* (Appendix 5).
- Interdisciplinary collaboration occurs through case conferences, patient care rounds, and patient/client family meetings.
- Patient/client, family, significant other, and caregiver understanding of anticipated goals and expected outcomes is increased.
- Placement needs are determined.
- Referrals are made to other professionals or resources whenever necessary and appropriate.
- Resources are utilized in a cost-effective way.

Patient/Client-Related Instruction

Patient/client-related instruction may include:

Interventions

- Instruction, education and training of patients/clients and caregivers regarding:
  - current condition (pathology/pathophysiology [disease, disorder, or condition], impairments, functional limitations, or disabilities)
  - enhancement of performance
  - health, wellness, and fitness programs
  - plan of care
  - risk factors for pathology/pathophysiology (disease, disorder, or condition), impairments, functional limitations, or disabilities
  - transitions across settings
  - transitions to new roles

Anticipated Goals and Expected Outcomes

- Ability to perform physical actions, tasks, or activities is improved.
- Awareness and use of community resources are improved.
- Behaviors that foster healthy habits, wellness, and prevention are acquired.
- Decision making is enhanced regarding patient/client health and the use of health care resources by patient/client, family, significant others, and caregivers.
- Disability associated with acute or chronic illnesses is reduced.
- Functional independence in activities of daily living (ADL) and instrumental activities of daily living (IADL) is increased.
- Health status is improved.
- Intensity of care is decreased.
- Level of supervision required for task performance is decreased.
- Patient/client, family, significant other, and caregiver knowledge and awareness of the diagnosis, prognosis, interventions, and anticipated goals and expected outcomes are increased.
- Patient/client knowledge of personal and environmental factors associated with the condition is increased.
- Performance levels in self-care, home management, work (job/school/play), community, or leisure actions, tasks, or activities are improved.
- Physical function is improved.
- Risk of recurrence of condition is reduced.
- Risk of secondary impairment is reduced.
- Safety of patient/client, family, significant others, and caregivers is improved.
- Self-management of symptoms is improved.
- Utilization and cost of health care services are decreased.

Procedural Interventions

Procedural interventions for this pattern may include:

Therapeutic Exercise

Interventions

- Aerobic and endurance conditioning or reconditioning
  - aquatic programs
  - gait and locomotor training
  - increased workload over time
  - walking and wheelchair propulsion programs
- Balance, coordination, and agility training
  - motor function (motor control and motor learning) training or retraining
  - neuromuscular education or reeducation
  - perceptual training
  - posture awareness training
  - standardized, programmatic, complementary exercise approaches
  - sensory training or retraining
  - task-specific performance training
  - vestibular training
- Body mechanics and postural stabilization
  - body mechanics training
  - posture awareness training
  - postural control training
  - postural stabilization activities
- Flexibility exercises
  - muscle lengthening
  - range of motion
  - stretching
- Gait and locomotion training
  - developmental activities training
  - gait training
  - implement and device training
  - perceptual training
  - standardized, programmatic, complementary exercise approaches
  - wheelchair training
- Neuromotor development
  - developmental activities training
  - motor training
  - movement pattern training
  - neuromuscular education or reeducation
- Relaxation
  - breathing strategies
  - movement strategies
  - relaxation techniques
  - standardized, programmatic, complementary exercise approaches
- Strength, power, and endurance training for head, neck, limb, pelvic-floor, trunk, and ventilatory muscles
  - active assistive, active, and resistive exercises (including concentric, dynamic/isotonic, eccentric, isokinetic, isometric, and plyometric)
  - aquatic programs
  - standardized, programmatic, complementary exercise approaches
  - task-specific performance training

Anticipated Goals and Expected Outcomes

- Impact on pathology/pathophysiology (disease, disorder, or condition)
  - Joint swelling, inflammation, or restriction is reduced.
  - Nutrient delivery to tissue is increased.
  - Osteogenic effects of exercise are maximized.
  - Pain is decreased.
  - Physiological response to increased oxygen demand is improved.
  - Soft tissue swelling, inflammation, or restriction is reduced.
  - Tissue perfusion and oxygenation are enhanced.
- Impact on impairments:
  - Aerobic capacity is increased.
  - Balance is improved.
  - Endurance is increased.
  - Energy expenditure per unit of work is decreased.
  - Gait, locomotion, and balance are improved.
  - Joint integrity and mobility are improved.
  - Motor function (motor control and motor learning) is improved.
  - Muscle performance (strength, power, and endurance) is increased.
  - Postural control is improved.
  - Quality and quantity of movement between and across body segments are improved.
  - Range of motion is improved.
  - Relaxation is increased.
  - Sensory awareness is increased.
  - Weight-bearing status is improved.
  - Work of breathing is decreased.
- Impact on functional limitations
  - Ability to perform physical actions, tasks, or activities related to self-care, home management, work (job/school/play), community, and leisure is improved.
  - Level of supervision required for task performance is decreased.
  - Performance of and independence in activities of daily living (ADL) and instrumental activities of daily living (IADL) with or without devices and equipment are increased.
  - Tolerance of positions and activities is increased.
- Impact on disabilities
  - Ability to assume or resume required self-care, home management, work (job/school/play), community, and leisure roles is improved.
- Risk reduction/prevention
  - Risk factors are reduced.
  - Risk of secondary impairments is reduced.
  - Safety is improved.
  - Self-management of symptoms is improved.
- Impact on health, wellness, and fitness
  - Fitness is improved.
  - Health status is improved.
  - Physical capacity is increased.
  - Physical function is improved.
- Impact on societal resources
  - Utilization of physical therapy services is optimized.
  - Utilization of physical therapy services results in efficient use of health care dollars.
- Patient/client satisfaction
  - Access, availability, and services provided are acceptable to patient/client.
  - Administrative management of practice is acceptable to patient/client.
  - Clinical proficiency of physical therapist is acceptable to patient/client.
  - Coordination of care is acceptable to patient/client.
  - Cost of health care services is decreased.
  - Intensity of care is decreased.
  - Interpersonal skills of physical therapist are acceptable to patient/client, family, and significant others.
  - Sense of well-being is improved.
  - Stressors are decreased.

Functional Training in Self-Care and Home Management (Including Activities of Daily Living [ADL] and Instrumental Activities of Daily Living [IADL])

Interventions

- ADL training
  - bathing
  - bed mobility and transfer training
  - developmental activities
  - dressing
  - eating
  - grooming
  - gait and locomotion training
  - toileting
- Devices and equipment use and training
  - assistive and adaptive device or equipment training during ADL and IADL
  - orthotic, protective, or supportive device or equipment training during ADL and IADL
- Functional training programs
  - simulated environments and tasks
  - task adaptation
  - travel training
- IADL training
  - caring for dependents
  - home maintenance
  - household chores
  - shopping
  - structured play for infants and children
  - yard work
- Injury prevention or reduction
  - injury prevention education during self-care and home management
  - injury prevention or reduction with use of devices and equipment
  - safety awareness training during self-care and home management

Anticipated Goals and Expected Outcomes

- Impact on pathology/pathophysiology (disease, disorder, or condition)
  - Pain is decreased.
  - Physiological response to increased oxygen demand is improved.
- Impact on impairments
  - Balance is improved.
  - Endurance is increased.
  - Energy expenditure per unit of work is decreased.
  - Motor function (motor control and motor learning) is improved.
  - Muscle performance (strength, power, and endurance) is increased.
  - Postural control is improved.
  - Sensory awareness is increased.
  - Weight-bearing status is improved.
  - Work of breathing is decreased.
- Impact on functional limitations
  - Ability to perform physical actions, tasks, or activities related to self-care and home management is improved.
  - Level of supervision required for task performance is decreased.
  - Performance of and independence in ADL and IADL with or without devices and equipment are increased.
  - Tolerance of positions and activities is increased.
- Impact on disabilities
  - Ability to assume or resume roles in self-care and home management is improved.
- Risk reduction/prevention
  - Risk factors are reduced.
  - Risk of secondary impairments is reduced.
  - Safety is improved.
  - Self-management of symptoms is improved.
- Impact on health, wellness, and fitness
  - Health status is improved.
  - Physical capacity is increased.
  - Physical function is improved.
- Impact on societal resources
  - Utilization of physical therapy services is optimized.
  - Utilization of physical therapy services results in efficient use of health care dollars.
- Patient/client satisfaction
  - Access, availability, and services provided are acceptable to patient/client.
  - Administrative management of practice is acceptable to patient/client.
  - Clinical proficiency of physical therapist is acceptable to patient/client.
  - Coordination of care is acceptable to patient/client.
  - Cost of health care services is decreased.
  - Intensity of care is decreased.
  - Interpersonal skills of physical therapist are acceptable to patient/client, family, and significant others.
  - Sense of well-being is improved.
  - Stressors are decreased.

Functional Training in Work (Job/School/Play), Community, and Leisure Integration or Reintegration (Including Instrumental Activities of Daily Living [IADL] and Work Conditioning)

Interventions

- Devices and equipment use and training
  - assistive and adaptive device or equipment training during IADL
  - orthotic, protective, or supportive device or equipment training during IADL
  - prosthetic device or equipment training during IADL
- Functional training programs
  - job coaching
  - simulated environments and tasks
  - task adaptation
  - task training
  - travel training
- IADL training
  - community service training involving instruments
  - school and play activities training including tools and instruments
  - work training with tools
- Injury prevention or reduction
  - injury prevention education during work (job/school/play), community, and leisure integration or reintegration
  - injury prevention or reduction with use of devices and equipment
  - safety awareness training during work (job/school/play), community, and leisure integration or reintegration
- Leisure and play activities training

Anticipated Goals and Expected Outcomes

- Impact on pathology/pathophysiology (disease, disorder, or condition)
  - Pain is decreased.
  - Physiological response to increased oxygen demand is improved.
- Impact on impairments
  - Balance is improved.
  - Endurance is increased.
  - Energy expenditure per unit of work is decreased.
  - Motor function (motor control and motor learning) is improved.
  - Muscle performance (strength, power, and endurance) is increased.
  - Postural control is improved.
  - Sensory awareness is increased.
  - Weight-bearing status is improved.
  - Work of breathing is decreased.
- Impact on functional limitations
  - Ability to perform physical actions, tasks, or activities related to work (job/school/play), community, and leisure integration or reintegration is improved.
  - Level of supervision required for task performance is decreased.
  - Performance of and independence in IADL with or without devices and equipment are increased.
  - Tolerance of positions and activities is increased.
- Impact on disabilities
  - Ability to assume or resume required work (job/school/play), community, and leisure roles is improved.
- Risk reduction/prevention
  - Risk factors are reduced.
  - Risk of secondary impairment is reduced.
  - Safety is improved.
  - Self-management of symptoms is improved.

Impact on health, wellness, and fitness
  - Fitness is improved.
  - Health status is improved.
  - Physical capacity is increased.
  - Physical function is improved.
- Impact on societal resources
  - Costs of work-related injury or disability are reduced.
  - Utilization of physical therapy services is optimized.
  - Utilization of physical therapy services results in efficient use of health care dollars.
- Patient/client satisfaction
  - Access, availability, and services provided are acceptable to patient/client.
  - Administrative management of practice is acceptable to patient/client.
  - Clinical proficiency of physical therapist is acceptable to patient/client.
  - Coordination of care is acceptable to patient/client.
  - Cost of health care services is decreased.
  - Intensity of care is decreased.
  - Interpersonal skills of physical therapist are acceptable to patient/client, family, and significant others.
  - Sense of well-being is improved.
  - Stressors are decreased.

Manual Therapy Techniques (Including Mobilization/Manipulation)

Interventions

- Manual traction
- Massage
  - connective tissue massage
  - therapeutic massage
- Mobilization/manipulation
  - soft tissue
- Passive range of motion

Anticipated Goals and Expected Outcomes

- Impact on pathology/pathophysiology (disease, disorder, or condition)
  - Edema, lymphedema, or effusion is reduced.
  - Joint swelling, inflammation, or restriction is reduced.
  - Pain is decreased.
  - Soft tissue swelling, inflammation, or restriction is reduced.
- Impact on impairments
  - Balance is improved.
  - Energy expenditure per unit of work is decreased.
  - Gait, locomotion, and balance are improved.
  - Integumentary integrity is improved.
  - Joint integrity and mobility are improved.
  - Muscle performance (strength, power, and endurance) is increased.
  - Postural control is improved.
  - Quality and quantity of movement between and across body segments are improved.
  - Range of motion is improved.
  - Relaxation is increased.
  - Sensory awareness is increased.
  - Weight-bearing status is improved.
  - Work of breathing is decreased.
- Impact on functional limitations
  - Ability to perform movement tasks is improved.
  - Ability to perform physical actions, tasks, or activities related to self-care, home management, work (job/school/play), community, and leisure is improved.
  - Tolerance of positions and activities is increased.
- Impact on disabilities
  - Ability to assume or resume required self-care, home management, work (job/school/play), community, and leisure roles is improved.
- Risk reduction/prevention
  - Risk factors are reduced.
  - Risk of secondary impairment is reduced.
  - Self-management of symptoms is improved.
- Impact on health, wellness, and fitness
  - Physical capacity is increased.
  - Physical function is improved.
- Impact on societal resources
  - Utilization of physical therapy services is optimized.
  - Utilization of physical therapy services results in efficient use of health care dollars.
- Patient/client satisfaction
  - Access, availability, and services provided are acceptable to patient/client.
  - Administrative management of practice is acceptable to patient/client.
  - Clinical proficiency of physical therapist is acceptable to patient/client.
  - Coordination of care is acceptable to patient/client.
  - Cost of health care services is decreased.
  - Intensity of care is decreased.
  - Interpersonal skills of physical therapist are acceptable to patient/client, family, and significant others.
  - Sense of well-being is improved.
  - Stressors are decreased.

Prescription, Application, and, as Appropriate, Fabrication of Devices and Equipment (Assistive, Adaptive, Orthotic, Protective, Supportive, and Prosthetic)

Interventions

- Adaptive devices
  - environmental controls
  - hospital beds
  - raised toilet seats
  - seating systems
- Assistive devices
  - canes
  - crutches
  - long-handled reachers
  - power devices
  - static and dynamic splints
  - walkers
  - wheelchairs
- Orthotic devices
  - braces
  - casts
  - shoe inserts
  - splints
- Protective devices
  - braces
  - cushions
  - helmets
  - protective taping
- Supportive devices
  - compression garments
  - corsets
  - elastic wraps
  - neck collars
  - serial casts
  - slings
  - supplemental oxygen
  - supportive taping

Anticipated Goals and Expected Outcomes

- Impact on pathology/pathophysiology (disease, disorder, or condition)
  - Edema, lymphedema, or effusion is reduced.
  - Joint swelling, inflammation, or restriction is reduced.
  - Pain is decreased.
  - Physiological response to increased oxygen demand is improved.
  - Soft tissue swelling, inflammation, or restriction is reduced.
- Impact on impairments
  - Balance is improved.
  - Endurance is increased.
  - Energy expenditure per unit of work is decreased.
  - Gait, locomotion, and balance are improved.
  - Integumentary integrity is improved.
  - Joint stability is improved.
  - Motor function (motor control and motor learning) is improved.
  - Muscle performance (strength, power, and endurance) is increased.
  - Optimal joint alignment is achieved.
  - Optimal loading on a body part is achieved.
  - Postural control is improved.
  - Quality and quantity of movement between and across body segments are improved.
  - Range of motion is improved.
  - Weight-bearing status is improved.
- Impact on functional limitations
  - Ability to perform physical actions, tasks, or activities related to self-care, home management, work (job/school/play), community, and leisure is improved.
  - Level of supervision required for task performance is decreased.
  - Performance of and independence in activities of daily living (ADL) and instrumental activities of daily living (IADL) with or without devices and equipment are increased.
  - Tolerance of positions and activities is improved.
- Impact on disabilities
  - Ability to assume or resume required self-care, home management, work (job/school/play), community, and leisure roles is improved.
- Risk reduction/prevention
  - Pressure on body tissues is reduced.
  - Protection of body parts is increased.
  - Risk factors are reduced.
  - Risk of secondary impairment is reduced.
  - Safety is improved.
  - Self-management of symptoms is improved.
- Impact on health, wellness, and fitness
  - Health status is improved.
  - Physical capacity is increased.
  - Physical function is improved.
- Impact on societal resources
  - Utilization of physical therapy services is optimized.
  - Utilization of physical therapy services results in efficient use of health care dollars.
- Patient/client satisfaction
  - Access, availability, and services provided are acceptable to patient/client.
  - Administrative management of practice is acceptable to patient/client.
  - Clinical proficiency of physical therapist is acceptable to patient/client.
  - Coordination of care is acceptable to patient/client.
  - Cost of health care services is decreased.
  - Intensity of care is decreased.
  - Interpersonal skills of physical therapist are acceptable to patient/client, family, and significant others.
  - Sense of well-being is improved.
  - Stressors are decreased.

Airway Clearance Techniques

Interventions

- Breathing strategies
  - active cycle of breathing or forced expiratory techniques
  - assisted cough/huff techniques
  - autogenic drainage
  - paced breathing
  - pursed lip breathing
  - techniques to maximize ventilation (eg, maximum inspiratory hold, staircase breathing, manual hyperinflation)
- Positioning
  - positioning to alter work of breathing
  - positioning to maximize ventilation and perfusion
  - pulmonary postural drainage

Anticipated Goals and Expected Outcomes

- Impact on pathology/pathophysiology (disease, disorder, or condition)
  - Nutrient delivery to tissue is increased.
  - Physiological response to increased oxygen demand is improved.
  - Symptoms associated with increased oxygen demand are decreased.
  - Tissue perfusion and oxygenation are enhanced.
- Impact on impairments
  - Airway clearance is improved.
  - Cough is improved.
  - Endurance is increased.
  - Energy expenditure per unit of work is decreased.
  - Muscle performance (strength, power, and endurance) is increased.
  - Ventilation and respiration/gas exchange are improved.
  - Work of breathing is decreased.
- Impact on functional limitations
  - Ability to perform physical actions, tasks, or activities related to self-care, home management, community, work (job/ school/ play), and leisure is improved.
  - Performance of and independence in activities of daily living (ADL) and instrumental activities of daily living (IADL) with or without devices and equipment are increased.
  - Tolerance of positions and activities is increased.
- Impact on disabilities
  - Ability to assume or resume required self-care, home management, work (job/school/play), community, and leisure roles is improved.
- Risk reduction/prevention
  - Risk factors are reduced.
  - Risk of secondary impairment is reduced.
  - Safety is improved.
  - Self-management of symptoms is improved.
- Impact on health, wellness, and fitness
  - Health status is improved.
  - Physical capacity is increased.
  - Physical function is improved.
- Impact on societal resources
  - Utilization of physical therapy services is optimized.
  - Utilization of physical therapy services results in efficient use of health care dollars.
- Patient/client satisfaction
  - Access, availability, and services provided are acceptable to patient/client.
  - Administrative management of practice is acceptable to patient/client.
  - Clinical proficiency of physical therapist is acceptable to patient/client.
  - Coordination of care is acceptable to patient/client.
  - Cost of health care services is decreased.
  - Intensity of care is decreased.
  - Interpersonal skills of physical therapist are acceptable to patient/client, family, and significant others.
  - Sense of well-being is improved.
  - Stressors are decreased.

Electrotherapeutic Modalities

Interventions

- Biofeedback
- Electrical stimulation
  - functional electrical stimulation (FES)
  - neuromuscular electrical stimulation (NMES)
  - transcutaneous electrical nerve stimulation (TENS)

Anticipated Goals and Expected Outcomes

- Impact on pathology/pathophysiology (disease, disorder, or condition)
  - Edema, lymphedema, or effusion is reduced.
  - Joint swelling, inflammation, or restriction is reduced.
  - Nutrient delivery to tissue is increased.
  - Osteogenic effects are enhanced..
  - Pain is decreased.
  - Soft tissue swelling, inflammation, or restriction is reduced.
  - Tissue perfusion and oxygenation are enhanced.
- Impact on impairments
  - Motor function (motor control and motor learning) is improved.
  - Muscle performance (strength, power, and endurance) is increased.
  - Postural control is improved.
  - Quality and quantity of movement between and across body segments are improved.
  - Range of motion is improved.
  - Sensory awareness is increased.
- Impact on functional limitations
  - Ability to perform physical actions, tasks, or activities related to self-care, home management, community, work (job/ school/ play), and leisure is improved.
  - Level of supervision required for task performance is decreased.
  - Performance of and independence in activities of daily living (ADL) and instrumental activities of daily living (IADL) with or without devices and equipment are increased.
  - Tolerance of positions and activities is increased.
- Impact on disabilities
  - Ability to assume or resume required self-care, home management, work (job/school/play), community, and leisure roles is improved.
- Risk reduction/prevention
  - Complications of immobility are reduced.
  - Risk factors are reduced.
  - Risk of secondary impairment is reduced.
  - Self-management of symptoms is improved.
- Impact on health, wellness, and fitness
  - Physical function is improved.
- Impact on societal resources
  - Utilization of physical therapy services is optimized.
  - Utilization of physical therapy services results in efficient use of health care dollars.
- Patient/client satisfaction
  - Access, availability, and services provided are acceptable to patient/client.
  - Administrative management of practice is acceptable to patient/client.
  - Clinical proficiency of physical therapist is acceptable to patient/client.
  - Coordination of care is acceptable to patient/client.
  - Interpersonal skills of physical therapist are acceptable to patient/client, family, and significant others.
  - Sense of well-being is improved.
  - Stressors are decreased.

Physical Agents and Mechanical Modalities

Interventions

Mechanical modalities may include:

- Compression therapies
  - compression bandaging
  - compression garments
  - taping
  - total contact casting
  - vasopneumatic compression devices
- Gravity-assisted compression devices
  - standing frame
  - tilt table

Anticipated Goals and Expected Outcomes

- Impact on pathology/pathophysiology (disease, disorder, or condition)
  - Edema, lymphedema, or effusion is reduced.
  - Joint swelling, inflammation, or restriction is reduced.
  - Nutrient delivery to tissue is increased.
  - Osteogenic effects are enhanced..
  - Pain is decreased.
  - Soft tissue swelling, inflammation, or restriction is reduced.
  - Tissue perfusion and oxygenation are enhanced.
- Impact on impairments:
  - Integumentary integrity is improved.
  - Muscle performance (strength, power, and endurance) is increased.
  - Range of motion is improved.
  - Weight-bearing status is improved.
- Impact on functional limitations
  - Ability to perform physical actions, tasks, or activities related to self-care, home management, work (job/school/play), community, and leisure is improved.
  - Performance of and independence in activities of daily living (ADL) and instrumental activities of daily living (IADL) with or without devices and equipment are increased.
  - Tolerance of positions and activities is increased.
- Impact on disabilities
  - Ability to assume or resume required self-care, home management, work (job/school/play), community, and leisure roles is improved.
- Risk reduction/prevention
  - Complications of soft tissue and circulatory disorders are decreased.
  - Risk of secondary impairments is reduced.
  - Self-management of symptoms is improved.
- Impact on health, wellness, and fitness
  - Physical function is improved.
- Impact on societal resources
  - Utilization of physical therapy services is optimized.
- Patient/client satisfaction
  - Access, availability, and services provided are acceptable to patient/client.
  - Administrative management of practice is acceptable to patient/client.
  - Clinical proficiency of physical therapist is acceptable to patient/client.
  - Coordination of care is acceptable to patient/client.
  - Interpersonal skills of physical therapist are acceptable to patient/client, family, and significant others.
  - Sense of well-being is improved.
  - Stressors are decreased.

Reexamination

Reexamination is the process of performing selected tests and measures after the initial examination to evaluate progress and to modify or redirect interventions. Reexamination may be indicated more than once during a single episode of care. It also may be performed over the course of a disease, disorder, or condition, which for some patients/clients may be over the life span. Indications for reexamination include new clinical findings or failure to respond to physical therapy interventions.

Global Outcomes for Patients/Clients in This Pattern

Throughout the entire episode of care, the physical therapist determines the anticipated goals and expected outcomes for each intervention. These anticipated goals and expected outcomes are delineated in shaded boxes that accompany the lists of interventions in each preferred practice pattern. As the patient/client reaches the termination of physical therapy services and the end of the episode of care, the physical therapist measures the global outcomes of the physical therapy services by characterizing or quantifying the impact of the physical therapy interventions in the following domains:

- Pathology/pathophysiology (disease, disorder, or condition)
- Impairments
- Functional limitations
- Disabilities
- Risk reduction/prevention
- Health, wellness, and fitness
- Societal resources
- Patient/client satisfaction

In some instances, a particular anticipated goal or expected outcome is thoroughly achieved through implementation of a single form of intervention. More commonly, however, the anticipated goals and expected outcomes are achieved as a result of the combined effects of several forms of interventions, leading to enhancement of both health status and health-related quality of life.

Criteria for Termination of Physical Therapy Services

Discharge is the process of ending physical therapy services that have been provided during a single episode of care. It occurs when the anticipated goals and expected outcomes have been achieved. Discharge does *not* occur with a *transfer* (defined as the time when a patient is moved from one site to another site within the same setting or across settings during a single episode of care). Although there may be facility-specific or payer-specific requirements for documentation regarding the conclusion of physical therapy services, *discharge occurs based on the physical therapist's analysis of the achievement of anticipated goals and expected outcomes.*

Discontinuation is the process of ending physical therapy services that have been provided during a single episode of care when (1) the patient/client, caregiver, or legal guardian declines to continue intervention; (2) the patient/client is unable to continue to progress toward outcomes because of medical or psychosocial complications or because financial/insurance resources have been expended; or (3) the physical therapist determines that the patient/client will no longer benefit from physical therapy. When physical therapy services are terminated prior to achievement of anticipated goals and expected outcomes, patient/client status and the rationale for termination are documented.

For patients/clients who require multiple episodes of care, periodic follow-up is needed over the life span to ensure safety and effective adaptation following changes in physical status, caregivers, environment, or task demands. In consultation with appropriate individuals, and in consideration of the outcomes, the physical therapist plans for discharge or discontinuation and provides for appropriate follow-up or referral.

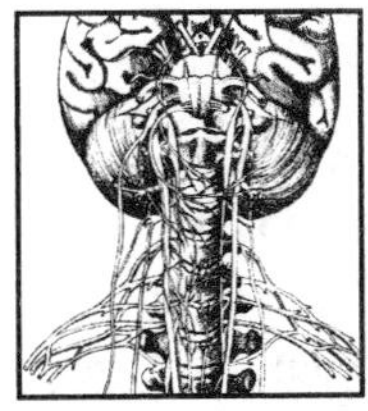

Impaired Motor Function and Sensory Integrity Associated With Nonprogressive Disorders of the Central Nervous System—Acquired in Adolescence or Adulthood

This preferred practice pattern describes the generally accepted elements of patient/client management that physical therapists provide for patients/clients who are classified in this pattern. The pattern title reflects the diagnosis made by the physical therapist. APTA emphasizes that preferred practice patterns are the boundaries within which a physical therapist may select any of a number of clinical alternatives, based on consideration of a wide variety of factors, such as individual patient/client needs; the profession's code of ethics and standards of practice; and patient/client age, culture, gender roles, race, sex, sexual orientation, and socioeconomic status.

Patient/Client Diagnostic Classification

Patients/clients will be classified into this pattern—for impaired motor function and sensory integrity associated with nonprogressive disorders of the central nervous system (acquired in adolescence or adulthood)—as a result of the physical therapist's evaluation of the examination data. The findings from the examination (history, systems review, and tests and measures) may indicate the presence or risk of pathology/pathophysiology (disease, disorder, or condition), impairments, functional limitations, or disabilities or the need for health, wellness, or fitness programs. The physical therapist integrates, synthesizes, and interprets the data to determine the diagnostic classification.

Inclusion

The following examples of examination findings may support the inclusion of patients/clients in this pattern:

Risk Factors or Consequences of Pathology/Pathophysiology (Disease, Disorder, or Condition)

- Aneurysm
- Anoxia or hypoxia
- Bell palsy
- Cerebrovascular accident
- Infectious disease that affects the central nervous system
- Intracranial neurosurgical procedures
- Neoplasm
- Seizures
- Traumatic brain injury

Impairments, Functional Limitations, or Disabilities

- Difficulty negotiating terrains
- Difficulty planning movements
- Difficulty with manipulation skills
- Difficulty with positioning
- Frequent falls
- Impaired affect
- Impaired arousal, attention, and cognition
- Impaired expressive or receptive communication
- Impaired motor function
- Loss of balance during daily activities
- Inability to keep up with peers
- Inability to perform work (job/school/play) activities

Note:

Some risk factors or consequences of pathology/pathophysiology—such as *traumatic brain injury*—may be severe and complex; *however, they do not necessarily exclude patients/clients from this pattern.* Severe and complex risk factors or consequences may require modification of the frequency of visits and duration of care. (See "Evaluation, Diagnosis, and Prognosis," page 363.)

Exclusion or Multiple-Pattern Classification

The following examples of examination findings may support exclusion from this pattern or classification into additional patterns. Depending on the level of severity or complexity of the examination findings, the physical therapist may determine that the patient/client would be more appropriately managed through (1) classification in an entirely different pattern or (2) classification in both this and another pattern.

Findings That May Require Classification in a Different Pattern

- Amputation
- Coma

Findings That May Require Classification in Additional Patterns

- Fracture
- Multisystem trauma

ICD-9-CM Codes

The listing below contains the current (as of press time) and most typical 3- and 4-digit ICD-9-CM codes related to this preferred practice pattern. Because patient/client diagnostic classification is based on impairments, functional limitations, and disabilities—not on codes—patients/clients may be classified into the pattern even though the codes listed with the pattern may not apply to those clients.

This listing is intended for general information only and should not be used for coding purposes. The codes should be confirmed by referring to the World Health Organization's *International Classification of Diseases, 9th Revision, Clinical Modification (ICD-9-CM 2001)*, Volumes 1 and 3 (Chicago, Ill:American Medical Association; 2000) or subsequent revisions or by referring to other ICD-9-CM coding manuals that contain exclusion notes and instructions regarding fifth-digit requirements.

049 Other non-arthropod-borne viral diseases of central nervous system
- **049.9** Unspecified non-arthropod-borne viral diseases of central nervous system
  - Viral encephalitis, not otherwise specified

225 Benign neoplasm of brain and other parts of nervous system
- **225.1** Cranial nerves

320 Bacterial meningitis
- **320.9** Meningitis due to unspecified bacterium

321 Meningitis due to other organisms
- **321.8** Meningitis due to other nonbacterial organisms classified elsewhere*

322 Meningitis of unspecified cause
- **322.9** Meningitis, unspecified

323 Encephalitis, myelitis, and encephalomyelitis
- **323.4** Other encephalitis due to infection classified elsewhere*
- **323.5** Encephalitis following immunization procedures
- **323.6** Postinfectious encephalitis*
- **323.8** Other causes of encephalitis
- **323.9** Unspecified cause of encephalitis

331 Other cerebral degenerations
- **331.3** Communicating hydrocephalus
- **331.4** Obstructive hydrocephalus

342 Hemiplegia and hemiparesis

345 Epilepsy
- **345.1** Generalized convulsive epilepsy
- **345.2** Petit mal status
- **345.3** Grand mal status
- **345.4** Partial epilepsy, with impairment of consciousness
  - Epilepsy:
    - partial:
      - secondarily generalized
- **345.5** Partial epilepsy, without mention of impairment of consciousness
  - Epilepsy:
    - sensory-induced
- **345.9** Epilepsy, unspecified

348 Other conditions of brain
- **348.0** Cerebral cysts
- **348.1** Anoxic brain damage
- **348.3** Encephalopathy, unspecified

350 Trigeminal nerve disorders
- **350.1** Trigeminal neuralgia

351 Facial nerve disorders
- **351.1** Bell's palsy

352 Disorders of other cranial nerves
- **352.4** Disorders of accessory [11th] nerve
- **352.5** Disorders of hypoglossal [12th] nerve
- **352.9** Unspecified disorder of cranial nerves

386 Vertiginous syndromes and other disorders of vestibular system
- **386.5** Labyrinthine dysfunction

431 Intracerebral hemorrhage

433 Occlusion and stenosis of precerebral arteries

434 Occlusion of cerebral arteries

435 Transient cerebral ischemia
- **435.1** Vertebral artery syndrome
- **435.8** Other specified transient cerebral ischemias

436 Acute, but ill-defined, cerebrovascular disease

437 Other and ill-defined cerebrovascular disease

442 Other aneurysm
- **442.8** Of other specified artery

444 Arterial embolism and thrombosis
- **444.9** Of unspecified artery

447 Other disorders of arteries and arterioles
- **447.1** Stricture of artery

780 General symptoms
- **780.3** Convulsions

781 Symptoms involving nervous and musculoskeletal systems
- **781.2** Abnormality of gait
  - Gait:
    - ataxic
- **781.3** Lack of coordination
  - Ataxia, not otherwise specified

799 Other ill-defined and unknown causes of morbidity and mortality
- **799.0** Asphyxia

800 Fracture of vault of skull

801 Fracture of base of skull

803 Other and unqualified skull fractures

804 Multiple fractures involving skull or face with other bones

850 Concussion

851 Cerebral laceration and contusion

852 Subarachnoid, subdural, and extradural hemorrhage, following injury

853 Other and unspecified intracranial hemorrhage following injury

854 Intracranial injury of other and unspecified nature

994 Effects of other external causes
- **994.1** Drowning and nonfatal submersion

* Not a primary diagnosis

Examination

Examination is a comprehensive screening and specific testing process that leads to a diagnostic classification or, when appropriate, to a referral to another practitioner. Examination is required prior to the initial intervention and is performed for all patients/clients. Through the examination, the physical therapist may identify impairments, functional limitations, disabilities, changes in physical function or overall health status, and needs related to restoration of health and to prevention, wellness, and fitness. The physical therapist synthesizes the examination findings to establish the diagnosis and the prognosis (including the plan of care). The patient/client, family, significant others, and caregivers may provide information during the examination process.

Examination has three components: the patient/client history, the systems review, and tests and measures. The *history* is a systematic gathering of past and current information (often from the patient/client) related to why the patient/client is seeking the services of the physical therapist. The *systems review* is a brief or limited examination of (1) the anatomical and physiological status of the cardiovascular/pulmonary, integumentary, musculoskeletal, and neuromuscular systems and (2) the communication ability, affect, cognition, language, and learning style of the patient/client. *Tests and measures* are the means of gathering data about the patient/client.

The selection of examination procedures and the depth of the examination vary based on patient/client age; severity of the problem; stage of recovery (acute, subacute, chronic); phase of rehabilitation (early, intermediate, late, return to activity); home, work (job/school/play), or community situation; and other relevant factors. *For clinical indications in selecting tests and measures and for listings of tests and measures, tools used to gather data, and the types of data generated by tests and measures, refer to Chapter 2.*

Patient/Client History

The history may include:

General Demographics
- Age
- Sex
- Race/ethnicity
- Primary language
- Education

Social History
- Cultural beliefs and behaviors
- Family and caregiver resources
- Social interactions, social activities, and support systems

Employment/Work (Job/School/Play)
- Current and prior work (job/school/play), community, and leisure actions, tasks, or activities

Growth and Development
- Developmental history
- Hand dominance

Living Environment
- Devices and equipment (eg, assistive, adaptive, orthotic, protective, supportive, prosthetic)
- Living environment and community characteristics
- Projected discharge destinations

General Health Status (Self-Report, Family Report, Caregiver Report)
- General health perception
- Physical function (eg, mobility, sleep patterns, restricted bed days)
- Psychological function (eg, memory, reasoning ability, depression, anxiety)
- Role function (eg, community, leisure, social, work)
- Social function (eg, social activity, social interaction, social support)

Social/Health Habits (Past and Current)
- Behavioral health risks (eg, smoking, drug abuse)
- Level of physical fitness

Family History
- Familial health risks

Medical/Surgical History
- Cardiovascular
- Endocrine/metabolic
- Gastrointestinal
- Genitourinary
- Gynecological
- Integumentary
- Musculoskeletal
- Neuromuscular
- Obstetrical
- Prior hospitalizations, surgeries, and preexisting medical and other health-related conditions
- Psychological
- Pulmonary

Current Condition(s)/Chief Complaint(s)
- Concerns that led patient/client to seek the services of a physical therapist
- Concerns or needs of patient/client who requires the services of a physical therapist
- Current therapeutic interventions
- Mechanisms of injury or disease, including date of onset and course of events
- Onset and pattern of symptoms
- Patient/client, family, significant other, and caregiver expectations and goals for the therapeutic intervention
- Patient/client, family, significant other, and caregiver perceptions of patient's/client's emotional response to the current clinical situation
- Previous occurrence of chief complaint(s)
- Prior therapeutic interventions

Functional Status and Activity Level
- Current and prior functional status in self-care and home management activities, including activities of daily living (ADL) and instrumental activities of daily living (IADL)
- Current and prior functional status in work (job/school/play), community, and leisure actions, tasks, or activities

Medications
- Medications for current condition
- Medications previously taken for current condition
- Medications for other conditions

Other Clinical Tests
- Laboratory and diagnostic tests
- Review of available records (eg, medical, education, surgical)
- Review of other clinical findings (eg, nutrition and hydration)

Systems Review

The systems review may include:

Anatomical and Physiological Status

- Cardiovascular/Pulmonary
  - Blood pressure
  - Edema
  - Heart rate
  - Respiratory rate
- Integumentary
  - Pliability (texture)
  - Presence of scar formation
  - Skin color
  - Skin integrity
- Musculoskeletal
  - Gross range of motion
  - Gross strength
  - Gross symmetry
  - Height
  - Weight
- Neuromuscular
  - Gross coordinated movements (eg, balance, gait, locomotion, transfers, transitions)
  - Motor function (motor control, motor learning)

Communication, Affect, Cognition, Language, and Learning Style

- Ability to make needs known
- Consciousness
- Expected emotional/behavioral responses
- Learning preferences (eg, education needs, learning barriers)
- Orientation (person, place, time)

Tests and Measures

Test and measures for this pattern may include those that characterize or quantify:

Aerobic Capacity and Endurance

- Aerobic capacity during functional activities (eg, activities of daily living [ADL] scales, indexes, instrumental activities of daily living [IADL] scales, observations)
- Aerobic capacity during standardized exercise test protocols (eg, ergometry, step tests, time/distance walk/run tests, treadmill tests, wheelchair tests)

Anthropometric Characteristics

- Body composition (eg, body mass index, impedance measurement, skinfold thickness measurement)
- Body dimensions (eg, girth measurement, length measurement)
- Edema (eg, girth measurement, palpation, scales, volume measurement)

Arousal, Attention, and Cognition

- Arousal and attention (eg, adaptability tests, arousal and awareness scales, indexes, profiles, questionnaires)
- Cognition, including ability to process commands (eg, developmental inventories, indexes, interviews, mental state scales, observations, questionnaires, safety checklists)
- Communication (eg, functional communication profiles, interviews, inventories, observations, questionnaires)
- Motivation (eg, adaptive behavior scales)
- Orientation to time, person, place, and situation (eg, attention tests, learning profiles, mental state scales)
- Recall, including memory and retention (eg, assessment scales, interviews, questionnaires)

Assistive and Adaptive Devices

- Assistive or adaptive devices and equipment use during functional activities (eg, ADL scales, functional scales, IADL scales, interviews, observations)
- Components, alignment, fit, and ability to care for the assistive or adaptive devices and equipment (eg, interviews, logs, observations, pressure-sensing maps, reports)
- Remediation of impairments, functional limitations, or disabilities with use of assistive or adaptive devices and equipment (eg, activity status indexes, ADL scales, aerobic capacity tests, functional performance inventories, health assessment questionnaires, IADL scales, pain scales, play scales, videographic assessments)
- Safety during use of assistive or adaptive devices and equipment (eg, diaries, fall scales, interviews, logs, observations, reports)

Circulation (Arterial, Venous, and Lymphatic)

- Cardiovascular signs, including heart rate, rhythm, and sounds; pressures and flow; and superficial vascular responses (eg, auscultation, electrocardiography, girth measurement, observations, palpation, sphygmomanometry, thermography)
- Cardiovascular symptoms (eg, angina, claudication, and perceived exertion scales)
- Physiological responses to position change, including autonomic responses, central and peripheral pressures, heart rate and rhythm, respiratory rate and rhythm, ventilatory pattern (eg, auscultation, electrocardiography, observations, palpation, sphygmomanometry)

Cranial and Peripheral Nerve Integrity

- Electrophysiological integrity (eg, electroneuromyography)
- Motor distribution of the cranial nerves (eg, dynamometry, muscle tests, observations)
- Motor distribution of the peripheral nerves (eg, dynamometry, muscle tests, observations, thoracic outlet tests)
- Response to neural provocation (eg, tension tests, vertebral artery compression tests)
- Response to stimuli, including auditory, gustatory, olfactory, pharyngeal, vestibular, and visual (eg, observations, provocation tests)
- Sensory distribution of the cranial nerves (eg, discrimination tests; tactile tests, including coarse and light touch, cold and heat, pain, pressure, and vibration)
- Sensory distribution of the peripheral nerves (eg, discrimination tests; tactile tests, including coarse and light touch, cold and heat, pain, pressure, and vibration; thoracic outlet tests)

Environmental, Home, and Work (Job/School/Play) Barriers

- Current and potential barriers (eg, checklists, interviews, observations, questionnaires)
- Physical space and environment (eg, compliance standards, observations, photographic assessments, questionnaires, structural specifications, videographic assessments)

Ergonomics and Body Mechanics

Ergonomics

- Dexterity and coordination during work (job/school/play) (eg, hand function tests, impairment rating scales, manipulative ability tests)
- Functional capacity and performance during work actions, tasks, or activities (eg, accelerometry, dynamometry, electroneuromyography, endurance tests, force platform tests, goniometry, interviews, observations, photographic assessments, physical capacity tests, postural loading analyses, technology-assisted assessments, videographic assessments, work analyses)
- Safety in work environments (eg, hazard identification checklists, job severity indexes, lifting standards, risk assessment scales, standards for exposure limits)
- Specific work conditions or activities (eg, handling checklists, job simulations, lifting models, preemployment screenings, task analysis checklists, workstation checklists)
- Tools, devices, equipment, and workstations related to work actions, tasks, or activities (eg, observations, tool analysis checklists, vibration assessments)

Body mechanics

- Body mechanics during self-care, home management, work, community, or leisure actions, tasks, or activities (eg, ADL scales, IADL scales, observations, photographic assessments, technology-assisted assessments, videographic assessments)

Gait, Locomotion, and Balance

- Balance during functional activities with or without the use of assistive, adaptive, orthotic, protective, supportive, or prosthetic devices or equipment (eg, ADL scales, IADL scales, observations, videographic assessments)
- Balance (dynamic and static) with or without the use of assistive, adaptive, orthotic, protective, supportive, or prosthetic devices or equipment (eg, balance scales, dizziness inventories, dynamic posturography, fall scales, motor impairment tests, observations, photographic assessments, postural control tests)
- Gait and locomotion during functional activities with or without the use of assistive, adaptive, orthotic, protective, supportive, or prosthetic devices or equipment (eg, ADL scales, gait indexes, IADL scales, mobility skill profiles, observations, videographic assessments)
- Gait and locomotion with or without the use of assistive, adaptive, orthotic, protective, supportive, or prosthetic devices or equipment (eg, dynamometry, electroneuromyography, footprint analyses, gait indexes, mobility skill profiles, observations, photographic assessments, technology-assisted assessments, videographic assessments, weight-bearing scales, wheelchair mobility tests)
- Safety during gait, locomotion, and balance (eg, confidence scales, diaries, fall scales, functional assessment profiles, logs, reports)

Integumentary Integrity

Associated skin

- Activities, positioning, and postures that produce or relieve trauma to the skin (eg, observations, pressure-sensing maps, scales)
- Assistive, adaptive, orthotic, protective, supportive, or prosthetic devices and equipment that may produce or relieve trauma to the skin (eg, observations, pressure-sensing maps, risk assessment scales)
- Skin characteristics, including blistering, continuity of skin color, dermatitis, hair growth, mobility, nail growth, sensation, temperature, texture, and turgor (eg, observations, palpation, photographic assessments, thermography)

Joint Integrity and Mobility

- Joint integrity and mobility (eg, apprehension, compression and distraction, drawer, glide, impingement, shear, and valgus/varus stress tests; arthrometry; palpation)

Motor Function (Motor Control and Motor Learning)

- Dexterity, coordination, and agility (eg, coordination screens, motor impairment tests, motor proficiency tests, observations, videographic assessments)
- Electrophysiological integrity (eg, electroneuromyography)
- Hand function (eg, fine and gross motor control tests, finger dexterity tests, manipulative ability tests, observations)
- Initiation, modification, and control of movement patterns and voluntary postures (eg, activity indexes, developmental scales, gross motor function profiles, motor scales, movement assessment batteries, neuromotor tests, observations, physical performance tests, postural challenge tests, videographic assessments)

Muscle Performance (Including Strength, Power, and Endurance)

- Electrophysiological integrity (eg, electroneuromyography)
- Muscle strength, power, and endurance (eg, dynamometry, manual muscle tests, muscle performance tests, physical capacity tests, technology-assisted assessments, timed activity tests)
- Muscle strength, power, and endurance during functional activities (eg, ADL scales, functional muscle tests, IADL scales, observations, videographic assessments)
- Muscle tension (eg, palpation)

Neuromotor Development and Sensory Integration

- Acquisition and evolution of motor skills, including age-appropriate development (eg, activity indexes, developmental inventories and questionnaires, learning profiles, motor function tests, motor proficiency assessments, neuromotor assessments, reflex tests, screens, videographic assessments)
- Oral motor function, phonation, and speech production (eg, interviews, observations)
- Sensorimotor integration, including postural, equilibrium, and righting reactions (eg, behavioral assessment scales, motor and processing skill tests, observations, postural challenge tests, reflex tests, sensory profiles, visual perceptual skill tests)

Orthotic, Protective, and Supportive Devices

- Components, alignment, fit, and ability to care for orthotic, protective, and supportive devices and equipment (eg, interviews, logs, observations, pressure-sensing maps, reports)
- Orthotic, protective, and supportive devices and equipment use during functional activities (eg, ADL scales, functional scales, IADL scales, interviews, observations, profiles)
- Remediation of impairments, functional limitations, or disabilities with use of orthotic, protective, and supportive devices and equipment (eg, activity status indexes, ADL scales, aerobic capacity tests, functional performance inventories, health assessment questionnaires, IADL scales, pain scales, play scales, videographic assessments)
- Safety during use of orthotic, protective, and supportive devices and equipment (eg, diaries, fall scales, interviews, logs, observations, reports)

Pain

- Pain, soreness, and nociception (eg, analog scales, discrimination tests, pain drawings and maps, provocation tests, verbal and pictorial descriptor tests)
- Pain in specific body parts (eg, pain indexes, pain questionnaires, structural provocation tests)

Posture

- Postural alignment and position (static and dynamic), including symmetry and deviation from midline (eg, grid measurement, observations, photographic assessments, technology-assisted assessments, videographic assessments)
- Specific body parts (eg, angle assessments, forward-bending test, goniometry, observations, palpation, positional tests)

Range of Motion (ROM) (Including Muscle Length)

- Functional ROM (eg, observations, squat testing, toe touch tests)
- Joint active and passive movement (eg, goniometry, inclinometry, observations, photographic assessments, technology-assisted assessments, videographic assessments)
- Muscle length, soft tissue extensibility, and flexibility (eg, contracture tests, goniometry, inclinometry, ligamentous tests, linear measurement, multisegment flexibility tests, palpation)

Reflex Integrity

- Deep reflexes (eg, myotatic reflex scale, observations, reflex tests)
- Electrophysiological integrity (eg, electroneuromyography)
- Postural reflexes and reactions, including righting, equilibrium, and protective reactions (eg, observations, postural challenge tests, reflex profiles, videographic assessments)
- Primitive reflexes and reactions, including developmental (eg, reflex profiles, screening tests)
- Resistance to passive stretch (eg, tone scales)
- Superficial reflexes and reactions (eg, observations, provocation tests)

Self-Care and Home Management (Including ADL and IADL)

- Ability to gain access to home environments (eg, barrier identification, observations, physical performance tests)
- Ability to perform self-care and home management activities with or without assistive, adaptive, orthotic, protective, supportive, or prosthetic devices and equipment (eg, ADL scales, aerobic capacity tests, IADL scales, interviews, observations, profiles)
- Safety in self-care and home management activities and environments (eg, diaries, fall scales, interviews, logs, observations, reports, videographic assessments)

Sensory Integrity

- Combined/cortical sensations (eg, stereognosis, tactile discrimination tests)
- Deep sensations (eg, kinesthesiometry, observations, photographic assessments, vibration tests)
- Electrophysiological integrity (eg, electroneuromyography)

Ventilation and Respiration/Gas Exchange

- Pulmonary signs of respiration/gas exchange, including breath sounds (eg, gas analyses, observations, oximetry)
- Pulmonary signs of ventilatory function, including airway protection; breath and voice sounds; respiratory rate, rhythm, and pattern; ventilatory flow, forces, and volumes (eg, airway clearance tests, observations, palpation, pulmonary function tests, ventilatory muscle force tests)
- Pulmonary symptoms (eg, dyspnea and perceived exertion indexes and scales)

Work (Job/School/Play), Community, and Leisure Integration or Reintegration (Including IADL)

- Ability to assume or resume work (job/school/play), community, and leisure activities with or without assistive, adaptive, orthotic, protective, supportive, or prosthetic devices and equipment (eg, activity profiles, disability indexes, functional status questionnaires, IADL scales, observations, physical capacity tests)
- Ability to gain access to work (job/school/play), community, and leisure environments (eg, barrier identification, interviews, observations, physical capacity tests, transportation assessments)
- Safety in work (job/school/play), community, and leisure activities and environments (eg, diaries, fall scales, interviews, logs, observations, videographic assessments)

Evaluation, Diagnosis, and Prognosis (Including Plan of Care)

Physical therapists perform *evaluations* (make clinical judgments) based on the data gathered from the history, systems review, and tests and measures. In the evaluation process, physical therapists synthesize the examination data to establish the diagnosis and prognosis (including the plan of care). Factors that influence the complexity of the evaluation include the clinical findings, extent of loss of function, chronicity or severity of the problem, possibility of multisite or multisystem involvement, preexisting condition(s), potential discharge destination, social considerations, physical function, and overall health status.

A *diagnosis* is a label encompassing a cluster of signs and symptoms, syndromes, or categories. It is the result of the systematic diagnostic process, which includes integrating and evaluating the data from the examination. The diagnostic label indicates the primary dysfunction(s) toward which the therapist will direct interventions. The *prognosis* is the determination of the predicted optimal level of improvement in function and the amount of time needed to reach that level and may also include a prediction of levels of improvement that may be reached at various intervals during the course of therapy. During the prognostic process, the physical therapist develops the plan of care. The *plan of care* identifies specific interventions, proposed frequency and duration of the interventions, anticipated goals, expected outcomes, and discharge plans. The plan of care identifies realistic anticipated goals and expected outcomes, taking into consideration the expectations of the patient/client and appropriate others. These anticipated goals and expected outcomes should be measureable and time limited.

The frequency of visits and duration of the episode of care may vary from a short episode with a high intensity of intervention to a longer episode with a diminishing intensity of intervention. Frequency and duration may vary greatly among patients/clients based on a variety of factors that the physical therapist considers throughout the evaluation process, such as anatomical and physiological changes related to growth and development; caregiver consistency or expertise; chronicity or severity of the current condition; living environment; multisite or multisystem involvement; social support; potential discharge destinations; probability of prolonged impairment, functional limitation, or disability; and stability of the condition.

Prognosis

Over the course of 12 months, patient/client will demonstrate optimal motor function and sensory integrity and the highest level of functioning in home, work (job/school/play), community, and leisure environments, within the context of the impairments, functional limitations, and disabilities.

During the episode of care, patient/client will achieve (1) the anticipated goals and expected outcomes of the interventions that are described in the plan of care and (2) the global outcomes for patients/clients who are classified in this pattern.

Expected Range of Number of Visits Per Episode of Care

10 to 60

This range represents the lower and upper limits of the number of physical therapist visits required to achieve anticipated goals and expected outcomes. *It is anticipated that 80% of patients/clients who are classified into this pattern will achieve the anticipated goals and expected outcomes within 10 to 60 visits during a single continuous episode of care.* Frequency of visits and duration of the episode of care should be determined by the physical therapist to maximize effectiveness of care and efficiency of service delivery.

Note:

These patients/clients may require multiple episodes of care over the lifetime to ensure safety and effective adaptation following changes in physical status, caregivers, environment, or task demands. Factors that may lead to these additional episodes of care include:

- Cognitive maturation
- Periods of rapid growth

Factors That May Require New Episode of Care or That May Modify Frequency of Visits/Duration of Care

- Accessibility and availability of resources
- Adherence to the intervention program
- Age
- Anatomical and physiological changes related to growth and development
- Caregiver consistency or expertise
- Chronicity or severity of the current condition
- Cognitive status
- Comorbitities, complications, or secondary impairments
- Concurrent medical, surgical, and therapeutic interventions
- Decline in functional independence
- Level of impairment
- Level of physical function
- Living environment
- Multisite or multisystem involvement
- Nutritional status
- Overall health status
- Potential discharge destinations
- Premorbid conditions
- Probability of prolonged impairment, functional limitation, or disability
- Psychological and socioeconomic factors
- Psychomotor abilities
- Social support
- Stability of the condition

Intervention

Intervention is the purposeful interaction of the physical therapist with the patient/client and, when appropriate, with other individuals involved in patient/client care, using various physical therapy procedures and techniques to produce changes in the condition consistent with the diagnosis and prognosis. Decisions about interventions are contingent on the timely monitoring of patient/client response and the progress made toward achieving the anticipated goals and expected outcomes.

Communication, coordination, and documentation and patient/client-related instruction are provided for all patients/clients across all settings. Procedural interventions are selected or modified based on the examination data and the evaluation, the diagnosis and the prognosis, and the anticipated goals and expected outcomes for a particular patient/client. *For clinical considerations in selecting interventions, listings of interventions, and listings of anticipated goals and expected outcomes, refer to Chapter 3.*

Coordination, Communication, and Documentation

Coordination, communication, and documentation may include:

Interventions

- Addressing required functions
  - advance directives
  - individualized family service plans (IFSPs) or individualized education plans (IEPs)
  - informed consent
  - mandatory communication and reporting (eg, patient advocacy and abuse reporting)
- Admission and discharge planning
- Case management
- Collaboration and coordination with agencies, including:
  - equipment suppliers
  - home care agencies
  - payer groups
  - schools
  - transportation agencies
- Communication across settings, including:
  - case conferences
  - documentation
  - education plans
- Cost-effective resource utilization
- Data collection, analysis, and reporting
  - outcome data
  - peer review findings
  - record reviews
- Documentation across settings, following APTA's *Guidelines for Physical Therapy Documentation* (Appendix 5), including:
  - changes in impairments, functional limitations, and disabilities
  - changes in interventions
  - elements of patient/client management (examination, evaluation, diagnosis, prognosis, intervention)
  - outcomes of intervention
- Interdisciplinary teamwork
  - case conferences
  - patient care rounds
  - patient/client family meetings
- Referrals to other professionals or resources

Anticipated Goals and Expected Outcomes

- Accountability for services is increased.
- Admission data and discharge planning are completed.
- Advance directives, individualized family service plans (IFSPs) or individualized education plans (IEPs), informed consent, and mandatory communication and reporting (eg, patient advocacy and abuse reporting) are obtained or completed.
- Available resources are maximally utilized.
- Care is coordinated with patient/client, family, significant others, caregivers, and other professionals.
- Case is managed throughout the episode of care.
- Collaboration and coordination occurs with agencies, including equipment suppliers, home care agencies, payer groups, schools, and transportation agencies.
- Communication enhances risk reduction and prevention.
- Communication occurs across settings through case conferences, education plans, and documentation.
- Data are collected, analyzed, and reported, including outcome data, peer review findings, and record reviews.
- Decision making is enhanced regarding health, wellness, and fitness needs.
- Decision making is enhanced regarding patient/client health and the use of health care resources by patient/client, family, significant others, and caregivers.
- Documentation occurs throughout patient/client management and across settings and follows APTA's *Guidelines for Physical Therapy Documentation* (Appendix 5).
- Interdisciplinary collaboration occurs through case conferences, patient care rounds, and patient/client family meetings.
- Patient/client, family, significant other, and caregiver understanding of anticipated goals and expected outcomes is increased.
- Placement needs are determined.
- Referrals are made to other professionals or resources whenever necessary and appropriate.
- Resources are utilized in a cost-effective way.

Patient/Client-Related Instruction

Patient/client-related instruction may include:

Interventions

- Instruction, education and training of patients/clients and caregivers regarding:
  - current condition (pathology/pathophysiology [disease, disorder, or condition], impairments, functional limitations, or disabilities)
  - enhancement of performance
  - health, wellness, and fitness programs
  - plan of care
  - risk factors for pathology/pathophysiology (disease, disorder, or condition), impairments, functional limitations, or disabilities
  - transitions across settings
  - transitions to new roles

Anticipated Goals and Expected Outcomes

- Ability to perform physical actions, tasks, or activities is improved.
- Awareness and use of community resources are improved.
- Behaviors that foster healthy habits, wellness, and prevention are acquired.
- Decision making is enhanced regarding patient/client health and the use of health care resources by patient/client, family, significant others, and caregivers.
- Disability associated with acute or chronic illnesses is reduced.
- Functional independence in activities of daily living (ADL) and instrumental activities of daily living (IADL) is increased.
- Health status is improved.
- Intensity of care is decreased.
- Level of supervision required for task performance is decreased.
- Patient/client, family, significant other, and caregiver knowledge and awareness of the diagnosis, prognosis, interventions, and anticipated goals and expected outcomes are increased.
- Patient/client knowledge of personal and environmental factors associated with the condition is increased.
- Performance levels in self-care, home management, work (job/school/play), community, or leisure actions, tasks, or activities are improved.
- Physical functio is improved.
- Risk of recurrence of condition is reduced.
- Risk of secondary impairment is reduced.
- Safety of patient/client, family, significant others, and caregivers is improved.
- Self-management of symptoms is improved.
- Utilization and cost of health care services are decreased.

Procedural interventions for this pattern may include:

Therapeutic Exercise

Interventions

- Aerobic and endurance conditioning or reconditioning
  - aquatic programs
  - gait and locomotor training
  - increased workload over time
  - walking and wheelchair propulsion programs
- Balance, coordination, and agility training
  - developmental activities training
  - motor function (motor control and motor learning) training or retraining
  - neuromuscular education or reeducation
  - perceptual training
  - posture awareness training
  - standardized, programmatic, complementary exercise approaches
  - sensory training or retraining
  - task-specific performance training
  - vestibular training
- Body mechanics and postural stabilization
  - body mechanics training
  - posture awareness training
  - postural control training
  - postural stabilization activities
- Flexibility exercises
  - muscle lengthening
  - range of motion
  - stretching
- Gait and locomotion training
  - developmental activities training
  - gait training
  - implement and device training
  - perceptual training
  - standardized, programmatic, complementary exercise approaches
  - wheelchair training
- Neuromotor development training
  - developmental activities training
  - motor training
  - movement pattern training
  - neuromuscular education or reeducation
- Relaxation
  - breathing strategies
  - movement strategies
  - relaxation techniques
  - standardized, programmatic, complementary exercise approaches
- Strength, power, and endurance training for head, neck, limb, pelvic-floor, trunk, and ventilatory muscles
  - active assistive, active, and resistive exercises (including concentric, dynamic/isotonic, eccentric, isokinetic, isometric, and plyometric)
  - aquatic programs
  - standardized, programmatic, complementary exercise approaches
  - task-specific performance training

Anticipated Goals and Expected Outcomes

- Impact on pathology/pathophysiology (disease, disorder, or condition)
  - Joint swelling, inflammation, or restriction is reduced.
  - Nutrient delivery to tissue is increased.
  - Osteogenic effects of exercise are maximized.
  - Pain is decreased.
  - Physiological response to increased oxygen demand is improved.
  - Soft tissue swelling, inflammation, or restriction is reduced.
  - Tissue perfusion and oxygenation are enhanced.
- Impact on impairments
  - Aerobic capacity is increased.
  - Balance is improved.
  - Endurance is increased.
  - Energy expenditure per unit of work is decreased.
  - Gait, locomotion, and balance are improved.
  - Integumentary integrity is improved.
  - Joint integrity and mobility are improved.
  - Motor function (motor control and motor learning) is improved.
  - Muscle performance (strength, power, and endurance) is increased.
  - Postural control is improved.
  - Quality and quantity of movement between and across body segments are improved.
  - Range of motion is improved.
  - Relaxation is increased.
  - Sensory awareness is increased.
  - Weight-bearing status is improved.
  - Work of breathing is decreased.
- Impact on functional limitations
  - Ability to perform physical actions, tasks, or activities related to self-care, home management, work (job/school/play), community, and leisure is improved.
  - Level of supervision required for task performance is decreased.
  - Performance of and independence in activities of daily living (ADL) and instrumental activities of daily living (IADL) with or without devices and equipment are increased.
  - Tolerance of positions and activities is increased.
- Impact on disabilities
  - Ability to assume or resume required self-care, home management, work (job/school/play), community, and leisure roles is improved.
- Risk reduction/prevention
  - Preoperative and postoperative complications are reduced.
  - Risk factors are reduced.
  - Risk of recurrence of condition is reduced.
  - Risk of secondary impairment is reduced.
  - Safety is improved.
  - Self-management of symptoms is improved.
- Impact on health, wellness, and fitness
  - Fitness is improved.
  - Health status is improved.
  - Physical capacity is increased.
  - Physical function is improved.
- Impact on societal resources
  - Utilization of physical therapy services is optimized.
  - Utilization of physical therapy services results in efficient use of health care dollars.
- Patient/client satisfaction
  - Access, availability, and services provided are acceptable to patient/client.
  - Administrative management of practice is acceptable to patient/client.
  - Clinical proficiency of physical therapist is acceptable to patient/client.
  - Coordination of care is acceptable to patient/client.
  - Cost of health care services is decreased.
  - Intensity of care is decreased.
  - Interpersonal skills of physical therapist are acceptable to patient/client, family, and significant others.
  - Sense of well-being is improved.
  - Stressors are decreased.

Functional Training in Self-Care and Home Management (Including Activities of Daily Living (ADL) and Instrumental Activities of Daily Living(IADL)

Interventions

- ADL training
  - bathing
  - bed mobility and transfer training
  - developmental activities
  - dressing
  - eating
  - grooming
  - toileting
- Devices and equipment use and training
  - assistive and adaptive device or equipment training during activities of daily living (ADL) and instrumental activities of daily living (IADL)
  - orthotic, protective, or supportive device or equipment training during ADL and IADL
  - prosthetic device or equipment training during ADL and IADL
- Functional training programs
  - simulated environments and tasks
  - task adaptation
  - travel training
- IADL training
  - caring for dependents
  - home maintenance
  - household chores
  - shopping
  - yard work
- Injury prevention or reduction
  - injury prevention education during self-care and home management
  - injury prevention or reduction with use of devices and equipment
  - safety awareness training during self-care and home management

Anticipated Goals and Expected Outcomes

- Impact on pathology/pathophysiology (disease, disorder, or condition)
  - Pain is decreased.
  - Physiological response to increased oxygen demand is improved.
  - Symptoms associated with increased oxygen demand are decreased.
- Impact on impairments
  - Balance is improved.
  - Endurance is increased.
  - Energy expenditure per unit of work is decreased.
  - Motor function (motor control and motor learning) is improved.
  - Muscle performance (strength, power, and endurance) is increased.
  - Postural control is improved.
  - Sensory awareness is increased.
  - Weight-bearing status is improved.
  - Work of breathing is decreased.
- Impact on functional limitations
  - Ability to perform physical actions, tasks, or activities related to self-care and home management is improved.
  - Level of supervision required for task performance is decreased.
  - Performance of and independence in ADL and IADL with or without devices and equipment are increased.
  - Tolerance of positions and activities is increased.
- Impact on disabilities
  - Ability to assume or resume required self-care and home management roles is improved.
- Risk reduction/prevention
  - Risk factors are reduced.
  - Risk of secondary impairments is reduced.
  - Safety is improved.
  - Self-management of symptoms is improved.
- Impact on health, wellness, and fitness
  - Health status is improved.
  - Physical capacity is increased.
  - Physical function is improved.
- Impact on societal resources
  - Utilization of physical therapy services is optimized.
  - Utilization of physical therapy services results in efficient use of health care dollars.
- Patient/client satisfaction
  - Access, availability, and services provided are acceptable to patient/client.
  - Administrative management of practice is acceptable to patient/client.
  - Clinical proficiency of physical therapist is acceptable to patient/client.
  - Coordination of care is acceptable to patient/client.
  - Cost of health care services is decreased.
  - Intensity of care is decreased.
  - Interpersonal skills of physical therapist are acceptable to patient/client, family, and significant others.
  - Sense of well-being is improved.
  - Stressors are decreased.

Functional Training in Work (Job/School/Play), Community, and Leisure Integration or Reintegration (Including Instrumental Activities of Daily Living [IADL] and Work Conditioning)

Interventions

- Devices and equipment use and training
  - assistive and adaptive device or equipment training during IADL
  - orthotic, protective, or supportive device or equipment training during IADL
- Functional training programs
  - back schools
  - job coaching
  - simulated environments and tasks
  - task adaptation
  - task training
  - travel training
- IADL training
  - community service training involving instruments
  - school and play activities training including tools and instruments
  - work training with tools
- Injury prevention or reduction
  - injury prevention education during work (job/school/play), community, and leisure integration or reintegration
  - injury prevention or reduction with use of devices and equipment
  - safety awareness training during work (job/school/play), community, and leisure integration or reintegration
- Leisure and play activities training

Anticipated Goals and Expected Outcomes

- Impact on pathology/pathophysiology (disease, disorder, or condition)
  - Pain is decreased.
  - Physiological response to increased oxygen demand is improved.
  - Symptoms associated with increased oxygen demand are decreased.
- Impact on impairments
  - Balance is improved.
  - Endurance is increased.
  - Energy expenditure per unit of work is decreased.
  - Motor function (motor control and motor learning) is improved.
  - Muscle performance (strength, power, and endurance) is increased.
  - Postural control is improved.
  - Sensory awareness is increased.
  - Weight-bearing status is improved.
  - Work of breathing is decreased.
- Impact on functional limitations
  - Ability to perform physical actions, tasks, or activities related to work (job/school/play), community, and leisure integration or reintegration is improved.
  - Level of supervision required for task performance is decreased.
  - Performance of and independence in IADL with or without devices and equipment are increased.
  - Tolerance of positions and activities is increased.
- Impact on disabilities
  - Ability to assume or resume required work (job/school/play), community, and leisure roles is improved.
- Risk reduction/prevention
  - Risk factors are reduced.
  - Risk of secondary impairment is reduced.
  - Safety is improved.
  - Self-management of symptoms is improved.
- Impact on health, wellness, and fitness
  - Fitness is improved.
  - Health status is improved.
  - Physical capacity is increased.
  - Physical function is improved.
- Impact on societal resources
  - Costs of work-related injury or disability are reduced.
  - Utilization of physical therapy services is optimized.
  - Utilization of physical therapy services results in efficient use of health care dollars.
- Patient/client satisfaction
  - Access, availability, and services provided are acceptable to patient/client.
  - Administrative management of practice is acceptable to patient/client.
  - Clinical proficiency of physical therapist is acceptable to patient/client.
  - Coordination of care is acceptable to patient/client.
  - Cost of health care services is decreased.
  - Intensity of care is decreased.
  - Interpersonal skills of physical therapist are acceptable to patient/client, family, and significant others.
  - Sense of well-being is improved.
  - Stressors are decreased.

Manual Therapy Techniques (Including Mobilization/Manipulation)

Interventions

- Massage
  - connective tissue massage
  - therapeutic massage
- Mobilization/manipulation
  - soft tissue
- Passive range of motion

Anticipated Goals and Expected Outcomes

- Impact on pathology/pathophysiology (disease, disorder, or condition)
  - Edema, lymphedema, or effusion is reduced.
  - Joint swelling, inflammation, or restriction is reduced.
  - Pain is decreased.
  - Soft tissue swelling, inflammation, or restriction is reduced.
- Impact on impairments
  - Balance is improved.
  - Energy expenditure per unit of work is decreased.
  - Gait, locomotion, and balance are improved.
  - Integumentary integrity is improved.
  - Muscle performance (strength, power, and endurance) is increased.
  - Postural control is improved.
  - Quality and quantity of movement between and across body segments are improved.
  - Range of motion is improved.
  - Relaxation is increased.
  - Sensory awareness is increased.
  - Weight-bearing status is improved.
  - Work of breathing is decreased.
- Impact on functional limitations
  - Ability to perform movement tasks is improved.
  - Ability to perform physical actions, tasks, or activities related to self-care, home management, work (job/school/play), community, and leisure is improved.
  - Tolerance of positions and activities is increased.
- Impact on disabilities
  - Ability to assume or resume required self-care, home management, work (job/school/play), community, and leisure roles is improved.
- Risk reduction/prevention
  - Risk factors are reduced.
  - Risk of secondary impairment is reduced.
  - Self-management of symptoms is improved.
- Impact on health, wellness, and fitness
  - Physical capacity is increased.
  - Physical function is improved.
- Impact on societal resources
  - Utilization of physical therapy services is optimized.
  - Utilization of physical therapy services results in efficient use of health care dollars.
- Patient/client satisfaction
  - Access, availability, and services provided are acceptable to patient/client.
  - Administrative management of practice is acceptable to patient/client.
  - Clinical proficiency of physical therapist is acceptable to patient/client.
  - Coordination of care is acceptable to patient/client.
  - Cost of health care services is decreased.
  - Intensity of care is decreased.
  - Interpersonal skills of physical therapist are acceptable to patient/client, family, and significant others.
  - Sense of well-being is improved.
  - Stressors are decreased.

Prescription, Application, and, as Appropriate, Fabrication of Devices and Equipment (Assistive, Adaptive, Orthotic, Protective, Supportive, and Prosthetic)

Interventions

- Adaptive devices
  - environmental controls
  - hospital beds
  - raised toilet seats
  - seating systems
- Assistive devices
  - canes
  - crutches
  - long-handled reachers
  - power devices
  - static and dynamic splints
  - walkers
  - wheelchairs
- Orthotic devices
  - braces
  - casts
  - shoe inserts
  - splints
- Protective devices
  - braces
  - cushions
  - helmets
  - protective taping
- Supportive devices
  - compression garments
  - corsets
  - elastic wraps
  - neck collars
  - serial casts
  - slings
  - supplemental oxygen
  - supportive taping

Anticipated Goals and Expected Outcomes

- Impact on pathology/pathophysiology (disease, disorder, or condition)
  - Edema, lymphedema, or effusion is reduced.
  - Joint swelling, inflammation, or restriction is reduced.
  - Pain is decreased.
  - Physiological response to increased oxygen demand is improved.
  - Soft tissue swelling, inflammation, or restriction is reduced.
  - Symptoms associated with increased oxygen demand are decreased.
- Impact on impairments
  - Balance is improved.
  - Endurance is increased.
  - Energy expenditure per unit of work is decreased.
  - Gait, locomotion, and balance are improved.
  - Integumentary integrity is improved.
  - Joint stability is improved.
  - Motor function (motor control and motor learning) is improved.
  - Muscle performance (strength, power, and endurance) is increased.
  - Optimal joint alignment is achieved.
  - Optimal loading on a body part is achieved.
  - Postural control is improved.
  - Quality and quantity of movement between and across body segments are improved.
  - Range of motion is improved.
  - Weight-bearing status is improved.
  - Work of breathing is decreased.
- Impact on functional limitations
  - Ability to perform physical actions, tasks, or activities related to self-care, home management, work (job/school/play), community, and leisure is improved.
  - Level of supervision required for task performance is decreased.
  - Performance of and independence in activities of daily living (ADL) and instrumental activities of daily living (IADL) with or without devices and equipment are increased.
  - Tolerance of positions and activities is increased.
- Impact on disabilities
  - Ability to assume or resume required self-care, home management, work (job/school/play), community, and leisure roles is improved.
- Risk reduction/prevention
  - Pressure on body tissues is reduced.
  - Protection of body parts is increased.
  - Risk factors are reduced.
  - Risk of secondary impairment is reduced.
  - Safety is improved.
  - Self-management of symptoms is improved.
  - Stresses precipitating injury are decreased.
- Impact on health, wellness, and fitness
  - Health status is improved.
  - Physical capacity is increased.
  - Physical function is improved.
- Impact on societal resources
  - Utilization of physical therapy services is optimized.
  - Utilization of physical therapy services results in efficient use of health care dollars.
- Patient/client satisfaction
  - Access, availability, and services provided are acceptable to patient/client.
  - Administrative management of practice is acceptable to patient/client.
  - Clinical proficiency of physical therapist is acceptable to patient/client.
  - Coordination of care is acceptable to patient/client.
  - Cost of health care services is decreased.
  - Intensity of care is decreased.
  - Interpersonal skills of physical therapist are acceptable to patient/client, family, and significant others.
  - Sense of well-being is improved.
  - Stressors are decreased.

Airway Clearance Techniques

Interventions

- Breathing strategies
  - active cycle of breathing or forced expiratory techniques
  - assisted cough/huff techniques
  - autogenic drainage
  - paced breathing
  - pursed lip breathing
  - techniques to maximize ventilation (eg, maximum inspiratory hold, staircase breathing, manual hyperinflation)
- Manual/mechanical techniques
  - assistive devices
  - chest percussion, vibration, and shaking
  - chest wall manipulation
  - suctioning
  - ventilatory aids
- Positioning
  - positioning to alter work of breathing
  - positioning to maximize ventilation and perfusion
  - pulmonary postural drainage

Anticipated Goals and Expected Outcomes

- Impact on pathology/pathophysiology (disease, disorder, or condition)
  - Atelectasis is decreased.
  - Nutrient delivery to tissue is increased.
  - Physiological response to increased oxygen demand is improved.
  - Symptoms associated with increased oxygen demand are decreased.
  - Tissue perfusion and oxygenation are enhanced.
- Impact on impairments
  - Aerobic capacity is increased.
  - Airway clearance is improved.
  - Cough is improved.
  - Endurance is increased.
  - Energy expenditure per unit of work is decreased.
  - Exercise tolerance is improved.
  - Muscle performance (strength, power, and endurance) is increased.
  - Ventilation and respiration/gas exchange are improved.
  - Work of breathing is decreased.
- Impact on functional limitations
  - Ability to perform physical actions, tasks, or activities related to self-care, home management, work (job/school/play), community, and leisure is improved.
  - Performance of and independence in activities of daily living (ADL) and instrumental activities of daily living (IADL) with or without devices and equipment are increased.
  - Tolerance of positions and activities is increased.
- Impact on disabilities
  - Ability to assume or resume required self-care, home management, work (job/school/play), community, and leisure roles is improved.
- Risk reduction/prevention
  - Preoperative and postoperative complications are reduced.
  - Risk factors are reduced.
  - Risk of recurrence of condition is reduced.
  - Risk of secondary impairment is reduced.
  - Safety is improved.
  - Self-management of symptoms is improved.
- Impact on health, wellness, and fitness
  - Fitness is improved.
  - Health status is improved.
  - Physical capacity is increased.
  - Physical function is improved.
- Impact on societal resources
  - Utilization of physical therapy services is optimized.
  - Utilization of physical therapy services results in efficient use of health care dollars.
- Patient/client satisfaction
  - Access, availability, and services provided are acceptable to patient/client.
  - Administrative management of practice is acceptable to patient/client.
  - Clinical proficiency of physical therapist is acceptable to patient/client.
  - Coordination of care is acceptable to patient/client.
  - Cost of health care services is decreased.
  - Intensity of care is decreased.
  - Interpersonal skills of physical therapist are acceptable to patient/client, family, and significant others.
  - Sense of well-being is improved.
  - Stressors are decreased.

Electrotherapeutic Modalities

Interventions

- Biofeedback
- Electrical stimulation
  - electrical muscle stimulation (EMS)
  - functional electrical stimulation (FES)
  - transcutaneous electrical nerve stimulation (TENS)

Anticipated Goals and Expected Outcomes

- Impact on pathology/pathophysiology (disease, disorder, or condition)
  - Edema, lymphedema, or effusion is reduced.
  - Joint swelling, inflammation, or restriction is reduced.
  - Nutrient delivery to tissue is increased.
  - Osteogenic effects are enhanced.
  - Pain is decreased.
  - Soft tissue swelling, inflammation, or restriction is reduced.
  - Tissue perfusion and oxygenation are enhanced.
- Impact on impairments
  - Integumentary integrity is improved.
  - Motor function (motor control and motor learning) is improved.
  - Muscle performance (strength, power, and endurance) is increased.
  - Postural control is improved.
  - Quality and quantity of movement between and across body segments are improved.
  - Range of motion is improved.
  - Relaxation is increased.
  - Sensory awareness is increased.
- Impact on functional limitations
  - Ability to perform physical actions, tasks, or activities related to self-care, home management, work (job/school/play), community, and leisure is improved.
  - Level of supervision required for task performance is decreased.
  - Performance of and independence in activities of daily living (ADL) and instrumental activities of daily living (IADL) with or without devices and equipment are increased.
  - Tolerance of positions and activities is increased.
- Impact on disabilities
  - Ability to assume or resume required self-care, home management, work (job/school/play), community, and leisure roles is improved.
- Risk reduction/prevention
  - Complications of immobility are reduced.
  - Preoperative and postoperative complications are reduced.
  - Risk factors are reduced.
  - Risk of secondary impairment is reduced.
  - Self-management of symptoms is improved.
- Impact on health, wellness, and fitness
  - Physical capacity is increased.
  - Physical function is improved.
- Impact on societal resources
  - Utilization of physical therapy services is optimized.
  - Utilization of physical therapy services results in efficient use of health care dollars.
- Patient/client satisfaction
  - Access, availability, and services provided are acceptable to patient/client.
  - Administrative management of practice is acceptable to patient/client.
  - Clinical proficiency of physical therapist is acceptable to patient/client.
  - Coordination of care is acceptable to patient/client.
  - Interpersonal skills of physical therapist are acceptable to patient/client, family, and significant others.
  - Sense of well-being is improved.
  - Stressors are decreased.

Physical Agents and Mechanical Modalities

Interventions

Physical agents may include:

- Cryotherapy
  - cold packs
  - ice massage
  - vapocoolant spray
- Hydrotherapy
  - whirlpool tanks
  - pools
- Sound agents
  - phonophoresis
  - ultrasound
- Thermotherapy
  - dry heat
  - hot packs
  - paraffin baths

Mechanical modalities may include:

- Compression therapies
  - compression bandaging
  - compression garments
  - taping
- Gravity-assisted compression devices
  - standing frame
  - tilt table

Anticipated Goals and Expected Outcomes

- Impact on pathology/pathophysiology (disease, disorder, or condition)
  - Edema, lymphedema, or effusion is reduced.
  - Joint swelling, inflammation, or restriction is reduced.
  - Nutrient delivery to tissue is increased.
  - Pain is decreased.
  - Soft tissue swelling, inflammation, or restriction is reduced.
  - Tissue perfusion and oxygenation are enhanced.
- Impact on impairments
  - Integumentary integrity is improved.
  - Muscle performance (strength, power, and endurance) is increased.
  - Range of motion is improved.
  - Weight-bearing status is improved.
- Impact on functional limitations
  - Ability to perform physical actions, tasks, or activities related to self-care, home management, work (job/school/play), community, and leisure is improved.
  - Performance of and independence in activities of daily living (ADL) and instrumental activities of daily living (IADL) with or without devices and equipment are increased.
  - Tolerance of positions and activities is increased.
- Impact on disabilities
  - Ability to assume or resume required self-care, home management, work (job/school/play), community, and leisure roles is improved.
- Risk reduction/prevention
  - Complications of soft tissue and circulatory disorders are decreased.
  - Risk of secondary impairment is reduced.
  - Self-management of symptoms is improved.
  - Stresses precipitating injury are decreased.
- Impact on health, wellness, and fitness
  - Physical function is improved.
- Impact on societal resources
  - Utilization of physical therapy services is optimized.
- Patient/client satisfaction
  - Access, availability, and services provided are acceptable to patient/client.
  - Administrative management of practice is acceptable to patient/client.
  - Clinical proficiency of physical therapist is acceptable to patient/client.
  - Coordination of care is acceptable to patient/client.
  - Interpersonal skills of physical therapist are acceptable to patient/client, family, and significant others.
  - Sense of well-being is improved.
  - Stressors are decreased.

Reexamination

Reexamination is the process of performing selected tests and measures after the initial examination to evaluate progress and to modify or redirect interventions. Reexamination may be indicated more than once during a single episode of care. It also may be performed over the course of a disease, disorder, or condition, which for some patients/clients may be over the life span. Indications for reexamination include new clinical findings or failure to respond to physical therapy interventions.

Global Outcomes for Patients/Clients in This Pattern

Throughout the entire episode of care, the physical therapist determines the anticipated goals and expected outcomes for each intervention. These anticipated goals and expected outcomes are delineated in shaded boxes that accompany the lists of interventions in each preferred practice pattern. As the patient/client reaches the termination of physical therapy services and the end of the episode of care, the physical therapist measures the global outcomes of the physical therapy services by characterizing or quantifying the impact of the physical therapy interventions in the following domains:

- Pathology/pathophysiology (disease, disorder, or condition)
- Impairments
- Functional limitations
- Disabilities
- Risk reduction/prevention
- Health, wellness, and fitness
- Societal resources
- Patient/client satisfaction

In some instances, a particular anticipated goal or expected outcome is thoroughly achieved through implementation of a single form of intervention. More commonly, however, the anticipated goals and expected outcomes are achieved as a result of the combined effects of several forms of interventions, leading to enhancement of both health status and health-related quality of life.

Criteria for Termination of Physical Therapy Services

Discharge is the process of ending physical therapy services that have been provided during a single episode of care. It occurs when the anticipated goals and expected outcomes have been achieved. Discharge does *not* occur with a *transfer* (defined as the time when a patient is moved from one site to another site within the same setting or across settings during a single episode of care). Although there may be facility-specific or payer-specific requirements for documentation regarding the conclusion of physical therapy services, *discharge occurs based on the physical therapist's analysis of the achievement of anticipated goals and expected outcomes.*

Discontinuation is the process of ending physical therapy services that have been provided during a single episode of care when (1) the patient/client, caregiver, or legal guardian declines to continue intervention; (2) the patient/client is unable to continue to progress toward outcomes because of medical or psychosocial complications or because financial/insurance resources have been expended; or (3) the physical therapist determines that the patient/client will no longer benefit from physical therapy. When physical therapy services are terminated prior to achievement of anticipated goals and expected outcomes, patient/client status and the rationale for termination are documented.

For patients/clients who require multiple episodes of care, periodic follow-up is needed over the life span to ensure safety and effective adaptation following changes in physical status, caregivers, environment, or task demands. In consultation with appropriate individuals, and in consideration of the outcomes, the physical therapist plans for discharge or discontinuation and provides for appropriate follow-up or referral.

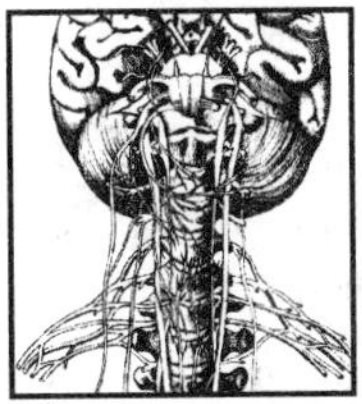

Impaired Motor Function and Sensory Integrity Associated With Progressive Disorders of the Central Nervous System

This preferred practice pattern describes the generally accepted elements of patient/client management that physical therapists provide for patients/clients who are classified in this pattern. The pattern title reflects the diagnosis made by the physical therapist. APTA emphasizes that preferred practice patterns are the boundaries within which a physical therapist may select any of a number of clinical alternatives, based on consideration of a wide variety of factors, such as individual patient/client needs; the profession's code of ethics and standards of practice; and patient/client age, culture, gender roles, race, sex, sexual orientation, and socioeconomic status.

Patient/Client Diagnostic Classification

Patients/clients will be classified into this pattern—for impaired motor function and sensory integrity associated with progressive disorders of the central nervous system—as a result of the physical therapist's evaluation of the examination data. The findings from the examination (history, systems review, and tests and measures) may indicate the presence or risk of pathology/ pathophysiology, impairments, functional limitations, or disabilities or the need for health, wellness, or fitness programs. The physical therapist integrates, synthesizes, and interprets the data to determine the diagnostic classification.

Inclusion

The following examples of examination findings may support the inclusion of patients/clients in this pattern:

Risk Factors or Consequences of Pathology/Pathophysiology (Disease, Disorder, or Condition)

- Acquired immune deficiency syndrome
- Alcoholic ataxia
- Alzheimer disease
- Amyotrophic lateral sclerosis
- Basal ganglia disease
- Cerebellar ataxia
- Cerebellar disease
- Huntington disease
- Idiopathic progressive cortical disease
- Intracranial neurosurgical procedures
- Multiple sclerosis
- Neoplasm
- Parkinson disease
- Primary lateral palsy
- Progressive muscular atrophy
- Seizures

Impairments, Functional Limitations, or Disabilities

- Difficulty coordinating movement
- Difficulty with manipulation skills
- Difficulty negotiating terrains
- Frequent falls
- Impaired affect
- Impaired arousal, attention, and cognition
- Impaired endurance
- Impaired motor function
- Impaired sensory integrity
- Loss of balance during daily activities
- Progressive loss of function
- Inability to keep up with peers
- Inability to negotiate community environment
- Inability to perform job/school activities
- Lack of safety in home environment

Note:

Some risk factors or consequences of pathology/pathophysiology—such as *neoplasm*—may be severe and complex; *however, they do not necessarily exclude patients/clients from this pattern*. Severe and complex risk factors or consequences may require modification of the frequency of visits and duration of care. (See "Evaluation, Diagnosis, and Prognosis," page 381.)

Exclusion or Multiple-Pattern Classification

The following examples of examination findings may support exclusion from this pattern or classification into additional patterns. Depending on the level of severity or complexity of the examination findings, the physical therapist may determine that the patient/client would be more appropriately managed through (1) classification in an entirely different pattern or (2) classification in both this and another pattern.

Findings That May Require Classification in a Different Pattern

- Amputation
- Coma

Findings That May Require Classification in Additional Patterns

- Amyotrophic lateral sclerosis with pneumonia
- Parkinson disease with arthritis

ICD-9-CM Codes

The listing below contains the current (as of press time) and most typical 3- and 4-digit ICD-9-CM codes related to this preferred practice pattern. Because patient/client diagnostic classification is based on impairments, functional limitations, and disabilities—not on codes—patients/clients may be classified into the pattern even though the codes listed with the pattern may not apply to those clients.

This listing is intended for general information only and should not be used for coding purposes. The codes should be confirmed by referring to the World Health Organization's *International Classification of Diseases, 9th Revision, Clinical Modification (ICD-9-CM 2001)*, Volumes 1 and 3 (Chicago, Ill: American Medical Association; 2000) or subsequent revisions or by referring to other ICD-9-CM coding manuals that contain exclusion notes and instructions regarding fifth-digit requirements.

042 Human immunodeficiency virus [HIV] disease

191 Malignant neoplasm of brain

192 Malignant neoplasm of other and unspecified parts of nervous system

237 Neoplasm of uncertain behavior of endocrine glands and nervous system

- **237.5** Brain and spinal cord

303 Alcohol dependence syndrome

- **303.9** Ataxia

331 Other cerebral degenerations

- **331.0** Alzheimer's disease
- **331.3** Communicating hydrocephalus
- **331.4** Obstructive hydrocephalus

332 Parkinson's disease

333 Other extrapyramidal disease and abnormal movement disorders

- **333.0** Other degenerative diseases of the basal ganglia
- **333.3** Tics of organic origin
- **333.4** Huntington's chorea
- **333.9** Other and unspecified extrapyramidal diseases and abnormal movement disorders

334 Spinocerebellar disease

- **334.2** Primary cerebellar degeneration
- **334.3** Other cerebellar ataxia
- **334.8** Other spinocerebellar diseases

335 Anterior horn cell disease

- **335.0** Werdnig-Hoffmann disease
- **335.1** Spinal muscular atrophy
- **335.2** Motor neuron disease

336 Other diseases of spinal cord

- **336.0** Syringomyelia and syringobulbia

340 Multiple sclerosis

341 Other demyelinating diseases of central nervous system

- **341.8** Other demyelinating diseases of central nervous system
  Central demyelination of corpus callosum
- **341.9** Demyelinating disease of central nervous system, unspecified

345 Epilepsy

- **345.4** Partial epilepsy, with impairment of consciousness
  Epilepsy:
    partial:
      secondarily generalized
- **345.5** Partial epilepsy, without mention of impairment of consciousness
  Epilepsy:
    sensory-induced

348 Other conditions of brain

- **348.9** Unspecified condition of brain

780 General symptoms

- **780.3** Convulsions

781 Symptoms involving nervous and musculoskeletal systems

- **781.2** Abnormality of gait
  Gait:
    ataxic
- **781.3** Lack of coordination
  Ataxia, not otherwise specified

Examination

Examination is a comprehensive screening and specific testing process that leads to a diagnostic classification or, when appropriate, to a referral to another practitioner. Examination is required prior to the initial intervention and is performed for all patients/clients. Through the examination, the physical therapist may identify impairments, functional limitations, disabilities, changes in physical function or overall health status, and needs related to restoration of health and to prevention, wellness, and fitness. The physical therapist synthesizes the examination findings to establish the diagnosis and the prognosis (including the plan of care). The patient/client, family, significant others, and caregivers may provide information during the examination process.

Examination has three components: the patient/client history, the systems review, and tests and measures. The *history* is a systematic gathering of past and current information (often from the patient/client) related to why the patient/client is seeking the services of the physical therapist. The *systems review* is a brief or limited examination of (1) the anatomical and physiological status of the cardiovascular/pulmonary, integumentary, musculoskeletal, and neuromuscular systems and (2) the communication ability, affect, cognition, language, and learning style of the patient/client. *Tests and measures* are the means of gathering data about the patient/client.

The selection of examination procedures and the depth of the examination vary based on patient/client age; severity of the problem; stage of recovery (acute, subacute, chronic); phase of rehabilitation (early, intermediate, late, return to activity); home, work (job/school/play), or community situation; and other relevant factors. *For clinical indications in selecting tests and measures and for listings of tests and measures, tools used to gather data, and the types of data generated by tests and measures, refer to Chapter 2.*

Patient/Client History

The history may include:

General Demographics

- Age
- Sex
- Race/ethnicity
- Primary language
- Education

Social History

- Cultural beliefs and behaviors
- Family and caregiver resources
- Social interactions, social activities, and support systems

Employment/Work (Job/School/Play)

- Current and prior work (job/school/play), community, and leisure actions, tasks, or activities

Growth and Development

- Developmental history
- Hand dominance

Living Environment

- Devices and equipment (eg, assistive, adaptive, orthotic, protective, supportive, prosthetic)
- Living environment and community characteristics
- Projected discharge destinations

General Health Status (Self-Report, Family Report, Caregiver Report)

- General health perception
- Physical function (eg, mobility, sleep patterns, restricted bed days)
- Psychological function (eg, memory, reasoning ability, depression, anxiety)
- Role function (eg, community, leisure, social, work)
- Social function (eg, social activity, social interaction, social support)

Social/Health Habits (Past and Current)

- Behavioral health risks (eg, smoking, drug abuse)
- Level of physical fitness

Family History

- Familial health risks

Medical/Surgical History

- Cardiovascular
- Endocrine/metabolic
- Gastrointestinal
- Genitourinary
- Gynecological
- Integumentary
- Musculoskeletal
- Neuromuscular
- Obstetrical
- Prior hospitalizations, surgeries, and preexisting medical and other health-related conditions
- Psychological
- Pulmonary

Current Condition(s)/Chief Complaint(s)

- Concerns that led patient/client to seek the services of a physical therapist
- Concerns or needs of patient/client who requires the services of a physical therapist
- Current therapeutic interventions
- Mechanisms of injury or disease, including date of onset and course of events
- Onset and pattern of symptoms
- Patient/client, family, significant other, and caregiver expectations and goals for the therapeutic intervention
- Patient/client, family, significant other, and caregiver perceptions of patient's/client's emotional response to the current clinical situation
- Previous occurrence of chief complaint(s)
- Prior therapeutic interventions

Functional Status and Activity Level

- Current and prior functional status in self-care and home management activities, including activities of daily living (ADL) and instrumental activities of daily living (IADL)
- Current and prior functional status in work (job/school/play), community, and leisure actions, tasks, or activities

Medications

- Medications for current condition
- Medications previously taken for current condition
- Medications for other conditions

Other Clinical Tests

- Laboratory and diagnostic tests
- Review of available records (eg, medical, education, surgical)
- Review of other clinical findings (eg, nutrition and hydration)

Systems Review

The systems review may include:

Anatomical and Physiological Status

- Cardiovascular/Pulmonary
  - Blood pressure
  - Edema
  - Heart rate
  - Respiratory rate
- Integumentary
  - Pliability (texture)
  - Presence of scar formation
  - Skin color
  - Skin integrity
- Musculoskeletal
  - Gross range of motion
  - Gross strength
  - Gross symmetry
  - Height
  - Weight
- Neuromuscular
  - Gross coordinated movements (eg, balance, gait, locomotion, transfers, transitions)
  - Motor function (motor control, motor learning)

Communication, Affect, Cognition, Language, and Learning Style

- Ability to make needs known
- Consciousness
- Expected emotional/behavioral responses
- Learning preferences (eg, education needs, learning barriers)
- Orientation (person, place, time)

Tests and Measures

Test and measures for this pattern may include those that characterize or quantify:

Aerobic Capacity and Endurance

- Aerobic capacity during functional activities (eg, activities of daily living [ADL] scales, indexes, instrumental activities of daily living [IADL] scales, observations)
- Aerobic capacity during standardized exercise test protocols (eg, ergometry, step tests, time/distance walk/run tests, treadmill tests, wheelchair tests)
- Cardiovascular signs and symptoms in response to increased oxygen demand with exercise or activity, including pressures and flow; heart rate, rhythm, and sounds; and superficial vascular responses (eg, angina, claudication, and exertion scales; electrocardiography; observations; palpation; sphygmomanometry)
- Pulmonary signs and symptoms in response to increased oxygen demand with exercise or activity, including breath and voice sounds; cyanosis; gas exchange; respiratory pattern, rate, and rhythm; and ventilatory flow, force, and volume (eg, auscultation, dyspnea and exertion scales, gas analyses, observations, oximetry, palpation, pulmonary function tests)

Anthropometric Characteristics

- Body dimensions (eg, girth measurement, length measurement)
- Edema (eg, girth measurement, palpation, scales, volume measurement)

Arousal, Attention, and Cognition

- Arousal and attention (eg, adaptability tests, arousal and awareness scales, indexes, profiles, questionnaires)
- Cognition, including ability to process commands (eg, developmental inventories, indexes, interviews, mental state scales, observations, questionnaires, safety checklists)
- Communication (eg, functional communication profiles, interviews, inventories, observations, questionnaires)
- Motivation (eg, adaptive behavior scales)
- Orientation to time, person, place, and situation (eg, attention tests, learning profiles, mental state scales)
- Recall, including memory and retention (eg, assessment scales, interviews, questionnaires)

Assistive and Adaptive Devices

- Assistive or adaptive devices and equipment use during functional activities (eg, ADL scales, functional scales, IADL scales, interviews, observations)
- Components, alignment, fit, and ability to care for the assistive or adaptive devices and equipment (eg, interviews, logs, observations, pressure-sensing maps, reports)
- Remediation of impairments, functional limitations, or disabilities with use of assistive or adaptive devices and equipment (eg, activity status indexes, ADL scales, aerobic capacity tests, functional performance inventories, health assessment questionnaires, IADL scales, pain scales, play scales, videographic assessments)
- Safety during use of assistive or adaptive devices and equipment (eg, diaries, fall scales, interviews, logs, observations, reports)

Circulation (Arterial, Venous, and Lymphatic)

- Physiological responses to position change, including autonomic responses, central and peripheral pressures, heart rate and rhythm, respiratory rate and rhythm, ventilatory pattern (eg, auscultation, electrocardiography, observations, palpation, sphygmomanometry)

Cranial and Peripheral Nerve Integrity

- Electrophysiological integrity (eg, electroneuromyography)
- Motor distribution of the cranial nerves (eg, dynamometry, muscle tests, observations)
- Motor distribution of the peripheral nerves (eg, dynamometry, muscle tests, observations, thoracic outlet tests)
- Response to neural provocation (eg, tension tests, vertebral artery compression tests)
- Response to stimuli, including auditory, gustatory, olfactory, pharyngeal, vestibular, and visual (eg, observations, provocation tests)
- Sensory distribution of the cranial nerves (eg, discrimination tests; tactile tests, including coarse and light touch, cold and heat, pain, pressure, and vibration)
- Sensory distribution of the peripheral nerves (eg, discrimination tests; tactile tests, including coarse and light touch, cold and heat, pain, pressure, and vibration; thoracic outlet tests)

Environmental, Home, and Work (Job/School/Play) Barriers

- Current and potential barriers (eg, checklists, interviews, observations, questionnaires)
- Physical space and environment (eg, compliance standards, observations, photographic assessments, questionnaires, structural specifications, videographic assessments)

Ergonomics and Body Mechanics

Ergonomics

- Dexterity and coordination during work (job/school/play) (eg, hand function tests, impairment rating scales, manipulative ability tests)
- Safety in work environments (eg, hazard identification checklists, job severity indexes, lifting standards, risk assessment scales, standards for exposure limits)
- Specific work conditions or activities (eg, handling checklists, job simulations, lifting models, preemployment screenings, task analysis checklists, workstation checklists)
- Tools, devices, equipment, and workstations related to work actions, tasks, or activities (eg, observations, tool analysis checklists, vibration assessments)

Body mechanics

- Body mechanics during self-care, home management, work, community, or leisure actions, tasks, or activities (eg, ADL scales, IADL scales, observations, photographic assessments, technology-assisted assessments, videographic assessments)

Gait, Locomotion, and Balance

- Balance during functional activities with or without the use of assistive, adaptive, orthotic, protective, supportive, or prosthetic devices or equipment (eg, ADL scales, IADL scales, observations, videographic assessments)
- Balance (dynamic and static) with or without the use of assistive, adaptive, orthotic, protective, supportive, or prosthetic devices or equipment (eg, balance scales, dizziness inventories, dynamic posturography, fall scales, motor impairment tests, observations, photographic assessments, postural control tests)
- Gait and locomotion during functional activities with or without the use of assistive, adaptive, orthotic, protective, supportive, or prosthetic devices or equipment (eg, ADL scales, gait indexes, IADL scales, mobility skill profiles, observations, videographic assessments)
- Gait and locomotion with or without the use of assistive, adaptive, orthotic, protective, supportive, or prosthetic devices or equipment (eg, dynamometry, electroneuromyography, footprint analyses, gait indexes, mobility skill profiles, observations, photographic assessments, technology-assisted assessments, videographic assessments, weight-bearing scales, wheelchair mobility tests)
- Safety during gait, locomotion, and balance (eg, confidence scales, diaries, fall scales, functional assessment profiles, logs, reports)

Integumentary Integrity

Associated skin

- Activities, positioning, and postures that produce or relieve trauma to the skin (eg, observations, pressure-sensing maps, scales)
- Assistive, adaptive, orthotic, protective, supportive, or prosthetic devices and equipment that may produce or relieve trauma to the skin (eg, observations, pressure-sensing maps, risk assessment scales)
- Skin characteristics, including blistering, continuity of skin color, dermatitis, hair growth, mobility, nail growth, sensation, temperature, texture, and turgor (eg, observations, palpation, photographic assessments, thermography)

Motor Function (Motor Learning and Motor Control)

- Dexterity, coordination, and agility (eg, coordination screens, motor impairment tests, motor proficiency tests, observations, videographic assessments)
- Electrophysiological integrity (eg, electroneuromyography)
- Hand function (eg, fine and gross motor control tests, finger dexterity tests, manipulative ability tests, observations)
- Initiation, modification, and control of movement patterns and voluntary postures (eg, activity indexes, developmental scales, gross motor function profiles, motor scales, movement assessment batteries, neuromotor tests, observations, physical performance tests, postural challenge tests, videographic assessments)

Muscle Performance (Including Strength, Power, and Endurance)

- Electrophysiological integrity (eg, electroneuromyography)
- Muscle strength, power, and endurance (eg, dynamometry, manual muscle tests, muscle performance tests, physical capacity tests, technology-assisted assessments, timed activity tests)
- Muscle strength, power, and endurance during functional activities (eg, ADL scales, functional muscle tests, IADL scales, observations, videographic assessments)
- Muscle tension (eg, palpation)

Neuromotor Development and Sensory Integration
- Acquisition and evolution of motor skills, including age-appropriate development (eg, activity indexes, developmental inventories and questionnaires, infant and toddler motor assessments, learning profiles, motor function tests, motor proficiency assessments, neuromotor assessments, reflex tests, screens, videographic assessments)
- Oral motor function, phonation, and speech production (eg, interviews, observations)
- Sensorimotor integration, including postural, equilibrium, and righting reactions (eg, behavioral assessment scales, motor and processing skill tests, observations, postural challenge tests, reflex tests, sensory profiles, visual perceptual skill tests)

Orthotic, Protective, and Supportive Devices
- Components, alignment, fit, and ability to care for orthotic, protective, and supportive devices and equipment (eg, interviews, logs, observations, pressure-sensing maps, reports)
- Orthotic, protective, and supportive devices and equipment use during functional activities (eg, ADL scales, functional scales, IADL scales, interviews, observations, profiles)
- Remediation of impairments, functional limitations, or disabilities with use of orthotic, protective, and supportive devices and equipment (eg, activity status indexes, ADL scales, aerobic capacity tests, functional performance inventories, health assessment questionnaires, IADL scales, pain scales, play scales, videographic assessments)
- Safety during use of orthotic, protective, and supportive devices and equipment (eg, diaries, fall scales, interviews, logs, observations, reports)

Pain
- Pain, soreness, and nociception (eg, analog scales, discrimination tests, pain drawings and maps, provocation tests, verbal and pictorial descriptor tests)
- Pain in specific body parts (eg, pain indexes, pain questionnaires, structural provocation tests)

Posture
- Postural alignment and position (static and dynamic), including symmetry and deviation from midline (eg, grid measurement, observations, photographic assessments, technology-assisted assessments, videographic assessments)
- Specific body parts (eg, angle assessments, forward-bending test, goniometry, observations, palpation, positional tests)

Range of Motion (ROM) (Including Muscle Length)
- Functional ROM (eg, observations, squat testing, toe touch tests)
- Joint active and passive movement (eg, goniometry, inclinometry, observations, photographic assessments, technology-assisted assessments, videographic assessments)
- Muscle length, soft tissue extensibility, and flexibility (eg, contracture tests, goniometry, inclinometry, ligamentous tests, linear measurement, multisegment flexibility tests, palpation)

Reflex Integrity
- Deep reflexes (eg, myotatic reflex scale, observations, reflex tests)
- Electrophysiological integrity (eg, electroneuromyography)
- Postural reflexes and reactions, including righting, equilibrium, and protective reactions (eg, observations, postural challenge tests, reflex profiles, videographic assessments)
- Primitive reflexes and reactions, including developmental (eg, reflex profiles, screening tests)
- Resistance to passive stretch (eg, tone scales)
- Superficial reflexes and reactions (eg, observations, provocation tests)

Self-Care and Home Management (Including ADL and IADL)
- Ability to gain access to home environments (eg, barrier identification, observations, physical performance tests)
- Ability to perform self-care and home management activities with or without assistive, adaptive, orthotic, protective, supportive, or prosthetic devices and equipment (eg, ADL scales, aerobic capacity tests, IADL scales, interviews, observations, profiles)
- Safety in self-care and home management activities and environments (eg, diaries, fall scales, interviews, logs, observations, reports, videographic assessments)

Sensory Integrity
- Combined/cortical sensations (eg, stereognosis tests, tactile discrimination tests)
- Deep sensations (eg, kinesthesiometry, observations, photographic assessments, vibration tests)
- Electrophysiological integrity (eg,electroneuromyography)

Ventilation and Respiration/Gas Exchange
- Pulmonary signs of respiration/gas exchange, including breath sounds (eg, gas analyses, observations, oximetry)
- Pulmonary signs of ventilatory function, including airway protection; breath and voice sounds; respiratory rate, rhythm, and pattern; ventilatory flow, forces, and volumes (eg, airway clearance tests, observations, palpation, pulmonary function tests, ventilatory muscle force tests)
- Pulmonary symptoms (eg, dyspnea and perceived exertion indexes and scales)

Work (Job/School/Play), Community, and Leisure Integration or Reintegration (Including IADL)
- Ability to assume or resume work (job/school/play), community, and leisure activities with or without assistive, adaptive, orthotic, protective, supportive, or prosthetic devices and equipment (eg, activity profiles, disability indexes, functional status questionnaires, IADL scales, observations, physical capacity tests)
- Ability to gain access to work (job/school/play), community, and leisure environments (eg, barrier identification, interviews, observations, physical capacity tests, transportation assessments)
- Safety in work (job/school/play), community, and leisure activities and environments (eg, diaries, fall scales, interviews, logs, observations, videographic assessments)

Evaluation, Diagnosis, and Prognosis (Including Plan of Care)

Physical therapists perform *evaluations* (make clinical judgments) based on the data gathered from the history, systems review, and tests and measures. In the evaluation process, physical therapists synthesize the examination data to establish the diagnosis and prognosis (including the plan of care). Factors that influence the complexity of the evaluation include the clinical findings, extent of loss of function, chronicity or severity of the problem, possibility of multisite or multisystem involvement, preexisting condition(s), potential discharge destination, social considerations, physical function, and overall health status.

A *diagnosis* is a label encompassing a cluster of signs and symptoms, syndromes, or categories. It is the result of the systematic diagnostic process, which includes integrating and evaluating the data from the examination. The diagnostic label indicates the primary dysfunction(s) toward which the therapist will direct interventions. The *prognosis* is the determination of the predicted optimal level of improvement in function and the amount of time needed to reach that level and may also include a prediction of levels of improvement that may be reached at various intervals during the course of therapy. During the prognostic process, the physical therapist develops the plan of care. The *plan of care* identifies specific interventions, proposed frequency and duration of the interventions, anticipated goals, expected outcomes, and discharge plans. The plan of care identifies realistic anticipated goals and expected outcomes, taking into consideration the expectations of the patient/client and appropriate others. These anticipated goals and expected outcomes should be measureable and time limited.

The frequency of visits and duration of the episode of care may vary from a short episode with a high intensity of intervention to a longer episode with a diminishing intensity of intervention. Frequency and duration may vary greatly among patients/clients based on a variety of factors that the physical therapist considers throughout the evaluation process, such as anatomical and physiological changes related to growth and development; caregiver consistency or expertise; chronicity or severity of the current condition; living environment; multisite or multisystem involvement; social support; potential discharge destinations; probability of prolonged impairment, functional limitation, or disability; and stability of the condition.

Prognosis

Over the course of 12 months, patient/client will demonstrate optimal motor function and sensory integrity and the highest level of functioning in home, work (job/school/play), community, and leisure environments, within the context of the impairments, functional limitations, and disabilities.

During the episode of care, patient/client will achieve (1) the anticipated goals and expected outcomes of the interventions that are described in the plan of care and (2) the global outcomes for patients/clients who are classified in this pattern.

Expected Range of Number of Visits Per Episode of Care

6 to 50

This range represents the lower and upper limits of the number of physical therapist visits required to achieve anticipated goals and expected outcomes. *It is anticipated that 80% of patients/clients who are classified into this pattern will achieve the anticipated goals and expected outcomes within 6 to 50 visits during a single continuous episode of care.* Frequency of visits and duration of the episode of care should be determined by the physical therapist to maximize effectiveness of care and efficiency of service delivery.

Factors That May Require New Episode of Care or That May Modify Frequency of Visits/Duration of Care

- Accessibility and availability of resources
- Adherence to the intervention program
- Age
- Anatomical and physiological changes related to growth and development
- Caregiver consistency or expertise
- Chronicity or severity of the current condition
- Cognitive status
- Comorbitities, complications, or secondary impairments
- Concurrent medical, surgical, and therapeutic interventions
- Decline in functional independence
- Level of impairment
- Level of physical function
- Living environment
- Multisite or multisystem involvement
- Nutritional status
- Overall health status
- Potential discharge destinations
- Premorbid conditions
- Probability of prolonged impairment, functional limitation, or disability
- Psychological and socioeconomic factors
- Psychomotor abilities
- Social support
- Stability of the condition

Intervention

Intervention is the purposeful interaction of the physical therapist with the patient/client and, when appropriate, with other individuals involved in patient/client care, using various physical therapy procedures and techniques to produce changes in the condition consistent with the diagnosis and prognosis. Decisions about interventions are contingent on the timely monitoring of patient/client response and the progress made toward achieving the anticipated goals and expected outcomes.

Communication, coordination, and documentation and patient/client-related instruction are provided for all patients/clients across all settings. Procedural interventions are selected or modified based on the examination data and the evaluation, the diagnosis and the prognosis, and the anticipated goals and expected outcomes for a particular patient/client. *For clinical considerations in selecting interventions, listings of interventions, and listings of anticipated goals and expected outcomes, refer to Chapter 3.*

Coordination, Communication, and Documentation

Coordination, communication, and documentation may include:

Interventions

- Addressing required functions
  - advance directives
  - individualized family service plans (IFSPs) or individualized education plans (IEPs)
  - informed consent
  - mandatory communication and reporting (eg, patient advocacy and abuse reporting)
- Admission and discharge planning
- Case management
- Collaboration and coordination with agencies, including:
  - equipment suppliers
  - home care agencies
  - payer groups
  - schools
  - transportation agencies
- Communication across settings, including:
  - case conferences
  - documentation
  - education plans
- Cost-effective resource utilization
- Data collection, analysis, and reporting
  - outcome data
  - peer review findings
  - record reviews
- Documentation across settings, following APTA's *Guidelines for Physical Therapy Documentation* (Appendix 5), including:
  - changes in impairments, functional limitations, and disabilities
  - changes in interventions
  - elements of patient/client management (examination, evaluation, diagnosis, prognosis, intervention)
  - outcomes of intervention
- Interdisciplinary teamwork
  - case conferences
  - patient care rounds
  - patient/client family meetings
- Referrals to other professionals or resources

Anticipated Goals and Expected Outcomes

- Accountability for services is increased.
- Admission data and discharge planning are completed.
- Advance directives, individualized family service plans (IFSPs) or individualized education plans (IEPs), informed consent, and mandatory communication and reporting (eg, patient advocacy and abuse reporting) are obtained or completed.
- Available resources are maximally utilized.
- Care is coordinated with patient/client, family, significant others, caregivers, and other professionals.
- Case is managed throughout the episode of care.
- Collaboration and coordination occurs with agencies, including equipment suppliers, home care agencies, payer groups, schools, and transportation agencies.
- Communication enhances risk reduction and prevention.
- Communication occurs across settings through case conferences, education plans, and documentation.
- Data are collected, analyzed, and reported, including outcome data, peer review findings, and record reviews.
- Decision making is enhanced regarding on health, wellness, and fitness needs.
- Decision making is enhanced regarding patient/client health and the use of health care resources by patient/client, family, significant others, and caregivers.
- Documentation occurs throughout patient/client management and across settings and follows APTA's *Guidelines for Physical Therapy Documentation* (Appendix 5).
- Interdisciplinary collaboration occurs through case conferences, patient care rounds, and patient/client family meetings.
- Patient/client, family, significant other, and caregiver understanding of anticipated goals and expected outcomes is increased.
- Placement needs are determined.
- Referrals are made to other professionals or resources whenever necessary and appropriate.
- Resources are utilized in a cost-effective way.

Patient/Client-Related Instruction

Patient/client-related instruction may include:

Interventions

- Instruction, education and training of patients/clients and caregivers regarding:
  - current condition (pathology/pathophysiology [disease, disorder, or condition], impairments, functional limitations, or disabilities)
  - enhancement of performance
  - health, wellness, and fitness programs
  - plan of care
  - risk factors for pathology/pathophysiology (disease, disorder, or condition), impairments, functional limitations, or disabilities
  - transitions across settings
  - transitions to new roles

Anticipated Goals and Expected Outcomes

- Ability to perform physical actions, tasks, or activities is improved.
- Awareness and use of community resources are improved.
- Behaviors that foster healthy habits, wellness, and prevention are acquired.
- Decision making is enhanced regarding patient/client health and the use of health care resources by patient/client, family, significant others, and caregivers.
- Disability associated with acute or chronic illnesses is reduced.
- Functional independence in activities of daily living (ADL) and instrumental activities of daily living (IADL) is increased.
- Health status is improved.
- Intensity of care is decreased.
- Level of supervision required for task performance is decreased.
- Patient/client, family, significant other, and caregiver knowledge and awareness of the diagnosis, prognosis, interventions, and anticipated goals and expected outcomes are increased.
- Patient/client knowledge of personal and environmental factors associated with the condition is increased.
- Performance levels in self-care, home management, work (job/school/play), community, or leisure actions, tasks, or activities are improved.
- Physical function is improved.
- Risk of recurrence of condition is reduced.
- Risk of secondary impairment is reduced.
- Safety of patient/client, family, significant others, and caregivers is improved.
- Self-management of symptoms is improved.
- Utilization and cost of health care services are decreased.

Procedural Interventions

Procedural interventions for this pattern may include:

Therapeutic Exercise

Interventions

- Aerobic and endurance conditioning or reconditioning
  - aquatic programs
  - gait and locomotor training
  - increased workload over time
  - walking and wheelchair propulsion programs
- Balance, coordination, and agility training
  - developmental activities training
  - motor function (motor control and motor learning) training or retraining
  - neuromuscular education or reeducation
  - perceptual training
  - posture awareness training
  - standardized, programmatic, complementary exercise approaches
  - sensory training or retraining
  - task-specific performance training
  - vestibular training
- Body mechanics and postural stabilization
  - body mechanics training
  - posture awareness training
  - postural control training
  - postural stabilization activities
- Flexibility exercises
  - muscle lengthening
  - range of motion
  - stretching
- Gait and locomotion training
  - developmental activities training
  - gait training
  - implement and device training
  - perceptual training
  - standardized, programmatic, complementary exercise approaches
  - wheelchair training
- Neuromotor development
  - developmental activities training
  - motor training
  - movement pattern training
  - neuromuscular education or reeducation
- Relaxation
  - breathing strategies
  - movement strategies
  - relaxation techniques
  - standardized, programmatic, complementary exercise approaches
- Strength, power, and endurance training for head, neck, limb, pelvic-floor, trunk, and ventilatory muscles
  - active assistive, active, and resistive exercises (including concentric, dynamic/isotonic, eccentric, isokinetic, isometric, and plyometric)
  - aquatic programs
  - standardized, programmatic, complementary exercise approaches
  - task-specific performance training

Anticipated Goals and Expected Outcomes

- Impact on pathology/pathophysiology (disease, disorder, or condition)
  - Joint swelling, inflammation, or restriction is reduced.
  - Nutrient delivery to tissue is increased.
  - Osteogenic effects of exercise are maximized.
  - Pain is decreased.
  - Physiological response to increased oxygen demand is improved.
  - Soft tissue swelling, inflammation, or restriction is reduced.
  - Symptoms associated with increased oxygen demand are decreased.
  - Tissue perfusion and oxygenation are enhanced.
- Impact on impairments:
  - Aerobic capacity is increased.
  - Balance is improved.
  - Endurance is increased.
  - Energy expenditure per unit of work is decreased.
  - Gait, locomotion, and balance are improved.
  - Integumentary integrity is improved.
  - Joint integrity and mobility are improved.
  - Motor function (motor control and motor learning) is improved.
  - Muscle performance (strength, power, and endurance) is increased.
  - Postural control is improved.
  - Quality and quantity of movement between and across body segments are improved.
  - Range of motion is improved.
  - Relaxation is increased.
  - Sensory awareness is increased.
  - Weight-bearing status is improved.
  - Work of breathing is decreased.
- Impact on functional limitations
  - Ability to perform physical actions, tasks, or activities related to self-care, home management, work (job/school/play), community, and leisure is improved.
  - Level of supervision required for task performance is decreased.
  - Performance of and independence in activities of daily living (ADL) and instrumental activities of daily living (IADL) with or without devices and equipment are increased.
  - Tolerance of positions and activities is increased.
- Impact on disabilities
  - Ability to assume or resume required self-care, home management, work (job/school/play), community, and leisure roles is improved.
- Risk reduction/prevention
  - Risk factors are reduced.
  - Risk of secondary impairments is reduced.
  - Safety is improved.
  - Self-management of symptoms is improved.
- Impact on health, wellness, and fitness
  - Fitness is improved.
  - Health status is improved.
  - Physical capacity is increased.
  - Physical function is improved.
- Impact on societal resources
  - Utilization of physical therapy services is optimized.
  - Utilization of physical therapy services results in efficient use of health care dollars.
- Patient/client satisfaction
  - Access, availability, and services provided are acceptable to patient/client.
  - Administrative management of practice is acceptable to patient/client.
  - Clinical proficiency of physical therapist is acceptable to patient/client.
  - Coordination of care is acceptable to patient/client.
  - Cost of health care services is decreased.
  - Intensity of care is decreased.
  - Interpersonal skills of physical therapist are acceptable to patient/client, family, and significant others.
  - Sense of well-being is improved.
  - Stressors are decreased.

Functional Training in Self-Care and Home Management (Including Activities of Daily Living [ADL] and Instrumental Activities of Daily Living [IADL])

Interventions

- ADL training
  - bathing
  - bed mobility and transfer training
  - developmental activities
  - dressing
  - eating
  - grooming
  - toileting
- Devices and equipment use and training
  - assistive and adaptive device or equipment training during ADL and IADL
  - orthotic, protective, or supportive device or equipment training during ADL and IADL
- Functional training programs
  - simulated environments and tasks
  - task adaptation
  - travel training
- IADL training
  - caring for dependents
  - home maintenance
  - household chores
  - shopping
  - structured play for infants and children
  - yard work
- Injury prevention or reduction
  - injury prevention education during self-care and home management
  - injury prevention or reduction with use of devices and equipment
  - safety awareness training during self-care and home management

Anticipated Goals and Expected Outcomes

- Impact on pathology/pathophysiology (disease, disorder, or condition)
  - Pain is decreased.
  - Physiological response to increased oxygen demand is improved.
  - Symptoms associated with increased oxygen demand are decreased.
- Impact on impairments
  - Balance is improved.
  - Endurance is increased.
  - Energy expenditure per unit of work is decreased.
  - Motor function (motor control and motor learning) is improved.
  - Muscle performance (strength, power, and endurance) is increased.
  - Postural control is improved.
  - Sensory awareness is increased.
  - Weight-bearing status is improved.
  - Work of breathing is decreased.
- Impact on functional limitations
  - Ability to perform physical actions, tasks, or activities related to self-care and home management is improved.
  - Level of supervision required for task performance is decreased.
  - Performance of and independence in ADL and IADL with or without devices and equipment are increased.
  - Tolerance of positions and activities is increased.
- Impact on disabilities
  - Ability to assume or resume required self-care and home management roles is improved.
- Risk reduction/prevention
  - Risk factors are reduced.
  - Risk of secondary impairments is reduced.
  - Safety is improved.
  - Self-management of symptoms is improved.
- Impact on health, wellness, and fitness
  - Health status is improved.
  - Physical capacity is increased.
  - Physical function is improved.
- Impact on societal resources
  - Utilization of physical therapy services is optimized.
  - Utilization of physical therapy services results in efficient use of health care dollars.
- Patient/client satisfaction
  - Access, availability, and services provided are acceptable to patient/client.
  - Administrative management of practice is acceptable to patient/client.
  - Clinical proficiency of physical therapist is acceptable to patient/client.
  - Coordination of care is acceptable to patient/client.
  - Cost of health care services is decreased.
  - Intensity of care is decreased.
  - Interpersonal skills of physical therapist are acceptable to patient/client, family, and significant others.
  - Sense of well-being is improved.
  - Stressors are decreased.

Functional Training in Work (Job/School/Play), Community, and Leisure Integration or Reintegration (Including Instrumental Activities of Daily Living [IADL], Work Hardening, and Work Conditioning)

Interventions

- Devices and equipment use and training
  - assistive and adaptive device or equipment training during IADL
  - orthotic, protective, or supportive device or equipment training during IADL
- Functional training programs
  - job coaching
  - simulated environments and tasks
  - task adaptation
  - task training
  - travel training
- IADL training
  - community service training involving instruments
  - school and play activities training including tools and instruments
  - work training with tools
- Injury prevention or reduction
  - injury prevention education during work (job/school/play), community, and leisure integration or reintegration
  - injury prevention or reduction with use of devices and equipment
  - safety awareness training during work (job/school/play), community, and leisure integration or reintegration
- Leisure and play activities training

Anticipated Goals and Expected Outcomes

- Impact on pathology/pathophysiology (disease, disorder, or condition)
  - Pain is decreased.
  - Physiological response to increased oxygen demand is improved.
  - Symptoms associated with increased oxygen demand are decreased.
- Impact on impairments
  - Balance is improved.
  - Endurance is increased.
  - Energy expenditure per unit of work is decreased.
  - Motor function (motor control and motor learning) is improved.
  - Muscle performance (strength, power, and endurance) is increased.
  - Postural control is improved.
  - Sensory awareness is increased.
  - Weight bearing status is improved.
  - Work of breathing is decreased.
- Impact on functional limitations
  - Ability to perform physical actions, tasks, or activities related to work (job/school/play), community, and leisure integration or reintegration is improved.
  - Level of supervision required for task performance is decreased.
  - Performance of and independence in IADL with or without devices and equipment are increased.
  - Tolerance of positions and activities is increased.
- Impact on disabilities
  - Ability to assume or resume required work (job/school/play), community, and leisure roles is improved.
- Risk reduction/prevention
  - Risk factors are reduced.
  - Risk of secondary impairment is reduced.
  - Safety is improved.
  - Self-management of symptoms is improved.
- Impact on health, wellness, and fitness
  - Fitness is improved.
  - Health status is improved.
  - Physical capacity is increased.
  - Physical function is improved.
- Impact on societal resources
  - Costs of work-related injury or disability are reduced.
  - Utilization of physical therapy services is optimized.
  - Utilization of physical therapy services results in efficient use of health care dollars.
- Patient/client satisfaction
  - Access, availability, and services provided are acceptable to patient/client.
  - Administrative management of practice is acceptable to patient/client.
  - Clinical proficiency of physical therapist is acceptable to patient/client.
  - Coordination of care is acceptable to patient/client.
  - Cost of health care services is decreased.
  - Intensity of care is decreased.
  - Interpersonal skills of physical therapist are acceptable to patient/client, family, and significant others.
  - Sense of well-being is improved.
  - Stressors are decreased.

Manual Therapy Techniques (Including Mobilization/Manipulation)

Interventions

- Manual traction
- Massage
  - connective tissue massage
  - therapeutic massage
- Mobilization/manipulation
  - soft tissue
- Passive range of motion

Anticipated Goals and Expected Outcomes

- Impact on pathology/pathophysiology (disease, disorder, or condition)
  - Edema, lymphedema, or effusion is reduced.
  - Joint swelling, inflammation, or restriction is reduced.
  - Pain is decreased.
  - Soft tissue swelling, inflammation, or restriction is reduced.
- Impact on impairments
  - Balance is improved.
  - Energy expenditure per unit of work is decreased.
  - Gait, locomotion, and balance are improved.
  - Integumentary integrity is improved.
  - Muscle performance (strength, power, and endurance) is increased.
  - Postural control is improved.
  - Quality and quantity of movement between and across body segments are improved.
  - Range of motion is improved.
  - Relaxation is increased.
  - Sensory awareness is increased.
  - Weight-bearing status is improved.
  - Work of breathing is decreased.
- Impact on functional limitations
  - Ability to perform movement tasks is improved.
  - Ability to perform physical actions, tasks, or activities related to self-care, home management, work (job/school/play), community, and leisure is improved.
  - Tolerance of positions and activities is increased.
- Impact on disabilities
  - Ability to assume or resume required self-care, home management, work (job/school/play), community, and leisure roles is improved.
- Risk reduction/prevention
  - Risk factors are reduced.
  - Risk of secondary impairment is reduced.
  - Self-management of symptoms is improved.
- Impact on health, wellness, and fitness
  - Physical function is improved.
- Impact on societal resources
  - Utilization of physical therapy services is optimized.
- Patient/client satisfaction
  - Access, availability, and services provided are acceptable to patient/client.
  - Administrative management of practice is acceptable to patient/client.
  - Clinical proficiency of physical therapist is acceptable to patient/client.
  - Coordination of care is acceptable to patient/client.
  - Cost of health care services is decreased.
  - Intensity of care is decreased.
  - Interpersonal skills of physical therapist are acceptable to patient/client, family, and significant others.
  - Sense of well-being is improved.
  - Stressors are decreased.

Prescription, Application, and, as Appropriate, Fabrication of Devices and Equipment (Assistive, Adaptive, Orthotic, Protective, Supportive, and Prosthetic)

Interventions

- Adaptive devices
  - environmental controls
  - hospital beds
  - raised toilet seats
  - seating systems
- Assistive devices
  - canes
  - crutches
  - long-handled reachers
  - power devices
  - static and dynamic splints
  - walkers
  - wheelchairs
- Orthotic devices
  - braces
  - casts
  - shoe inserts
  - splints
- Protective devices
  - braces
  - cushions
  - helmets
  - protective taping
- Supportive devices
  - compression garments
  - corsets
  - elastic wraps
  - mechanical ventilators
  - neck collars
  - serial casts
  - slings
  - supplemental oxygen
  - supportive taping

Anticipated Goals and Expected Outcomes

- Impact on pathology/pathophysiology (disease, disorder, or condition)
  - Edema, lymphedema, or effusion is reduced.
  - Joint swelling, inflammation, or restriction is reduced.
  - Pain is decreased.
  - Physiological response to increased oxygen demand is improved.
  - Soft tissue swelling, inflammation, or restriction is reduced.
  - Symptoms associated with increased oxygen demand are decreased.
- Impact on impairments
  - Balance is improved.
  - Endurance is increased.
  - Energy expenditure per unit of work is decreased.
  - Gait, locomotion, and balance are improved.
  - Integumentary integrity is improved.
  - Joint stability is increased
  - Motor function (motor control and motor learning) is improved.
  - Muscle performance (strength, power, and endurance) is increased.
  - Optimal joint alignment is achieved.
  - Optimal loading on a body part is achieved.
  - Postural control is improved.
  - Quality and quantity of movement between and across body segments are improved.
  - Range of motion is improved.
  - Weight-bearing status is improved.
  - Work of breathing is decreased.
- Impact on functional limitations
  - Ability to perform physical actions, tasks, or activities related to self-care, home management, work (job/school/play), community, and leisure is improved.
  - Level of supervision required for task performance is decreased.
  - Performance of and independence in activities of daily living (ADL) and instrumental activities of daily living (IADL) with or without devices and equipment are increased.
  - Tolerance of positions and activities is improved.
- Impact on disabilities
  - Ability to assume or resume required self-care, home management, work (job/school/play), community, and leisure roles is improved.
- Risk reduction/prevention
  - Pressure on body tissues is reduced.
  - Protection of body parts is increased.
  - Risk factors are reduced.
  - Risk of secondary impairment is reduced.
  - Safety is improved.
  - Self-management of symptoms is improved.
  - Stresses precipitating injury are decreased.
- Impact on health, wellness, and fitness
  - Health status is improved.
  - Physical capacity is increased.
  - Physical function is improved.
- Impact on societal resources
  - Utilization of physical therapy services is optimized.
  - Utilization of physical therapy services results in efficient use of health care dollars.
- Patient/client satisfaction
  - Access, availability, and services provided are acceptable to patient/client.
  - Administrative management of practice is acceptable to patient/client.
  - Clinical proficiency of physical therapist is acceptable to patient/client.
  - Coordination of care is acceptable to patient/client.
  - Cost of health care services is decreased.
  - Intensity of care is decreased.
  - Interpersonal skills of physical therapist are acceptable to patient/client, family, and significant others.
  - Sense of well-being is improved.
  - Stressors are decreased.

Airway Clearance Techniques

Interventions

- Breathing strategies
  - active cycle of breathing or forced expiratory techniques
  - assisted cough/huff techniques
  - autogenic drainage
  - paced breathing
  - pursed lip breathing
  - techniques to maximize ventilation (eg, maximum inspiratory hold, staircase breathing, manual hyperinflation)
- Manual/mechanical techniques
  - assistive devices
  - chest percussion, vibration, and shaking
  - chest wall manipulation
  - suctioning
  - ventilatory aids
- Positioning
  - positioning to alter work of breathing
  - positioning to maximize ventilation and perfusion
  - pulmonary postural drainage

Anticipated Goals and Expected Outcomes

- Impact on pathology/pathophysiology (disease, disorder, or condition)
  - Atelectasis is decreased.
  - Nutrient delivery to tissue is increased.
  - Physiological response to increased oxygen demand is improved.
  - Symptoms associated with increased oxygen demand are decreased.
  - Tissue perfusion and oxygenation are enhanced.
- Impact on impairments
  - Airway clearance is improved.
  - Cough is improved.
  - Endurance is increased.
  - Energy expenditure per unit of work is decreased.
  - Exercise tolerance is improved.
  - Muscle performance (strength, power, and endurance) is increased.
  - Ventilation and respiration/gas exchange are improved.
  - Work of breathing is decreased.
- Impact on functional limitations
  - Ability to perform physical actions, tasks, or activities related to self-care, home management, work (job/ school/ play), community, and leisure is improved.
  - Performance of and independence in activities of daily living (ADL) and instrumental activities of daily living (IADL) with or without devices and equipment are increased.
  - Tolerance of positions and activities is increased.
- Impact on disabilities
  - Ability to assume or resume required self-care, home management, work (job/school/play), community, and leisure roles is improved.
- Risk reduction/prevention
  - Risk factors are reduced.
  - Risk of secondary impairment is reduced.
  - Safety is improved.
  - Self-management of symptoms is improved.
- Impact on health, wellness, and fitness
  - Health status is improved.
  - Physical function is improved.
- Impact on societal resources
  - Utilization of physical therapy services is optimized.
  - Utilization of physical therapy services results in efficient use of health care dollars.
- Patient/client satisfaction
  - Access, availability, and services provided are acceptable to patient/client.
  - Administrative management of practice is acceptable to patient/client.
  - Clinical proficiency of physical therapist is acceptable to patient/client.
  - Coordination of care is acceptable to patient/client.
  - Cost of health care services is decreased.
  - Intensity of care is decreased.
  - Interpersonal skills of physical therapist are acceptable to patient/client, family, and significant others.
  - Sense of well-being is improved.
  - Stressors are decreased.

Electrotherapeutic Modalities

Interventions

- Electrotherapeutic delivery of medications
  - iontophoresis
- Electrical stimulation
  - electrical muscle stimulation (EMS)
  - functional electrical stimulation (FES)
  - neuromuscular electrical stimulation (NMES)
  - transcutaneous electrical nerve stimulation (TENS)

Anticipated Goals and Expected Outcomes

- Impact on pathology/pathophysiology
  - Edema, lymphedema, or effusion is reduced.
  - Joint swelling, inflammation, or restriction is reduced.
  - Nutrient delivery to tissue is increased.
  - Osteogenic effects are enhanced.
  - Pain is decreased.
  - Soft tissue swelling, inflammation, or restriction is reduced.
  - Tissue perfusion and oxygenation are enhanced.
- Impact on impairments
  - Integumentary integrity is improved.
  - Motor function (motor control and motor learning) is improved.
  - Muscle performance (strength, power, and endurance) is increased.
  - Postural control is improved.
  - Quality and quantity of movement between and across body segments are improved.
  - Range of motion is improved.
  - Relaxation is increased.
  - Sensory awareness is increased.
- Impact on functional limitations
  - Ability to perform physical actions, tasks, or activities related to self-care, home management, community, work (job/ school/play), and leisure is improved.
  - Level of supervision required for task performance is decreased.
  - Performance of and independence in activities of daily living (ADL) and instrumental activities of daily living (IADL) with or without devices and equipment are increased.
  - Tolerance of positions and activities is increased.
- Impact on disabilities
  - Ability to assume or resume required self-care, home management, work (job/school/play), community, and leisure roles is improved.
- Risk reduction/prevention
  - Complications of immobility are reduced.
  - Risk factors are reduced.
  - Risk of secondary impairment is reduced.
  - Self-management of symptoms is improved.
- Impact on health, wellness, and fitness
  - Physical capacity is increased.
  - Physical function is improved.
- Impact on societal resources
  - Utilization of physical therapy services is optimized.
  - Utilization of physical therapy services results in efficient use of health care dollars.
- Patient/client satisfaction
  - Access, availability, and services provided are acceptable to patient/client.
  - Administrative management of practice is acceptable to patient/client.
  - Clinical proficiency of physical therapist is acceptable to patient/client.
  - Coordination of care is acceptable to patient/client.
  - Interpersonal skills of physical therapist are acceptable to patient/client, family, and significant others.
  - Sense of well-being is improved.
  - Stressors are decreased.

Physical Agents and Mechanical Modalities

Interventions

Physical agents may include:

- Cryotherapy
  - cold packs
  - ice massage
  - vapocoolant spray
- Hydrotherapy
  - whirlpool tanks
  - pools
- Thermotherapy
  - dry heat
  - hot packs
  - paraffin baths

Mechanical modalities may include:

- Compression therapies
  - compression bandaging
  - compression garments
  - taping
- Gravity-assisted compression devices
  - standing frame
  - tilt table

Anticipated Goals and Expected Outcomes

- Impact on pathology/pathophysiology (disease, disorder, or condition)
  - Edema, lymphedema, or effusion is reduced.
  - Joint swelling, inflammation, or restriction is reduced.
  - Nutrient delivery to tissue is increased.
  - Pain is decreased.
  - Soft tissue swelling, inflammation, or restriction is reduced.
  - Tissue perfusion and oxygenation are enhanced.
- Impact on impairments:
  - Integumentary integrity is improved.
  - Muscle performance (strength, power, and endurance) is increased.
  - Range of motion is improved.
  - Weight-bearing status is improved.
- Impact on functional limitations
  - Ability to perform physical actions, tasks, or activities related to self-care, home management, work (job/school/play), community, and leisure is improved.
  - Performance of and independence in activities of daily living (ADL) and instrumental activities of daily living (IADL) with or without devices and equipment are increased.
  - Tolerance of positions and activities is increased.
- Impact on disabilities
  - Ability to assume or resume required self-care, home management, work (job/school/play), community, and leisure roles is improved.
- Risk reduction/prevention
  - Complications of soft tissue and circulatory disorders are decreased.
  - Risk of secondary impairments is reduced.
  - Self-management of symptoms is improved.
- Impact on societal resources
  - Utilization of physical therapy services is optimized.
- Patient/client satisfaction
  - Access, availability, and services provided are acceptable to patient/client.
  - Administrative management of practice is acceptable to patient/client.
  - Clinical proficiency of physical therapist is acceptable to patient/client.
  - Coordination of care is acceptable to patient/client.
  - Interpersonal skills of physical therapist are acceptable to patient/client, family, and significant others.
  - Sense of well-being is improved.
  - Stressors are decreased.

Reexamination

Reexamination is the process of performing selected tests and measures after the initial examination to evaluate progress and to modify or redirect interventions. Reexamination may be indicated more than once during a single episode of care. It also may be performed over the course of a disease, disorder, or condition, which for some patients/clients may be over the life span. Indications for reexamination include new clinical findings or failure to respond to physical therapy interventions.

Global Outcomes for Patients/Clients in This Pattern

Throughout the entire episode of care, the physical therapist determines the anticipated goals and expected outcomes for each intervention. These anticipated goals and expected outcomes are delineated in shaded boxes that accompany the lists of interventions in each preferred practice pattern. As the patient/client reaches the termination of physical therapy services and the end of the episode of care, the physical therapist measures the global outcomes of the physical therapy services by characterizing or quantifying the impact of the physical therapy interventions in the following domains:

- Pathology/pathophysiology (disease, disorder, or condition)
- Impairments
- Functional limitations
- Disabilities
- Risk reduction/prevention
- Health, wellness, and fitness
- Societal resources
- Patient/client satisfaction

In some instances, a particular anticipated goal or expected outcome is thoroughly achieved through implementation of a single form of intervention. More commonly, however, the anticipated goals and expected outcomes are achieved as a result of the combined effects of several forms of interventions, leading to enhancement of both health status and health-related quality of life.

Criteria for Termination of Physical Therapy Services

Discharge is the process of ending physical therapy services that have been provided during a single episode of care. It occurs when the anticipated goals and expected outcomes have been achieved. Discharge does *not* occur with a *transfer* (defined as the time when a patient is moved from one site to another site within the same setting or across settings during a single episode of care). Although there may be facility-specific or payer-specific requirements for documentation regarding the conclusion of physical therapy services, *discharge occurs based on the physical therapist's analysis of the achievement of anticipated goals and expected outcomes.*

Discontinuation is the process of ending physical therapy services that have been provided during a single episode of care when (1) the patient/client, caregiver, or legal guardian declines to continue intervention; (2) the patient/client is unable to continue to progress toward outcomes because of medical or psychosocial complications or because financial/insurance resources have been expended; or (3) the physical therapist determines that the patient/client will no longer benefit from physical therapy. When physical therapy services are terminated prior to achievement of anticipated goals and expected outcomes, patient/client status and the rationale for termination are documented.

For patients/clients who require multiple episodes of care, periodic follow-up is needed over the life span to ensure safety and effective adaptation following changes in physical status, caregivers, environment, or task demands. In consultation with appropriate individuals, and in consideration of the outcomes, the physical therapist plans for discharge or discontinuation and provides for appropriate follow-up or referral.

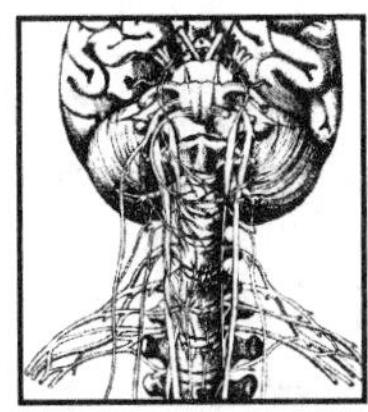

Impaired Peripheral Nerve Integrity and Muscle Performance Associated With Peripheral Nerve Injury

This preferred practice pattern describes the generally accepted elements of patient/client management that physical therapists provide for patients/clients who are classified in this pattern. The pattern title reflects the diagnosis made by the physical therapist. APTA emphasizes that preferred practice patterns are the boundaries within which a physical therapist may select any of a number of clinical alternatives, based on consideration of a wide variety of factors, such as individual patient/client needs; the profession's code of ethics and standards of practice; and patient/client age, culture, gender roles, race, sex, sexual orientation, and socioeconomic status.

Patient/Client Diagnostic Classification

Patients/clients will be classified into this pattern—for impaired peripheral nerve integrity and muscle performance associated with peripheral nerve injury—as a result of the physical therapist's evaluation of the examination data. The findings from the examination (history, systems review, and tests and measures) may indicate the presence or risk of pathology/pathophysiology (disease, disorder, or condition), impairments, functional limitations, or disabilities or the need for health, wellness, or fitness programs. The physical therapist integrates, synthesizes, and interprets the data to determine the diagnostic classification.

Inclusion

The following examples of examination findings may support the inclusion of patients/clients in this pattern:

Risk Factors or Consequences of Pathology/Pathophysiology (Disease, Disorder, or Condition)

- Neuropathies
  - Carpal tunnel syndrome
  - Cubital tunnel syndrome
  - Erb palsy
  - Radial tunnel syndrome
  - Tarsal tunnel syndrome
- Peripheral vestibular disorders
  - Labyrinthitis
  - Paroxysmal positional vertigo
- Surgical nerve lesions
- Traumatic nerve lesions

Impairments, Functional Limitations, or Disabilities

- Difficulty with manipulation skills
- Decreased muscle strength
- Impaired peripheral nerve integrity
- Impaired proprioception
- Impaired sensory integrity
- Loss of balance during daily activities
- Inability to negotiate community environment
- Lack of safety in home environment

Note:

Some risk factors or consequences of pathology/pathophysiology—such as *peripheral vascular disease*—may be severe and complex; *however, they do not necessarily exclude patients/clients from this pattern.* Severe and complex risk factors or consequences may require modification of the frequency of visits and duration of care. (See "Evaluation, Diagnosis, and Prognosis," page 399.)

Exclusion or Multiple-Pattern Classification

The following examples of examination findings may support exclusion from this pattern or classification into additional patterns. Depending on the level of severity or complexity of the examination findings, the physical therapist may determine that the patient/client would be more appropriately managed through (1) classification in an entirely different pattern or (2) classification in both this and another pattern.

Findings That May Require Classification in a Different Pattern

- Impairments associated with Bell palsy
- Impairments associated with demyelinating disease
- Radiculopathies

Findings That May Require Classification in Additional Patterns

- Decubitis ulcer
- Reflex sympathetic dystrophy syndrome

ICD-9-CM Codes

The listing below contains the current (as of press time) and most typical 3- and 4-digit ICD-9-CM codes related to this preferred practice pattern. Because patient/client diagnostic classification is based on impairments, functional limitations, and disabilities—not on codes—patients/clients may be classified into the pattern even though the codes listed with the pattern may not apply to those clients.

This listing is intended for general information only and should not be used for coding purposes. The codes should be confirmed by referring to the World Health Organization's *International Classification of Diseases, 9th Revision, Clinical Modification (ICD-9-CM 2001)*, Volumes 1 and 3 (Chicago, Ill: American Medical Association; 2000) or subsequent revisions or by referring to other ICD-9-CM coding manuals that contain exclusion notes and instructions regarding fifth-digit requirements.

353 Nerve root and plexus disorders
- **353.0** Brachial plexus lesions
- **353.1** Lumbosacral plexus lesions
- **353.6** Phantom limb (syndrome)

354 Mononeuritis of upper limb and mononeuritis multiplex
- **354.0** Carpal tunnel syndrome
- **354.2** Lesion of ulnar nerve
- **354.3** Lesion of radial nerve

355 Mononeuritis of lower limb

357 Inflammatory and toxic neuropathy
- **357.1** Polyneuropathy in collagen vascular disease*

386 Vertiginous syndromes and other disorders of vestibular system
- **386.0** Ménière's disease
  - **386.03** Active Ménière's disease, vestibular
- **386.1** Other and unspecified peripheral vertigo
- **386.3** Labyrinthitis

767 Birth trauma
- **767.6** Injury to brachial plexus
  Palsy or paralysis:
  Erb (Duchenne)

* Not a primary diagnosis

Examination

Examination is a comprehensive screening and specific testing process that leads to a diagnostic classification or, when appropriate, to a referral to another practitioner. Examination is required prior to the initial intervention and is performed for all patients/clients. Through the examination, the physical therapist may identify impairments, functional limitations, disabilities, changes in physical function or overall health status, and needs related to restoration of health and to prevention, wellness, and fitness. The physical therapist synthesizes the examination findings to establish the diagnosis and the prognosis (including the plan of care). The patient/client, family, significant others, and caregivers may provide information during the examination process.

Examination has three components: the patient/client history, the systems review, and tests and measures. The *history* is a systematic gathering of past and current information (often from the patient/client) related to why the patient/client is seeking the services of the physical therapist. The *systems review* is a brief or limited examination of (1) the anatomical and physiological status of the cardiovascular/pulmonary, integumentary, musculoskeletal, and neuromuscular systems and (2) the communication ability, affect, cognition, language, and learning style of the patient/client. *Tests and measures* are the means of gathering data about the patient/client.

The selection of examination procedures and the depth of the examination vary based on patient/client age; severity of the problem; stage of recovery (acute, subacute, chronic); phase of rehabilitation (early, intermediate, late, return to activity); home, work (job/school/play), or community situation; and other relevant factors. *For clinical indications in selecting tests and measures and for listings of tests and measures, tools used to gather data, and the types of data generated by tests and measures, refer to Chapter 2.*

Patient/Client History

The history may include:

General Demographics
- Age
- Sex
- Race/ethnicity
- Primary language
- Education

Social History
- Cultural beliefs and behaviors
- Family and caregiver resources
- Social interactions, social activities, and support systems

Employment/Work (Job/School/Play)
- Current and prior work (job/school/play), community, and leisure actions, tasks, or activities

Growth and Development
- Developmental history
- Hand dominance

Living Environment
- Devices and equipment (eg, assistive, adaptive, orthotic, protective, supportive, prosthetic)
- Living environment and community characteristics
- Projected discharge destinations

General Health Status (Self-Report, Family Report, Caregiver Report)
- General health perception
- Physical function (eg, mobility, sleep patterns, restricted bed days)
- Psychological function (eg, memory, reasoning ability, depression, anxiety)
- Role function (eg, community, leisure, social, work)
- Social function (eg, social activity, social interaction, social support)

Social/Health Habits (Past and Current)
- Behavioral health risks (eg, smoking, drug abuse)
- Level of physical fitness

Family History
- Familial health risks

Medical/Surgical History
- Cardiovascular
- Endocrine/metabolic
- Gastrointestinal
- Genitourinary
- Gynecological
- Integumentary
- Musculoskeletal
- Neuromuscular
- Obstetrical
- Prior hospitalizations, surgeries, and preexisting medical and other health-related conditions
- Psychological
- Pulmonary

Current Condition(s)/Chief Complaint(s)
- Concerns that led patient/client to seek the services of a physical therapist
- Concerns or needs of patient/client who requires the services of a physical therapist
- Current therapeutic interventions
- Mechanisms of injury or disease, including date of onset and course of events
- Onset and pattern of symptoms
- Patient/client, family, significant other, and caregiver expectations and goals for the therapeutic intervention
- Patient/client, family, significant other, and caregiver perceptions of patient's/client's emotional response to the current clinical situation
- Previous occurrence of chief complaint(s)
- Prior therapeutic interventions

Functional Status and Activity Level
- Current and prior functional status in self-care and home management activities, including activities of daily living (ADL) and instrumental activities of daily living (IADL)
- Current and prior functional status in work (job/school/play), community, and leisure actions, tasks, or activities

Medications
- Medications for current condition
- Medications previously taken for current condition
- Medications for other conditions

Other Clinical Tests
- Laboratory and diagnostic tests
- Review of available records (eg, medical, education, surgical)
- Review of other clinical findings (eg, nutrition and hydration)

Systems Review

The systems review may include:

Anatomical and Physiological Status

- Cardiovascular/Pulmonary
  - Blood pressure
  - Edema
  - Heart rate
  - Respiratory rate
- Integumentary
  - Pliability (texture)
  - Presence of scar formation
  - Skin color
  - Skin integrity
- Musculoskeletal
  - Gross range of motion
  - Gross strength
  - Gross symmetry
  - Height
  - Weight
- Neuromuscular
  - Gross coordinated movements (eg, balance, gait, locomotion, transfers, transitions)
  - Motor function (motor control, motor learning)

Communication, Affect, Cognition, Language, and Learning Style

- Ability to make needs known
- Consciousness
- Expected emotional/behavioral responses
- Learning preferences (eg, education needs, learning barriers)
- Orientation (person, place, time)

Tests and Measures

Test and measures for this pattern may include those that characterize or quantify:

Aerobic Capacity and Endurance

- Aerobic capacity during functional activities (eg, activities of daily living [ADL] scales, indexes, instrumental activities of daily living [IADL] scales, observations)

Anthropometric Characteristics

- Body dimensions (eg, girth measurement, length measurement)
- Edema (eg, girth measurement, palpation, scales, volume measurement)

Assistive and Adaptive Devices

- Assistive or adaptive devices and equipment use during functional activities (eg, ADL scales, functional scales, IADL scales, interviews, observations)
- Components, alignment, fit, and ability to care for the assistive or adaptive devices and equipment (eg, interviews, logs, observations, pressure-sensing maps, reports)
- Remediation of impairments, functional limitations, or disabilities with use of assistive or adaptive devices and equipment (eg, activity status indexes, ADL scales, aerobic capacity tests, functional performance inventories, health assessment questionnaires, IADL scales, pain scales, play scales, videographic assessments)
- Safety during use of assistive or adaptive devices and equipment (eg, diaries, fall scales, interviews, logs, observations, reports)

Circulation (Arterial, Venous, and Lymphatic)

- Cardiovascular signs, including heart rate, rhythm, and sounds; pressures and flow; and superficial vascular responses (eg, auscultation, electrocardiography, girth measurement, observations, palpation, sphygmomanometry, thermography)
- Physiological responses to position change, including autonomic responses, central and peripheral pressures, heart rate and rhythm, respiratory rate and rhythm, ventilatory pattern (eg, auscultation, electrocardiography, observations, palpation, sphygmomanometry)

Cranial and Peripheral Nerve Integrity

- Electrophysiological integrity (eg, electroneuromyography)
- Motor distribution of the cranial nerves (eg, dynamometry, muscle tests, observations)
- Motor distribution of the peripheral nerves (eg, dynamometry, muscle tests, observations, thoracic outlet tests)
- Response to neural provocation (eg, tension tests, vertebral artery compression tests)
- Response to stimuli, including auditory, gustatory, olfactory, pharyngeal, vestibular, and visual (eg, observations, provocation tests)
- Sensory distribution of the cranial nerves (eg, discrimination tests; tactile tests, including coarse and light touch, cold and heat, pain, pressure, and vibration)
- Sensory distribution of the peripheral nerves (eg, discrimination tests; tactile tests, including coarse and light touch, cold and heat, pain, pressure, and vibration; thoracic outlet tests)

Environmental, Home, and Work (Job/School/Play) Barriers

- Current and potential barriers (eg, checklists, interviews, observations, questionnaires)

Ergonomics and Body Mechanics

Ergonomics

- Dexterity and coordination during work (job/school/play) (eg, hand function tests, impairment rating scales, manipulative ability tests)
- Functional capacity and performance during work actions, tasks, or activities (eg, accelerometry, dynamometry, electroneuromyography, endurance tests, force platform tests, goniometry, interviews, observations, photographic assessments, physical capacity tests, postural loading analyses, technology-assisted assessments, videographic assessments, work analyses)
- Safety in work environments (eg, hazard identification checklists, job severity indexes, lifting standards, risk assessment scales, standards for exposure limits)
- Specific work conditions or activities (eg, handling checklists, job simulations, lifting models, preemployment screenings, task analysis checklists, workstation checklists)
- Tools, devices, equipment, and workstations related to work actions, tasks, or activities (eg, observations, tool analysis checklists, vibration assessments)

Body mechanics

- Body mechanics during self-care, home management, work, community, or leisure actions, tasks, or activities (eg, ADL scales, IADL scales, observations, photographic assessments, technology-assisted assessments, videographic assessments)

Gait, Locomotion, and Balance

- Balance during functional activities with or without the use of assistive, adaptive, orthotic, protective, supportive, or prosthetic devices or equipment (eg, ADL scales, IADL scales, observations, videographic assessments)
- Balance (dynamic and static) with or without the use of assistive, adaptive, orthotic, protective, supportive, or prosthetic devices or equipment (eg, balance scales, dizziness inventories, dynamic posturography, fall scales, motor impairment tests, observations, photographic assessments, postural control tests)
- Gait and locomotion during functional activities with or without the use of assistive, adaptive, orthotic, protective, supportive, or prosthetic devices or equipment (eg, ADL scales, gait indexes, IADL scales, mobility skill profiles, observations, videographic assessments)
- Gait and locomotion with or without the use of assistive, adaptive, orthotic, protective, supportive, or prosthetic devices or equipment (eg, dynamometry, electroneuromyography, footprint analyses, gait indexes, mobility skill profiles, observations, photographic assessments, technology-assisted assessments, videographic assessments, weight-bearing scales, wheelchair mobility tests)
- Safety during gait, locomotion, and balance (eg, confidence scales, diaries, fall scales, functional assessment profiles, logs, reports)

Integumentary Integrity

Associated skin

- Activities, positioning, and postures that produce or relieve trauma to the skin (eg, observations, pressure-sensing maps, scales)
- Assistive, adaptive, orthotic, protective, supportive, or prosthetic devices and equipment that may produce or relieve trauma to the skin (eg, observations, pressure-sensing maps, risk assessment scales)
- Skin characteristics, including blistering, continuity of skin color, dermatitis, hair growth, mobility, nail growth, sensation, temperature, texture, and turgor (eg, observations, palpation, photographic assessments, thermography)

Joint Integrity and Mobility

- Joint integrity and mobility (eg, apprehension, compression and distraction, drawer, glide, impingement, shear, and valgus/varus stress tests; arthrometry; palpation)

Motor Function (Motor Control and Motor Learning)

- Dexterity, coordination, and agility (eg, coordination screens, motor impairment tests, motor proficiency tests, observations, videographic assessments)
- Hand function (eg, fine and gross motor control tests, finger dexterity tests, manipulative ability tests, observations)
- Initiation, modification, and control of movement patterns and voluntary postures (eg, activity indexes, developmental scales, gross motor function profiles, motor scales, movement assessment batteries, neuromotor tests, observations, physical performance tests, postural challenge tests, videographic assessments)

Muscle Performance (Including Strength, Power, and Endurance)

- Electrophysiological integrity (eg, electroneuromyography)
- Muscle strength, power, and endurance (eg, dynamometry, manual muscle tests, muscle performance tests, physical capacity tests, technology-assisted assessments, timed activity tests)
- Muscle strength, power, and endurance during functional activities (eg, ADL scales, functional muscle tests, IADL scales, observations, videographic assessments)
- Muscle tension (eg, palpation)

Orthotic, Protective, and Supportive Devices

- Components, alignment, fit, and ability to care for orthotic, protective, and supportive devices and equipment (eg, interviews, logs, observations, pressure-sensing maps, reports)
- Orthotic, protective, and supportive devices and equipment use during functional activities (eg, ADL scales, functional scales, IADL scales, interviews, observations, profiles)
- Remediation of impairments, functional limitations, or disabilities with use of orthotic, protective, and supportive devices and equipment (eg, activity status indexes, ADL scales, aerobic capacity tests, functional performance inventories, health assessment questionnaires, IADL scales, pain scales, play scales, videographic assessments)
- Safety during use of orthotic, protective, and supportive devices and equipment (eg, diaries, fall scales, interviews, logs, observations, reports)

Pain

- Pain, soreness, and nociception (eg, analog scales, discrimination tests, pain drawings and maps, provocation tests, verbal and pictorial descriptor tests,)
- Pain in specific body parts (eg, pain indexes, pain questionnaires, structural provocation tests)

Posture

- Postural alignment and position (static and dynamic), including symmetry and deviation from midline (eg, grid measurement, observations, photographic assessments, technology-assisted assessments, videographic assessments)
- Specific body parts (eg, angle assessments, forward-bending test, goniometry, observations, palpation, positional tests)

Range of Motion (ROM) (Including Muscle Length)

- Functional ROM (eg, observations, squat testing, toe touch tests)
- Joint active and passive movement (eg, goniometry, inclinometry, observations, photographic assessments, technology-assisted assessments, videographic assessments)
- Muscle length, soft tissue extensibility, and flexibility (eg, contracture tests, goniometry, inclinometry, ligamentous tests, linear measurement, multisegment flexibility tests, palpation)

Reflex Integrity

- Deep reflexes (eg, myotatic reflex scale, observations, reflex tests)
- Electrophysiological integrity (eg, electroneuromyography)
- Postural reflexes and reactions, including righting, equilibrium, and protective reactions (eg, observations, postural challenge tests, reflex profiles, videographic assessments)
- Superficial reflexes and reactions (eg, observations, provocation tests)

Self-Care and Home Management (Including ADL and IADL)

- Ability to gain access to home environments (eg, barrier identification, observations, physical performance tests)
- Ability to perform self-care and home management activities with or without assistive, adaptive, orthotic, protective, supportive, or prosthetic devices and equipment (eg, ADL scales, aerobic capacity tests, IADL scales, interviews, observations, profiles)
- Safety in self-care and home management activities and environments (eg, diaries, fall scales, interviews, logs, observations, reports, videographic assessments)

Sensory Integrity

- Combined/cortical sensations (eg, stereognosis, tactile discrimination tests)
- Deep sensations (eg, kinesthesiometry, observations, photographic assessments, vibration tests)
- Electrophysiological integrity (eg, electroneuromyography)

Work (Job/School/Play), Community, and Leisure Integration or Reintegration (Including IADL)

- Ability to assume or resume work (job/school/play), community, and leisure activities with or without assistive, adaptive, orthotic, protective, supportive, or prosthetic devices and equipment (eg, activity profiles, disability indexes, functional status questionnaires, IADL scales, observations, physical capacity tests)
- Ability to gain access to work (job/school/play), community, and leisure environments (eg, barrier identification, interviews, observations, physical capacity tests, transportation assessments)
- Safety in work (job/school/play), community, and leisure activities and environments (eg, diaries, fall scales, interviews, logs, observations, videographic assessments)

Evaluation, Diagnosis, and Prognosis (Including Plan of Care)

Physical therapists perform *evaluations* (make clinical judgments) based on the data gathered from the history, systems review, and tests and measures. In the evaluation process, physical therapists synthesize the examination data to establish the diagnosis and prognosis (including the plan of care). Factors that influence the complexity of the evaluation include the clinical findings, extent of loss of function, chronicity or severity of the problem, possibility of multisite or multisystem involvement, preexisting condition(s), potential discharge destination, social considerations, physical function, and overall health status.

A *diagnosis* is a label encompassing a cluster of signs and symptoms, syndromes, or categories. It is the result of the systematic diagnostic process, which includes integrating and evaluating the data from the examination. The diagnostic label indicates the primary dysfunction(s) toward which the therapist will direct interventions. The *prognosis* is the determination of the predicted optimal level of improvement in function and the amount of time needed to reach that level and may also include a prediction of levels of improvement that may be reached at various intervals during the course of therapy. During the prognostic process, the physical therapist develops the plan of care. The *plan of care* identifies specific interventions, proposed frequency and duration of the interventions, anticipated goals, expected outcomes, and discharge plans. The plan of care identifies realistic anticipated goals and expected outcomes, taking into consideration the expectations of the patient/client and appropriate others. These anticipated goals and expected outcomes should be measureable and time limited.

The frequency of visits and duration of the episode of care may vary from a short episode with a high intensity of intervention to a longer episode with a diminishing intensity of intervention. Frequency and duration may vary greatly among patients/clients based on a variety of factors that the physical therapist considers throughout the evaluation process, such as anatomical and physiological changes related to growth and development; caregiver consistency or expertise; chronicity or severity of the current condition; living environment; multisite or multisystem involvement; social support; potential discharge destinations; probability of prolonged impairment, functional limitation, or disability; and stability of the condition.

Prognosis

Over the course of 4 to 8 months, patient/client will demonstrate optimal peripheral nerve integrity and muscle performance and the highest level of functioning in home, work (job/school/play), community, and leisure environments, within the context of the impairments, functional limitations, and disabilities.

During the episode of care, patient/client will achieve (1) the anticipated goals and expected outcomes of the interventions that are described in the plan of care and (2) the global outcomes for patients/clients who are classified in this pattern.

Expected Range of Number of Visits Per Episode of Care

12 to 56

This range represents the lower and upper limits of the number of physical therapist visits required to achieve anticipated goals and expected outcomes. *It is anticipated that 80% of patients/clients who are classified into this pattern will achieve the anticipated goals and expected outcomes within 12 to 56 visits during a single continuous episode of care.* Frequency of visits and duration of the episode of care should be determined by the physical therapist to maximize effectiveness of care and efficiency of service delivery.

Factors That May Require New Episode of Care or That May Modify Frequency of Visits/Duration of Care

- Accessibility and availability of resources
- Adherence to the intervention program
- Age
- Anatomical and physiological changes related to growth and development
- Caregiver consistency or expertise
- Chronicity or severity of the current condition
- Cognitive status
- Comorbitities, complications, or secondary impairments
- Concurrent medical, surgical, and therapeutic interventions
- Decline in functional independence
- Level of impairment
- Level of physical function
- Living environment
- Multisite or multisystem involvement
- Nutritional status
- Overall health status
- Potential discharge destinations
- Premorbid conditions
- Probability of prolonged impairment, functional limitation, or disability
- Psychological and socioeconomic factors
- Psychomotor abilities
- Social support
- Stability of the condition

Intervention

Intervention is the purposeful interaction of the physical therapist with the patient/client and, when appropriate, with other individuals involved in patient/client care, using various physical therapy procedures and techniques to produce changes in the condition consistent with the diagnosis and prognosis. Decisions about interventions are contingent on the timely monitoring of patient/client response and the progress made toward achieving the anticipated goals and expected outcomes.

Communication, coordination, and documentation and patient/client-related instruction are provided for all patients/clients across all settings. Procedural interventions are selected or modified based on the examination data and the evaluation, the diagnosis and the prognosis, and the anticipated goals and expected outcomes for a particular patient/client. *For clinical considerations in selecting interventions, listings of interventions, and listings of anticipated goals and expected outcomes, refer to Chapter 3.*

Coordination, Communication, and Documentation

Coordination, communication, and documentation may include:

Interventions

- Addressing required functions
  - advance directives
  - individualized family service plans (IFSPs) or individualized education plans (IEPs)
  - informed consent
  - mandatory communication and reporting (eg, patient advocacy and abuse reporting)
- Admission and discharge planning
- Case management
- Collaboration and coordination with agencies, including:
  - equipment suppliers
  - home care agencies
  - payer groups
  - schools
  - transportation agencies
- Communication across settings, including:
  - case conferences
  - documentation
  - education plans
- Cost-effective resource utilization
- Data collection, analysis, and reporting
  - outcome data
  - peer review findings
  - record reviews
- Documentation across settings, following APTA's *Guidelines for Physical Therapy Documentation* (Appendix 5), including:
  - changes in impairments, functional limitations, and disabilities
  - changes in interventions
  - elements of patient/client management (examination, evaluation, diagnosis, prognosis, intervention)
  - outcomes of intervention
- Interdisciplinary teamwork
  - case conferences
  - patient care rounds
  - patient/client family meetings
- Referrals to other professionals or resources

Anticipated Goals and Expected Outcomes

- Accountability for services is increased.
- Admission data and discharge planning are completed.
- Advance directives, individualized family service plans (IFSPs) or individualized education plans (IEPs), informed consent, and mandatory communication and reporting (eg, patient advocacy and abuse reporting) are obtained or completed.
- Available resources are maximally utilized.
- Care is coordinated with patient/client, family, significant others, caregivers, and other professionals.
- Case is managed throughout the episode of care.
- Collaboration and coordination occurs with agencies, including equipment suppliers, home care agencies, payer groups, schools, and transportation agencies.
- Communication enhances risk reduction and prevention.
- Communication occurs across settings through case conferences, education plans, and documentation.
- Data are collected, analyzed, and reported, including outcome data, peer review findings, and record reviews.
- Decision making is enhanced regarding on health, wellness, and fitness needs.
- Decision making is enhanced regarding patient/client health and the use of health care resources by patient/client, family, significant others, and caregivers.
- Documentation occurs throughout patient/client management and across settings and follows APTA's *Guidelines for Physical Therapy Documentation* (Appendix 5).
- Interdisciplinary collaboration occurs through case conferences, patient care rounds, and patient/client family meetings.
- Patient/client, family, significant other, and caregiver understanding of anticipated goals and expected outcomes is increased.
- Placement needs are determined.
- Referrals are made to other professionals or resources whenever necessary and appropriate.
- Resources are utilized in a cost-effective way.

Patient/Client-Related Instruction

Patient/client-related instruction may include:

Interventions

- Instruction, education and training of patients/clients and caregivers regarding:
  - current condition (pathology/pathophysiology [disease, disorder, or condition], impairments, functional limitations, or disabilities)
  - enhancement of performance
  - health, wellness, and fitness programs
  - plan of care
  - risk factors for pathology/pathophysiology (disease, disorder, or condition), impairments, functional limitations, or disabilities
  - transitions across settings
  - transitions to new roles

Anticipated Goals and Expected Outcomes

- Ability to perform physical actions, tasks, or activities is improved.
- Awareness and use of community resources are improved.
- Behaviors that foster healthy habits, wellness, and prevention are acquired.
- Decision making is enhanced regarding patient/client health and the use of health care resources by patient/client, family, significant others, and caregivers.
- Disability associated with acute or chronic illnesses is reduced.
- Functional independence in activities of daily living (ADL) and instrumental activities of daily living (IADL) is increased.
- Health status is improved.
- Intensity of care is decreased.
- Level of supervision required for task performance is decreased.
- Patient/client, family, significant other, and caregiver knowledge and awareness of the diagnosis, prognosis, interventions, and anticipated goals and expected outcomes are increased.
- Patient/client knowledge of personal and environmental factors associated with the condition is increased.
- Performance levels in self-care, home management, work (job/school/play), community, or leisure actions, tasks, or activities are improved.
- Physical function is improved.
- Risk of recurrence of condition is reduced.
- Risk of secondary impairment is reduced.
- Safety of patient/client, family, significant others, and caregivers is improved.
- Self-management of symptoms is improved.
- Utilization and cost of health care services are decreased.

Procedural Interventions

Procedural interventions for this pattern may include:

Therapeutic Exercise

Interventions

- Aerobic and endurance conditioning or reconditioning
  - aquatic programs
  - gait and locomotor training
  - increased workload over time
  - walking and wheelchair propulsion programs
- Balance, coordination, and agility training
  - developmental activities training
  - motor function (motor control and motor learning) training or retraining
  - neuromuscular education or reeducation
  - perceptual training
  - posture awareness training
  - standardized, programmatic, complementary exercise approaches
  - sensory training or retraining
  - task-specific performance training
  - vestibular training
- Body mechanics and postural stabilization
  - body mechanics training
  - posture awareness training
  - postural control training
  - postural stabilization activities
- Flexibility exercises
  - muscle lengthening
  - range of motion
  - stretching
- Gait and locomotion training
  - developmental activities training
  - gait training
  - implement and device training
  - perceptual training
  - standardized, programmatic, complementary exercise approaches
  - wheelchair training
- Strength, power, and endurance training for head, neck, limb, pelvic-floor, trunk, and ventilatory muscles
  - active assistive, active, and resistive exercises (including concentric, dynamic/isotonic, eccentric, isokinetic, isometric, and plyometric)
  - aquatic programs
  - standardized, programmatic, complementary exercise approaches
  - task-specific performance training
- Relaxation
  - breathing strategies
  - movement strategies
  - relaxation techniques

Anticipated Goals and Expected Outcomes

- Impact on pathology/pathophysiology (disease, disorder, or condition)
  - Joint swelling, inflammation, or restriction is reduced.
  - Nutrient delivery to tissue is increased.
  - Osteogenic effects of exercise are maximized.
  - Pain is decreased.
  - Physiological response to increased oxygen demand is improved.
  - Soft tissue swelling, inflammation, or restriction is reduced.
  - Tissue perfusion and oxygenation are enhanced.
- Impact on impairments
  - Aerobic capacity is increased.
  - Balance is improved.
  - Endurance is increased.
  - Energy expenditure per unit of work is decreased.
  - Gait, locomotion, and balance are improved.
  - Integumentary integrity is improved.
  - Joint integrity and mobility are improved.
  - Motor function (motor control and motor learning) is improved.
  - Muscle performance (strength, power, and endurance) is increased.
  - Postural control is improved.
  - Quality and quantity of movement between and across body segments are improved.
  - Range of motion is improved.
  - Relaxation is increased.
  - Sensory awareness is increased.
  - Weight-bearing status is improved.
  - Work of breathing is decreased.
- Impact on functional limitations
  - Ability to perform physical actions, tasks, or activities related to self-care, home management, work (job/school/play), community, and leisure is improved.
  - Level of supervision required for task performance is decreased.
  - Performance of and independence in activities of daily living (ADL) and instrumental activities of daily living (IADL) with or without devices and equipment are increased.
  - Tolerance of positions and activities is increased.
- Impact on disabilities
  - Ability to assume or resume required self-care, home management, work (job/school/play), community, and leisure roles is improved.
- Risk reduction/prevention
  - Preoperative and postoperative complications are reduced.
  - Risk factors are reduced.
  - Risk of recurrence of condition is reduced.
  - Risk of secondary impairment is reduced.
  - Safety is improved.
  - Self-management of symptoms is improved.
- Impact on health, wellness, and fitness
  - Fitness is improved.
  - Health status is improved.
  - Physical capacity is increased.
  - Physical function is improved.
- Impact on societal resources
  - Utilization of physical therapy services is optimized.
  - Utilization of physical therapy services results in efficient use of health care dollars.
- Patient/client satisfaction
  - Access, availability, and services provided are acceptable to patient/client.
  - Administrative management of practice is acceptable to patient/client.
  - Clinical proficiency of physical therapist is acceptable to patient/client.
  - Coordination of care is acceptable to patient/client.
  - Cost of health care services is decreased.
  - Intensity of care is decreased.
  - Interpersonal skills of physical therapist are acceptable to patient/client, family, and significant others.
  - Sense of well-being is improved.
  - Stressors are decreased.

Functional Training in Self-Care and Home Management (Including Activities of Daily Living [ADL] and Instrumental Activities of Daily Living [IADL])

Interventions

- ADL training
  - bathing
  - bed mobility and transfer training
  - developmental activities
  - dressing
  - eating
  - grooming
  - toileting
- Functional training programs
  - simulated environments and tasks
  - task adaptation
  - travel training
- IADL training
  - caring for dependents
  - home maintenance
  - household chores
  - shopping
  - structured play for infants and children
  - yard work
- Injury prevention or reduction
  - injury prevention education during self-care and home management
  - injury prevention or reduction with use of devices and equipment
  - safety awareness training during self-care and home management

Anticipated Goals and Expected Outcomes

- Impact on pathology/pathophysiology (disease, disorder, or condition)
  - Pain is decreased.
  - Physiological response to increased oxygen demand is improved.
- Impact on impairments
  - Balance is improved.
  - Endurance is increased.
  - Energy expenditure per unit of work is decreased.
  - Motor function (motor control and motor learning) is improved.
  - Muscle performance (strength, power, and endurance) is increased.
  - Postural control is improved.
  - Sensory awareness is increased.
  - Weight-bearing status is improved.
  - Work of breathing is decreased.
- Impact on functional limitations
  - Ability to perform physical actions, tasks, or activities related to self-care and home management is improved.
  - Level of supervision required for task performance is decreased.
  - Performance of and independence in ADL and IADL with or without devices and equipment are increased.
  - Tolerance of positions and activities is increased.
- Impact on disabilities
  - Ability to assume or resume required self-care and home management roles is improved.
- Risk reduction/prevention
  - Risk factors are reduced.
  - Risk of secondary impairments is reduced.
  - Safety is improved.
  - Self-management of symptoms is improved.
- Impact on health, wellness, and fitness
  - Health status is improved.
  - Physical capacity is increased.
  - Physical function is improved.
- Impact on societal resources
  - Utilization of physical therapy services is optimized.
  - Utilization of physical therapy services results in efficient use of health care dollars.
- Patient/client satisfaction
  - Access, availability, and services provided are acceptable to patient/client.
  - Administrative management of practice is acceptable to patient/client.
  - Clinical proficiency of physical therapist is acceptable to patient/client.
  - Coordination of care is acceptable to patient/client.
  - Cost of health care services is decreased.
  - Intensity of care is decreased.
  - Interpersonal skills of physical therapist are acceptable to patient/client, family, and significant others.
  - Sense of well-being is improved.
  - Stressors are decreased.

Functional Training in Work (Job/School/Play), Community, and Leisure Integration or Reintegration (Including Instrumental Activities of Daily Living [IADL], Work Hardening, and Work Conditioning)

Interventions

- Functional training programs
  - back schools
  - job coaching
  - simulated environments and tasks
  - task adaptation
  - task training
  - travel training
- IADL training
  - community service training involving instruments
  - school and play activities training including tools and instruments
  - work training with tools
- Injury prevention or reduction
  - injury prevention education during work (job/school/play), community, and leisure integration or reintegration
  - injury prevention or reduction with use of devices and equipment
  - safety awareness training during work (job/school/play), community, and leisure integration or reintegration
- Leisure and play activities training

Anticipated Goals and Expected Outcomes

- Impact on pathology/pathophysiology (disease, disorder, or condition)
  - Pain is decreased.
  - Physiological response to increased oxygen demand is improved.
- Impact on impairments
  - Balance is improved.
  - Endurance is increased.
  - Energy expenditure per unit of work is decreased.
  - Motor function (motor control and motor learning) is improved.
  - Muscle performance (strength, power, and endurance) is increased.
  - Postural control is improved.
  - Sensory awareness is increased.
  - Weight-bearing status is improved.
  - Work of breathing is decreased.
- Impact on functional limitations
  - Ability to perform physical actions, tasks, or activities related to work (job/school/play), community, and leisure integration or reintegration is improved.
  - Level of supervision required for task performance is decreased.
  - Performance of and independence in IADL with or without devices and equipment are increased.
  - Tolerance of positions and activities is increased.
- Impact on disabilities
  - Ability to assume or resume required work (job/school/play), community, and leisure roles is improved.
- Risk reduction/prevention
  - Risk factors are reduced.
  - Risk of secondary impairment is reduced.
  - Safety is improved.
  - Self-management of symptoms is improved.
- Impact on health, wellness, and fitness
  - Fitness is improved.
  - Health status is improved.
  - Physical capacity is increased.
  - Physical function is improved.
- Impact on societal resources
  - Costs of work-related injury or disability are reduced.
  - Utilization of physical therapy services is optimized.
  - Utilization of physical therapy services results in efficient use of health care dollars.
- Patient/client satisfaction
  - Access, availability, and services provided are acceptable to patient/client.
  - Administrative management of practice is acceptable to patient/client.
  - Clinical proficiency of physical therapist is acceptable to patient/client.
  - Coordination of care is acceptable to patient/client.
  - Cost of health care services is decreased.
  - Intensity of care is decreased.
  - Interpersonal skills of physical therapist are acceptable to patient/client, family, and significant others.
  - Sense of well-being is improved.
  - Stressors are decreased.

Manual Therapy Techniques (Including Mobilization/Manipulation)

Interventions

- Massage
  - connective tissue massage
  - therapeutic massage
- Mobilization/manipulation
  - soft tissue
- Passive range of motion

Anticipated Goals and Expected Outcomes

- Impact on pathology/pathophysiology (disease, disorder, or condition)
  - Edema, lymphedema, or effusion is reduced.
  - Joint swelling, inflammation, or restriction is reduced.
  - Pain is decreased.
  - Soft tissue swelling, inflammation, or restriction is reduced.
- Impact on impairments
  - Balance is improved.
  - Energy expenditure per unit of work is decreased.
  - Gait, locomotion, and balance are improved.
  - Integumentary integrity is improved.
  - Muscle performance (strength, power, and endurance) is increased.
  - Postural control is improved.
  - Quality and quantity of movement between and across body segments are improved.
  - Range of motion is improved.
  - Relaxation is increased.
  - Sensory awareness is increased.
  - Weight-bearing status is improved.
  - Work of breathing is decreased.
- Impact on functional limitations
  - Ability to perform movement tasks is improved.
  - Ability to perform physical actions, tasks, or activities related to self-care, home management, work (job/school/play), community, and leisure is improved.
  - Tolerance of positions and activities is increased.
- Impact on disabilities
  - Ability to assume or resume required self-care, home management, work (job/school/play), community, and leisure roles is improved.
- Risk reduction/prevention
  - Risk factors are reduced.
  - Risk of recurrence of condition is reduced.
  - Risk of secondary impairment is reduced.
  - Self-management of symptoms is improved.
- Impact on health, wellness, and fitness
  - Physical capacity is increased.
  - Physical function is improved.
- Impact on societal resources
  - Utilization of physical therapy services is optimized.
  - Utilization of physical therapy services results in efficient use of health care dollars.
  - Access, availability, and services provided are acceptable to patient/client.
  - Administrative management of practice is acceptable to patient/client.
  - Clinical proficiency of physical therapist is acceptable to patient/client.
  - Coordination of care is acceptable to patient/client.
  - Cost of health care services is decreased.
  - Intensity of care is decreased.
  - Interpersonal skills of physical therapist are acceptable to patient/client, family, and significant others.
  - Sense of well-being is improved.
  - Stressors are decreased.

Prescription, Application, and, as Appropriate, Fabrication of Devices and Equipment (Assistive, Adaptive, Orthotic, Protective, Supportive, and Prosthetic)

Interventions

- Adaptive devices
  - environmental controls
  - raised toilet seats
  - seating systems
- Assistive devices
  - canes
  - crutches
  - long-handled reachers
  - power devices
  - static and dynamic splints
  - walkers
  - wheelchairs
- Orthotic devices
  - braces
  - casts
  - shoe inserts
  - splints
- Prosthetic devices (lower-extremity and upper-extremity)
- Protective devices
  - braces
  - cushions
  - helmets
  - protective taping
- Supportive devices
  - compression garments
  - corsets
  - elastic wraps
  - neck collars
  - serial casts
  - slings
  - supplemental oxygen
  - supportive taping

Anticipated Goals and Expected Outcomes

- Impact on pathology/pathophysiology (disease, disorder, or condition)
  - Edema, lymphedema, or effusion is reduced.
  - Joint swelling, inflammation, or restriction is reduced.
  - Pain is decreased.
  - Physiological response to increased oxygen demand is improved.
  - Soft tissue swelling, inflammation, or restriction is reduced.
- Impact on impairments
  - Balance is improved.
  - Endurance is increased.
  - Energy expenditure per unit of work is decreased.
  - Gait, locomotion, and balance are improved.
  - Integumentary integrity is improved.
  - Joint stability is improved.
  - Motor function (motor control and motor learning) is improved.
  - Muscle performance (strength, power, and endurance) is increased.
  - Optimal joint alignment is achieved.
  - Optimal loading on a body part is achieved.
  - Postural control is improved.
  - Quality and quantity of movement between and across body segments are improved.
  - Range of motion is improved.
  - Weight-bearing status is improved.
  - Work of breathing is decreased.
- Impact on functional limitations
  - Ability to perform physical actions, tasks, or activities related to self-care, home management, work (job/school/play), community, and leisure is improved.
  - Level of supervision required for task performance is decreased.
  - Performance of and independence in activities of daily living (ADL) and instrumental activities of daily living (IADL) with or without devices and equipment are increased.
  - Tolerance of positions and activities is increased.
- Impact on disabilities
  - Ability to assume or resume required self-care, home management, work (job/school/play), community, and leisure roles is improved.
- Risk reduction/prevention
  - Pressure on body tissues is reduced.
  - Protection of body parts is increased.
  - Risk factors are reduced.
  - Risk of recurrence of condition is reduced.
  - Risk of secondary impairment is reduced.
  - Safety is improved.
  - Self-management of symptoms is improved.
  - Stresses precipitating injury are decreased.
- Impact on health, wellness, and fitness
  - Health status is improved.
  - Physical capacity is increased.
  - Physical function is improved.
- Impact on societal resources
  - Utilization of physical therapy services is optimized.
  - Utilization of physical therapy services results in efficient use of health care dollars.
- Patient/client satisfaction
  - Access, availability, and services provided are acceptable to patient/client.
  - Administrative management of practice is acceptable to patient/client.
  - Clinical proficiency of physical therapist is acceptable to patient/client.
  - Coordination of care is acceptable to patient/client.
  - Cost of health care services is decreased.
  - Intensity of care is decreased.
  - Interpersonal skills of physical therapist are acceptable to patient/client, family, and significant others.
  - Sense of well-being is improved.
  - Stressors are decreased.

Electrotherapeutic Modalities

Interventions

- Biofeedback
- Electrical stimulation
  - electrical muscle stimulation (EMS)
  - functional electrical stimulation (FES)
  - high voltage pulsed current (HVPC)
  - neuromuscular electrical stimulation (NMES)
  - transcutaneous electrical nerve stimulation (TENS)

Anticipated Goals and Expected Outcomes

- Impact on pathology/pathophysiology (disease, disorder, or condition)
  - Edema, lymphedema, or effusion is reduced.
  - Joint swelling, inflammation, or restriction is reduced.
  - Nutrient delivery to tissue is increased.
  - Osteogenic effects are enhanced.
  - Pain is decreased.
  - Soft tissue or wound healing is enhanced.
  - Soft tissue swelling, inflammation, or restriction is reduced.
  - Tissue perfusion and oxygenation are enhanced.
- Impact on impairments
  - Integumentary integrity is improved.
  - Motor function (motor control and motor learning) is improved.
  - Muscle performance (strength, power, and endurance) is increased.
  - Postural control is improved.
  - Quality and quantity of movement between and across body segments are improved.
  - Range of motion is improved.
  - Relaxation is increased.
  - Sensory awareness is increased.
- Impact on functional limitations
  - Ability to perform physical actions, tasks, or activities related to self-care, home management, work (job/school/play), community, and leisure is improved.
  - Level of supervision required for task performance is decreased.
  - Performance of and independence in activities of daily living (ADL) and instrumental activities of daily living (IADL) with or without devices and equipment are increased.
  - Tolerance of positions and activities is increased.
- Impact on disabilities
  - Ability to assume or resume required self-care, home management, work (job/school/play), community, and leisure roles is improved.
- Risk reduction/prevention
  - Preoperative and postoperative complications are reduced.
  - Risk factors are reduced.
  - Risk of recurrence of condition is reduced.
  - Risk of secondary impairment is reduced.
  - Self-management of symptoms is improved.
- Impact on health, wellness, and fitness
  - Physical capacity is increased.
  - Physical function is improved.
- Impact on societal resources
  - Utilization of physical therapy services is optimized.
  - Utilization of physical therapy services results in efficient use of health care dollars.
- Patient/client satisfaction
  - Access, availability, and services provided are acceptable to patient/client.
  - Administrative management of practice is acceptable to patient/client.
  - Clinical proficiency of physical therapist is acceptable to patient/client.
  - Coordination of care is acceptable to patient/client.
  - Interpersonal skills of physical therapist are acceptable to patient/client, family, and significant others.
  - Sense of well-being is improved.
  - Stressors are decreased.

Physical Agents and Mechanical Modalities

Interventions

Physical agents may include:

- Athermal agents
  - pulsed electromagnetic fields
- Cryotherapy
  - cold packs
  - ice massage
- Hydrotherapy
  - whirlpool tanks
  - contrast bath
- Sound agents
  - phonophoresis
  - ultrasound
- Thermotherapy
  - hot packs

Anticipated Goals and Expected Outcomes

- Impact on pathology/pathophysiology (disease, disorder, or condition)
  - Edema, lymphedema, or effusion is reduced.
  - Joint swelling, inflammation, or restriction is reduced.
  - Nutrient delivery to tissue is increased.
  - Pain is decreased.
  - Soft tissue swelling, inflammation, or restriction is reduced.
  - Tissue perfusion and oxygenation are enhanced.
- Impact on impairments
  - Integumentary integrity is improved.
  - Muscle performance (strength, power, and endurance) is increased.
  - Range of motion is improved.
  - Weight-bearing status is improved.
- Impact on functional limitations
  - Ability to perform physical actions, tasks, or activities related to self-care, home management, work (job/school/play), community, and leisure is increased.
  - Performance of and independence in activities of daily living (ADL) and instrumental activities of daily living (IADL) with or without devices and equipment are increased.
  - Tolerance of positions and activities is increased.
- Impact on disabilities
  - Ability to assume or resume required self-care, home management, work (job/school/play), community, and leisure roles is improved.
- Risk reduction/prevention
  - Complications of soft tissue and circulatory disorders are decreased.
  - Risk of secondary impairment is reduced.
  - Self-management of symptoms is improved.
  - Stresses precipitating injury are decreased.
- Impact on health, wellness, and fitness
  - Physical function is improved.
- Impact on societal resources
  - Utilization of physical therapy services is optimized.
- Patient/client satisfaction
  - Access, availability, and services provided are acceptable to patient/client.
  - Administrative management of practice is acceptable to patient/client.
  - Clinical proficiency of physical therapist is acceptable to patient/client.
  - Coordination of care is acceptable to patient/client.
  - Interpersonal skills of physical therapist are acceptable to patient/client, family, and significant others.
  - Sense of well-being is improved.
  - Stressors are decreased.

Reexamination

Reexamination is the process of performing selected tests and measures after the initial examination to evaluate progress and to modify or redirect interventions. Reexamination may be indicated more than once during a single episode of care. It also may be performed over the course of a disease, disorder, or condition, which for some patients/clients may be over the life span. Indications for reexamination include new clinical findings or failure to respond to physical therapy interventions.

Global Outcomes for Patients/Clients in This Pattern

Throughout the entire episode of care, the physical therapist determines the anticipated goals and expected outcomes for each intervention. These anticipated goals and expected outcomes are delineated in shaded boxes that accompany the lists of interventions in each preferred practice pattern. As the patient/client reaches the termination of physical therapy services and the end of the episode of care, the physical therapist measures the global outcomes of the physical therapy services by characterizing or quantifying the impact of the physical therapy interventions in the following domains:

- Pathology/pathophysiology (disease, disorder, or condition)
- Impairments
- Functional limitations
- Disabilities
- Risk reduction/prevention
- Health, wellness, and fitness
- Societal resources
- Patient/client satisfaction

In some instances, a particular anticipated goal or expected outcome is thoroughly achieved through implementation of a single form of intervention. More commonly, however, the anticipated goals and expected outcomes are achieved as a result of the combined effects of several forms of interventions, leading to enhancement of both health status and health-related quality of life.

Criteria for Termination of Physical Therapy Services

Discharge is the process of ending physical therapy services that have been provided during a single episode of care. It occurs when the anticipated goals and expected outcomes have been achieved. Discharge does *not* occur with a *transfer* (defined as the time when a patient is moved from one site to another site within the same setting or across settings during a single episode of care). Although there may be facility-specific or payer-specific requirements for documentation regarding the conclusion of physical therapy services, *discharge occurs based on the physical therapist's analysis of the achievement of anticipated goals and expected outcomes.*

Discontinuation is the process of ending physical therapy services that have been provided during a single episode of care when (1) the patient/client, caregiver, or legal guardian declines to continue intervention; (2) the patient/client is unable to continue to progress toward outcomes because of medical or psychosocial complications or because financial/insurance resources have been expended; or (3) the physical therapist determines that the patient/client will no longer benefit from physical therapy. When physical therapy services are terminated prior to achievement of anticipated goals and expected outcomes, patient/client status and the rationale for termination are documented.

For patients/clients who require multiple episodes of care, periodic follow-up is needed over the life span to ensure safety and effective adaptation following changes in physical status, caregivers, environment, or task demands. In consultation with appropriate individuals, and in consideration of the outcomes, the physical therapist plans for discharge or discontinuation and provides for appropriate follow-up or referral.

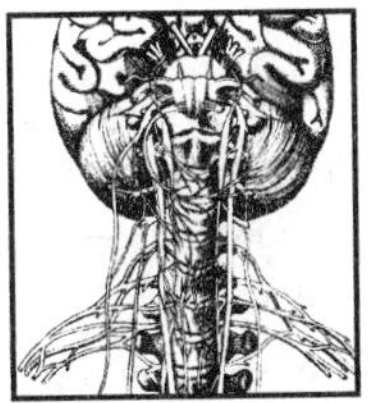

Impaired Motor Function and Sensory Integrity Associated With Acute or Chronic Polyneuropathies

This preferred practice pattern describes the generally accepted elements of patient/client management that physical therapists provide for patients/clients who are classified in this pattern. The pattern title reflects the diagnosis made by the physical therapist. APTA emphasizes that preferred practice patterns are the boundaries within which a physical therapist may select any of a number of clinical alternatives, based on consideration of a wide variety of factors, such as individual patient/client needs; the profession's code of ethics and standards of practice; and patient/client age, culture, gender roles, race, sex, sexual orientation, and socioeconomic status.

Patient/Client Diagnostic Classification

Patients/clients will be classified into this pattern—for impaired motor function and sensory integrity associated with acute or chronic polyneuropathies—as a result of the physical therapist's evaluation of the examination data. The findings from the examination (history, systems review, and tests and measures) may indicate the presence or risk of pathology/pathophysiology (disease, disorder, or condition), impairments, functional limitations, or disabilities or the need for health, wellness, or fitness programs. The physical therapist integrates, synthesizes, and interprets the data to determine the diagnostic classification.

Inclusion

The following examples of examination findings may support the inclusion of patients/clients in this pattern:

Risk Factors or Consequences of Pathology/Pathophysiology (Disease, Disorder, or Condition)

- Amputation
- Axonal polyneuropathies
  - Alcoholic
  - Diabetic
  - Renal
- Dysfunction of the autonomic nervous system
- Guillian-Barré syndrome
- Leprosy
- Post-polio syndrome

Impairments, Functional Limitations, or Disabilities

- Decreased endurance
- Decreased independence in activities of daily living
- Difficulty with manipulation skills
- Impaired motor function
- Impaired peripheral nerve integrity
- Impaired proprioception
- Impaired sensory integrity
- Inability to negotiate work environment
- Lack of safety in community environment
- Loss of balance during daily activities

Note:

Some risk factors or consequences of pathology/pathophysiology—such as *Guillain-Barré syndrome with aspiration pneumonia*—may be severe and complex; *however, they do not necessarily exclude patients/clients from this pattern.* Severe and complex risk factors or consequences may require modification of the frequency of visits and duration of care. (See "Evaluation, Diagnosis, and Prognosis," page 417.)

Exclusion or Multiple-Pattern Classification

The following examples of examination findings may support exclusion from this pattern or classification into additional patterns. Depending on the level of severity or complexity of the examination findings, the physical therapist may determine that the patient/client would be more appropriately managed through (1) classification in an entirely different pattern or (2) classification in both this and another pattern.

Findings That May Require Classification in a Different Pattern

- Coma
- Impairments associated with compression or traumatic neuropathies
- Impairments associated with multisystem trauma

Findings That May Require Classification in Additional Patterns

- Decubitis ulcer

ICD-9-CM Codes

The listing below contains the current (as of press time) and most typical 3- and 4-digit ICD-9-CM codes related to this preferred practice pattern. Because patient/client diagnostic classification is based on impairments, functional limitations, and disabilities—not on codes—patients/clients may be classified into the pattern even though the codes listed with the pattern may not apply to those clients.

This listing is intended for general information only and should not be used for coding purposes. The codes should be confirmed by referring to the World Health Organization's *International Classification of Diseases, 9th Revision, Clinical Modification (ICD-9-CM 2001)*, Volumes 1 and 3 (Chicago, Ill: American Medical Association; 2000) or subsequent revisions or by referring to other ICD-9-CM coding manuals that contain exclusion notes and instructions regarding fifth-digit requirements.

030 Leprosy

138 Late effects of acute poliomyelitis

250 Diabetes mellitus

- **250.6** Diabetes with neurological manifestations

337 Disorders of the autonomic nervous system

- **337.0** Idiopathic peripheral autonomic neuropathy
- **337.1** Peripheral autonomic neuropathy in disorders classified elsewhere *
- **337.2** Reflex sympathetic dystrophy

356 Hereditary and idiopathic peripheral neuropathy

- **356.4** Idiopathic progressive polyneuropathy
- **356.9** Unspecified

357 Inflammatory and toxic neuropathy

- **357.0** Acute infective polyneuritis
  - Guillain-Barré syndrome
- **357.2** Polyneuropathy in diabetes *
- **357.4** Polyneuropathy in other diseases classified elsewhere *
  - Uremia
- **357.5** Alcoholic polyneuropathy
- **357.7** Polyneuropathy due to other toxic agents

588 Disorders resulting from impaired renal function

- **588.1** Nephrogenic diabetes insipidus
- **588.8** Other specified disorders resulting from impaired renal function

* Not a primary diagnosis

Examination

Examination is a comprehensive screening and specific testing process that leads to a diagnostic classification or, when appropriate, to a referral to another practitioner. Examination is required prior to the initial intervention and is performed for all patients/clients. Through the examination, the physical therapist may identify impairments, functional limitations, disabilities, changes in physical function or overall health status, and needs related to restoration of health and to prevention, wellness, and fitness. The physical therapist synthesizes the examination findings to establish the diagnosis and the prognosis (including the plan of care). The patient/client, family, significant others, and caregivers may provide information during the examination process.

Examination has three components: the patient/client history, the systems review, and tests and measures. The *history* is a systematic gathering of past and current information (often from the patient/client) related to why the patient/client is seeking the services of the physical therapist. The *systems review* is a brief or limited examination of (1) the anatomical and physiological status of the cardiovascular/pulmonary, integumentary, musculoskeletal, and neuromuscular systems and (2) the communication ability, affect, cognition, language, and learning style of the patient/client. *Tests and measures* are the means of gathering data about the patient/client.

The selection of examination procedures and the depth of the examination vary based on patient/client age; severity of the problem; stage of recovery (acute, subacute, chronic); phase of rehabilitation (early, intermediate, late, return to activity); home, work (job/school/play), or community situation; and other relevant factors. *For clinical indications in selecting tests and measures and for listings of tests and measures, tools used to gather data, and the types of data generated by tests and measures, refer to Chapter 2.*

Patient/Client History

The history may include:

General Demographics

- Age
- Sex
- Race/ethnicity
- Primary language
- Education

Social History

- Cultural beliefs and behaviors
- Family and caregiver resources
- Social interactions, social activities, and support systems

Employment/Work (Job/School/Play)

- Current and prior work (job/school/play), community, and leisure actions, tasks, or activities

Growth and Development

- Developmental history
- Hand dominance

Living Environment

- Devices and equipment (eg, assistive, adaptive, orthotic, protective, supportive, prosthetic)
- Living environment and community characteristics
- Projected discharge destinations

General Health Status (Self-Report, Family Report, Caregiver Report)

- General health perception
- Physical function (eg, mobility, sleep patterns, restricted bed days)
- Psychological function (eg, memory, reasoning ability, depression, anxiety)
- Role function (eg, community, leisure, social, work)
- Social function (eg, social activity, social interaction, social support)

Social/Health Habits (Past and Current)

- Behavioral health risks (eg, smoking, drug abuse)
- Level of physical fitness

Family History

- Familial health risks

Medical/Surgical History

- Cardiovascular
- Endocrine/metabolic
- Gastrointestinal
- Genitourinary
- Gynecological
- Integumentary
- Musculoskeletal
- Neuromuscular
- Obstetrical
- Prior hospitalizations, surgeries, and preexisting medical and other health-related conditions
- Psychological
- Pulmonary

Current Condition(s)/Chief Complaint(s)

- Concerns that led patient/client to seek the services of a physical therapist
- Concerns or needs of patient/client who requires the services of a physical therapist
- Current therapeutic interventions
- Mechanisms of injury or disease, including date of onset and course of events
- Onset and pattern of symptoms
- Patient/client, family, significant other, and caregiver expectations and goals for the therapeutic intervention
- Patient/client, family, significant other, and caregiver perceptions of patient's/client's emotional response to the current clinical situation
- Previous occurrence of chief complaint(s)
- Prior therapeutic interventions

Functional Status and Activity Level

- Current and prior functional status in self-care and home management activities, including activities of daily living (ADL) and instrumental activities of daily living (IADL)
- Current and prior functional status in work (job/school/play), community, and leisure actions, tasks, or activities

Medications

- Medications for current condition
- Medications previously taken for current condition
- Medications for other conditions

Other Clinical Tests

- Laboratory and diagnostic tests
- Review of available records (eg, medical, education, surgical)
- Review of other clinical findings (eg, nutrition and hydration)

Systems Review

The systems review may include:

Anatomical and Physiological Status

- Cardiovascular/Pulmonary
  - Blood pressure
  - Edema
  - Heart rate
  - Respiratory rate
- Integumentary
  - Pliability (texture)
  - Presence of scar formation
  - Skin color
  - Skin integrity
- Musculoskeletal
  - Gross range of motion
  - Gross strength
  - Gross symmetry
  - Height
  - Weight
- Neuromuscular
  - Gross coordinated movements (eg, balance, gait, locomotion, transfers, transitions)
  - Motor function (motor control, motor learning)

Communication, Affect, Cognition, Language, and Learning Style

- Ability to make needs known
- Consciousness
- Expected emotional/behavioral responses
- Learning preferences (eg, education needs, learning barriers)
- Orientation (person, place, time)

Tests and Measures

Test and measures for this pattern may include those that characterize or quantify:

Aerobic Capacity and Endurance

- Aerobic capacity during functional activities (eg, activities of daily living [ADL] scales, indexes, instrumental activities of daily living [IADL] scales, observations)
- Aerobic capacity during standardized exercise test protocols (eg, ergometry, step tests, time/distance walk/run tests, treadmill tests, wheelchair tests)
- Cardiovascular signs and symptoms in response to increased oxygen demand with exercise or activity, including pressures and flow; heart rate, rhythm, and sounds; and superficial vascular responses (eg, angina, claudication, and exertion scales; electrocardiography; observations; palpation; sphygmomanometry)
- Pulmonary signs and symptoms in response to increased oxygen demand with exercise or activity, including breath and voice sounds; cyanosis; gas exchange; respiratory pattern, rate, and rhythm; and ventilatory flow, force, and volume (eg, auscultation, dyspnea and exertion scales, gas analyses, observations, oximetry, palpation, pulmonary function tests)

Anthropometric Characteristics

- Body composition (eg, body mass index, impedance measurement, skinfold thickness measurement)
- Body dimensions (eg, girth measurement, length measurement)
- Edema (eg, girth measurement, palpation, scales, volume measurement)

Assistive and Adaptive Devices

- Assistive or adaptive devices and equipment use during functional activities (eg, ADL scales, functional scales, IADL scales, interviews, observations)
- Components, alignment, fit, and ability to care for the assistive or adaptive devices and equipment (eg, interviews, logs, observations, pressure-sensing maps, reports)
- Remediation of impairments, functional limitations, or disabilities with use of assistive or adaptive devices and equipment (eg, activity status indexes, ADL scales, aerobic capacity tests, functional performance inventories, health assessment questionnaires, IADL scales, pain scales, play scales, videographic assessments)
- Safety during use of assistive or adaptive devices and equipment (eg, diaries, fall scales, interviews, logs, observations, reports)

Circulation (Arterial, Venous, and Lymphatic)

- Cardiovascular signs, including heart rate, rhythm, and sounds; pressures and flow; and superficial vascular responses (eg, auscultation, electrocardiography, girth measurement, observations, palpation, sphygmomanometry, thermography)
- Cardiovascular symptoms (eg, angina, claudication, dyspnea, and perceived exertion scales)
- Physiological responses to position change, including autonomic responses, central and peripheral pressures, heart rate and rhythm, respiratory rate and rhythm, ventilatory pattern (eg, auscultation, electrocardiography, observations, palpation, sphygmomanometry)

Cranial and Peripheral Nerve Integrity

- Electrophysiological integrity (eg, electroneuromyography)
- Motor distribution of the cranial nerves (eg, dynamometry, muscle tests, observations)
- Motor distribution of the peripheral nerves (eg, dynamometry, muscle tests, observations, thoracic outlet tests)
- Response to neural provocation (eg, tension tests, vertebral artery compression tests)
- Response to stimuli, including auditory, gustatory, olfactory, pharyngeal, vestibular, and visual (eg, observations, provocation tests)
- Sensory distribution of the cranial nerves (eg, discrimination tests; tactile tests, including coarse and light touch, cold and heat, pain, pressure, and vibration)
- Sensory distribution of the peripheral nerves (eg, discrimination tests; tactile tests, including coarse and light touch, cold and heat, pain, pressure, and vibration; thoracic outlet tests)

Environmental, Home, and Work (Job/School/Play) Barriers

- Current and potential barriers (eg, checklists, interviews, observations, questionnaires)
- Physical space and environment (eg, compliance standards, observations, photographic assessments, questionnaires, structural specifications, videographic assessments)

Ergonomics and Body Mechanics

Ergonomics

- Dexterity and coordination during work (job/school/play) (eg, hand function tests, impairment rating scales, manipulative ability tests)
- Functional capacity and performance during work actions, tasks, or activities (eg, accelerometry, dynamometry, electroneuromyography, endurance tests, force platform tests, goniometry, interviews, observations, photographic assessments, physical capacity tests, postural loading analyses, technology-assisted assessments, videographic assessments, work analyses)
- Safety in work environments (eg, hazard identification checklists, job severity indexes, lifting standards, risk assessment scales, standards for exposure limits)
- Specific work conditions or activities (eg, handling checklists, job simulations, lifting models, preemployment screenings, task analysis checklists, workstation checklists)
- Tools, devices, equipment, and workstations related to work actions, tasks, or activities (eg, observations, tool analysis checklists, vibration assessments)

Body mechanics

- Body mechanics during self-care, home management, work, community, or leisure actions, tasks, or activities (eg, ADL scales, IADL scales, observations, photographic assessments, technology-assisted assessments, videographic assessments)

Gait, Locomotion, and Balance

- Balance during functional activities with or without the use of assistive, adaptive, orthotic, protective, supportive, or prosthetic devices or equipment (eg, ADL scales, IADL scales, observations, videographic assessments)
- Balance (dynamic and static) with or without the use of assistive, adaptive, orthotic, protective, supportive, or prosthetic devices or equipment (eg, balance scales, dizziness inventories, dynamic posturography, fall scales, motor impairment tests, observations, photographic assessments, postural control tests)
- Gait and locomotion during functional activities with or without the use of assistive, adaptive, orthotic, protective, supportive, or prosthetic devices or equipment (eg, ADL scales, gait indexes, IADL scales, mobility skill profiles, observations, videographic assessments)
- Gait and locomotion with or without the use of assistive, adaptive, orthotic, protective, supportive, or prosthetic devices or equipment (eg, dynamometry, electroneuromyography, footprint analyses, gait indexes, mobility skill profiles, observations, photographic assessments, technology-assisted assessments, videographic assessments, weight-bearing scales, wheelchair mobility tests)
- Safety during gait, locomotion, and balance (eg, confidence scales, diaries, fall scales, functional assessment profiles, logs, reports)

Integumentary Integrity

Associated skin

- Activities, positioning, and postures that produce or relieve trauma to the skin (eg, observations, pressure-sensing maps, scales)
- Assistive, adaptive, orthotic, protective, supportive, or prosthetic devices and equipment that may produce or relieve trauma to the skin (eg, observations, pressure-sensing maps, risk assessment scales)
- Skin characteristics, including blistering, continuity of skin color, dermatitis, hair growth, mobility, nail growth, sensation, temperature, texture, and turgor (eg, observations, palpation, photographic assessments, thermography)

Joint Integrity and Mobility

- Joint integrity and mobility (eg, apprehension, compression and distraction, drawer, glide, impingement, shear, and valgus/varus stress tests; arthrometry; palpation)

Motor Function (Motor Control and Motor Learning)

- Dexterity, coordination, and agility (eg, coordination screens, motor impairment tests, motor proficiency tests, observations, videographic assessments)
- Electrophysiological integrity (eg, electroneuromyography)
- Hand function (eg, fine and gross motor control tests, finger dexterity tests, manipulative ability tests, observations)

Muscle Performance (Including Strength, Power, and Endurance)

- Electrophysiological integrity (eg, electroneuromyography)
- Muscle strength, power, and endurance (eg, dynamometry, manual muscle tests, muscle performance tests, physical capacity tests, technology-assisted assessments, timed activity tests)
- Muscle strength, power, and endurance during functional activities (eg, ADL scales, functional muscle tests, IADL scales, observations, videographic assessments)

Orthotic, Protective, and Supportive Devices

- Components, alignment, fit, and ability to care for orthotic, protective, and supportive devices and equipment (eg, interviews, logs, observations, pressure-sensing maps, reports)
- Orthotic, protective, and supportive devices and equipment use during functional activities (eg, ADL scales, functional scales, IADL scales, interviews, observations)
- Remediation of impairments, functional limitations, or disabilities with use of orthotic, protective, and supportive devices and equipment (eg, activity status indexes, ADL scales, aerobic capacity tests, functional performance inventories, health assessment questionnaires, IADL scales, pain scales, play scales, videographic assessments)
- Safety during use of orthotic, protective, and supportive devices and equipment (eg, diaries, fall scales, interviews, logs, observations, reports)

Pain

- Pain, soreness, and nociception (eg, analog scales, angina scales, discrimination tests, pain drawings and maps, provocation tests, verbal and pictorial descriptor tests)
- Pain in specific body parts (eg, pain indexes, pain questionnaires, structural provocation tests)

Posture

- Postural alignment and position (static and dynamic), including symmetry and deviation from midline (eg, grid measurement, observations, photographic assessments, technology-assisted assessments, videographic assessments)
- Specific body parts (eg, angle assessments, forward-bending test, goniometry, observations, palpation, positional tests)

Range of Motion (ROM) (Including Muscle Length)

- Functional ROM (eg, observations, squat testing, toe touch tests)
- Joint active and passive movement (eg, goniometry, inclinometry, observations, photographic assessments, technology-assisted assessments, videographic assessments)
- Muscle length, soft tissue extensibility, and flexibility (eg, contracture tests, goniometry, inclinometry, ligamentous tests, linear measurement, multisegment flexibility tests, palpation)

Reflex Integrity

- Deep reflexes (eg, myotatic reflex scale, observations, reflex tests)
- Electrophysiological integrity (eg, electroneuromyography)
- Superficial reflexes and reactions (eg, observations, provocation tests)

Self-Care and Home Management (Including ADL and IADL)

- Ability to gain access to home environments (eg, barrier identification, observations, physical performance tests)
- Ability to perform self-care and home management activities with or without assistive, adaptive, orthotic, protective, supportive, or prosthetic devices and equipment (eg, ADL scales, aerobic capacity tests, IADL scales, interviews, observations, profiles)
- Safety in self-care and home management activities and environments (eg, diaries, fall scales, interviews, logs, observations, reports, videographic assessments)

Sensory Integrity

- Combined/cortical sensations (eg, stereognosis tests, tactile discrimination tests)
- Deep sensations (eg, kinesthesiometry, observations, photographic assessments, vibration tests)
- Electrophysiological integrity (eg,electroneuromyography)

Ventilation and Respiration/Gas Exchange

- Pulmonary signs of respiration/gas exchange, including breath sounds (eg, gas analyses, observations, oximetry)
- Pulmonary signs of ventilatory function, including airway protection; breath and voice sounds; respiratory rate, rhythm, and pattern; ventilatory flow, forces, and volumes (eg, airway clearance tests, observations, palpation, pulmonary function tests, ventilatory muscle force tests)
- Pulmonary symptoms (eg, dyspnea and perceived exertion indexes and scales)

Work (Job/School/Play), Community, and Leisure Integration or Reintegration (Including IADL)

- Ability to assume or resume work (job/school/play), community, and leisure activities with or without assistive, adaptive, orthotic, protective, supportive, or prosthetic devices and equipment (eg, activity profiles, disability indexes, functional status questionnaires, IADL scales, observations, physical capacity tests)
- Ability to gain access to work (job/school/play), community, and leisure environments (eg, barrier identification, interviews, observations, physical capacity tests, transportation assessments)
- Safety in work (job/school/play), community, and leisure activities and environments (eg, diaries, fall scales, interviews, logs, observations, videographic assessments)

Evaluation, Diagnosis, and Prognosis (Including Plan of Care)

Physical therapists perform *evaluations* (make clinical judgments) based on the data gathered from the history, systems review, and tests and measures. In the evaluation process, physical therapists synthesize the examination data to establish the diagnosis and prognosis (including the plan of care). Factors that influence the complexity of the evaluation include the clinical findings, extent of loss of function, chronicity or severity of the problem, possibility of multisite or multisystem involvement, preexisting condition(s), potential discharge destination, social considerations, physical function, and overall health status.

A *diagnosis* is a label encompassing a cluster of signs and symptoms, syndromes, or categories. It is the result of the systematic diagnostic process, which includes integrating and evaluating the data from the examination. The diagnostic label indicates the primary dysfunction(s) toward which the therapist will direct interventions. The *prognosis* is the determination of the predicted optimal level of improvement in function and the amount of time needed to reach that level and may also include a prediction of levels of improvement that may be reached at various intervals during the course of therapy. During the prognostic process, the physical therapist develops the plan of care. The *plan of care* identifies specific interventions, proposed frequency and duration of the interventions, anticipated goals, expected outcomes, and discharge plans. The plan of care identifies realistic anticipated goals and expected outcomes, taking into consideration the expectations of the patient/client and appropriate others. These anticipated goals and expected outcomes should be measureable and time limited.

The frequency of visits and duration of the episode of care may vary from a short episode with a high intensity of intervention to a longer episode with a diminishing intensity of intervention. Frequency and duration may vary greatly among patients/clients based on a variety of factors that the physical therapist considers throughout the evaluation process, such as anatomical and physiological changes related to growth and development; caregiver consistency or expertise; chronicity or severity of the current condition; living environment; multisite or multisystem involvement; social support; potential discharge destinations; probability of prolonged impairment, functional limitation, or disability; and stability of the condition.

Prognosis

Over the course of 3 to 6 months, patient/client will demonstrate optimal motor function and sensory integrity and the highest level of functioning in home, work (job/school/play), community, and leisure environments, within the context of the impairments, functional limitations, and disabilities.

During the episode of care, patient/client will achieve (1) the anticipated goals and expected outcomes of the interventions that are described in the plan of care and (2) the global outcomes for patients/clients who are classified in this pattern.

Expected Range of Number of Visits Per Episode of Care

6 to 24

This range represents the lower and upper limits of the number of physical therapist visits required to achieve anticipated goals and expected outcomes. *It is anticipated that 80% of patients/clients who are classified into this pattern will achieve the anticipated goals and expected outcomes within 6 to 24 visits during a single continuous episode of care.* Frequency of visits and duration of the episode of care should be determined by the physical therapist to maximize effectiveness of care and efficiency of service delivery.

Factors That May Require New Episode of Care or That May Modify Frequency of Visits/Duration of Care

- Accessibility and availability of resources
- Adherence to the intervention program
- Age
- Anatomical and physiological changes related to growth and development
- Caregiver consistency or expertise
- Chronicity or severity of the current condition
- Cognitive status
- Comorbitities, complications, or secondary impairments
- Concurrent medical, surgical, and therapeutic interventions
- Decline in functional independence
- Level of impairment
- Level of physical function
- Living environment
- Multisite or multisystem involvement
- Nutritional status
- Overall health status
- Potential discharge destinations
- Premorbid conditions
- Probability of prolonged impairment, functional limitation, or disability
- Psychological and socioeconomic factors
- Psychomotor abilities
- Social support
- Stability of the condition

Intervention

Intervention is the purposeful interaction of the physical therapist with the patient/client and, when appropriate, with other individuals involved in patient/client care, using various physical therapy procedures and techniques to produce changes in the condition consistent with the diagnosis and prognosis. Decisions about interventions are contingent on the timely monitoring of patient/client response and the progress made toward achieving the anticipated goals and expected outcomes.

Communication, coordination, and documentation and patient/client-related instruction are provided for all patients/clients across all settings. Procedural interventions are selected or modified based on the examination data and the evaluation, the diagnosis and the prognosis, and the anticipated goals and expected outcomes for a particular patient/client. *For clinical considerations in selecting interventions, listings of interventions, and listings of anticipated goals and expected outcomes, refer to Chapter 3.*

Coordination, Communication, and Documentation

Coordination, communication, and documentation may include:

Interventions

- Addressing required functions
  - advance directives
  - individualized family service plans (IFSPs) or individualized education plans (IEPs)
  - informed consent
  - mandatory communication and reporting (eg, patient advocacy and abuse reporting)
- Admission and discharge planning
- Case management
- Collaboration and coordination with agencies, including:
  - equipment suppliers
  - home care agencies
  - payer groups
  - schools
  - transportation agencies
- Communication across settings, including:
  - case conferences
  - documentation
  - education plans
- Cost-effective resource utilization
- Data collection, analysis, and reporting
  - outcome data
  - peer review findings
  - record reviews
- Documentation across settings, following APTA's *Guidelines for Physical Therapy Documentation* (Appendix 5), including:
  - changes in impairments, functional limitations, and disabilities
  - changes in interventions
  - elements of patient/client management (examination, evaluation, diagnosis, prognosis, intervention)
  - outcomes of intervention
- Interdisciplinary teamwork
  - case conferences
  - patient care rounds
  - patient/client family meetings
- Referrals to other professionals or resources

Anticipated Goals and Expected Outcomes

- Accountability for services is increased.
- Admission data and discharge planning are completed.
- Advance directives, individualized family service plans (IFSPs) or individualized education plans (IEPs), informed consent, and mandatory communication and reporting (eg, patient advocacy and abuse reporting) are obtained or completed.
- Available resources are maximally utilized.
- Care is coordinated with patient/client, family, significant others, caregivers, and other professionals.
- Case is managed throughout the episode of care.
- Collaboration and coordination occurs with agencies, including equipment suppliers, home care agencies, payer groups, schools, and transportation agencies.
- Communication enhances risk reduction and prevention.
- Communication occurs across settings through case conferences, education plans, and documentation.
- Data are collected, analyzed, and reported, including outcome data, peer review findings, and record reviews.
- Decision making is enhanced regarding on health, wellness, and fitness needs.
- Decision making is enhanced regarding patient/client health and the use of health care resources by patient/client, family, significant others, and caregivers.
- Documentation occurs throughout patient/client management and across settings and follows APTA's *Guidelines for Physical Therapy Documentation* (Appendix 5).
- Interdisciplinary collaboration occurs through case conferences, patient care rounds, and patient/client family meetings.
- Patient/client, family, significant other, and caregiver understanding of anticipated goals and expected outcomes is increased.
- Placement needs are determined.
- Referrals are made to other professionals or resources whenever necessary and appropriate.
- Resources are utilized in a cost-effective way.

Patient/Client-Related Instruction

Patient/client-related instruction may include:

Interventions

- Instruction, education and training of patients/clients and caregivers regarding:
  - current condition (pathology/pathophysiology [disease, disorder, or condition], impairments, functional limitations, or disabilities)
  - enhancement of performance
  - health, wellness, and fitness programs
  - plan of care
  - risk factors for pathology/pathophysiology (disease, disorder, or condition), impairments, functional limitations, or disabilities
  - transitions across settings
  - transitions to new roles

Anticipated Goals and Expected Outcomes

- Ability to perform physical actions, tasks, or activities is improved.
- Awareness and use of community resources are improved.
- Behaviors that foster healthy habits, wellness, and prevention are acquired.
- Decision making is enhanced regarding patient/client health and the use of health care resources by patient/client, family, significant others, and caregivers.
- Disability associated with acute or chronic illnesses is reduced.
- Functional independence in activities of daily living (ADL) and instrumental activities of daily living (IADL) is increased.
- Health status is improved.
- Intensity of care is decreased.
- Level of supervision required for task performance is decreased.
- Patient/client, family, significant other, and caregiver knowledge and awareness of the diagnosis, prognosis, interventions, and anticipated goals and expected outcomes are increased.
- Patient/client knowledge of personal and environmental factors associated with the condition is increased.
- Performance levels in self-care, home management, work (job/school/play), community, or leisure actions, tasks, or activities are improved.
- Physical functionis improved.
- Risk of recurrence of condition is reduced.
- Risk of secondary impairment is reduced.
- Safety of patient/client, family, significant others, and caregivers is improved.
- Self-management of symptoms is improved.
- Utilization and cost of health care services are decreased.

Procedural Interventions

Procedural interventions for this pattern may include:

Therapeutic Exercise

Interventions

- Aerobic and endurance conditioning or reconditioning
  - aquatic programs
  - gait and locomotor training
  - increased workload over time
  - walking and wheelchair propulsion programs
- Balance, coordination, and agility training
  - developmental activities training
  - motor function (motor control and motor learning) training or retraining
  - neuromuscular education or reeducation
  - perceptual training
  - posture awareness training
  - standardized, programmatic, complementary exercise approaches
  - sensory training or retraining
  - task-specific performance training
  - vestibular training
- Body mechanics and postural stabilization
  - body mechanics training
  - posture awareness training
  - postural control training
  - postural stabilization activities
- Flexibility exercises
  - muscle lengthening
  - range of motion
  - stretching
- Gait and locomotion training
  - developmental activities training
  - gait training
  - implement and device training
  - perceptual training
  - standardized, programmatic, complementary exercise approaches
  - wheelchair training
- Relaxation
  - breathing strategies
  - movement strategies
  - relaxation techniques
  - standardized, programmatic, complementary exercise approaches
- Strength, power, and endurance training for head, neck, limb, pelvic-floor, trunk, and ventilatory muscles
  - active assistive, active, and resistive exercises (including concentric, dynamic/isotonic, eccentric, isokinetic, isometric, and plyometric)
  - aquatic programs
  - standardized, programmatic, complementary exercise approaches
  - task-specific performance training

Anticipated Goals and Expected Outcomes

- Impact on pathology/pathophysiology (disease, disorder, or condition)
  - Joint swelling, inflammation, or restriction is reduced.
  - Nutrient delivery to tissue is increased.
  - Osteogenic effects of exercise are maximized.
  - Pain is decreased.
  - Physiological response to increased oxygen demand is improved.
  - Soft tissue swelling, inflammation, or restriction is reduced.
  - Symptoms associated with increased oxygen demand are decreased.
  - Tissue perfusion and oxygenation are enhanced.
- Impact on impairments
  - Aerobic capacity is increased.
  - Balance is improved.
  - Endurance is increased.
  - Energy expenditure per unit of work is decreased.
  - Gait, locomotion, and balance are improved.
  - Integumentary integrity is improved.
  - Joint integrity and mobility are improved.
  - Motor function (motor control and motor learning) is improved.
  - Muscle performance (strength, power, and endurance) is increased.
  - Postural control is improved.
  - Quality and quantity of movement between and across body segments are improved.
  - Range of motion is improved.
  - Relaxation is increased.
  - Sensory awareness is increased.
  - Weight-bearing status is improved.
  - Work of breathing is decreased.
- Impact on functional limitations
  - Ability to perform physical actions, tasks, or activities related to self-care, home management, work (job/school/play), community, and leisure is improved.
  - Level of supervision required for task performance is decreased.
  - Performance of and independence in activities of daily living (ADL) and instrumental activities of daily living (IADL) with or without devices and equipment are increased.
  - Tolerance of positions and activities is increased.
- Impact on disabilities
  - Ability to assume or resume required self-care, home management, work (job/school/play), community, and leisure roles is improved.
- Risk reduction/prevention
  - Risk factors are reduced.
  - Risk of secondary impairment is reduced.
  - Safety is improved.
  - Self-management of symptoms is improved.
- Impact on health, wellness, and fitness
  - Fitness is improved.
  - Health status is improved.
  - Physical capacity is increased.
  - Physical function is improved.
- Impact on societal resources
  - Utilization of physical therapy services is optimized.
  - Utilization of physical therapy services results in efficient use of health care dollars.
- Patient/client satisfaction
  - Access, availability, and services provided are acceptable to patient/client.
  - Administrative management of practice is acceptable to patient/client.
  - Clinical proficiency of physical therapist is acceptable to patient/client.
  - Coordination of care is acceptable to patient/client.
  - Cost of health care services is decreased.
  - Intensity of care is decreased.
  - Interpersonal skills of physical therapist are acceptable to patient/client, family, and significant others.
  - Sense of well-being is improved.
  - Stressors are decreased.

Functional Training in Self-Care and Home Management (Including Activities of Daily Living [ADL] and Instrumental Activities of Daily Living [IADL])

Interventions

- ADL training
  - bathing
  - bed mobility and transfer training
  - developmental activities
  - dressing
  - eating
  - gait and locomotion training
  - grooming
  - toileting
- Devices and equipment use and training
  - assistive and adaptive device or equipment training during ADL and IADL
  - orthotic, protective, or supportive device or equipment training during ADL and IADL
  - prosthetic device or equipment training during ADL and IADL
- Functional training programs
  - simulated environments and tasks
  - task adaptation
  - travel training
- IADL training
  - caring for dependents
  - home maintenance
  - household chores
  - shopping
  - structured play for infants and children
  - yard work
- Injury prevention or reduction
  - injury prevention education during self-care and home management
  - injury prevention or reduction with use of devices and equipment
  - safety awareness training during self-care and home management

Anticipated Goals and Expected Outcomes

- Impact on pathology/pathophysiology (disease, disorder, or condition)
  - Pain is decreased.
  - Physiological response to increased oxygen demand is improved.
  - Symptoms associated with increased oxygen demand are decreased.
- Impact on impairments
  - Balance is improved.
  - Endurance is increased.
  - Energy expenditure per unit of work is decreased.
  - Motor function (motor control and motor learning) is improved.
  - Muscle performance (strength, power, and endurance) is increased.
  - Postural control is improved.
  - Sensory awareness is increased.
  - Weight-bearing status is improved.
  - Work of breathing is decreased.
- Impact on functional limitations
  - Ability to perform physical actions, tasks, or activities related to self-care and home management is improved.
  - Level of supervision required for task performance is decreased.
  - Performance of and independence in ADL and IADL with or without devices and equipment are increased.
  - Tolerance of positions and activities is increased.
- Impact on disabilities
  - Ability to assume or resume required self-care and home management roles is improved.
- Risk reduction/prevention
  - Risk factors are reduced.
  - Risk of secondary impairments is reduced.
  - Safety is improved.
  - Self-management of symptoms is improved.
- Impact on health, wellness, and fitness
  - Health status is improved.
  - Physical capacity is increased.
  - Physical function is improved.
- Impact on societal resources
  - Utilization of physical therapy services is optimized.
  - Utilization of physical therapy services results in efficient use of health care dollars.
- Patient/client satisfaction
  - Access, availability, and services provided are acceptable to patient/client.
  - Administrative management of practice is acceptable to patient/client.
  - Clinical proficiency of physical therapist is acceptable to patient/client.
  - Coordination of care is acceptable to patient/client.
  - Cost of health care services is decreased.
  - Intensity of care is decreased.
  - Interpersonal skills of physical therapist are acceptable to patient/client, family, and significant others.
  - Sense of well-being is improved.
  - Stressors are decreased.

Functional Training in Work (Job/School/Play), Community, and Leisure Integration or Reintegration (Including Instrumental Activities of Daily Living [IADL] and Work Conditioning)

Interventions

- Devices and equipment use and training
  - assistive and adaptive device or equipment training during IADL
  - orthotic, protective, or supportive device or equipment training during IADL
  - prosthetic device or equipment training during IADL
- Functional training programs
  - job coaching
  - simulated environments and tasks
  - task adaptation
  - task training
  - travel training
- IADL training
  - community service training involving instruments
  - school and play activities training including tools and instruments
  - work training with tools
- Injury prevention or reduction
  - injury prevention education during work (job/school/play), community, and leisure integration or reintegration
  - injury prevention or reduction with use of devices and equipment
  - safety awareness training during work (job/school/play), community, and leisure integration or reintegration
- Leisure and play activities training

Anticipated Goals and Expected Outcomes

- Impact on pathology/pathophysiology (disease, disorder, or condition)
  - Pain is decreased.
  - Physiological response to increased oxygen demand is improved.
  - Symptoms associated with increased oxygen demand are decreased.
- Impact on impairments
  - Balance is improved.
  - Endurance is increased.
  - Energy expenditure per unit of work is decreased.
  - Motor function (motor control and motor learning) is improved.
  - Muscle performance (strength, power, and endurance) is increased.
  - Postural control is improved.
  - Sensory awareness is increased.
  - Weight-bearing status is improved.
  - Work of breathing is decreased.
- Impact on functional limitations
  - Ability to perform physical actions, tasks, or activities related to work (job/school/play), community, and leisure integration or reintegration is improved.
  - Level of supervision required for task performance is decreased.
  - Performance of and independence in IADL with or without devices and equipment are increased.
  - Tolerance of positions and activities is increased.
- Impact on disabilities
  - Ability to assume or resume required work (job/school/play), community, and leisure roles is improved.
- Risk reduction/prevention
  - Risk factors are reduced.
  - Risk of secondary impairment is reduced.
  - Safety is improved.
  - Self-management of symptoms is improved.
- Impact on health, wellness, and fitness
  - Fitness is improved.
  - Health status is improved.
  - Physical capacity is increased.
  - Physical function is improved.
- Impact on societal resources
  - Costs of work-related injury or disability are reduced.
  - Utilization of physical therapy services is optimized.
  - Utilization of physical therapy services results in efficient use of health care dollars.
- Patient/client satisfaction
  - Access, availability, and services provided are acceptable to patient/client.
  - Administrative management of practice is acceptable to patient/client.
  - Clinical proficiency of physical therapist is acceptable to patient/client.
  - Coordination of care is acceptable to patient/client.
  - Cost of health care services is decreased.
  - Intensity of care is decreased.
  - Interpersonal skills of physical therapist are acceptable to patient/client, family, and significant others.
  - Sense of well-being is improved.
  - Stressors are decreased.

Manual Therapy Techniques (Including Mobilization/Manipulation)

Interventions

- Manual traction
- Massage
  - connective tissue massage
  - therapeutic massage
- Mobilization/manipulation
  - soft tissue
- Passive range of motion

Anticipated Goals and Expected Outcomes

- Impact on pathology/pathophysiology (disease, disorder, or condition)
  - Edema, lymphedema, or effusion is reduced.
  - Joint swelling, inflammation, or restriction is reduced.
  - Pain is decreased.
  - Soft tissue swelling, inflammation, or restriction is reduced.
- Impact on impairments
  - Balance is improved.
  - Energy expenditure per unit of work is decreased.
  - Gait, locomotion, and balance are improved.
  - Integumentary integrity is improved.
  - Muscle performance (strength, power, and endurance) is increased.
  - Postural control is improved.
  - Quality and quantity of movement between and across body segments are improved.
  - Range of motion is improved.
  - Relaxation is increased.
  - Sensory awareness is increased.
  - Weight-bearing status is improved.
  - Work of breathing is decreased.
- Impact on functional limitations
  - Ability to perform movement tasks is improved.
  - Ability to perform physical actions, tasks, or activities related to self-care, home management, work (job/school/play), community, and leisure is improved.
  - Tolerance of positions and activities is increased.
- Impact on disabilities
  - Ability to assume or resume required self-care, home management, work (job/school/play), community, and leisure roles is improved.
- Risk reduction/prevention
  - Risk factors are reduced.
  - Risk of secondary impairment is reduced.
  - Self-management of symptoms is improved.
- Impact on health, wellness, and fitness
  - Physical capacity is increased.
  - Physical function is improved.
- Impact on societal resources
  - Utilization of physical therapy services is optimized.
  - Utilization of physical therapy services results in efficient use of health care dollars.
- Patient/client satisfaction
  - Access, availability, and services provided are acceptable to patient/client.
  - Administrative management of practice is acceptable to patient/client.
  - Clinical proficiency of physical therapist is acceptable to patient/client.
  - Coordination of care is acceptable to patient/client.
  - Cost of health care services is decreased.
  - Intensity of care is decreased.
  - Interpersonal skills of physical therapist are acceptable to patient/client, family, and significant others.
  - Sense of well-being is improved.
  - Stressors are decreased.

Prescription, Application, and, as Appropriate, Fabrication of Devices and Equipment (Assistive, Adaptive, Orthotic, Protective, Supportive, and Prosthetic)

Interventions

- Adaptive devices
  - environmental controls
  - hospital beds
  - raised toilet seats
  - seating systems
- Assistive devices
  - canes
  - crutches
  - long-handled reachers
  - power devices
  - static and dynamic splints
  - walkers
  - wheelchairs
- Orthotic devices
  - braces
  - casts
  - shoe inserts
  - splints
- Prosthetic devices (lower-extremity and upper-extremity)
- Protective devices
  - braces
  - cushions
  - helmets
  - protective taping
- Supportive devices
  - compression garments
  - corsets
  - elastic wraps
  - neck collars
  - serial casts
  - slings
  - supplemental oxygen
  - supportive taping

Anticipated Goals and Expected Outcomes

- Impact on pathology/pathophysiology (disease, disorder, or condition)
  - Edema, lymphedema, or effusion is reduced.
  - Joint swelling, inflammation, or restriction is reduced.
  - Pain is decreased.
  - Physiological response to increased oxygen demand is improved.
  - Soft tissue swelling, inflammation, or restriction is reduced.
  - Symptoms associated with increased oxygen demand are decreased.
- Impact on impairments
  - Balance is improved.
  - Endurance is increased.
  - Energy expenditure per unit of work is decreased.
  - Gait, locomotion, and balance are improved.
  - Integumentary integrity is improved.
  - Joint stability is improved.
  - Motor function (motor control and motor learning) is improved.
  - Muscle performance (strength, power, and endurance) is increased.
  - Optimal joint alignment is achieved.
  - Optimal loading on a body part is achieved.
  - Postural control is improved.
  - Prosthetic fit is achieved.
  - Quality and quantity of movement between and across body segments are improved.
  - Range of motion is improved.
  - Weight-bearing status is improved.
  - Work of breathing is decreased.
- Impact on functional limitations
  - Ability to perform physical actions, tasks, or activities related to self-care, home management, work (job/school/play), community, and leisure is improved.
  - Level of supervision required for task performance is decreased.
  - Performance of and independence in activities of daily living (ADL) and instrumental activities of daily living (IADL) with or without devices and equipment are increased.
  - Tolerance of positions and activities is increased.
- Impact on disabilities
  - Ability to assume or resume required self-care, home management, work (job/school/play), community, and leisure roles is improved.
- Risk reduction/prevention
  - Pressure on body tissues is reduced.
  - Protection of body parts is increased.
  - Risk factors are reduced.
  - Risk of recurrence of condition is reduced.
  - Risk of secondary impairment is reduced.
  - Safety is improved.
  - Self-management of symptoms is improved.
  - Stresses precipitating injury are decreased.
- Impact on health, wellness, and fitness
  - Fitness is improved.
  - Health status is improved.
  - Physical capacity is increased.
  - Physical function is improved.
- Impact on societal resources
  - Utilization of physical therapy services is optimized.
  - Utilization of physical therapy services results in efficient use of health care dollars.
- Patient/client satisfaction
  - Access, availability, and services provided are acceptable to patient/client.
  - Administrative management of practice is acceptable to patient/client.
  - Clinical proficiency of physical therapist is acceptable to patient/client.
  - Coordination of care is acceptable to patient/client.
  - Cost of health care services is decreased.
  - Intensity of care is decreased.
  - Interpersonal skills of physical therapist are acceptable to patient/client, family, and significant others.
  - Sense of well-being is improved.
  - Stressors are decreased.

Airway Clearance Techniques

Interventions

- Breathing strategies
  - active cycle of breathing or forced expiratory techniques
  - assisted cough/huff techniques
  - autogenic drainage
  - paced breathing
  - pursed lip breathing
  - techniques to maximize ventilation (eg, maximum inspiratory hold, staircase breathing, manual hyper-inflation)
- Manual/mechanical techniques
  - assistive devices
  - chest percussion, vibration, and shaking
  - chest wall manipulation
  - suctioning
  - ventilatory aids
- Positioning
  - positioning to alter work of breathing
  - positioning to maximize ventilation and perfusion
  - pulmonary postural drainage

Anticipated Goals and Expected Outcomes

- Impact on pathology/pathophysiology (disease, disorder, or condition)
  - Atelectasis is decreased.
  - Nutrient delivery to tissue is increased.
  - Physiological response to increased oxygen demand is improved.
  - Symptoms associated with increased oxygen demand are decreased.
  - Tissue perfusion and oxygenation are enhanced.
- Impact on impairments
  - Airway clearance is improved.
  - Balance is improved.
  - Cough is improved.
  - Endurance is increased.
  - Energy expenditure per unit of work is decreased.
  - Exercise tolerance is improved.
  - Muscle performance (strength, power, and endurance) is increased.
  - Ventilation and respiration/gas exchange are improved.
  - Work of breathing is decreased.
- Impact on functional limitations
  - Ability to perform physical actions, tasks, or activities related to self-care, home management, work (job/school/play), community, and leisure is improved.
  - Performance of and independence in activities of daily living (ADL) and instrumental activities of daily living (IADL) with or without devices and equipment are increased.
  - Tolerance of positions and activities is increased.
- Impact on disabilities
  - Ability to assume or resume required self-care, home management, work (job/school/play), community, and leisure roles is improved.
- Risk reduction/prevention
  - Risk factors are reduced.
  - Risk of recurrence of condition is reduced.
  - Risk of secondary impairment is reduced.
  - Safety is improved.
  - Self-management of symptoms is improved.
- Impact on health, wellness, and fitness
  - Health status is improved.
  - Physical capacity is increased.
  - Physical function is improved.
- Impact on societal resources
  - Utilization of physical therapy services is optimized.
  - Utilization of physical therapy services results in efficient use of health care dollars.
- Patient/client satisfaction
  - Access, availability, and services provided are acceptable to patient/client.
  - Administrative management of practice is acceptable to patient/client.
  - Clinical proficiency of physical therapist is acceptable to patient/client.
  - Coordination of care is acceptable to patient/client.
  - Cost of health care services is decreased.
  - Intensity of care is decreased.
  - Interpersonal skills of physical therapist are acceptable to patient/client, family, and significant others.
  - Sense of well-being is improved.
  - Stressors are decreased.

Interventions

- Biofeedback
- Electrical stimulation
  - electrical muscle stimulation (EMS)

Anticipated Goals and Expected Outcomes

- Impact on pathology/pathophysiology (disease, disorder, or condition)
  - Edema, lymphedema, or effusion is reduced.
  - Joint swelling, inflammation, or restriction is reduced.
  - Nutrient delivery to tissue is increased.
  - Osteogenic effects are enhanced.
  - Pain is decreased.
  - Soft tissue swelling, inflammation, or restriction is reduced.
  - Tissue perfusion and oxygenation are enhanced.
- Impact on impairments
  - Integumentary integrity is improved.
  - Motor function (motor control and motor learning) is improved.
  - Muscle performance (strength, power, and endurance) is increased.
  - Postural control is improved.
  - Quality and quantity of movement between and across body segments are improved.
  - Range of motion is improved.
  - Relaxation is increased.
  - Sensory awareness is increased.
- Impact on functional limitations
  - Ability to perform physical actions, tasks, or activities related to self-care, home management, work (job/school/play), community, and leisure is improved.
  - Level of supervision required for task performance is decreased.
  - Performance of and independence in activities of daily living (ADL) and instrumental activities of daily living (IADL) with or without devices and equipment are increased.
  - Tolerance of positions and activities is increased.
- Impact on disabilities
  - Ability to assume or resume required self-care, home management, work (job/school/play), community, and leisure roles is improved.
- Risk reduction/prevention
  - Complications of immobility are reduced.
  - Risk factors are reduced.
  - Risk of recurrence of condition is reduced.
  - Risk of secondary impairment is reduced.
  - Self-management of symptoms is improved.
- Impact on health, wellness, and fitness
  - Physical capacity is increased.
  - Physical function is improved.
- Impact on societal resources
  - Utilization of physical therapy services is optimized.
  - Utilization of physical therapy services results in efficient use of health care dollars.
- Patient/client satisfaction
  - Access, availability, and services provided are acceptable to patient/client.
  - Administrative management of practice is acceptable to patient/client.
  - Clinical proficiency of physical therapist is acceptable to patient/client.
  - Coordination of care is acceptable to patient/client.
  - Interpersonal skills of physical therapist are acceptable to patient/client, family, and significant others.
  - Sense of well-being is improved.
  - Stressors are decreased.

Physical Agents and Mechanical Modalities

Interventions

Physical agents may include:

- Athermal agents
  - pulsed electromagnetic fields
- Cryotherapy
  - cold packs
  - ice massage
  - vapocoolant spray
- Sound agents
  - phonophoresis
  - ultrasound

Mechanical modalities may include:

- Compression therapies
  - compression bandaging
  - compression garments
  - vasopneumatic compression devices
- Gravity-assisted compression devices
  - standing frame
  - tilt table

Anticipated Goals and Expected Outcomes

- Impact on pathology/pathophysiology (disease, disorder, or condition)
  - Edema, lymphedema, or effusion is reduced.
  - Joint swelling, inflammation, or restriction is reduced.
  - Nutrient delivery to tissue is increased.
  - Osteogenic effects of exercise are maximized.
  - Pain is decreased.
  - Soft tissue swelling, inflammation, or restriction is reduced.
  - Tissue perfusion and oxygenation are enhanced.
- Impact on impairments
  - Integumentary integrity is improved.
  - Muscle performance (strength, power, and endurance) is increased.
  - Range of motion is improved.
  - Weight-bearing status is improved.
- Impact on functional limitations
  - Ability to perform physical actions, tasks, or activities related to self-care, home management, work (job/school/play), community, and leisure is increased.
  - Performance of and independence in activities of daily living (ADL) and instrumental activities of daily living (IADL) with or without devices and equipment are increased.
  - Tolerance of positions and activities is increased.
- Impact on disabilities
  - Ability to assume or resume required self-care, home management, work (job/school/play), community, and leisure roles is improved.
- Risk reduction/prevention
  - Complications of soft tissue and circulatory disorders are decreased.
  - Risk factors are reduced.
  - Risk of secondary impairment is reduced.
  - Self-management of symptoms is improved.
  - Stresses precipitating injury are decreased.
- Impact on health, wellness, and fitness
  - Physical function is improved.
- Impact on societal resources
  - Utilization of physical therapy services is optimized.
- Patient/client satisfaction
  - Access, availability, and services provided are acceptable to patient/client.
  - Administrative management of practice is acceptable to patient/client.
  - Clinical proficiency of physical therapist is acceptable to patient/client.
  - Coordination of care is acceptable to patient/client.
  - Interpersonal skills of physical therapist are acceptable to patient/client, family, and significant others.
  - Sense of well-being is improved.
  - Stressors are decreased.

Reexamination

Reexamination is the process of performing selected tests and measures after the initial examination to evaluate progress and to modify or redirect interventions. Reexamination may be indicated more than once during a single episode of care. It also may be performed over the course of a disease, disorder, or condition, which for some patients/clients may be over the life span. Indications for reexamination include new clinical findings or failure to respond to physical therapy interventions.

Global Outcomes for Patients/Clients in This Pattern

Throughout the entire episode of care, the physical therapist determines the anticipated goals and expected outcomes for each intervention. These anticipated goals and expected outcomes are delineated in shaded boxes that accompany the lists of interventions in each preferred practice pattern. As the patient/client reaches the termination of physical therapy services and the end of the episode of care, the physical therapist measures the global outcomes of the physical therapy services by characterizing or quantifying the impact of the physical therapy interventions in the following domains:

- Pathology/pathophysiology (disease, disorder, or condition)
- Impairments
- Functional limitations
- Disabilities
- Risk reduction/prevention
- Health, wellness, and fitness
- Societal resources
- Patient/client satisfaction

In some instances, a particular anticipated goal or expected outcome is thoroughly achieved through implementation of a single form of intervention. More commonly, however, the anticipated goals and expected outcomes are achieved as a result of the combined effects of several forms of interventions, leading to enhancement of both health status and health-related quality of life.

Criteria for Termination of Physical Therapy Services

Discharge is the process of ending physical therapy services that have been provided during a single episode of care. It occurs when the anticipated goals and expected outcomes have been achieved. Discharge does *not* occur with a *transfer* (defined as the time when a patient is moved from one site to another site within the same setting or across settings during a single episode of care). Although there may be facility-specific or payer-specific requirements for documentation regarding the conclusion of physical therapy services, *discharge occurs based on the physical therapist's analysis of the achievement of anticipated goals and expected outcomes.*

Discontinuation is the process of ending physical therapy services that have been provided during a single episode of care when (1) the patient/client, caregiver, or legal guardian declines to continue intervention; (2) the patient/client is unable to continue to progress toward outcomes because of medical or psychosocial complications or because financial/insurance resources have been expended; or (3) the physical therapist determines that the patient/client will no longer benefit from physical therapy. When physical therapy services are terminated prior to achievement of anticipated goals and expected outcomes, patient/client status and the rationale for termination are documented.

For patients/clients who require multiple episodes of care, periodic follow-up is needed over the life span to ensure safety and effective adaptation following changes in physical status, caregivers, environment, or task demands. In consultation with appropriate individuals, and in consideration of the outcomes, the physical therapist plans for discharge or discontinuation and provides for appropriate follow-up or referral.

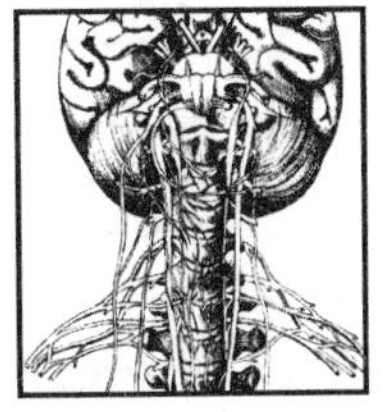

Impaired Motor Function, Peripheral Nerve Integrity, and Sensory Integrity Associated With Nonprogressive Disorders of the Spinal Cord

This preferred practice pattern describes the generally accepted elements of patient/client management that physical therapists provide for patients/clients who are classified in this pattern. The pattern title reflects the diagnosis made by the physical therapist. APTA emphasizes that preferred practice patterns are the boundaries within which a physical therapist may select any of a number of clinical alternatives, based on consideration of a wide variety of factors, such as individual patient/client needs; the profession's code of ethics and standards of practice; and patient/client age, culture, gender roles, race, sex, sexual orientation, and socioeconomic status.

Patient/Client Diagnostic Classification

Patients/clients will be classified into this pattern—for impaired motor function, peripheral nerve integrity, and sensory integrity associated with nonprogressive disorders of the spinal cord—as a result of the physical therapist's evaluation of the examination data. The findings from the examination (history, systems review, and tests and measures) may indicate the presence or risk of pathology/pathophysiology (disease, disorder, or condition), impairments, functional limitations, or disabilities or the need for health, wellness, or fitness programs. The physical therapist integrates, synthesizes, and interprets the data to determine the diagnostic classification.

Inclusion

The following examples of examination findings may support the inclusion of patients/clients in this pattern:

Risk Factors or Consequences of Pathology/Pathophysiology (Disease, Disorder, or Condition)

- Benign spinal neoplasm
- Complete and incomplete spinal cord lesions
- Infectious diseases affecting the spinal cord
- Spinal cord compression
  - Degenerative spinal joint disease
  - Herniated intervertebral disk
  - Osteomyelitis
  - Spondylosis

Impairments, Functional Limitations, or Disabilities

- Decreased aerobic capacity
- Difficulty accessing community
- Difficulty with activities of daily living
- Difficulty with instrumental activities of daily living
- Impaired ventilation
- Impaired motor function
- Impaired muscle performance
- Impaired peripheral nerve integrity
- Inability to keep up with peers
- Inability to perform work (job/school/play)

Note:

Some risk factors or consequences of pathology/pathophysiology—such as *abdominal trauma* and *autonomic dysreflexia*—may be severe and complex; *however, they do not necessarily exclude patients/clients from this pattern.* Severe and complex risk factors or consequences may require modification of the frequency of visits and duration of care. (See "Evaluation, Diagnosis, and Prognosis," page 435.)

Exclusion or Multiple-Pattern Classification

The following examples of examination findings may support exclusion from this pattern or classification into additional patterns. Depending on the level of severity or complexity of the examination findings, the physical therapist may determine that the patient/client would be more appropriately managed through (1) classification in an entirely different pattern or (2) classification in both this and another pattern.

Findings That May Require Classification in a Different Pattern

- Impairments associated with Guillian-Barré syndrome
- Meningocele
- Nerve root compression due to lumbar radiculopathy
- Tethered cord

Findings That May Require Classification in Additional Patterns

- Decubitis ulcer
- Impairments associated with ventilator dependency

ICD-9-CM Codes

The listing below contains the current (as of press time) and most typical 3- and 4-digit ICD-9-CM codes related to this preferred practice pattern. Because patient/client diagnostic classification is based on impairments, functional limitations, and disabilities—not on codes—patients/clients may be classified into the pattern even though the codes listed with the pattern may not apply to those clients.

This listing is intended for general information only and should not be used for coding purposes. The codes should be confirmed by referring to the World Health Organization's *International Classification of Diseases, 9th Revision, Clinical Modification (ICD-9-CM 2001)*, Volumes 1 and 3 (Chicago, Ill: American Medical Association; 2000) or subsequent revisions or by referring to other ICD-9-CM coding manuals that contain exclusion notes and instructions regarding fifth-digit requirements.

225 Benign neoplasm of brain and other parts of nervous system
- **225.3** Spinal cord
  - Cauda equina

237 Neoplasm of uncertain behavior of endocrine glands and nervous system
- **237.5** Brain and spinal cord

239 Neoplasms of unspecified nature
- **239.7** Endocrine glands and other parts of nervous system

320 Bacterial meningitis

321 Meningitis due to other organisms

336 Other diseases of spinal cord

344 Other paralytic syndromes
- **344.0** Quadriplegia and quadriparesis
- **344.1** Paraplegia
- **344.8** Other specified paralytic syndromes

721 Spondylosis and allied disorders
- **721.1** Cervical spondylosis with myelopathy
- **721.4** Thoracic or lumbar spondylosis with myelopathy
- **721.9** Spondylosis of unspecified site
  - **721.91** With myelopathy

722 Intervertebral disk disorders
- **722.1** Displacement of thoracic or lumbar intervertebral disk without myelopathy
- **722.7** Intervertebral disk disorder with myelopathy

730 Osteomyelitis, periostitis, and other infections involving bone
- **730.2** Unspecified osteomyelitis

733 Other disorders of bone and cartilage
- **733.1** Pathologic fracture

806 Fracture of vertebral column with spinal cord injury

839 Other, multiple, and ill-defined dislocations
- **839.0** Cervical vertebra, closed
- **839.1** Cervical vertebra, open
- **839.2** Thoracic and lumbar vertebra, closed
- **839.3** Thoracic and lumbar vertebra, open
- **839.4** Other vertebra, closed
- **839.5** Other vertebra, open
- **839.6** Other location, closed
- **839.7** Other location, open
- **839.8** Multiple and ill-defined, closed
- **839.9** Multiple and ill-defined, open

952 Spinal cord injury without evidence of spinal bone injury
- **952.0** Cervical
- **952.1** Dorsal [thoracic]
- **952.2** Lumbar

Examination

Examination is a comprehensive screening and specific testing process that leads to a diagnostic classification or, when appropriate, to a referral to another practitioner. Examination is required prior to the initial intervention and is performed for all patients/clients. Through the examination, the physical therapist may identify impairments, functional limitations, disabilities, changes in physical function or overall health status, and needs related to restoration of health and to prevention, wellness, and fitness. The physical therapist synthesizes the examination findings to establish the diagnosis and the prognosis (including the plan of care). The patient/client, family, significant others, and caregivers may provide information during the examination process.

Examination has three components: the patient/client history, the systems review, and tests and measures. The *history* is a systematic gathering of past and current information (often from the patient/client) related to why the patient/client is seeking the services of the physical therapist. The *systems review* is a brief or limited examination of (1) the anatomical and physiological status of the cardiovascular/pulmonary, integumentary, musculoskeletal, and neuromuscular systems and (2) the communication ability, affect, cognition, language, and learning style of the patient/client. *Tests and measures* are the means of gathering data about the patient/client.

The selection of examination procedures and the depth of the examination vary based on patient/client age; severity of the problem; stage of recovery (acute, subacute, chronic); phase of rehabilitation (early, intermediate, late, return to activity); home, work (job/school/play), or community situation; and other relevant factors. *For clinical indications in selecting tests and measures and for listings of tests and measures, tools used to gather data, and the types of data generated by tests and measures, refer to Chapter 2.*

Patient/Client History

The history may include:

General Demographics
- Age
- Sex
- Race/ethnicity
- Primary language
- Education

Social History
- Cultural beliefs and behaviors
- Family and caregiver resources
- Social interactions, social activities, and support systems

Employment/Work (Job/School/Play)
- Current and prior work (job/school/play), community, and leisure actions, tasks, or activities

Growth and Development
- Developmental history
- Hand dominance

Living Environment
- Devices and equipment (eg, assistive, adaptive, orthotic, protective, supportive, prosthetic)
- Living environment and community characteristics
- Projected discharge destinations

General Health Status (Self-Report, Family Report, Caregiver Report)
- General health perception
- Physical function (eg, mobility, sleep patterns, restricted bed days)
- Psychological function (eg, memory, reasoning ability, depression, anxiety)
- Role function (eg, community, leisure, social, work)
- Social function (eg, social activity, social interaction, social support)

Social/Health Habits (Past and Current)
- Behavioral health risks (eg, smoking, drug abuse)
- Level of physical fitness

Family History
- Familial health risks

Medical/Surgical History
- Cardiovascular
- Endocrine/metabolic
- Gastrointestinal
- Genitourinary
- Gynecological
- Integumentary
- Musculoskeletal
- Neuromuscular
- Obstetrical
- Prior hospitalizations, surgeries, and preexisting medical and other health-related conditions
- Psychological
- Pulmonary

Current Condition(s)/Chief Complaint(s)
- Concerns that led patient/client to seek the services of a physical therapist
- Concerns or needs of patient/client who requires the services of a physical therapist
- Current therapeutic interventions
- Mechanisms of injury or disease, including date of onset and course of events
- Onset and pattern of symptoms
- Patient/client, family, significant other, and caregiver expectations and goals for the therapeutic intervention
- Patient/client, family, significant other, and caregiver perceptions of patient's/client's emotional response to the current clinical situation
- Previous occurrence of chief complaint(s)
- Prior therapeutic interventions

Functional Status and Activity Level
- Current and prior functional status in self-care and home management activities, including activities of daily living (ADL) and instrumental activities of daily living (IADL)
- Current and prior functional status in work (job/school/play), community, and leisure actions, tasks, or activities

Medications
- Medications for current condition
- Medications previously taken for current condition
- Medications for other conditions

Other Clinical Tests
- Laboratory and diagnostic tests
- Review of available records (eg, medical, education, surgical)
- Review of other clinical findings (eg, nutrition and hydration)

Systems Review

The systems review may include:

Anatomical and Physiological Status

- Cardiovascular/Pulmonary
  - Blood pressure
  - Edema
  - Heart rate
  - Respiratory rate
- Integumentary
  - Pliability (texture)
  - Presence of scar formation
  - Skin color
  - Skin integrity
- Musculoskeletal
  - Gross range of motion
  - Gross strength
  - Gross symmetry
  - Height
  - Weight
- Neuromuscular
  - Gross coordinated movements (eg, balance, gait, locomotion, transfers, transitions)
  - Motor function (motor control, motor learning)

Communication, Affect, Cognition, Language, and Learning Style

- Ability to make needs known
- Consciousness
- Expected emotional/behavioral responses
- Learning preferences (eg, education needs, learning barriers)
- Orientation (person, place, time)

Tests and Measures

Test and measures for this pattern may include those that characterize or quantify:

Aerobic Capacity and Endurance

- Aerobic capacity during functional activities (eg, activities of daily living [ADL] scales, indexes, instrumental activities of daily living [IADL] scales, observations)
- Aerobic capacity during standardized exercise test protocols (eg, ergometry, step tests, time/distance walk/run tests, treadmill tests, wheelchair tests)
- Cardiovascular signs and symptoms in response to increased oxygen demand with exercise or activity, including pressures and flow; heart rate, rhythm, and sounds; and superficial vascular responses (eg, electrocardiography, exertion scales, observations, palpation, sphygmomanometry)
- Pulmonary signs and symptoms in response to increased oxygen demand with exercise or activity, including breath and voice sounds; cyanosis; gas exchange; respiratory pattern, rate, and rhythm; ventilatory flow, force, and volume (eg, auscultation, dyspnea and exertion scales, gas analyses, observations, oximetry, palpation, pulmonary function tests)

Anthropometric Characteristics

- Body composition (eg, body mass index, impedance measurement, skinfold thickness measurement)
- Body dimensions (eg, girth measurement, length measurement)
- Edema (eg, girth measurement, palpation, scales, volume measurement)

Arousal, Attention, and Cognition

- Arousal and attention (eg, adaptability tests, arousal and awareness scales, indexes, profiles, questionnaires)
- Cognition, including ability to process commands (eg, developmental inventories, indexes, interviews, mental state scales, observations, questionnaires, safety checklists)
- Motivation (eg, adaptive behavior scales)
- Orientation to time, person, place, and situation (eg, attention tests, learning profiles, mental state scales)
- Recall, including memory and retention (eg, assessment scales, interviews, questionnaires)

Assistive and Adaptive Devices

- Assistive or adaptive devices and equipment use during functional activities (eg, ADL scales, functional scales, IADL scales, interviews, observations)
- Components, alignment, fit, and ability to care for the assistive or adaptive devices and equipment (eg, interviews, logs, observations, pressure-sensing maps, reports)
- Remediation of impairments, functional limitations, or disabilities with use of assistive or adaptive devices and equipment (eg, activity status indexes, ADL scales, aerobic capacity tests, functional performance inventories, health assessment questionnaires, IADL scales, pain scales, play scales, videographic assessments)
- Safety during use of assistive or adaptive devices and equipment (eg, diaries, fall scales, interviews, logs, observations, reports)

Circulation (Arterial, Venous, and Lymphatic)

- Cardiovascular signs, including heart rate, rhythm, and sounds; pressures and flow; and superficial vascular responses (eg, auscultation, electrocardiography, girth measurement, observations, palpation, sphygmomanometry, thermography)
- Cardiovascular symptoms (eg, angina, claudication, dyspnea, and perceived exertion scales)
- Physiological responses to position change, including autonomic responses, central and peripheral pressures, heart rate and rhythm, respiratory rate and rhythm, ventilatory pattern (eg, auscultation, electrocardiography, observations, palpation, sphygmomanometry)

Cranial and Peripheral Nerve Integrity

- Electrophysiological integrity (eg, electroneuromyography)
- Motor distribution of the cranial nerves (eg, dynamometry, muscle tests, observations)
- Motor distribution of the peripheral nerves (eg, dynamometry, muscle tests, observations, thoracic outlet tests)
- Response to neural provocation (eg, tension tests, vertebral artery compression tests)
- Sensory distribution of the cranial nerves (eg, discrimination tests; tactile tests, including coarse and light touch, cold and heat, pain, pressure, and vibration)
- Sensory distribution of the peripheral nerves (eg, discrimination tests; tactile tests, including coarse and light touch, cold and heat, pain, pressure, and vibration; thoracic outlet tests)

Environmental, Home, and Work (Job/School/Play) Barriers

- Current and potential barriers (eg, checklists, interviews, observations, questionnaires)
- Physical space and environment (eg, compliance standards, observations, photographic assessments, questionnaires, structural specifications, videographic assessments)

Ergonomics and Body Mechanics

Ergonomics

- Dexterity and coordination during work (job/school/play) (eg, hand function tests, impairment rating scales, manipulative ability tests)
- Functional capacity and performance during work actions, tasks, or activities (eg, accelerometry, dynamometry, electroneuromyography, endurance tests, force platform tests, goniometry, interviews, observations, photographic assessments, physical capacity tests, postural loading analyses, technology-assisted assessments, videographic assessments, work analyses)
- Safety in work environments (eg, hazard identification checklists, job severity indexes, lifting standards, risk assessment scales, standards for exposure limits)
- Specific work conditions or activities (eg, handling checklists, job simulations, lifting models, preemployment screenings, task analysis checklists, workstation checklists)
- Tools, devices, equipment, and workstations related to work actions, tasks, or activities (eg, observations, tool analysis checklists, vibration assessments)

Body mechanics

- Body mechanics during self-care, home management, work, community, or leisure actions, tasks, or activities (eg, ADL scales, IADL scales, observations, photographic assessments, technology-assisted assessments, videographic assessments)

Gait, Locomotion, and Balance

- Balance during functional activities with or without the use of assistive, adaptive, orthotic, protective, supportive, or prosthetic devices or equipment (eg, ADL scales, IADL scales, observations, videographic assessments)
- Balance (dynamic and static) with or without the use of assistive, adaptive, orthotic, protective, supportive, or prosthetic devices or equipment (eg, balance scales, dizziness inventories, dynamic posturography, fall scales, motor impairment tests, observations, photographic assessments, postural control tests)
- Gait and locomotion during functional activities with or without the use of assistive, adaptive, orthotic, protective, supportive, or prosthetic devices or equipment (eg, ADL scales, gait indexes, IADL scales, mobility skill profiles, observations, videographic assessments)
- Gait and locomotion with or without the use of assistive, adaptive, orthotic, protective, supportive, or prosthetic devices or equipment (eg, dynamometry, electroneuromyography, footprint analyses, gait indexes, mobility skill profiles, observations, photographic assessments, technology-assisted assessments, videographic assessments, weight-bearing scales, wheelchair mobility tests)
- Safety during gait, locomotion, and balance (eg, confidence scales, diaries, fall scales, functional assessment profiles, logs, reports)

Integumentary Integrity

Associated skin

- Activities, positioning, and postures that produce or relieve trauma to the skin (eg, observations, pressure-sensing maps, scales)
- Assistive, adaptive, orthotic, protective, supportive, or prosthetic devices and equipment that may produce or relieve trauma to the skin (eg, observations, pressure-sensing maps, risk assessment scales)
- Skin characteristics, including blistering, continuity of skin color, dermatitis, hair growth, mobility, nail growth, sensation, temperature, texture, and turgor (eg, observations, palpation, photographic assessments, thermography)

Joint Integrity and Mobility

- Joint integrity and mobility (eg, apprehension, compression and distraction, drawer, glide, impingement, shear, and valgus/varus stress tests; arthrometry; palpation)

Motor Function (Motor Control and Motor Learning)

- Dexterity, coordination, and agility (eg, coordination screens, motor impairment tests, motor proficiency tests, observations, videographic assessments)
- Electrophysiological integrity (eg, electroneuromyography)
- Hand function (eg, fine and gross motor control tests, finger dexterity tests, manipulative ability tests, observations)
- Initiation, modification, and control of movement patterns and voluntary postures (eg, activity indexes, gross motor function profiles, motor scales, movement assessment batteries, neuromotor tests, observations, physical performance tests, postural challenge tests, videographic assessments)

Muscle Performance (Including Strength, Power, and Endurance)

- Electrophysiological integrity (eg, electroneuromyography)
- Muscle strength, power, and endurance (eg, dynamometry, manual muscle tests, muscle performance tests, physical capacity tests, technology-assisted assessments, timed activity tests)
- Muscle strength, power, and endurance during functional activities (eg, ADL scales, functional muscle tests, IADL scales, observations, videographic assessments)
- Muscle tension (eg, palpation)

Neuromotor Development and Sensory Integration

- Acquisition and evolution of motor skills, including age-appropriate development (eg, activity indexes, developmental inventories and questionnaires, infant and toddler motor assessments, learning profiles, motor function tests, motor proficiency assessments, neuromotor assessments, reflex tests, screens, videographic assessments)
- Oral motor function, phonation, and speech production (eg, interviews, observations)

Orthotic, Protective, and Supportive Devices

- Components, alignment, fit, and ability to care for orthotic, protective, and supportive devices and equipment (eg, interviews, logs, observations, pressure-sensing maps, reports)
- Orthotic, protective, and supportive devices and equipment use during functional activities (eg, ADL scales, functional scales, IADL scales, interviews, observations, profiles)
- Remediation of impairments, functional limitations, or disabilities with use of orthotic, protective, and supportive devices and equipment (eg, activity status indexes, ADL scales, aerobic capacity tests, functional performance inventories, health assessment questionnaires, IADL scales, pain scales, play scales, videographic assessments)
- Safety during use of orthotic, protective, and supportive devices and equipment (eg, diaries, fall scales, interviews, logs, observations, reports)

Pain

- Pain, soreness, and nociception (eg, analog scales, discrimination tests, pain drawings and maps, provocation tests, verbal and pictorial descriptor tests)
- Pain in specific body parts (eg, pain indexes, pain questionnaires, structural provocation tests)

Posture

- Postural alignment and position (static and dynamic), including symmetry and deviation from midline (eg, grid measurement, observations, photographic assessments, technology-assisted assessments, videographic assessments)
- Specific body parts (eg, angle assessments, forward-bending test, goniometry, observations, palpation, positional tests)

Range of Motion (ROM) (Including Muscle Length)

- Functional ROM (eg, observations, squat testing, toe touch tests)
- Joint active and passive movement (eg, goniometry, inclinometry, observations, photographic assessments, technology-assisted assessments, videographic assessments)
- Muscle length, soft tissue extensibility, and flexibility (eg, contracture tests, goniometry, inclinometry, ligamentous tests, linear measurement, multisegment flexibility tests, palpation)

Reflex Integrity

- Deep reflexes (eg, myotatic reflex scale, observations, reflex tests)
- Electrophysiological integrity (eg, electroneuromyography)
- Postural reflexes and reactions, including righting, equilibrium, and protective reactions (eg, observations, postural challenge tests, reflex profiles, videographic assessments)
- Resistance to passive stretch (eg, tone scales)
- Superficial reflexes and reactions (eg, observations, provocation tests)

Self-Care and Home Management (Including ADL and IADL)

- Ability to gain access to home environments (eg, barrier identification, observations, physical performance tests)
- Ability to perform self-care and home management activities with or without assistive, adaptive, orthotic, protective, supportive, or prosthetic devices and equipment (eg, ADL scales, aerobic capacity tests, IADL scales, interviews, observations, profiles)
- Safety in self-care and home management activities and environments (eg, diaries, fall scales, interviews, logs, observations, reports, videographic assessments)

Sensory Integrity

- Combined/cortical sensations (eg, stereognosis tests, tactile discrimination tests)
- Deep sensations (eg, kinesthesiometry, observations, photographic assessments, vibration tests)
- Electrophysiological integrity (eg, electroneuromyography)

Ventilation and Respiration/Gas Exchange

- Pulmonary signs of respiration/gas exchange, including breath sounds (eg, gas analyses, observations, oximetry)
- Pulmonary signs of ventilatory function, including airway protection; breath and voice sounds; respiratory rate, rhythm, and pattern; ventilatory flow, forces, and volumes (eg, airway clearance testing, observations, palpation, pulmonary function tests, ventilatory muscle force tests)
- Pulmonary symptoms (eg, dyspnea and perceived exertion indexes and scales)

Work (Job/School/Play), Community, and Leisure Integration or Reintegration (Including IADL)

- Ability to assume or resume work (job/school/play), community, and leisure activities with or without assistive, adaptive, orthotic, protective, supportive, or prosthetic devices and equipment (eg, activity profiles, disability indexes, functional status questionnaires, IADL scales, observations, physical capacity tests)
- Ability to gain access to work (job/school/play), community, and leisure environments (eg, barrier identification, interviews, observations, physical capacity tests, transportation assessments)
- Safety in work (job/school/play), community, and leisure activities and environments (eg, diaries, fall scales, interviews, logs, observations, videographic assessments)

Evaluation, Diagnosis, and Prognosis (Including Plan of Care)

Physical therapists perform *evaluations* (make clinical judgments) based on the data gathered from the history, systems review, and tests and measures. In the evaluation process, physical therapists synthesize the examination data to establish the diagnosis and prognosis (including the plan of care). Factors that influence the complexity of the evaluation include the clinical findings, extent of loss of function, chronicity or severity of the problem, possibility of multisite or multisystem involvement, preexisting condition(s), potential discharge destination, social considerations, physical function, and overall health status.

A *diagnosis* is a label encompassing a cluster of signs and symptoms, syndromes, or categories. It is the result of the systematic diagnostic process, which includes integrating and evaluating the data from the examination.The diagnostic label indicates the primary dysfunction(s) toward which the therapist will direct interventions. The *prognosis* is the determination of the predicted optimal level of improvement in function and the amount of time needed to reach that level and may also include a prediction of levels of improvement that may be reached at various intervals during the course of therapy. During the prognostic process, the physical therapist develops the plan of care. The *plan of care* identifies specific interventions, proposed frequency and duration of the interventions, anticipated goals, expected outcomes, and discharge plans. The plan of care identifies realistic anticipated goals and expected outcomes, taking into consideration the expectations of the patient/client and appropriate others.These anticipated goals and expected outcomes should be measureable and time limited.

The frequency of visits and duration of the episode of care may vary from a short episode with a high intensity of intervention to a longer episode with a diminishing intensity of intervention. Frequency and duration may vary greatly among patients/clients based on a variety of factors that the physical therapist considers throughout the evaluation process, such as anatomical and physiological changes related to growth and development; caregiver consistency or expertise; chronicity or severity of the current condition; living environment; multisite or multisystem involvement; social support; potential discharge destinations; probability of prolonged impairment, functional limitation, or disability; and stability of the condition.

Prognosis

Over the course of 9 months, patient/client will demonstrate optimal motor function, peripheral nerve integrity, and sensory integrity and the highest level of functioning in home, work (job/school/play), community, and leisure environments, within the context of the impairments, functional limitations, and disabilities.

During the episode of care, patient/client will achieve (1) the anticipated goals and expected outcomes of the interventions that are described in the plan of care and (2) the global outcomes for patients/clients who are classified in this pattern.

Expected Range of Number of Visits Per Episode of Care

4 to 150

This range represents the lower and upper limits of the number of physical therapist visits required to achieve anticipated goals and expected outcomes. *It is anticipated that 80% of patients/clients who are classified into this pattern will achieve the anticipated goals and expected outcomes within 4 to 150 visits during a single continuous episode of care.* Frequency of visits and duration of the episode of care should be determined by the physical therapist to maximize effectiveness of care and efficiency of service delivery.

Note:

These patients/clients may require multiple episodes of care over the lifetime to ensure safety and effective adaptation following changes in physical status, caregivers, environment, or task demands. Factors that may lead to these additional episodes of care include:

- Cognitive maturation
- Periods of rapid growth

Factors That May Require New Episode of Care or That May Modify Frequency of Visits/Duration of Care

- Accessibility and availability of resources
- Adherence to the intervention program
- Age
- Anatomical and physiological changes related to growth and development
- Caregiver consistency or expertise
- Chronicity or severity of the current condition
- Cognitive status
- Comorbitities, complications, or secondary impairments
- Concurrent medical, surgical, and therapeutic interventions
- Decline in functional independence
- Level of impairment
- Level of physical function
- Living environment
- Multisite or multisystem involvement
- Nutritional status
- Overall health status
- Potential discharge destinations
- Premorbid conditions
- Probability of prolonged impairment, functional limitation, or disability
- Psychological and socioeconomic factors
- Psychomotor abilities
- Social support
- Stability of the condition

Intervention

Intervention is the purposeful interaction of the physical therapist with the patient/client and, when appropriate, with other individuals involved in patient/client care, using various physical therapy procedures and techniques to produce changes in the condition consistent with the diagnosis and prognosis. Decisions about interventions are contingent on the timely monitoring of patient/client response and the progress made toward achieving the anticipated goals and expected outcomes.

Communication, coordination, and documentation and patient/client-related instruction are provided for all patients/clients across all settings. Procedural interventions are selected or modified based on the examination data and the evaluation, the diagnosis and the prognosis, and the anticipated goals and expected outcomes for a particular patient/client. *For clinical considerations in selecting interventions, listings of interventions, and listings of anticipated goals and expected outcomes, refer to Chapter 3.*

Coordination, Communication, and Documentation

Coordination, communication, and documentation may include:

Interventions

- Addressing required functions
  - advance directives
  - individualized family service plans (IFSPs) or individualized education plans (IEPs)
  - informed consent
  - mandatory communication and reporting (eg, patient advocacy and abuse reporting)
- Admission and discharge planning
- Case management
- Collaboration and coordination with agencies, including:
  - equipment suppliers
  - home care agencies
  - payer groups
  - schools
  - transportation agencies
- Communication across settings, including:
  - case conferences
  - documentation
  - education plans
- Cost-effective resource utilization
- Data collection, analysis, and reporting
  - outcome data
  - peer review findings
  - record reviews
- Documentation across settings, following APTA's *Guidelines for Physical Therapy Documentation* (Appendix 5), including:
  - changes in impairments, functional limitations, and disabilities
  - changes in interventions
  - elements of patient/client management (examination, evaluation, diagnosis, prognosis, intervention)
  - outcomes of intervention
- Interdisciplinary teamwork
  - case conferences
  - patient care rounds
  - patient/client family meetings
- Referrals to other professionals or resources

Anticipated Goals and Expected Outcomes

- Accountability for services is increased.
- Admission data and discharge planning are completed.
- Advance directives, individualized family service plans (IFSPs) or individualized education plans (IEPs), informed consent, and mandatory communication and reporting (eg, patient advocacy and abuse reporting) are obtained or completed.
- Available resources are maximally utilized.
- Care is coordinated with patient/client, family, significant others, caregivers, and other professionals.
- Case is managed throughout the episode of care.
- Collaboration and coordination occurs with agencies, including equipment suppliers, home care agencies, payer groups, schools, and transportation agencies.
- Communication enhances risk reduction and prevention.
- Communication occurs across settings through case conferences, education plans, and documentation.
- Data are collected, analyzed, and reported, including outcome data, peer review findings, and record reviews.
- Decision making is enhanced regarding health, wellness, and fitness needs.
- Decision making is enhanced regarding patient/client health and the use of health care resources by patient/client, family, significant others, and caregivers.
- Documentation occurs throughout patient/client management and across settings and follows APTA's *Guidelines for Physical Therapy Documentation* (Appendix 5).
- Interdisciplinary collaboration occurs through case conferences, patient care rounds, and patient/client family meetings.
- Patient/client, family, significant other, and caregiver understanding of anticipated goals and expected outcomes is increased.
- Placement needs are determined.
- Referrals are made to other professionals or resources whenever necessary and appropriate.
- Resources are utilized in a cost-effective way.

Patient/Client-Related Instruction

Patient/client-related instruction may include:

Interventions

- Instruction, education and training of patients/clients and caregivers regarding:
- current condition (pathology/pathophysiology [disease, disorder, or condition], impairments, functional limitations, or disabilities)
  - enhancement of performance
  - health, wellness, and fitness programs
  - plan of care
  - risk factors for pathology/pathophysiology (disease, disorder, or condition), impairments, functional limitations, or disabilities
  - transitions across settings
  - transitions to new roles

Anticipated Goals and Expected Outcomes

- Ability to perform physical actions, tasks, or activities is improved.
- Awareness and use of community resources are improved.
- Behaviors that foster healthy habits, wellness, and prevention are acquired.
- Decision making is enhanced regarding patient/client health and the use of health care resources by patient/client, family, significant others, and caregivers.
- Disability associated with acute or chronic illnesses is reduced.
- Functional independence in activities of daily living (ADL) and instrumental activities of daily living (IADL) is increased.
- Health status is improved.
- Intensity of care is decreased.
- Level of supervision required for task performance is decreased.
- Patient/client, family, significant other, and caregiver knowledge and awareness of the diagnosis, prognosis, interventions, and anticipated goals and expected outcomes are increased.
- Patient/client knowledge of personal and environmental factors associated with the condition is increased.
- Performance levels in self-care, home management, work (job/school/play), community, or leisure actions, tasks, or activities are improved.
- Physical function is improved.
- Risk of recurrence of condition is reduced.
- Risk of secondary impairment is reduced.
- Safety of patient/client, family, significant others, and caregivers is improved.
- Self-management of symptoms is improved.
- Utilization and cost of health care services are decreased.

Procedural Interventions

Procedural interventions for this pattern may include:

Therapeutic Exercise

Interventions

- Aerobic and endurance conditioning or reconditioning
  - aquatic programs
  - gait and locomotor training
  - increased workload over time
  - walking and wheelchair propulsion programs
- Balance, coordination, and agility training
  - developmental activities training
  - motor function (motor control and motor learning) training or retraining
  - neuromuscular education or reeducation
  - perceptual training
  - posture awareness training
  - standardized, programmatic, complementary exercise approaches
  - sensory training or retraining
  - task-specific performance training
- Body mechanics and postural stabilization
  - body mechanics training
  - posture awareness training
  - postural control training
  - postural stabilization activities
- Flexibility exercises
  - muscle lengthening
  - range of motion
  - stretching
- Gait and locomotion training
  - developmental activities training
  - gait training
  - implement and device training
  - perceptual training
  - standardized, programmatic, complementary exercise approaches
  - wheelchair training
- Relaxation
  - breathing strategies
  - movement strategies
  - relaxation techniques
  - standardized, programmatic, complementary exercise approaches
- Strength, power, and endurance training for head, neck, limb, pelvic-floor, trunk, and ventilatory muscles
  - active assistive, active, and resistive exercises (including concentric, dynamic/isotonic, eccentric, isokinetic, isometric, and plyometric)
  - aquatic programs
  - standardized, programmatic, complementary exercise approaches
  - task-specific performance training

Anticipated Goals and Expected Outcomes

- Impact on pathology/pathophysiology (disease, disorder, or condition)
  - Joint swelling, inflammation, or restriction is reduced.
  - Nutrient delivery to tissue is increased.
  - Osteogenic effects of exercise are maximized.
  - Pain is decreased.
  - Physiological response to increased oxygen demand is improved.
  - Soft tissue swelling, inflammation, or restriction is reduced.
  - Symptoms associated with increased oxygen demand are decreased.
  - Tissue perfusion and oxygenation are enhanced.
- Impact on impairments
  - Aerobic capacity is increased.
  - Airway clearance is improved.
  - Balance is improved.
  - Endurance is increased.
  - Energy expenditure per unit of work is decreased.
  - Gait, locomotion, and balance are improved.
  - Integumentary integrity is improved.
  - Joint integrity and mobility are improved.
  - Motor function (motor control and motor learning) is improved.
  - Muscle performance (strength, power, and endurance) is increased.
  - Postural control is improved.
  - Quality and quantity of movement between and across body segments are improved.
  - Range of motion is improved.
  - Relaxation is increased.
  - Sensory awareness is increased.
  - Weight-bearing status is improved.
  - Work of breathing is decreased.
- Impact on functional limitations
  - Ability to perform physical actions, tasks, or activities related to self-care, home management, work (job/school/play), community, and leisure is improved.
  - Level of supervision required for task performance is decreased.
  - Performance of and independence in activities of daily living (ADL) and instrumental activities of daily living (IADL) with or without devices and equipment are increased.
  - Tolerance of positions and activities is increased.
- Impact on disabilities
  - Ability to assume or resume required self-care, home management, work (job/school/play), community, and leisure roles is improved.
- Risk reduction/prevention
  - Preoperative and postoperative complications are reduced.
  - Risk factors are reduced.
  - Safety is improved.
  - Self-management of symptoms is improved.
- Impact on health, wellness, and fitness
  - Fitness is improved.
  - Health status is improved.
  - Physical capacity is increased.
  - Physical function is improved.
- Impact on societal resources
  - Utilization of physical therapy services is optimized.
  - Utilization of physical therapy services results in efficient use of health care dollars.
- Patient/client satisfaction
  - Access, availability, and services provided are acceptable to patient/client.
  - Administrative management of practice is acceptable to patient/client.
  - Clinical proficiency of physical therapist is acceptable to patient/client.
  - Coordination of care is acceptable to patient/client.
  - Cost of health care services is decreased.
  - Intensity of care is decreased.
  - Interpersonal skills of physical therapist are acceptable to patient/client, family, and significant others.
  - Sense of well-being is improved.
  - Stressors are decreased.

Functional Training in Self-Care and Home Management (Including Activities of Daily Living [ADL] and Instrumental Activities of Daily Living [IADL])

Interventions

- ADL training
  - bathing
  - bed mobility and transfer training
  - developmental activities
  - dressing
  - eating
  - grooming
  - toileting
- Devices and equipment use and training
  - assistive and adaptive device or equipment training during ADL and IADL
  - orthotic, protective, or supportive device or equipment training during ADL and IADL
  - prosthetic device or equipment training during ADL and IADL
- Functional training programs
  - simulated environments and tasks
  - task adaptation
  - travel training
- IADL training
  - caring for dependents
  - home maintenance
  - household chores
  - shopping
  - structured play for infants and children
  - yard work
- Injury prevention or reduction
  - injury prevention education during self-care and home management
  - injury prevention or reduction with use of devices and equipment
  - safety awareness training during self-care and home management

Anticipated Goals and Expected Outcomes

- Impact on pathology/pathophysiology (disease, disorder, or condition)
  - Pain is decreased.
  - Physiological response to increased oxygen demand is improved.
  - Symptoms associated with increased oxygen demand are decreased.
- Impact on impairments
  - Balance is improved.
  - Endurance is increased.
  - Energy expenditure per unit of work is decreased.
  - Motor function (motor control and motor learning) is improved.
  - Muscle performance (strength, power, and endurance) is increased.
  - Postural control is improved.
  - Sensory awareness is increased.
  - Weight-bearing status is improved.
  - Work of breathing is decreased.
- Impact on functional limitations
  - Ability to perform physical actions, tasks, or activities related to self-care and home management is improved.
  - Level of supervision required for task performance is decreased.
  - Performance of and independence in ADL and IADL with or without devices and equipment are increased.
  - Tolerance of positions and activities is increased.
- Impact on disabilities
  - Ability to assume or resume required self-care and home management roles is improved.
- Risk reduction/prevention
  - Risk factors are reduced.
  - Risk of secondary impairments is reduced.
  - Safety is improved.
  - Self-management of symptoms is improved.
- Impact on health, wellness, and fitness
  - Health status is improved.
  - Physical capacity is increased.
  - Physical function is improved.
- Impact on societal resources
  - Utilization of physical therapy services is optimized.
  - Utilization of physical therapy services results in efficient use of health care dollars.
- Patient/client satisfaction
  - Access, availability, and services provided are acceptable to patient/client.
  - Administrative management of practice is acceptable to patient/client.
  - Clinical proficiency of physical therapist is acceptable to patient/client.
  - Coordination of care is acceptable to patient/client.
  - Cost of health care services is decreased.
  - Intensity of care is decreased.
  - Interpersonal skills of physical therapist are acceptable to patient/client, family, and significant others.
  - Sense of well-being is improved.
  - Stressors are decreased.

Functional Training in Work (Job/School/Play), Community, and Leisure Integration or Reintegration (Including Instrumental Activities of Daily Living [IADL] and Work Conditioning)

Interventions

- Devices and equipment use and training
  - assistive and adaptive device or equipment training during IADL
  - orthotic, protective, or supportive device or equipment training during IADL
  - prosthetic device or equipment training during IADL
- Functional training programs
  - job coaching
  - simulated environments and tasks
  - task adaptation
  - task training
  - travel training
- IADL training
  - community service training involving instruments
  - school and play activities training including tools and instruments
  - work training with tools
- Injury prevention or reduction
  - injury prevention education during work (job/school/play), community, and leisure integration or reintegration
  - injury prevention or reduction with use of devices and equipment
  - safety awareness training during work (job/school/play), community, and leisure integration or reintegration
- Leisure and play activities training

Anticipated Goals and Expected Outcomes

- Impact on pathology/pathophysiology (disease, disorder, or condition)
  - Pain is decreased.
  - Physiological response to increased oxygen demand is improved.
  - Symptoms associated with increased oxygen demand are decreased.
- Impact on impairments
  - Balance is improved.
  - Endurance is increased.
  - Energy expenditure per unit of work is decreased.
  - Motor function (motor control and motor learning) is improved.
  - Muscle performance (strength, power, and endurance) is increased.
  - Postural control is improved.
  - Sensory awareness is increased.
  - Weight-bearing status is improved.
  - Work of breathing is decreased.
- Impact on functional limitations
  - Ability to perform physical actions, tasks, or activities related to work (job/school/play), community, and leisure integration or reintegration is improved.
  - Level of supervision required for task performance is decreased.
  - Performance of and independence in IADL with or without devices and equipment are increased.
  - Tolerance of positions and activities is increased.
- Impact on disabilities
  - Ability to assume or resume required work (job/school/play), community, and leisure roles is improved.
- Risk reduction/prevention
  - Risk factors are reduced.
  - Risk of secondary impairment is reduced.
  - Safety is improved
  - Self-management of symptoms is improved.
- Impact on health, wellness, and fitness
  - Fitness is improved.
  - Health status is improved.
  - Physical capacity is increased.
  - Physical function is improved.
- Impact on societal resources
  - Costs of work-related injury or disability are reduced.
  - Utilization of physical therapy services is optimized.
  - Utilization of physical therapy services results in efficient use of health care dollars.
- Patient/client satisfaction
  - Access, availability, and services provided are acceptable to patient/client.
  - Administrative management of practice is acceptable to patient/client.
  - Clinical proficiency of physical therapist is acceptable to patient/client.
  - Coordination of care is acceptable to patient/client.
  - Cost of health care services is decreased.
  - Intensity of care is decreased.
  - Interpersonal skills of physical therapist are acceptable to patient/client, family, and significant others.
  - Sense of well-being is improved.
  - Stressors are decreased.

Manual Therapy Techniques (Including Mobilization/Manipulation)

Interventions

- Massage
  - connective tissue massage
  - therapeutic massage
- Mobilization/manipulation
  - soft tissue
- Passive range of motion

Anticipated Goals and Expected Outcomes

- Impact on pathology/pathophysiology (disease, disorder, or condition)
  - Edema, lymphedema, or effusion is reduced.
  - Joint swelling, inflammation, or restriction is reduced.
  - Pain is decreased.
  - Soft tissue swelling, inflammation, or restriction is reduced.
- Impact on impairments
  - Balance is improved.
  - Energy expenditure per unit of work is decreased.
  - Gait, locomotion, and balance are improved.
  - Integumentary integrity is improved.
  - Muscle performance (strength, power, and endurance) is increased.
  - Postural control is improved.
  - Quality and quantity of movement between and across body segments are improved.
  - Range of motion is improved.
  - Relaxation is increased.
  - Sensory awareness is increased.
  - Weight-bearing status is improved.
  - Work of breathing is decreased.
- Impact on functional limitations
  - Ability to perform movement tasks is improved.
  - Ability to perform physical actions, tasks, or activities related to self-care, home management, work (job/school/play), community, and leisure is improved.
  - Tolerance of positions and activities is increased.
- Impact on disabilities
  - Ability to assume or resume required self-care, home management, work (job/school/play), community, and leisure roles is improved.
- Risk reduction/prevention
  - Risk factors are reduced.
  - Risk of secondary impairment is reduced.
  - Self-management of symptoms is improved.
- Impact on health, wellness, and fitness
  - Physical capacity is increased.
  - Physical function is improved.
- Impact on societal resources
  - Utilization of physical therapy services is optimized.
  - Utilization of physical therapy services results in efficient use of health care dollars.
- Patient/client satisfaction
  - Access, availability, and services provided are acceptable to patient/client.
  - Administrative management of practice is acceptable to patient/client.
  - Clinical proficiency of physical therapist is acceptable to patient/client.
  - Coordination of care is acceptable to patient/client.
  - Cost of health care services is decreased.
  - Intensity of care is decreased.
  - Interpersonal skills of physical therapist are acceptable to patient/client, family, and significant others.
  - Sense of well-being is improved.
  - Stressors are decreased.

Prescription, Application, and, as Appropriate, Fabrication of Devices and Equipment (Assistive, Adaptive, Orthotic, Protective, Supportive, and Prosthetic)

Interventions

- Adaptive devices
  - environmental controls
  - hospital beds
  - raised toilet seats
  - seating systems
- Assistive devices
  - canes
  - crutches
  - long-handled reachers
  - power devices
  - static and dynamic splints
  - walkers
  - wheelchairs
- Orthotic devices
  - braces
  - casts
  - shoe inserts
  - splints
- Protective devices
  - braces
  - cushions
  - helmets
  - protective taping
- Supportive devices
  - compression garments
  - corsets
  - elastic wraps
  - mechanical ventilators
  - neck collars
  - serial casts
  - slings
  - supplemental oxygen
  - supportive taping

Anticipated Goals and Expected Outcomes

- Impact on pathology/pathophysiology (disease, disorder, or condition)
  - Edema, lymphedema, or effusion is reduced.
  - Joint swelling, inflammation, or restriction is reduced.
  - Pain is decreased.
  - Physiological response to increased oxygen demand is improved.
  - Soft tissue swelling, inflammation, or restriction is reduced.
  - Symptoms associated with increased oxygen demand are decreased.
- Impact on impairments
  - Balance is improved.
  - Endurance is increased.
  - Energy expenditure per unit of work is decreased.
  - Gait, locomotion, and balance are improved.
  - Integumentary integrity is improved.
  - Joint stability is improved.
  - Motor function (motor control and motor learning) is improved.
  - Muscle performance (strength, power, and endurance) is increased.
  - Optimal joint alignment is achieved.
  - Optimal loading on a body part is achieved.
  - Postural control is improved.
  - Quality and quantity of movement between and across body segments are improved.
  - Range of motion is improved.
  - Weight-bearing status is improved.
  - Work of breathing is decreased.
- Impact on functional limitations
  - Ability to perform physical actions, tasks, or activities related to self-care, home management, work (job/school/play), community, and leisure is improved.
  - Level of supervision required for task performance is decreased.
  - Performance of and independence in activities of daily living (ADL) and instrumental activities of daily living (IADL) with or without devices and equipment are increased.
  - Tolerance of positions and activities is increased.
- Impact on disabilities
  - Ability to assume or resume required self-care, home management, work (job/school/play), community, and leisure roles is improved.
- Risk reduction/prevention
  - Pressure on body tissues is reduced.
  - Protection of body parts is increased.
  - Risk factors are reduced.
  - Risk of secondary impairment is reduced.
  - Safety is improved.
  - Self-management of symptoms is improved.
  - Stresses precipitating injury are decreased.
- Impact on health, wellness, and fitness
  - Health status is improved.
  - Physical capacity is increased.
  - Physical function is improved.
- Impact on societal resources
  - Utilization of physical therapy services is optimized.
  - Utilization of physical therapy services results in efficient use of health care dollars.
- Patient/client satisfaction
  - Access, availability, and services provided are acceptable to patient/client.
  - Administrative management of practice is acceptable to patient/client.
  - Clinical proficiency of physical therapist is acceptable to patient/client.
  - Coordination of care is acceptable to patient/client.
  - Cost of health care services is decreased.
  - Intensity of care is decreased.
  - Interpersonal skills of physical therapist are acceptable to patient/client, family, and significant others.
  - Sense of well-being is improved.
  - Stressors are decreased.

Airway Clearance Techniques

Interventions

- Breathing strategies
  - active cycle of breathing or forced expiratory techniques
  - assisted cough/huff techniques
  - autogenic drainage
  - paced breathing
  - pursed lip breathing
  - techniques to maximize ventilation (eg, maximum inspiratory hold, staircase breathing, manual hyperinflation)
- Manual/mechanical techniques
  - assistive devices
  - chest percussion, vibration, and shaking
  - chest wall manipulation
  - suctioning
  - ventilatory aids
- Positioning
  - positioning to alter work of breathing
  - positioning to maximize ventilation and perfusion
  - pulmonary postural drainage

Anticipated Goals and Expected Outcomes

- Impact on pathology/pathophysiology (disease, disorder, or condition)
  - Atelectasis is decreased.
  - Nutrient delivery to tissue is increased.
  - Physiological response to increased oxygen demand is improved.
  - Symptoms associated with increased oxygen demand are decreased.
  - Tissue perfusion and oxygenation are enhanced.
- Impact on impairments
  - Airway clearance is improved.
  - Cough is improved.
  - Endurance is increased.
  - Energy expenditure per unit of work is decreased.
  - Exercise tolerance is improved.
  - Muscle performance (strength, power, and endurance) is increased.
  - Ventilation and respiration/gas exchange are improved.
  - Work of breathing is decreased.
- Impact on functional limitations
  - Ability to perform physical actions, tasks, or activities related to self-care, home management, community, work (job/ school/ play), and leisure is improved.
  - Performance of and independence in activities of daily living (ADL) and instrumental activities of daily living (IADL) with or without devices and equipment are increased.
  - Tolerance of positions and activities is increased.
- Impact on disabilities
  - Ability to assume or resume required self-care, home management, work (job/school/play), community, and leisure roles is improved.
- Risk reduction/prevention
  - Preoperative and postoperative complications are reduced.
  - Risk factors are reduced.
  - Risk of secondary impairment is reduced.
  - Safety is improved.
  - Self-management of symptoms is improved.
- Impact on health, wellness, and fitness
  - Fitness is improved.
  - Health status is improved.
  - Physical capacity is increased.
  - Physical function is improved.
- Impact on societal resources
  - Utilization of physical therapy services is optimized.
  - Utilization of physical therapy services results in efficient use of health care dollars.
- Patient/client satisfaction
  - Access, availability, and services provided are acceptable to patient/client.
  - Administrative management of practice is acceptable to patient/client.
  - Clinical proficiency of physical therapist is acceptable to patient/client.
  - Coordination of care is acceptable to patient/client.
  - Cost of health care services is decreased.
  - Intensity of care is decreased.
  - Interpersonal skills of physical therapist are acceptable to patient/client, family, and significant others.
  - Sense of well-being is improved.
  - Stressors are decreased.

Electrotherapeutic Modalities

Interventions

- Electrical stimulation
  - electrical muscle stimulation (EMS)
  - functional electrical stimulation (FES)
  - high voltage pulsed current (HVPC)
  - transcutaneous electrical nerve stimulation (TENS)

Anticipated Goals and Expected Outcomes

- Impact on pathology/pathophysiology (disease, disorder, or condition)
  - Edema, lymphedema, or effusion is reduced.
  - Joint swelling, inflammation, or restriction is reduced.
  - Nutrient delivery to tissue is increased.
  - Osteogenic effects are enhanced.
  - Pain is decreased.
  - Soft tissue or wound healing is enhanced.
  - Soft tissue swelling, inflammation, or restriction is reduced.
  - Tissue perfusion and oxygenation are enhanced.
- Impact on impairments
  - Integumentary integrity is improved.
  - Motor function (motor control and motor learning) is improved.
  - Muscle performance (strength, power, and endurance) is increased.
  - Postural control is improved.
  - Quality and quantity of movement between and across body segments are improved.
  - Range of motion is improved.
  - Relaxation is increased.
  - Sensory awareness is increased.
- Impact on functional limitations
  - Ability to perform physical actions, tasks, or activities related to self-care, home management, work (job/school/play), community, and leisure is improved.
  - Level of supervision required for task performance is decreased.
  - Performance of and independence in activities of daily living (ADL) and instrumental activities of daily living (IADL) with or without devices and equipment are increased.
  - Tolerance of positions and activities is increased.
- Impact on disabilities
  - Ability to assume or resume required self-care, home management, work (job/school/play), community, and leisure roles is improved.
- Risk reduction/prevention
  - Complications of immobility are reduced.
  - Preoperative and postoperative complications are reduced.
  - Risk factors are reduced.
  - Risk of secondary impairment is reduced.
  - Self-management of symptoms is improved.
- Impact on health, wellness, and fitness
  - Physical capacity is increased.
  - Physical function is improved.
- Impact on societal resources
  - Utilization of physical therapy services is optimized.
  - Utilization of physical therapy services results in efficient use of health care dollars.
- Patient/client satisfaction
  - Access, availability, and services provided are acceptable to patient/client.
  - Administrative management of practice is acceptable to patient/client.
  - Clinical proficiency of physical therapist is acceptable to patient/client.
  - Coordination of care is acceptable to patient/client.
  - Interpersonal skills of physical therapist are acceptable to patient/client, family, and significant others.
  - Sense of well-being is improved.
  - Stressors are decreased.

Physical Agents and Mechanical Modalities

Interventions

Physical agents may include:

- Cryotherapy
  - cold packs
  - ice massage
  - vapocoolant spray
- Hydrotherapy
  - pools
- Sound agents
  - phonophoresis
  - ultrasound
- Thermotherapy
  - dry heat
  - hot packs
  - paraffin baths

Mechanical modalities may include:

- Gravity-assisted compression devices
  - standing frame
  - tilt table
- Compression therapies
  - compression bandaging
  - compression garments

Anticipated Goals and Expected Outcomes

- Impact on pathology/pathophysiology (disease, disorder, or condition)
  - Edema, lymphedema, or effusion is reduced.
  - Joint swelling, inflammation, or restriction is reduced.
  - Nutrient delivery to tissue is increased.
  - Pain is decreased.
  - Soft tissue swelling, inflammation, or restriction is reduced.
  - Tissue perfusion and oxygenation are enhanced.
- Impact on impairments
  - Integumentary integrity is improved.
  - Muscle performance (strength, power, and endurance) is increased.
  - Range of motion is improved.
  - Weight-bearing status is improved.
- Impact on functional limitations
  - Ability to perform physical actions, tasks, or activities related to self-care, home management, work (job/school/play), community, and leisure is improved.
  - Performance of and independence in activities of daily living (ADL) and instrumental activities of daily living (IADL) with or without devices and equipment are increased.
  - Tolerance of positions and activities is increased.
- Impact on disabilities
  - Ability to assume or resume required self-care, home management, work (job/school/play), community, and leisure roles is improved.
- Risk reduction/prevention
  - Complications of soft tissue and circulatory disorders are decreased.
  - Risk factors are reduced.
  - Risk of secondary impairment is reduced.
  - Safety is improved.
  - Self-management of symptoms is improved.
  - Stresses precipitating injury are decreased.
- Impact on health, wellness, and fitness
  - Physical function is improved.
- Impact on societal resources
  - Utilization of physical therapy services is optimized.
- Patient/client satisfaction
  - Access, availability, and services provided are acceptable to patient/client.
  - Administrative management of practice is acceptable to patient/client.
  - Clinical proficiency of physical therapist is acceptable to patient/client.
  - Coordination of care is acceptable to patient/client.
  - Interpersonal skills of physical therapist are acceptable to patient/client, family, and significant others.
  - Sense of well-being is improved.
  - Stressors are decreased.

Reexamination

Reexamination is the process of performing selected tests and measures after the initial examination to evaluate progress and to modify or redirect interventions. Reexamination may be indicated more than once during a single episode of care. It also may be performed over the course of a disease, disorder, or condition, which for some patients/clients may be over the life span. Indications for reexamination include new clinical findings or failure to respond to physical therapy interventions.

Global Outcomes for Patients/Clients in This Pattern

Throughout the entire episode of care, the physical therapist determines the anticipated goals and expected outcomes for each intervention. These anticipated goals and expected outcomes are delineated in shaded boxes that accompany the lists of interventions in each preferred practice pattern. As the patient/client reaches the termination of physical therapy services and the end of the episode of care, the physical therapist measures the global outcomes of the physical therapy services by characterizing or quantifying the impact of the physical therapy interventions in the following domains:

- Pathology/pathophysiology (disease, disorder, or condition)
- Impairments
- Functional limitations
- Disabilities
- Risk reduction/prevention
- Health, wellness, and fitness
- Societal resources
- Patient/client satisfaction

In some instances, a particular anticipated goal or expected outcome is thoroughly achieved through implementation of a single form of intervention. More commonly, however, the anticipated goals and expected outcomes are achieved as a result of the combined effects of several forms of interventions, leading to enhancement of both health status and health-related quality of life.

Criteria for Termination of Physical Therapy Services

Discharge is the process of ending physical therapy services that have been provided during a single episode of care. It occurs when the anticipated goals and expected outcomes have been achieved. Discharge does *not* occur with a *transfer* (defined as the time when a patient is moved from one site to another site within the same setting or across settings during a single episode of care). Although there may be facility-specific or payer-specific requirements for documentation regarding the conclusion of physical therapy services, *discharge occurs based on the physical therapist's analysis of the achievement of anticipated goals and expected outcomes.*

Discontinuation is the process of ending physical therapy services that have been provided during a single episode of care when (1) the patient/client, caregiver, or legal guardian declines to continue intervention; (2) the patient/client is unable to continue to progress toward outcomes because of medical or psychosocial complications or because financial/insurance resources have been expended; or (3) the physical therapist determines that the patient/client will no longer benefit from physical therapy. When physical therapy services are terminated prior to achievement of anticipated goals and expected outcomes, patient/client status and the rationale for termination are documented.

For patients/clients who require multiple episodes of care, periodic follow-up is needed over the life span to ensure safety and effective adaptation following changes in physical status, caregivers, environment, or task demands. In consultation with appropriate individuals, and in consideration of the outcomes, the physical therapist plans for discharge or discontinuation and provides for appropriate follow-up or referral.

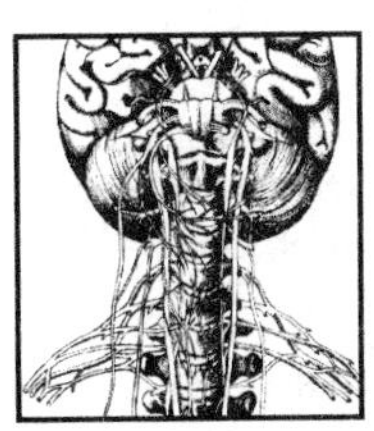

Impaired Arousal, Range of Motion, and Motor Control Associated With Coma, Near Coma, or Vegetative State

This preferred practice pattern describes the generally accepted elements of patient/client management that physical therapists provide for patients/clients who are classified in this pattern. The pattern title reflects the diagnosis made by the physical therapist. APTA emphasizes that preferred practice patterns are the boundaries within which a physical therapist may select any of a number of clinical alternatives, based on consideration of a wide variety of factors, such as individual patient/client needs; the profession's code of ethics and standards of practice; and patient/client age, culture, gender roles, race, sex, sexual orientation, and socioeconomic status.

Patient/Client Diagnostic Classification

Patients/clients will be classified into this pattern—for impaired arousal, range of motion, and motor control associated with coma, near coma, or vegetative state—as a result of the physical therapist's evaluation of the examination data. The findings from the examination (history, systems review, and tests and measures) may indicate the presence or risk of pathology/pathophysiology (disease, disorder, or condition), impairments, functional limitations, or disabilities or the need for health, wellness, or fitness programs. The physical therapist integrates, synthesizes, and interprets the data to determine the diagnostic classification.

Inclusion

The following examples of examination findings may support the inclusion of patients/clients in this pattern::

Risk Factors or Consequences of Pathology/Pathophysiology (Disease, Disorder, or Condition)

- Anoxia
- Birth trauma
- Cerebral vascular accident
- Infectious or inflammatory disease that affects the central nervous system
- Neoplasm
- Prematurity
- Traumatic brain injury

Impairments, Functional Limitations, or Disabilities

- Impaired arousal
- Impaired motor function
- Impaired range of motion
- Lack of response to stimuli
- Impaired sensory integrity

Note:

Some risk factors or consequences of pathology/pathophysiology—such as *pneumonia*—may be severe and complex; *however, they do not necessarily exclude patients/clients from this pattern.* Severe and complex risk factors or consequences may require modification of the frequency of visits and duration of care. (See "Evaluation, Diagnosis, and Prognosis," page 452.)

Multiple-Pattern Classification

The following examples of examination findings may support classification into additional patterns. Depending on the level of severity or complexity of the examination findings, the physical therapist may determine that the patient/client would be more appropriately managed through classification in both this and another pattern.

Findings That May Require Classification in Additional Patterns

- Decubitis ulcer
- Impairments associated with ventilator dependency

ICD-9-CM Codes

The listing below contains the current (as of press time) and most typical 3- and 4-digit ICD-9-CM codes related to this preferred practice pattern. Because patient/client diagnostic classification is based on impairments, functional limitations, and disabilities—not on codes—patients/clients may be classified into the pattern even though the codes listed with the pattern may not apply to those clients.

This listing is intended for general information only and should not be used for coding purposes. The codes should be confirmed by referring to the World Health Organization's *International Classification of Diseases, 9th Revision, Clinical Modification (ICD-9-CM 2001)*, Volumes 1 and 3 (Chicago, Ill: American Medical Association; 2000) or subsequent revisions or by referring to other ICD-9-CM coding manuals that contain exclusion notes and instructions regarding fifth-digit requirements.

049 Other non-arthropod-borne viral diseases of central nervous system
- **049.9** Unspecified non-arthropod-borne viral diseases of central nervous system
  - Viral encephalitis, not otherwise specified

191 Malignant neoplasm of brain

225 Benign neoplasm of brain and other parts of nervous system

322 Meningitis of unspecified cause

342 Hemiplegia and hemiparesis
- **342.0** Flaccid hemiplegia

348 Other conditions of brain
- **348.0** Cerebral cysts
- **348.1** Anoxic brain damage

431 Intracerebral hemorrhage

433 Occlusion and stenosis of precerebral arteries
- **433.0** Basilar artery

434 Occlusion of cerebral arteries

435 Transient cerebral ischemia
- **435.1** Vertebral artery syndrome
- **435.8** Other specified transient cerebral ischemias

436 Acute, but ill-defined, cerebrovascular disease

437 Other and ill-defined cerebrovascular disease

442 Other aneurysm
- **442.8** Of other specified artery

444 Arterial embolism and thrombosis
- **444.9** Of unspecified artery

447 Other disorders of arteries and arterioles
- **447.1** Stricture of artery

747 Other congenital anomalies of circulatory system
- **747.8** Other specified anomalies of circulatory system

765 Disorders relating to short gestation and unspecified low birth weight
- **765.1** Other preterm infants

767 Birth trauma
- **767.0** Subdural and cerebral hemorrhage
- **767.9** Birth trauma, unspecified

799 Other ill-defined and unknown causes of morbidity and mortality
- **799.0** Asphyxia

850 Concussion
- **850.5** With loss of consciousness of unspecified duration
- **850.9** Concussion, unspecified

851 Cerebral laceration and contusion

852 Subarachnoid, subdural, and extradural hemorrhage, following injury

853 Other and unspecified intracranial hemorrhage following injury
- **853.0** Without mention of open intracranial wound

854 Intracranial injury of other and unspecified nature

994 Effects of other external causes
- **994.1** Drowning and nonfatal submersion

Examination

Examination is a comprehensive screening and specific testing process that leads to a diagnostic classification or, when appropriate, to a referral to another practitioner. Examination is required prior to the initial intervention and is performed for all patients/clients. Through the examination, the physical therapist may identify impairments, functional limitations, disabilities, changes in physical function or overall health status, and needs related to restoration of health and to prevention, wellness, and fitness. The physical therapist synthesizes the examination findings to establish the diagnosis and the prognosis (including the plan of care). The patient/client, family, significant others, and caregivers may provide information during the examination process.

Examination has three components: the patient/client history, the systems review, and tests and measures. The *history* is a systematic gathering of past and current information (often from the patient/client) related to why the patient/client is seeking the services of the physical therapist. The *systems review* is a brief or limited examination of (1) the anatomical and physiological status of the cardiovascular/pulmonary, integumentary, musculoskeletal, and neuromuscular systems and (2) the communication ability, affect, cognition, language, and learning style of the patient/client. *Tests and measures* are the means of gathering data about the patient/client.

The selection of examination procedures and the depth of the examination vary based on patient/client age; severity of the problem; stage of recovery (acute, subacute, chronic); phase of rehabilitation (early, intermediate, late, return to activity); home, work (job/school/play), or community situation; and other relevant factors. *For clinical indications in selecting tests and measures and for listings of tests and measures, tools used to gather data, and the types of data generated by tests and measures, refer to Chapter 2.*

Patient/Client History

The history may include:

General Demographics
- Age
- Sex
- Race/ethnicity
- Primary language
- Education

Social History
- Cultural beliefs and behaviors
- Family and caregiver resources
- Social interactions, social activities, and support systems

Employment/Work (Job/School/Play)
- Current and prior work (job/school/play), community, and leisure actions, tasks, or activities

Growth and Development
- Developmental history
- Hand dominance

Living Environment
- Devices and equipment (eg, assistive, adaptive, orthotic, protective, supportive, prosthetic)
- Living environment and community characteristics
- Projected discharge destinations

General Health Status (Self-Report, Family Report, Caregiver Report)
- General health perception
- Physical function (eg, mobility, sleep patterns, restricted bed days)
- Psychological function (eg, memory, reasoning ability, depression, anxiety)
- Role function (eg, community, leisure, social, work)
- Social function (eg, social activity, social interaction, social support)

Social/Health Habits (Past and Current)
- Behavioral health risks (eg, smoking, drug abuse)
- Level of physical fitness

Family History
- Familial health risks

Medical/Surgical History
- Cardiovascular
- Endocrine/metabolic
- Gastrointestinal
- Genitourinary
- Gynecological
- Integumentary
- Musculoskeletal
- Neuromuscular
- Obstetrical
- Prior hospitalizations, surgeries, and preexisting medical and other health-related conditions
- Psychological
- Pulmonary

Current Condition(s)/Chief Complaint(s)
- Concerns that led patient/client to seek the services of a physical therapist
- Concerns or needs of patient/client who requires the services of a physical therapist
- Current therapeutic interventions
- Mechanisms of injury or disease, including date of onset and course of events
- Onset and pattern of symptoms
- Patient/client, family, significant other, and caregiver expectations and goals for the therapeutic intervention
- Patient/client, family, significant other, and caregiver perceptions of patient's/client's emotional response to the current clinical situation
- Previous occurrence of chief complaint(s)
- Prior therapeutic interventions

Functional Status and Activity Level
- Current and prior functional status in self-care and home management activities, including activities of daily living (ADL) and instrumental activities of daily living (IADL)
- Current and prior functional status in work (job/school/play), community, and leisure actions, tasks, or activities

Medications
- Medications for current condition
- Medications previously taken for current condition
- Medications for other conditions

Other Clinical Tests
- Laboratory and diagnostic tests
- Review of available records (eg, medical, education, surgical)
- Review of other clinical findings (eg, nutrition and hydration)

Systems Review

The systems review may include:

Anatomical and Physiological Status

- Cardiovascular/Pulmonary
  - Blood pressure
  - Edema
  - Heart rate
  - Respiratory rate
- Integumentary
  - Pliability (texture)
  - Presence of scar formation
  - Skin color
  - Skin integrity
- Musculoskeletal
  - Gross range of motion
  - Gross strength
  - Gross symmetry
  - Height
  - Weight
- Neuromuscular
  - Gross coordinated movements (eg, balance, gait, locomotion, transfers, transitions)
  - Motor function (motor control, motor learning)

Communication, Affect, Cognition, Language, and Learning Style

- Ability to make needs known
- Consciousness
- Expected emotional/behavioral responses
- Learning preferences (eg, education needs, learning barriers)
- Orientation (person, place, time)

Tests and Measures

Tests and measures for this pattern may include those that characterize or quantify:

Anthropometric Characteristics

- Edema (eg, girth measurement, palpation, scales, volume measurement)

Arousal, Attention, and Cognition

- Arousal and attention (eg, adaptability tests, arousal and awareness scales, indexes, profiles, questionnaires)
- Cognition, including ability to process commands (eg, developmental inventories, indexes, interviews, mental state scales, observations, questionnaires, safety checklists)
- Consciousness, including agitation and coma (eg, scales)

Assistive and Adaptive Devices

- Components, alignment, fit, and ability to care for the assistive or adaptive devices and equipment (eg, interviews, logs, observations, reports)
- Remediation of impairments, functional limitations, or disabilities with use of assistive or adaptive devices and equipment (eg, activity status indexes, ADL scales, aerobic capacity tests, functional performance inventories, health assessment questionnaires, IADL scales, pain scales, play scales, videographic assessments)
- Safety during use of assistive or adaptive devices and equipment (eg, diaries, logs, interviews, observations)

Circulation (Arterial, Venous, and Lymphatic)

- Cardiovascular signs, including heart rate, rhythm, and sounds; pressures and flow; and superficial vascular responses (eg, auscultation, electrocardiography, girth measurement, observations, palpation, sphygmomanometry, thermography)
- Physiological responses to position change, including autonomic responses, central and peripheral pressures, heart rate and rhythm, respiratory rate and rhythm, ventilatory pattern (eg, auscultation, electrocardiography, observations, palpation, sphygmomanometry)

Cranial and Peripheral Nerve Integrity

- Response to stimuli, including auditory, gustatory, olfactory, pharyngeal, vestibular, and visual (eg, observations, provocation tests)
- Sensory distribution of the cranial nerves (eg, discrimination tests; tactile tests, including coarse and light touch, cold and heat, pain, pressure, and vibration)
- Sensory distribution of the peripheral nerves (eg, discrimination tests; tactile tests, including coarse and light touch, cold and heat, pain, pressure, and vibration; thoracic outlet tests)

Environmental, Home, and Work (Job/School/Play) Barriers

- Current and potential barriers (eg, checklists, interviews, observations, questionnaires
- Physical space and environment (eg, compliance standards, observations, photographic assessments, questionnaires, structural specifications, videographic assessments)

Integumentary Integrity

Associated skin

- Activities, positioning, and postures that produce or relieve trauma to the skin (eg, observations, pressure-sensing maps, scales)
- Assistive, adaptive, orthotic, protective, supportive, or prosthetic devices and equipment that may produce or relieve trauma to the skin (eg, observations, pressure-sensing maps, risk assessment scales)
- Skin characteristics, including blistering, continuity of skin color, dermatitis, hair growth, mobility, nail growth, sensation, temperature, texture, and turgor (eg, observations, palpation, photographic assessments, thermography)

Motor Function (Motor Control and Motor Learning)

- Initiation, modification, and control of movement patterns and voluntary postures (eg, activity indexes, developmental scales, gross motor function profiles, motor scales, movement assessment batteries, neuromotor tests, observations, physical performance tests, postural challenge tests, videographic assessments)

Neuromotor Development and Sensory Integration

- Oral motor function, phonation and speech production (eg, interviews, observations)

Orthotic, Protective, and Supportive Devices

- Components, alignment, fit, and ability to care for orthotic, protective, and supportive devices and equipment (eg, interviews, logs, observations, reports)
- Remediation of impairments, functional limitations, or disabilities with use of orthotic, protective, and supportive devices and equipment (eg, ADL scales, pain scales)
- Safety during use of orthotic, protective, and supportive devices and equipment (eg, diaries, interviews, logs, observations, reports)

Pain

- Pain, soreness, and nociception (eg, angina scales, analog scales, discrimination tests, pain drawings and maps, provocation tests, verbal and pictorial descriptor tests)

Posture

- Postural alignment and position (static and dynamic), including symmetry and deviation from midline (eg, grid measurement, observations, photographic assessments, technology-assisted assessments, videographic assessments)
- Specific body parts (eg, angle assessments, forward-bending test, goniometry, observations, palpation, positional tests)

Range of Motion (ROM) (Including Muscle Length)

- Joint active and passive movement (eg, goniometry, inclinometry, observations, photographic assessments, technology-assisted assessments, videographic assessments)
- Muscle length, soft tissue extensibility, and flexibility (eg, contracture tests, goniometry, inclinometry, multisegment flexibility tests, palpation)

Reflex Integrity

- Deep reflexes (eg, myotatic reflex scale, observations, reflex tests)
- Primitive reflexes and reactions, including developmental (eg, reflex profiles, screening tests)
- Resistance to passive stretch (eg, tone scales)
- Superficial reflexes and reactions (eg, observations, provocation tests)

Self-Care and Home Management (Including ADL and IADL)

- Ability to gain access to home environments (eg, barrier identification, observations)
- Safety in self-care and home management activities and environments (eg, diaries, interviews, logs, observations, reports)

Ventilation and Respiration/Gas Exchange

- Pulmonary signs of respiration/gas exchange, including breath sounds (eg, gas analyses, observations, oximetry)
- Pulmonary signs of ventilatory function, including airway protection; breath and voice sounds; respiratory rate, rhythm, and pattern; ventilatory flow, forces, and volumes (eg, observations, palpation)
- Pulmonary symptoms (eg, dyspnea and perceived exertion indexes and scales)

Evaluation, Diagnosis, and Prognosis (Including Plan of Care)

Physical therapists perform *evaluations* (make clinical judgments) based on the data gathered from the history, systems review, and tests and measures. In the evaluation process, physical therapists synthesize the examination data to establish the diagnosis and prognosis (including the plan of care). Factors that influence the complexity of the evaluation include the clinical findings, extent of loss of function, chronicity or severity of the problem, possibility of multisite or multisystem involvement, preexisting condition(s), potential discharge destination, social considerations, physical function, and overall health status.

A *diagnosis* is a label encompassing a cluster of signs and symptoms, syndromes, or categories. It is the result of the systematic diagnostic process, which includes integrating and evaluating the data from the examination. The diagnostic label indicates the primary dysfunction(s) toward which the therapist will direct interventions. The *prognosis* is the determination of the predicted optimal level of improvement in function and the amount of time needed to reach that level and may also include a prediction of levels of improvement that may be reached at various intervals during the course of therapy. During the prognostic process, the physical therapist develops the plan of care. The *plan of care* identifies specific interventions, proposed frequency and duration of the interventions, anticipated goals, expected outcomes, and discharge plans. The plan of care identifies realistic anticipated goals and expected outcomes, taking into consideration the expectations of the patient/client and appropriate others. These anticipated goals and expected outcomes should be measureable and time limited.

The frequency of visits and duration of the episode of care may vary from a short episode with a high intensity of intervention to a longer episode with a diminishing intensity of intervention. Frequency and duration may vary greatly among patients/clients based on a variety of factors that the physical therapist considers throughout the evaluation process, such as anatomical and physiological changes related to growth and development; caregiver consistency or expertise; chronicity or severity of the current condition; living environment; multisite or multisystem involvement; social support; potential discharge destinations; probability of prolonged impairment, functional limitation, or disability; and stability of the condition.

Prognosis

Over the course of 3 months, patient/client will demonstrate optimal arousal, range of motion, and motor control and the minimization of secondary impairments.

During the episode of care, patient/client will achieve (1) the anticipated goals and expected outcomes of the interventions that are described in the plan of care and (2) the global outcomes for patients/clients who are classified in this pattern.

Expected Range of Number of Visits Per Episode of Care

5 to 20

This range represents the lower and upper limits of the number of physical therapist visits required to achieve anticipated goals and expected outcomes. *It is anticipated that 80% of patients who are classified into this pattern will achieve the anticipated goals and expected outcomes within 5 to 20 visits during a single continuous episode of care.* Frequency of visits and duration of the episode of care should be determined by the physical therapist to maximize effectiveness of care and efficiency of service delivery.

Factors That May Require New Episode of Care or That May Modify Frequency of Visits/Duration of Care

- Accessibility and availability of resources
- Adherence to the intervention program
- Age
- Anatomical and physiological changes related to growth and development
- Caregiver consistency or expertise
- Chronicity or severity of the current condition
- Cognitive status
- Comorbitities, complications, or secondary impairments
- Concurrent medical, surgical, and therapeutic interventions
- Decline in functional independence
- Level of impairment
- Level of physical function
- Living environment
- Multisite or multisystem involvement
- Nutritional status
- Overall health status
- Potential discharge destinations
- Premorbid conditions
- Probability of prolonged impairment, functional limitation, or disability
- Psychological and socioeconomic factors
- Psychomotor abilities
- Social support
- Stability of the condition

Intervention

Intervention is the purposeful interaction of the physical therapist with the patient/client and, when appropriate, with other individuals involved in patient/client care, using various physical therapy procedures and techniques to produce changes in the condition consistent with the diagnosis and prognosis. Decisions about interventions are contingent on the timely monitoring of patient/client response and the progress made toward achieving the anticipated goals and expected outcomes.

Communication, coordination, and documentation and patient/client-related instruction are provided for all patients/clients across all settings. Procedural interventions are selected or modified based on the examination data and the evaluation, the diagnosis and the prognosis, and the anticipated goals and expected outcomes for a particular patient/client. *For clinical considerations in selecting interventions, listings of interventions, and listings of anticipated goals and expected outcomes, refer to Chapter 3.*

Coordination, Communication, and Documentation

Coordination, communication, and documentation may include:

Interventions

- Addressing required functions
  - advance directives
  - informed consent (guardian consent)
  - mandatory communication and reporting (eg, patient advocacy and abuse reporting)
- Admission and discharge planning
- Case management
- Collaboration and coordination with agencies, including:
  - equipment suppliers
  - home care agencies
  - payer groups
  - schools
  - transportation agencies
- Communication across settings, including:
  - case conferences
  - documentation
  - education plans
- Cost-effective resource utilization
- Data collection, analysis, and reporting
  - outcome data
  - peer review findings
  - record reviews
- Documentation across settings, following APTA's *Guidelines for Physical Therapy Documentation* (Appendix 5), including:
  - changes in impairments, functional limitations, and disabilities
  - changes in interventions
  - elements of patient/client management (examination, evaluation, diagnosis, prognosis, intervention)
  - outcomes of intervention
- Interdisciplinary teamwork
  - case conferences
  - patient care rounds
  - patient/client family meetings
- Referrals to other professionals or resources

Anticipated Goals and Expected Outcomes

- Accountability for services is increased.
- Admission data and discharge planning are completed.
- Informed consent, and mandatory communication and reporting (eg, patient advocacy and abuse reporting) are obtained or completed.
- Available resources are maximally utilized.
- Care is coordinated with family, significant others, caregivers, and other professionals.
- Case is managed throughout the episode of care.
- Collaboration and coordination occurs with agencies, including equipment suppliers, home care agencies, payer groups, schools, and transportation agencies.
- Communication enhances risk reduction and prevention.
- Communication occurs across settings through case conferences, education plans, and documentation.
- Data are collected, analyzed, and reported, including outcome data, peer review findings, and record reviews.
- Decision making is enhanced regarding patient/client health and the use of health care resources by family, significant others, and caregivers.
- Documentation occurs throughout patient/client management and across settings and follows APTA's *Guidelines for Physical Therapy Documentation* (Appendix 5).
- Interdisciplinary collaboration occurs through case conferences, patient care rounds, and patient/client family meetings.
- Patient/client, family, significant other, and caregiver understanding of anticipated goals and expected outcomes is increased.
- Placement needs are determined.
- Referrals are made to other professionals or resources whenever necessary and appropriate.
- Resources are utilized in a cost-effective way.

Patient/Client-Related Instruction

Patient/client-related instruction may include:

Interventions

- Instruction, education and training of patients/clients and caregivers regarding:
  - current condition (pathology/pathophysiology [disease, disorder, or condition], impairments, functional limitations, or disabilities)
  - plan of care
  - risk factors for pathology/pathophysiology (disease, disorder, or condition), impairments, functional limitations, or disabilities
  - transitions across settings

Anticipated Goals and Expected Outcomes

- Ability to perform physical actions, tasks, or activities is improved.
- Awareness and use of community resources by family and caregivers are improved.
- Behaviors that foster healthy habits, wellness, and prevention are acquired.
- Decision making is enhanced regarding patient/client health and the use of health care resources by family, significant others, and caregivers.
- Disability associated with acute or chronic illnesses is reduced.
- Family, significant other, and caregiver knowledge and awareness of the diagnosis, prognosis, interventions, and anticipated goals and expected outcomes are increased.
- Health status is improved.
- Intensity of care is decreased.
- Level of supervision required for task performance by family or caregiver is decreased.
- Physical function is improved.
- Risk of recurrence of condition is reduced.
- Risk of secondary impairment is reduced.
- Safety of patient/client, family, significant others, and caregivers is improved.
- Utilization and cost of health care services are decreased.

Procedural Interventions

Procedural interventions for this pattern may include

Therapeutic Exercise

Interventions

- Flexibility exercises
  - muscle lengthening
  - range of motion
  - stretching

Anticipated Goals and Expected Outcomes

- Impact on pathology/pathophysiology (disease, disorder, or condition)
  - Joint swelling, inflammation, or restriction is reduced.
  - Nutrient delivery to tissue is increased.
  - Pain is decreased.
  - Soft tissue swelling, inflammation, or restriction is reduced.
  - Tissue perfusion and oxygenation are enhanced.
- Impact on impairments
  - Integumentary integrity is improved.
  - Joint integrity and mobility are improved.
  - Range of motion is improved.
  - Relaxation is increased.
  - Sensory awareness is increased.
  - Weight-bearing status is improved.
- Impact on functional limitations
  - Level of supervision required for task performance is decreased.
  - Tolerance of positions and activities is increased.
- Risk reduction/prevention
  - Caregiver management of symptoms is improved.
  - Preoperative and postoperative complications are reduced.
  - Risk factors are reduced.
  - Risk of secondary impairment is reduced.
- Impact on health, wellness, and fitness
  - Health status is improved.
  - Physical function is improved.
- Impact on societal resources
  - Utilization of physical therapy services is optimized.
  - Utilization of physical therapy services results in efficient use of health care dollars.
- Patient/client satisfaction
  - Access, availability, and services provided are acceptable to caregiver.
  - Administrative management of practice is acceptable to caregiver.
  - Caregiver's sense of well-being is improved.
  - Caregiver's stressors are decreased.
  - Clinical proficiency of physical therapist is acceptable to caregiver.
  - Coordination of care is acceptable to caregiver.
  - Cost of health care services is decreased.
  - Intensity of care is decreased.
  - Interpersonal skills of physical therapist are acceptable to caregiver.

Functional Training in Self-Care and Home Management (Including Activities of Daily Living [ADL] and Instrumental Activities of Daily Living [IADL])

Interventions

- ADL training
  - bathing
  - bed mobility and transfer training
  - dressing
  - grooming
  - toileting
- Devices and equipment use and training
  - assistive and adaptive device or equipment training during ADL
  - orthotic, protective, or supportive device or equipment training during ADL
- Injury prevention or reduction
  - injury prevention education during self-care and home management
  - injury prevention or reduction with use of devices and equipment
  - safety awareness training during self-care and home management

Anticipated Goals and Expected Outcomes

- Impact on pathology/pathophysiology (disease, disorder, or condition)
  - Pain is decreased.
- Impact on impairments
  - Endurance is increased
  - Sensory awareness is increased.
  - Weight-bearing status is improved.
  - Work of breathing is decreased.
- Impact on functional limitations
  - Ability of caregiver to perform physical actions, tasks, or activities related to home management is improved.
  - Performance of and independence in ADL by caregiver are increased.
  - Tolerance of positions and activities is increased.
- Risk reduction/prevention
  - Risk factors are reduced.
  - Risk of secondary impairments is reduced.
  - Safety is improved.
- Impact on health, wellness, and fitness
  - Health status is improved.
  - Physical function is improved.
- Impact on societal resources
  - Utilization of physical therapy services is optimized.
  - Utilization of physical therapy services results in efficient use of health care dollars.
- Patient/client satisfaction
  - Access, availability, and services provided are acceptable to caregiver.
  - Administrative management of practice is acceptable to caregiver.
  - Caregiver's sense of well-being is improved.
  - Caregiver's stressors are decreased.
  - Clinical proficiency of physical therapist is acceptable to caregiver.
  - Coordination of care is acceptable to caregiver.
  - Cost of health care services is decreased.
  - Intensity of care is decreased.
  - Interpersonal skills of physical therapist are acceptable to caregiver.

Manual Therapy Techniques (Including Mobilization/Manipulation)

Interventions

- Passive range of motion
- Mobilization/manipulation
  - soft tissue

Anticipated Goals and Expected Outcomes

- Impact on pathology/pathophysiology (disease, disorder, or condition)
  - Edema, lymphedema, or effusion is reduced.
  - Joint swelling, inflammation, or restriction is reduced.
  - Pain is decreased.
  - Soft tissue swelling, inflammation, or restriction is reduced.
- Impact on impairments
  - Integumentary integrity is improved.
  - Range of motion is improved.
  - Relaxation is increased.
  - Sensory awareness is increased.
  - Weight-bearing status is improved.
- Impact on functional limitations
  - Ability of caregiver to perform physical actions, tasks, or activities related to home management is improved.
  - Performance of and independence in activities of daily living (ADL) by caregiver are increased.
  - Tolerance of positions and activities is increased.
- Risk reduction/prevention
  - Risk factors are reduced.
  - Risk of secondary impairment is reduced.
- Impact on health, wellness, and fitness
  - Physical function is improved.
- Impact on societal resources
  - Utilization of physical therapy services is optimized.
  - Utilization of physical therapy services results in efficient use of health care dollars.
- Patient/client satisfaction
  - Access, availability, and services provided are acceptable to caregiver.
  - Administrative management of practice is acceptable to caregiver.
  - Caregiver's sense of well-being is improved.
  - Caregiver's stressors are decreased.
  - Clinical proficiency of physical therapist is acceptable to caregiver.
  - Coordination of care is acceptable to caregiver.
  - Cost of health care services is decreased.
  - Intensity of care is decreased.
  - Interpersonal skills of physical therapist are acceptable to caregiver.

Prescription, Application, and, as Appropriate, Fabrication of Devices and Equipment (Assistive, Adaptive, Orthotic, Protective, Supportive, and Prosthetic)

Interventions

- Adaptive devices
  - hospital beds
  - seating systems
- Assistive devices
  - wheelchairs
- Orthotic devices
  - braces
  - splints
- Protective devices
  - braces
  - cushions
  - helmets
  - protective taping
- Supportive devices
  - compression garments
  - corsets
  - elastic wraps
  - mechanical ventilators
  - neck collars
  - serial casts
  - slings
  - supplemental oxygen
  - supportive taping

Anticipated Goals and Expected Outcomes

- Impact on pathology/pathophysiology (disease, disorder, or condition)
  - Edema, lymphedema, or effusion is reduced.
  - Joint swelling, inflammation, or restriction is reduced.
  - Pain is decreased.
  - Physiological response to increased oxygen demand is improved.
  - Soft tissue swelling, inflammation, or restriction is reduced.
- Impact on impairments
  - Balance is improved.
  - Energy expenditure per unit of work is decreased.
  - Integumentary integrity is improved.
  - Joint stability is improved.
  - Optimal joint alignment is achieved.
  - Postural control is improved.
  - Range of motion is improved.
  - Weight-bearing status is improved.
  - Work of breathing is decreased.
- Impact on functional limitations
  - Level of supervision required for task performance is decreased.
  - Performance of and independence in activities of daily living (ADL) by caregiver are increased.
  - Tolerance of positions and activities is increased.
- Risk reduction/prevention
  - Pressure on body tissues is reduced.
  - Protection of body parts is increased.
  - Risk factors are reduced.
  - Risk of secondary impairment is reduced.
  - Safety is improved.
  - Stresses precipitating injury are decreased.
- Impact on health, wellness, and fitness
  - Health status is improved.
  - Physical function is improved.
- Impact on societal resources
  - Utilization of physical therapy services is optimized.
  - Utilization of physical therapy services results in efficient use of health care dollars.
- Patient/client satisfaction
  - Access, availability, and services provided are acceptable to caregiver.
  - Administrative management of practice is acceptable to caregiver.
  - Caregiver's sense of well-being is improved.
  - Caregiver's stressors are decreased.
  - Clinical proficiency of physical therapist is acceptable to caregiver.
  - Coordination of care is acceptable to caregiver.
  - Cost of health care services is decreased.
  - Intensity of care is decreased.
  - Interpersonal skills of physical therapist are acceptable to caregiver.

Airway Clearance Techniques

Interventions

- Breathing strategies
  - techniques to maximize ventilation (eg, manual hyperinflation)
- Manual/mechanical techniques
  - assistive devices
  - chest percussion, vibration, and shaking
  - suctioning
- Positioning
  - positioning to maximize ventilation and perfusion
  - pulmonary postural drainage

Anticipated Goals and Expected Outcomes

- Impact on pathology/pathophysiology (disease, disorder, or condition)
  - Atelectasis is decreased.
  - Nutrient delivery to tissue is increased.
  - Symptoms associated with increased oxygen demand are decreased.
  - Tissue perfusion and oxygenation are enhanced.
- Impact on impairments
  - Airway clearance is improved.
  - Cough is improved.
  - Energy expenditure per unit of work is decreased.
  - Ventilation and respiration/gas exchange are improved.
  - Work of breathing is decreased.
- Impact on functional limitations
  - Performance of and independence in activities of daily living (ADL) by caregiver are increased.
  - Tolerance of positions and activities is increased.
- Risk reduction/prevention
  - Preoperative and postoperative complications are reduced.
  - Risk factors are reduced.
  - Risk of recurrence of condition is reduced.
  - Risk of secondary impairment is reduced.
  - Safety is improved.
- Impact on health, wellness, and fitness
  - Health status is improved.
  - Physical function is improved.
- Impact on societal resources
  - Utilization of physical therapy services is optimized.
  - Utilization of physical therapy services results in efficient use of health care dollars.
- Patient/client satisfaction
  - Access, availability, and services provided are acceptable to caregiver.
  - Administrative management of practice is acceptable to caregiver.
  - Caregiver's sense of well-being is improved.
  - Caregiver's stressors are decreased.
  - Clinical proficiency of physical therapist is acceptable to caregiver.
  - Coordination of care is acceptable to caregiver.
  - Cost of health care services is decreased.
  - Intensity of care is decreased.
  - Interpersonal skills of physical therapist are acceptable to caregiver.

Physical Agents and Mechanical Modalities

Interventions

Physical agents may include:

- Athermal agents
  - pulsed electromagnetic fields
- Cryotherapy
  - cold packs
  - ice massage
- Thermotherapy
  - dry heat
  - hot packs

Anticipated Goals and Expected Outcomes

- Impact on pathology/pathophysiology (disease, disorder, or condition)
  - Edema, lymphedema, or effusion is reduced.
  - Joint swelling, inflammation, or restriction is reduced.
  - Nutrient delivery to tissue is increased.
  - Pain is decreased.
  - Soft tissue swelling, inflammation, or restriction is reduced.
  - Tissue perfusion and oxygenation are enhanced.
- Impact on impairments
  - Integumentary integrity is improved.
  - Range of motion is improved.
  - Weight-bearing status is improved.
- Impact on functional limitations
  - Performance of and independence in activities of daily living (ADL) by caregiver are increased.
  - Tolerance of positions and activities is increased.
- Risk reduction/prevention
  - Complications of soft tissue and circulatory disorders are decreased.
  - Risk of secondary impairment is reduced.
  - Stresses precipitating injury are decreased.
- Impact on health, wellness, and fitness
  - Physical function is improved.
- Impact on societal resources
  - Utilization of physical therapy services is optimized.
- Patient/client satisfaction
  - Access, availability, and services provided are acceptable to caregiver.
  - Administrative management of practice is acceptable to caregiver.
  - Caregiver's sense of well-being is improved.
  - Caregiver's stressors are decreased.
  - Clinical proficiency of physical therapist is acceptable to caregiver.
  - Coordination of care is acceptable to caregiver.
  - Interpersonal skills of physical therapist are acceptable to caregiver.

Reexamination

Reexamination is the process of performing selected tests and measures after the initial examination to evaluate progress and to modify or redirect interventions. Reexamination may be indicated more than once during a single episode of care. It also may be performed over the course of a disease, disorder, or condition, which for some patients/clients may be over the life span. Indications for reexamination include new clinical findings or failure to respond to physical therapy interventions.

Global Outcomes for Patients/Clients in This Pattern

Throughout the entire episode of care, the physical therapist determines the anticipated goals and expected outcomes for each intervention. These anticipated goals and expected outcomes are delineated in shaded boxes that accompany the lists of interventions in each preferred practice pattern. As the patient/client reaches the termination of physical therapy services and the end of the episode of care, the physical therapist measures the global outcomes of the physical therapy services by characterizing or quantifying the impact of the physical therapy interventions in the following domains:

- Pathology/pathophysiology (disease, disorder, or condition)
- Impairments
- Functional limitations
- Disabilities
- Risk reduction/prevention
- Health, wellness, and fitness
- Societal resources
- Patient/client satisfaction

In some instances, a particular anticipated goal or expected outcome is thoroughly achieved through implementation of a single form of intervention. More commonly, however, the anticipated goals and expected outcomes are achieved as a result of the combined effects of several forms of interventions, leading to enhancement of both health status and health-related quality of life.

Criteria for Termination of Physical Therapy Services

Discharge is the process of ending physical therapy services that have been provided during a single episode of care. It occurs when the anticipated goals and expected outcomes have been achieved. Discharge does *not* occur with a *transfer* (defined as the time when a patient is moved from one site to another site within the same setting or across settings during a single episode of care). Although there may be facility-specific or payer-specific requirements for documentation regarding the conclusion of physical therapy services, *discharge occurs based on the physical therapist's analysis of the achievement of anticipated goals and expected outcomes.*

Discontinuation is the process of ending physical therapy services that have been provided during a single episode of care when (1) the patient/client, caregiver, or legal guardian declines to continue intervention; (2) the patient/client is unable to continue to progress toward outcomes because of medical or psychosocial complications or because financial/insurance resources have been expended; or (3) the physical therapist determines that the patient/client will no longer benefit from physical therapy. When physical therapy services are terminated prior to achievement of anticipated goals and expected outcomes, patient/client status and the rationale for termination are documented.

For patients/clients who require multiple episodes of care, periodic follow-up is needed over the life span to ensure safety and effective adaptation following changes in physical status, caregivers, environment, or task demands. In consultation with appropriate individuals, and in consideration of the outcomes, the physical therapist plans for discharge or discontinuation and provides for appropriate follow-up or referral.

Chapter 6

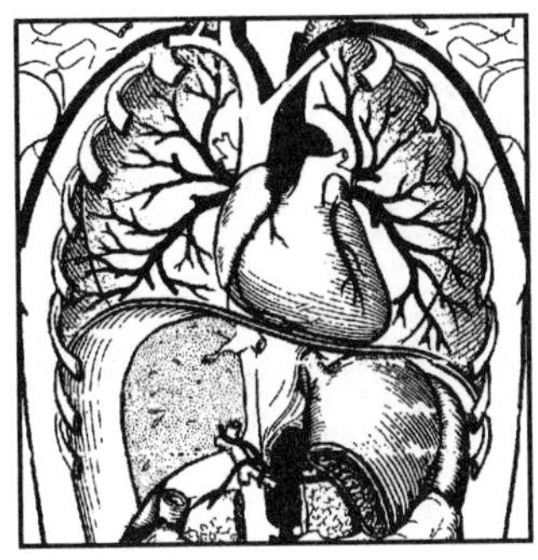

Preferred Physical Therapist Practice Patterns: Cardiovascular/Pulmonary

Preferred Physical Therapist Practice Patterns describe the five elements of patient/client management that are provided by physical therapists: examination (history, systems review, and tests and measures), evaluation, diagnosis, prognosis (including plan of care), and intervention (with anticipated goals and expected outcomes). Each pattern also addresses reexamination, global outcomes, and criteria for termination of physical therapy services. Examples of ICD-9-CM codes are included.

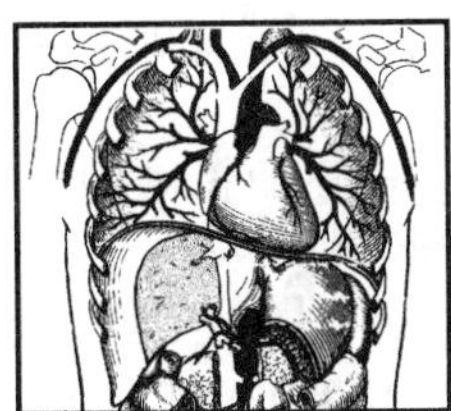

Primary Prevention/ Risk Reduction for Cardiovascular/Pulmonary Disorders

This preferred practice pattern describes the generally accepted elements of patient/client management that physical therapists provide for patients/clients who are classified in this pattern. The pattern title reflects the diagnosis made by the physical therapist. APTA emphasizes that preferred practice patterns are the boundaries within which a physical therapist may select any of a number of clinical alternatives, based on consideration of a wide variety of factors, such as individual patient/client needs; the profession's code of ethics and standards of practice; and patient/client age, culture, gender roles, race, sex, sexual orientation, and socioeconomic status.

Patient/Client Diagnostic Classification

Patients/clients will be classified into this primary prevention/risk reduction pattern as a result of the physical therapist's evaluation of the examination data. The findings from the examination (history, systems review, and tests and measures) may indicate the need for a prevention/risk reduction program. The physical therapist integrates, synthesizes, and interprets the data to determine inclusion in this diagnostic category.

Inclusion

The following examples of examination findings may support the inclusion of patients/clients in this pattern:

Risk Factors or Consequences of Pathology/Pathophysiology (Disease, Disorder, or Condition)

- Diabetes
- Family history of heart disease
- Hypercholesterolemia or hyperlipidemia
- Hypertension
- Obesity
- Sedentary lifestyle
- Smoking

Impairments, Functional Limitations, or Disabilities

- Decreased functional work capacity
- Decreased maximum aerobic capacity
- Dyspnea on exertion
- Sedentary job role

Note:

Prevention and risk reduction are inherent in all practice patterns. Patients/clients included in this pattern are in need of primary prevention/risk reduction only.

ICD-9-CM Codes

The listing below contains the current (as of press time) and most typical 3- and 4-digit ICD-9-CM codes related to this preferred practice pattern. Because patient/client diagnostic classification is based on impairments, functional limitations, and disabilities—not on codes—patients/clients may be classified into the pattern even though the codes listed with the pattern may not apply to those patients/clients.

This listing is intended for general information only and should not be used for coding purposes. The codes should be confirmed by referring to the World Health Organization's *International Classification of Diseases, 9th Revision, Clinical Modification (ICD-9-CM 2001)*, Volumes 1 and 3 (Chicago, Ill: American Medical Association; 2000) or subsequent revisions or by referring to other ICD-9-CM coding manuals that contain exclusion notes and instructions regarding fifth-digit requirements.

250 Diabetes mellitus

272 Disorders of lipoid metabolism

- **272.0** Pure hypercholesterolemia

278 Obesity and other hyperalimentation

- **278.0** Obesity

305 Nondependent abuse of drugs

- **305.1** Tobacco use disorder

401 Essential hypertension

Supplemental Classification of Factors Influencing Health Status and Contact With Health Services

V17 Family history of certain chronic disabling diseases

- **V17.4** Other cardiovascular diseases

Examination

Examination is a comprehensive screening and specific testing process that leads to a diagnostic classification or, when appropriate, to a referral to another practitioner. Examination is required prior to the initial intervention and is performed for all patients/clients. Through the examination, the physical therapist may identify impairments, functional limitations, disabilities, changes in physical function or overall health status, and needs related to restoration of health and to prevention, wellness, and fitness. The physical therapist synthesizes the examination findings to establish the diagnosis and the prognosis (including the plan of care). The patient/client, family, significant others, and caregivers may provide information during the examination process.

Examination has three components: the patient/client history, the systems review, and tests and measures. The *history* is a systematic gathering of past and current information (often from the patient/client) related to why the patient/client is seeking the services of the physical therapist. The *systems review* is a brief or limited examination of (1) the anatomical and physiological status of the cardiovascular/pulmonary, integumentary, musculoskeletal, and neuromuscular systems and (2) the communication ability, affect, cognition, language, and learning style of the patient/client. *Tests and measures* are the means of gathering data about the patient/client.

The selection of examination procedures and the depth of the examination vary based on patient/client age; severity of the problem; stage of recovery (acute, subacute, chronic); phase of rehabilitation (early, intermediate, late, return to activity); home, work (job/school/play), or community situation; and other relevant factors. *For clinical indications in selecting tests and measures and for listings of tests and measures, tools used to gather data, and the types of data generated by tests and measures, refer to Chapter 2.*

Patient/Client History

The history may include:

General Demographics

- Age
- Sex
- Race/ethnicity
- Primary language
- Education

Social History

- Cultural beliefs and behaviors
- Family and caregiver resources
- Social interactions, social activities, and support systems

Employment/Work (Job/School/Play)

- Current and prior work (job/school/play), community, and leisure actions, tasks, or activities

Growth and Development

- Developmental history
- Hand dominance

Living Environment

- Devices and equipment (eg, assistive, adaptive, orthotic, protective, supportive, prosthetic)
- Living environment and community characteristics
- Projected discharge destinations

General Health Status (Self-Report, Family Report, Caregiver Report)

- General health perception
- Physical function (eg, mobility, sleep patterns, restricted bed days)
- Psychological function (eg, memory, reasoning ability, depression, anxiety)
- Role function (eg, community, leisure, social, work)
- Social function (eg, social activity, social interaction, social support)

Social/Health Habits (Past and Current)

- Behavioral health risks (eg, smoking, drug abuse)
- Level of physical fitness

Family History

- Familial health risks

Medical/Surgical History

- Cardiovascular
- Endocrine/metabolic
- Gastrointestinal
- Genitourinary
- Gynecological
- Integumentary
- Musculoskeletal
- Neuromuscular
- Obstetrical
- Prior hospitalizations, surgeries, and preexisting medical and other health-related conditions
- Psychological
- Pulmonary

Current Condition(s)/Chief Complaint(s)

- Concerns that led patient/client to seek the services of a physical therapist
- Concerns or needs of patient/client who requires the services of a physical therapist
- Current therapeutic interventions
- Mechanisms of injury or disease, including date of onset and course of events
- Onset and pattern of symptoms
- Patient/client, family, significant other, and caregiver expectations and goals for the therapeutic intervention
- Patient/client, family, significant other, and caregiver perceptions of patient's/client's emotional response to the current clinical situation
- Previous occurrence of chief complaint(s)
- Prior therapeutic interventions

Functional Status and Activity Level

- Current and prior functional status in self-care and home management activities, including activities of daily living (ADL) and instrumental activities of daily living (IADL)
- Current and prior functional status in work (job/school/play), community, and leisure actions, tasks, or activities

Medications

- Medications for current condition
- Medications previously taken for current condition
- Medications for other conditions

Other Clinical Tests

- Laboratory and diagnostic tests
- Review of available records (eg, medical, education, surgical)
- Review of other clinical findings (eg, nutrition and hydration)

Systems Review

The systems review may include:

Anatomical and Physiological Status

- Cardiovascular/Pulmonary
  - Blood pressure
  - Edema
  - Heart rate
  - Respiratory rate
- Integumentary
  - Pliability (texture)
  - Presence of scar formation
  - Skin color
  - Skin integrity
- Musculoskeletal
  - Gross range of motion
  - Gross strength
  - Gross symmetry
  - Height
  - Weight
- Neuromuscular
  - Gross coordinated movements (eg, balance, gait, locomotion, transfers, transitions)
  - Motor function (motor control, motor learning)

Communication, Affect, Cognition, Language, and Learning Style

- Ability to make needs known
- Consciousness
- Expected emotional/behavioral responses
- Learning preferences (eg, education needs, learning barriers)
- Orientation (person, place, time)

Tests and Measures

Tests and measures for this pattern may include those that characterize or quantify:

Aerobic Capacity and Endurance

- Aerobic capacity during functional activities (eg, activities of daily living [ADL] scales, indexes, instrumental activities of daily living [IADL] scales, observations)
- Aerobic capacity during standardized exercise test protocols (eg, ergometry, step tests, time/distance walk/run tests, treadmill tests, wheelchair tests)

Anthropometric Characteristics

- Body composition (eg, body mass index, impedance measurement, skinfold thickness measurement)
- Body dimensions (eg, girth measurement, length measurement)

Arousal, Attention, and Cognition

- Motivation (eg, adaptive behavior scales)

Circulation (Arterial, Venous, and Lymphatic)

- Cardiovascular signs, including heart rate, rhythm, and sounds; pressures and flow; and superficial vascular responses (eg, auscultation, electrocardiography, palpation, sphygmomanometry, thermography)
- Physiological responses to position change, including autonomic responses, central and peripheral pressures, heart rate and rhythm, respiratory rate and rhythm, ventilatory pattern (eg, auscultation, electrocardiography, observations, palpation, sphygmomanometry)

Ergonomics and Body Mechanics

Ergonomics

- Safety in work environments (eg, hazard identification checklists, job severity indexes, lifting standards, risk assessment scales, standards for exposure limits)

Body Mechanics

- Body mechanics during self-care, home management, work, community, or leisure actions, tasks, or activities (eg, ADL and IADL scales, observations, photographic assessments, technology-assisted assessments, videographic assessments)

Muscle Performance (Including Strength, Power, and Endurance)

- Muscle strength, power, and endurance (eg, dynamometry, manual muscle tests, muscle performance tests, physical capacity tests, technology-assisted assessments, timed activity tests)
- Muscle strength, power, and endurance during functional activities (eg, ADL scales, functional muscle tests, IADL scales, observations, videographic assessments)

Posture

- Postural alignment and position (static and dynamic), including symmetry and deviation from midline (eg, grid measurement, observations, photographic assessments, videographic assessments)
- Specific body parts (eg, angle assessments, forward-bending test, goniometry, observations, palpation, positional tests)

Self-Care and Home Management (Including ADL and IADL)

- Ability to gain access to home environments (eg, barrier identification, observations, physical performance tests)
- Safety in self-care and home management activities and environments (eg, diaries, fall scales, interviews, logs, observations, reports, videographic assessments)

Ventilation and Respiration/Gas Exchange

- Pulmonary signs of respiration/gas exchange, including breath sounds (eg, gas analyses, observations, oximetry)
- Pulmonary symptoms (eg, dyspnea and perceived exertion indexes and scales)

Work (Job/School/Play), Community, and Leisure Integration or Reintegration (Including IADL)

- Ability to gain access to work (job/school/play), community, and leisure environments (eg, interviews, observations, physical capacity tests, transportation assessments)
- Safety in work (job/school/play), community, and leisure activities and environments (eg, diaries, fall scales, interviews, logs, observations, videographic assessments)

Evaluation, Diagnosis, and Prognosis (Including Plan of Care)

Physical therapists perform *evaluations* (make clinical judgments) based on the data gathered from the history, systems review, and tests and measures. In the evaluation process, physical therapists synthesize the examination data to establish the diagnosis and prognosis (including the plan of care). Factors that influence the complexity of the evaluation include the clinical findings, extent of loss of function, chronicity or severity of the problem, possibility of multisite or multisystem involvement, preexisting condition(s), potential discharge destination, social considerations, physical function, and overall health status.

A *diagnosis* is a label encompassing a cluster of signs and symptoms, syndromes, or categories. It is the result of the systematic diagnostic process, which includes integrating and evaluating the data from the examination.The diagnostic label indicates the primary dysfunction(s) toward which the therapist will direct interventions. The *prognosis* is the determination of the predicted optimal level of improvement in function and the amount of time needed to reach that level and may also include a prediction of levels of improvement that may be reached at various intervals during the course of therapy. During the prognostic process, the physical therapist develops the plan of care. The *plan of care* identifies specific interventions, proposed frequency and duration of the interventions, anticipated goals, expected outcomes, and discharge plans. The plan of care identifies realistic anticipated goals and expected outcomes, taking into consideration the expectations of the patient/client and appropriate others.These anticipated goals and expected outcomes should be measureable and time limited.

The frequency of visits and duration of the episode of care may vary from a short episode with a high intensity of intervention to a longer episode with a diminishing intensity of intervention. Frequency and duration may vary greatly among patients/clients based on a variety of factors that the physical therapist considers throughout the evaluation process, such as anatomical and physiological changes related to growth and development; caregiver consistency or expertise; chronicity or severity of the current condition; living environment; multisite or multisystem involvement; social support; potential discharge destinations; probability of prolonged impairment, functional limitation, or disability; and stability of the condition.

Prognosis

Patient/client will reduce risk for cardiovascular/pulmonary disorders through therapeutic exercise, aerobic conditioning, functional training, and lifestyle modification..

Expected Range of Number of Visits Per Episode of Care

1 to 6

This range represents the lower and upper limits of the number of physical therapist visits required to achieve anticipated goals and expected outcomes. *It is anticipated that 80% of patients/clients who are classified into this pattern will achieve the anticipated goals and expected outcomes within 1 to 6 visits during a single continuous episode of care.* Frequency of visits and duration of the episode of care should be determined by the physical therapist to maximize effectiveness of care and efficiency of service delivery.

Factors That May Modify Frequency of Visits

- Accessibility and availability of resources
- Adherence to the intervention program
- Age
- Anatomical and physiological changes related to growth and development
- Caregiver consistency or expertise
- Chronicity or severity of the current condition
- Cognitive status
- Comorbitities, complications, or secondary impairments
- Concurrent medical, surgical, and therapeutic interventions
- Decline in functional independence
- Level of impairment
- Level of physical function
- Living environment
- Multisite or multisystem involvement
- Nutritional status
- Overall health status
- Potential discharge destinations
- Premorbid conditions
- Probability of prolonged impairment, functional limitation, or disability
- Psychological and socioeconomic factors
- Psychomotor abilities
- Social support
- Stability of the condition

Intervention

Intervention is the purposeful interaction of the physical therapist with the patient/client and, when appropriate, with other individuals involved with the patient/client, using various physical therapy procedures and techniques to produce changes in the condition consistent with the diagnosis and prognosis. Decisions about interventions are contingent on the timely monitoring of patient/client response and the progress made toward achieving the anticipated goals and expected outcomes.

Communication, coordination, and documentation and patient/client-related instruction are provided for all patients/clients across all settings. Procedural interventions are selected or modified based on the examination data and the evaluation, the diagnosis and the prognosis, and the anticipated goals and expected outcomes for a particular patient/client. *For clinical considerations in selecting interventions, listings of interventions, and listings of anticipated goals and expected outcomes, refer to Chapter 3.*

Coordination, Communication, and Documentation

Coordination, communication, and documentation for primary prevention/risk reduction may include:

Interventions

- Addressing required functions
  - informed consent
  - mandatory communication and reporting (eg, patient/client advocacy and abuse reporting)
- Collaboration and coordination with agencies, including:
  - equipment suppliers
  - home care agencies
  - payer groups
  - schools
  - transportation agencies
- Communication, including:
  - education plans
  - documentation
- Data collection, analysis and reporting
  - outcome data
  - peer review findings
  - record reviews
- Documentation
  - elements of patient/client management (examination, evaluation, diagnosis, prognosis, intervention)
  - outcomes of intervention
- Referrals to other professionals or resources

Anticipated Goals and Expected Outcomes

- Accountability for services is increased.
- Available resources are maximally utilized.
- Informed consent and mandatory communication and reporting (eg, patient/client advocacy and abuse reporting) are obtained or completed.
- Collaboration and coordination occurs with agencies, including equipment suppliers, home care agencies, payer groups, schools, and transportation agencies.
- Communication occurs through education plans and documentation.
- Data are collected, analyzed, and reported, including outcome data, peer review findings, and record reviews.
- Decision making is enhanced regarding patient/client health and the use of health care resources by patient/client, family, significant others, and caregivers.
- Documentation occurs throughout patient/client management and follows APTA's *Guidelines for Physical Therapy Documentation* (Appendix 5).
- Patient/client, family, significant other, and caregiver understanding of anticipated goals and expected outcomes is increased.
- Referrals are made to other professionals or resources whenever necessary and appropriate.
- Resources are utilized in a cost-effective way.

Patient/Client-Related Instruction

Patient/client-related instruction may include:

Interventions

- Instruction, education, and training of patients/clients and caregivers regarding:
  - enhancement of performance
  - health, wellness, and fitness programs
  - plan for intervention
  - risk factors for pathology/pathophysiology (disease, disorder, or condition), impairments, functional limitations, or disabilities

Anticipated Goals and Expected Outcomes

- Ability to perform physical actions, tasks, or activities is improved.
- Awareness and use of community resources are improved.
- Behaviors that foster healthy habits, wellness, and prevention are acquired.
- Decision making is enhanced regarding patient/client health and the use of health care resources by patient/client, family, significant others, and caregivers.
- Health status is improved.
- Patient/client, family, significant other, and caregiver knowledge and awareness of the diagnosis, prognosis, interventions, and anticipated goals and expected outcomes are increased.
- Patient/client knowledge of personal and environmental factors associated with the condition is increased.
- Performance levels in self-care, home management, work (job/school/play), community, or leisure actions, tasks, or activities are improved.
- Physical function is improved.
- Risk of recurrence of condition is reduced.
- Safety of patient/client, family, significant others, and caregivers is improved.
- Utilization and cost of health care services are decreased.

Procedural Interventions

Procedural interventions for this pattern may include:

Therapeutic Exercise

Interventions

- Aerobic capacity/endurance conditioning or reconditioning
  - aquatic programs
  - gait and locomotor training
  - increased workload over time
  - task-specific performance training
  - walking and wheelchair propulsion programs
- Flexibility exercises
  - muscle lengthening
  - range of motion
  - stretching
- Relaxation
  - breathing strategies
  - movement strategies
  - relaxation techniques
  - standardized, programmatic, complementary exercise approaches
- Strength, power, and endurance training for head and neck, limb, pelvic-floor, trunk, and ventilatory muscles
  - active assistive, active, and resistive exercises (including concentric, dynamic/isotonic, isometric, and plyometric)
  - aquatic programs
  - standardized, programmatic, complementary exercise approaches
  - task-specific performance training

Anticipated Goals and Expected Outcomes

- Impact on pathology/pathophysiology (disease, disorder, or condition)
  - Nutrient delivery to tissue is increased.
  - Osteogenic effects of exercise are maximized.
  - Physiological response to increased oxygen demand is improved.
  - Tissue perfusion and oxygenation are enhanced.
- Impact on impairments
  - Aerobic capacity is increased.
  - Endurance is increased.
  - Energy expenditure per unit of work is decreased.
  - Joint integrity and mobility are improved.
  - Muscle performance (strength, power, and endurance) is increased.
  - Range of motion is improved.
  - Relaxation is increased.
- Impact on functional limitations
  - Ability to perform physical actions, tasks, or activities related to self-care, home management, work (job/school/play), community, and leisure is improved.
  - Performance of and independence in activities of daily living (ADL) and instrumental activities of daily living (IADL) with or without devices and equipment are increased.
  - Tolerance of positions and activities is increased.
- Impact on disabilities
  - Ability to assume or resume required self-care, home management, work (job/school/play), community, and leisure roles is improved.
- Risk reduction/prevention
  - Risk factors are reduced.
  - Safety is improved.
  - Self-management of symptoms is improved.
- Impact on health, wellness, and fitness
  - Fitness is improved.
  - Health status is improved.
  - Physical capacity is increased.
  - Physical function is improved.
- Impact on societal resources
  - Utilization of physical therapy services is optimized.
  - Utilization of physical therapy services results in efficient use of health care dollars.
- Patient/client satisfaction
  - Access, availability, and services provided are acceptable to patient/client.
  - Administrative management of practice is acceptable to patient/client.
  - Clinical proficiency of physical therapist is acceptable to patient/client.
  - Coordination of care is acceptable to patient/client.
  - Cost of health care services is decreased.
  - Interpersonal skills of physical therapist are acceptable to patient/client, family, and significant others.
  - Sense of well-being is improved.
  - Stressors are decreased.

Functional Training in Self-Care and Home Management (Including Activities of Daily Living [ADL] and Instrumental Activities of Daily Living [IADL])

Interventions

- Injury prevention or reduction
  - injury prevention education during self-care and home management
  - injury prevention or reduction with use of devices and equipment
  - safety awareness training during self-care and home management

Anticipated Goals and Expected Outcomes

- Impact on pathology/pathophysiology (disease, disorder, or condition)
  - Physiological response to increased oxygen demand is improved.
- Impact on impairments
  - Postural control is improved.
  - Weight-bearing status is improved.
  - Work of breathing is decreased.
- Impact on functional limitations
  - Ability to perform physical actions, tasks, or activities related to self-care and home management is improved.
  - Level of supervision required for task performance is decreased.
  - Performance of and independence in ADL and IADL with or without devices and equipment are increased.
  - Tolerance of positions and activities is increased.
- Impact on disabilities
  - Ability to assume or resume required self-care and home management roles is improved.
- Risk reduction/prevention
  - Risk factors are reduced.
  - Risk of secondary impairments is reduced.
  - Safety is improved.
  - Self-management of symptoms is improved.
- Impact on health, wellness, and fitness
  - Health status is improved.
  - Physical function is improved.
- Impact on societal resources
  - Utilization of physical therapy services is optimized.
  - Utilization of physical therapy services results in efficient use of health care dollars.
- Patient/client satisfaction
  - Access, availability, and services provided are acceptable to patient/client.
  - Administrative management of practice is acceptable to patient/client.
  - Clinical proficiency of physical therapist is acceptable to patient/client.
  - Coordination of care is acceptable to patient/client.
  - Cost of health care services is decreased.
  - Interpersonal skills of physical therapist are acceptable to patient/client, family, and significant others.
  - Sense of well-being is improved.
  - Stressors are decreased.

Functional Training in Work (Job/School/Play), Community, and Leisure Integration or Reintegration (Including Instrumental Activities of Daily Living [IADL], Work Hardening, and Work Conditioning)

Interventions

- Injury prevention or reduction
  - injury prevention education during work (job/school/play), community, and leisure integration or reintegration
  - injury prevention or reduction with use of devices and equipment
  - safety awareness training during work (job/school/play), community, and leisure integration or reintegration

Anticipated Goals and Expected Outcomes

- Impact on pathology/pathophysiology (disease, disorder, or condition)
  - Physiological response to increased oxygen demand is improved.
- Impact on impairments.
  - Endurance is increased.
  - Energy expenditure per unit of work is decreased.
  - Muscle performance (strength, power, and endurance) is increased.
- Impact on functional limitations
  - Ability to perform physical actions, tasks, or activities related to work (job/school/play), community, and leisure integration or reintegration is improved.
  - Performance of and independence in IADL with or without devices and equipment are increased.
  - Tolerance of positions and activities is increased.
- Impact on disabilities
  - Ability to assume or resume required work (job/school/play), community, and leisure roles is improved.
- Risk reduction/prevention
  - Risk factors are reduced.
  - Risk of secondary impairment is reduced.
  - Safety is improved.
  - Self-management of symptoms is improved.
- Impact on health, wellness, and fitness
  - Health status is improved.
  - Physical function is improved.
- Impact on societal resources
  - Utilization of physical therapy services is optimized.
  - Utilization of physical therapy services results in efficient use of health care dollars.
- Patient/client satisfaction
  - Access, availability, and services provided are acceptable to patient/client.
  - Administrative management of practice is acceptable to patient/client.
  - Clinical proficiency of physical therapist is acceptable to patient/client.
  - Coordination of care is acceptable to patient/client.
  - Cost of health care services is decreased.
  - Interpersonal skills of physical therapist are acceptable to patient/client, family, and significant others.
  - Sense of well-being is improved.
  - Stressors are decreased.

Reexamination

Reexamination is the process of performing selected tests and measures after the initial examination to evaluate progress and to modify or redirect interventions. Reexamination may be indicated more than once during a single episode of care. It also may be performed over the course of a disease, disorder, or condition, which for some patients/clients may be over the life span. Indications for reexamination include new clinical findings or failure to respond to physical therapy interventions.

Global Outcomes for Patients/Clients in This Pattern

Throughout the entire episode of care, the physical therapist determines the anticipated goals and expected outcomes for each intervention. These anticipated goals and expected outcomes are delineated in shaded boxes that accompany the lists of interventions in each preferred practice pattern. As the patient/client reaches the termination of physical therapy services and the end of the episode of care, the physical therapist measures the global outcomes of the physical therapy services by characterizing or quantifying the impact of the physical therapy interventions in the following domains:

- Pathology/pathophysiology (disease, disorder, or condition)
- Impairments
- Functional limitations
- Disabilities
- Risk reduction/prevention
- Health, wellness, and fitness
- Societal resources
- Patient/client satisfaction

In some instances, a particular anticipated goal or expected outcome is thoroughly achieved through implementation of a single form of intervention. More commonly, however, the anticipated goals and expected outcomes are achieved as a result of the combined effects of several forms of interventions, leading to enhancement of both health status and health-related quality of life.

Criteria for Termination of Physical Therapy Services

Discharge is the process of ending physical therapy services that have been provided during a single episode of care. It occurs when the anticipated goals and expected outcomes have been achieved. Discharge does *not* occur with a *transfer* (defined as the time when a patient is moved from one site to another site within the same setting or across settings during a single episode of care). Although there may be facility-specific or payer-specific requirements for documentation regarding the conclusion of physical therapy services, *discharge occurs based on the physical therapist's analysis of the achievement of anticipated goals and expected outcomes.*

Discontinuation is the process of ending physical therapy services that have been provided during a single episode of care when (1) the patient/client, caregiver, or legal guardian declines to continue intervention; (2) the patient/client is unable to continue to progress toward outcomes because of medical or psychosocial complications or because financial/insurance resources have been expended; or (3) the physical therapist determines that the patient/client will no longer benefit from physical therapy. When physical therapy services are terminated prior to achievement of anticipated goals and expected outcomes, patient/client status and the rationale for termination are documented.

For patients/clients who require multiple episodes of care, periodic follow-up is needed over the life span to ensure safety and effective adaptation following changes in physical status, caregivers, environment, or task demands. In consultation with appropriate individuals, and in consideration of the outcomes, the physical therapist plans for discharge or discontinuation and provides for appropriate follow-up or referral.

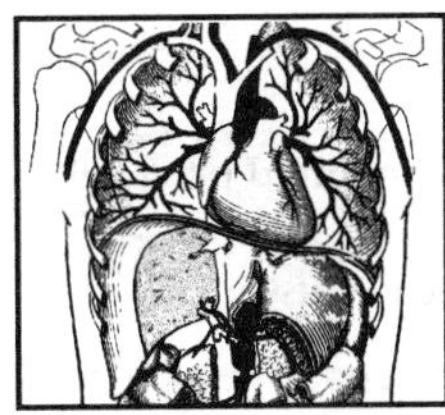

Impaired Aerobic Capacity/Endurance Associated With Deconditioning

This preferred practice pattern describes the generally accepted elements of patient/client management that physical therapists provide for patients/clients who are classified in this pattern. The pattern title reflects the diagnosis made by the physical therapist. APTA emphasizes that preferred practice patterns are the boundaries within which a physical therapist may select any of a number of clinical alternatives, based on consideration of a wide variety of factors, such as individual patient/client needs; the profession's code of ethics and standards of practice; and patient/client age, culture, gender roles, race, sex, sexual orientation, and socioeconomic status.

Patient/Client Diagnostic Classification

Patients/clients will be classified into this pattern—for impaired aerobic capacity/endurance associated with deconditioning—as a result of the physical therapist's evaluation of the examination data. The findings from the examination (history, systems review, and tests and measures) may indicate the presence or risk of pathology/pathophysiology (disease, disorder, or condition), impairments, functional limitations, or disabilities or the need for health, wellness, or fitness programs. The physical therapist integrates, synthesizes, and interprets the data to determine the diagnostic classification.

Inclusion

The following examples of examination findings may support the inclusion of patients/clients in this pattern:

Risk Factors or Consequences of Pathology/Pathophysiology (Disease, Disorder, or Condition)

- Acquired immune deficiency syndrome
- Cancer
- Cardiovascular disorders
- Chronic system failure
- Inactivity
- Multisystem impairments
- Musculoskeletal disorders
- Neuromuscular disorders
- Pulmonary disorders

Impairments, Functional Limitations, or Disabilities

- Decreased endurance
- Increased cardiovascular response to low level work loads
- Increased perceived exertion with functional activities
- Increased pulmonary response to low level work loads
- Inability to perform routine work tasks due to shortness of breath

Note:

Some risk factors or consequences of pathology/pathophysiology— such as *long-term mechanical ventilation* and *multisystem diseases or disorders*—may be severe and complex; *however, they do not necessarily exclude patients/clients from this pattern.* Severe and complex risk factors or consequences may require modification of the frequency of visits and duration of care. (See "Evaluation, Diagnosis, and Prognosis," page 480.)

Exclusion or Multiple-Pattern Classification

The following examples of examination findings may support exclusion from this pattern or classification into additional patterns. Depending on the level of severity or complexity of the examination findings, the physical therapist may determine that the patient/client would be more appropriately managed through (1) classification in an entirely different pattern or (2) classification in both this and another pattern.

Findings That May Require Classification in a Different Pattern

- Chronic obstructive pulmonary disease with acute exacerbation
- Impairments associated with acute cardiovascular pump dysfunction (eg, myocardial infarction)

Findings That May Require Classification in Additional Patterns

- Diabetes with wound
- Peripheral vascular disease with non-healing ulcer

ICD-9-CM Codes

The listing below contains the current (as of press time) and most typical 3- and 4-digit ICD-9-CM codes related to this preferred practice pattern. Because patient/client diagnostic classification is based on impairments, functional limitations, and disabilities—not on codes—patients/clients may be classified into the pattern even though the codes listed with the pattern may not apply to those clients.

This listing is intended for general information only and should not be used for coding purposes. The codes should be confirmed by referring to the World Health Organization's *International Classification of Diseases, 9th Revision, Clinical Modification (ICD-9-CM 2001)*, Volumes 1 and 3 (Chicago, Ill: American Medical Association; 2000) or subsequent revisions or by referring to other ICD-9-CM coding manuals that contain exclusion notes and instructions regarding fifth-digit requirements.

042 Human immunodeficiency virus [HIV] disease
  Acquired immune deficiency syndrome

250 Diabetes mellitus
  250.4 Diabetes with renal manifestations
  250.8 Diabetes with other specified manifestations
  250.9 Diabetes with unspecified complication

332 Parkinson's disease

333 Other extrapyramidal disease and abnormal movement disorders
  333.0 Other degenerative diseases of the basal ganglia
  333.3 Tics of organic origin
  333.4 Huntington's chorea
  333.9 Other and unspecified extrapyramidal diseases and abnormal movement disorders

334 Spinocerebellar disease
  334.2 Primary cerebellar degeneration

335 Anterior horn cell disease
  335.2 Motor neuron disease
    335.20 Amyotrophic lateral sclerosis

340 Multiple sclerosis

344 Other paralytic syndromes
  344.0 Quadriplegia and quadriparesis

357 Inflammatory and toxic neuropathy
  357.0 Acute infective polyneuritis
  Guillain-Barré syndrome

359 Muscular dystrophies and other myopathies
  359.1 Hereditary progressive muscular dystrophy

394 Diseases of mitral valve

396 Diseases of mitral and aortic valves

397 Diseases of other endocardial structures

398 Other rheumatic heart disease

402 Hypertensive heart disease

413 Angina pectoris

414 Other forms of chronic ischemic heart disease

416 Chronic pulmonary heart disease

424 Other diseases of endocardium

425 Cardiomyopathy

428 Heart failure
  428.0 Congestive heart failure

429 Ill-defined descriptions and complications of heart disease

440 Atherosclerosis

443 Other peripheral vascular disease
  443.9 Peripheral vascular disease, unspecified

482 Other bacterial pneumonia
  482.2 Pneumonia due to Hemophilus influenzae
  482.9 Bacterial pneumonia unspecified

491 Chronic bronchitis
  491.9 Unspecified chronic bronchitis

492 Emphysema
  492.8 Other emphysema

493 Asthma

494 Bronchiectasis

496 Chronic airway obstruction, not elsewhere classified
  Chronic obstructive pulmonary disease [COPD], not otherwise specified

508 Respiratory conditions due to other and unspecified external agents
  508.9 Respiratory conditions due to unspecified external agent

513 Abscess of lung and mediastinum
  513.0 Abscess of lung

514 Pulmonary congestion and hypostasis

516 Other alveolar and parietoalveolar pneumonopathy
  516.9 Unspecified alveolar and parietoalveolar pneumonopathy

517 Lung involvement in conditions classified elsewhere
  517.8 Lung involvement in other diseases classified elsewhere*

518 Other diseases of lung
  518.0 Pulmonary collapse
  518.8 Other diseases of lung

519 Other diseases of respiratory system
  519.4 Disorders of diaphragm

711 Arthropathy associated with infections

712 Crystal arthropathies

713 Arthropathy associated with other disorders classified elsewhere

714 Rheumatoid arthritis and other inflammatory polyarthropathies

715 Osteoarthrosis and allied disorders

786 Symptoms involving respiratory system and other chest symptoms
  786.0 Dyspnea and respiratory abnormalities

Note:

Patients/clients who have surgical procedures involving the abdomen, chest wall, diaphragm, mediastinum, and thorax also may be classified into this pattern.

* Not a primary diagnosis

Examination

Examination is a comprehensive screening and specific testing process that leads to a diagnostic classification or, when appropriate, to a referral to another practitioner. Examination is required prior to the initial intervention and is performed for all patients/clients. Through the examination, the physical therapist may identify impairments, functional limitations, disabilities, changes in physical function or overall health status, and needs related to restoration of health and to prevention, wellness, and fitness. The physical therapist synthesizes the examination findings to establish the diagnosis and the prognosis (including the plan of care). The patient/client, family, significant others, and caregivers may provide information during the examination process.

Examination has three components: the patient/client history, the systems review, and tests and measures. The *history* is a systematic gathering of past and current information (often from the patient/client) related to why the patient/client is seeking the services of the physical therapist. The *systems review* is a brief or limited examination of (1) the anatomical and physiological status of the cardiovascular/pulmonary, integumentary, musculoskeletal, and neuromuscular systems and (2) the communication ability, affect, cognition, language, and learning style of the patient/client. *Tests and measures* are the means of gathering data about the patient/client.

The selection of examination procedures and the depth of the examination vary based on patient/client age; severity of the problem; stage of recovery (acute, subacute, chronic); phase of rehabilitation (early, intermediate, late, return to activity); home, work (job/school/play), or community situation; and other relevant factors. *For clinical indications in selecting tests and measures and for listings of tests and measures, tools used to gather data, and the types of data generated by tests and measures, refer to Chapter 2.*

Patient/Client History

The history may include:

General Demographics
- Age
- Sex
- Race/ethnicity
- Primary language
- Education

Social History
- Cultural beliefs and behaviors
- Family and caregiver resources
- Social interactions, social activities, and support systems

Employment/Work (Job/School/Work)
- Current and prior work (job/school/play), community, and leisure actions, tasks, or activities

Growth and Development
- Developmental history
- Hand dominance

Living Environment
- Devices and equipment (eg, assistive, adaptive, orthotic, protective, supportive, prosthetic)
- Living environment and community characteristics
- Projected discharge destinations

General Health Status (Self-Report, Family Report, Caregiver Report)
- General health perception
- Physical function (eg, mobility, sleep patterns, restricted bed days)
- Psychological function (eg, memory, reasoning ability, depression, anxiety)
- Role function (eg, community, leisure, social, work)
- Social function (eg, social activity, social interaction, social support)

Social/Health Habits (Past and Current)
- Behavioral health risks (eg, smoking, drug abuse)
- Level of physical fitness

Family History
- Familial health risks

Medical/Surgical History
- Cardiovascular
- Endocrine/metabolic
- Gastrointestinal
- Genitourinary
- Gynecological
- Integumentary
- Musculoskeletal
- Neuromuscular
- Obstetrical
- Prior hospitalizations, surgeries, and preexisting medical and other health-related conditions
- Psychological
- Pulmonary

Current Condition(s)/Chief Complaint(s)
- Concerns that led patient/client to seek the services of a physical therapist
- Concerns or needs of patient/client who requires the services of a physical therapist
- Current therapeutic interventions
- Mechanisms of injury or disease, including date of onset and course of events
- Onset and pattern of symptoms
- Patient/client, family, significant other, and caregiver expectations and goals for the therapeutic intervention
- Patient/client, family, significant other, and caregiver perceptions of patient's/client's emotional response to the current clinical situation
- Previous occurrence of chief complaint(s)
- Prior therapeutic interventions

Functional Status and Activity Level
- Current and prior functional status in self-care and home management activities, including activities of daily living (ADL) and instrumental activities of daily living (IADL)
- Current and prior functional status in work (job/school/play), community, and leisure actions, tasks, or activities

Medications
- Medications for current condition
- Medications previously taken for current condition
- Medications for other conditions

Other Clinical Tests
- Laboratory and diagnostic tests
- Review of available records (eg, medical, education, surgical)
- Review of other clinical findings (eg, nutrition and hydration)

Systems Review

The systems review may include:

Anatomical and Physiological Status

- Cardiovascular/Pulmonary
  - Blood pressure
  - Edema
  - Heart rate
  - Respiratory rate
- Integumentary
  - Pliability (texture)
  - Presence of scar formation
  - Skin color
  - Skin integrity
- Musculoskeletal
  - Gross range of motion
  - Gross strength
  - Gross symmetry
  - Height
  - Weight
- Neuromuscular
  - Gross coordinated movements (eg, balance, gait, locomotion, transfers, transitions)
  - Motor function (motor control, motor learning)

Communication, Affect, Cognition, Language, and Learning Style

- Ability to make needs known
- Consciousness
- Expected emotional/behavioral responses
- Learning preferences (eg, education needs, learning barriers)
- Orientation (person, place, time)

Tests and Measures

Tests and measures for this pattern may include those that characterize or quantify:

Aerobic Capacity and Endurance

- Aerobic capacity during functional activities (eg, activities of daily living [ADL] scales, indexes, instrumental activities of daily living [IADL] scales, observations)
- Aerobic capacity during standardized exercise test protocols (eg, ergometry, step tests, time/distance walk/run tests, treadmill tests, wheelchair tests)
- Cardiovascular signs and symptoms in response to increased oxygen demand with exercise or activity, including pressures and flow; heart rate, rhythm, and sounds; and superficial vascular responses (eg, angina, claudication, and exertion scales; electrocardiography; observations; palpation; sphygmomanometry)
- Pulmonary signs and symptoms in response to increased oxygen demand with exercise or activity, including breath and voice sounds; cyanosis; gas exchange; respiratory pattern, rate, and rhythm; and ventilatory flow, force, and volume (eg, auscultation, dyspnea and exertion scales, gas analyses, observations, oximetry, palpation, pulmonary function tests)

Anthropometric Characteristics

- Body composition (eg, body mass index, impedance, measurement, skinfold thickness measurement)
- Body dimensions (eg, girth measurement, length measurement)

Arousal, Attention, and Cognition

- Arousal and attention (eg, adaptability tests, arousal and awareness scales, indexes, profiles, questionnaires)
- Cognition, including ability to process commands (eg, developmental inventories, indexes, interviews, mental state scales, observations, questionnaires, safety checklists)
- Motivation (eg, adaptive behavior scales)
- Orientation to time, person, place, and situation (eg, attention tests, learning profiles, mental state scales)
- Recall, including memory and retention (eg, assessment scales, interviews, questionnaires)

Assistive and Adaptive Devices

- Assistive or adaptive devices and equipment use during functional activities (eg, ADL scales, functional scales, IADL scales, interviews, observations)
- Safety during use of assistive or adaptive devices and equipment (eg, diaries, fall scales, interviews, logs, observations, reports)

Circulation (Arterial, Venous, and Lymphatic)

- Cardiovascular signs, including heart rate, rhythm, and sounds; pressures and flow; and superficial vascular responses (eg, auscultation, electrocardiography, palpation, sphygmomanometry, thermography)
- Cardiovascular symptoms (eg, angina, claudication, and perceived exertion scales)
- Physiological responses to position change, including autonomic responses, central and peripheral pressures, heart rate and rhythm, respiratory rate and rhythm, ventilatory pattern (eg, auscultation, electrocardiography, observations, palpation, sphygmomanometry)

Environmental, Home, and Work (Job/School/Play) Barriers

- Current and potential barriers (eg, checklists, interviews, observations, questionnaires)
- Physical space and environment (eg, compliance standards, observations, photographic assessments, questionnaires, structural specifications, videographic assessments)

Ergonomics and Body Mechanics

Ergonomics

- Dexterity and coordination during work (job/school/play) (eg, hand function tests, impairment rating scales, manipulative ability tests)
- Functional capacity and performance during work actions, tasks, or activities (eg, accelerometry, dynamometry, electroneuromyography, endurance tests, force platform tests, goniometry, interviews, observations, photographic assessments, physical capacity tests, postural loading analyses, technology-assisted assessments, videographic assessments, work analyses)

- Safety in work environments (eg, hazard identification checklists, job severity indexes, lifting standards, risk assessment scales, standards for exposure limits)
- Specific work conditions or activities (eg, handling checklists, job simulations, lifting models, preemployment screenings, task analysis checklists, workstation checklists)

Body mechanics

- Body mechanics during self-care, home management, work, community, or leisure actions, tasks, or activities (eg, ADL scales, IADL scales, observations, photographic assessments, technology-assisted assessments, videographic assessments)

Gait, Locomotion, and Balance

- Balance during functional activities with or without the use of assistive, adaptive, orthotic, protective, supportive, or prosthetic devices or equipment (eg, ADL scales, IADL scales, observations, videographic assessments)
- Balance (dynamic and static) with or without the use of assistive, adaptive, orthotic, protective, supportive, or prosthetic devices or equipment (eg, balance scales, dizziness inventories, dynamic posturography, fall scales, motor impairment tests, observations, photographic assessments, postural control tests)
- Gait and locomotion during functional activities with or without the use of assistive, adaptive, orthotic, protective, supportive, or prosthetic devices or equipment (eg, ADL scales, gait indexes, IADL scales, mobility skill profiles, observations, videographic assessments)
- Gait and locomotion with or without the use of assistive, adaptive, orthotic, protective, supportive, or prosthetic devices or equipment (eg, dynamometry, electroneuromyography, footprint analyses, gait indexes, mobility skill profiles, observations, photographic assessments, technology-assisted assessments, videographic assessments, weight-bearing scales, wheelchair mobility tests)
- Safety during gait, locomotion, and balance (eg, confidence scales, diaries, fall scales, functional assessment profiles, logs, reports)

Motor Function (Motor Control and Motor Learning)

- Initiation, modification, and control of movement patterns and voluntary postures (eg, activity indexes, observations, physical performance tests, postural challenge tests, videographic assessments)

Muscle Performance (Including Strength, Power, and Endurance)

- Muscle strength, power, and endurance (eg, dynamometry, manual muscle tests, muscle performance tests, physical capacity tests, technology-assisted assessments, timed activity tests)
- Muscle strength, power, and endurance during functional activities (eg, ADL scales, functional muscle tests, IADL scales, observations, videographic assessments)
- Muscle tension (eg, palpation)

Orthotic, Protective, and Supportive Devices

- Safety during use of orthotic, protective, and supportive devices and equipment (eg, diaries, fall scales, logs, interviews, observations, reports)

Pain

- Pain, soreness, and nociception (eg, angina scales, analog scales, discrimination tests, pain drawings and maps, provocation tests, verbal and pictorial descriptor tests)
- Pain in specific body parts (eg, pain indexes, pain questionnaires, structural provocation tests)

Posture

- Postural alignment and position (static and dynamic), including symmetry and deviation from midline (eg, grid measurement, observations, photographic assessments, technology-assisted assessments, videographic assessments)
- Specific body parts (eg, angle assessments, forward-bending test, goniometry, observations, palpation, positional tests)

Range of Motion (ROM) (Including Muscle Length)

- Functional ROM (eg, observations, squat tests, toe touch tests)
- Joint active and passive movement (eg, goniometry, inclinometry, observations, photographic assessments, technology-assisted assessments, videographic assessments)
- Muscle length, soft tissue extensibility, and flexibility (eg, contracture tests, goniometry, inclinometry, ligamentous tests, linear measurement, multisegment flexibility tests, palpation)

Self-Care and Home Management (Including ADL and IADL)

- Ability to gain access to home environments (eg, barrier identification, observations, physical performance tests)
- Ability to perform self-care and home management activities with or without assistive, adaptive, orthotic, protective, supportive, or prosthetic devices and equipment (eg, ADL scales, aerobic capacity tests, IADL scales, interviews, observations, profiles)
- Safety in self-care and home management activities and environments (eg, diaries, fall scales, interviews, logs, observations, reports, videographic assessments)

Sensory Integrity

- Deep sensations (eg, kinesthesiometry, observations, photographic assessments, vibration tests)

Ventilation and Respiration/Gas Exchange

- Pulmonary signs of respiration/gas exchange, including breath sounds (eg, gas analyses, observations, oximetry)
- Pulmonary signs of ventilatory function, including airway protection; breath and voice sounds; respiratory rate, rhythm, and pattern; ventilatory flow, forces, and volumes (eg, airway clearance tests, observations, palpation, pulmonary function tests, ventilatory muscle force tests)
- Pulmonary symptoms (eg, dyspnea and perceived exertion indexes and scales)

Work (Job/School/Play), Community, and Leisure Integration or Reintegration (Including IADL)

- Ability to assume or resume work (job/school/play), community, and leisure activities with or without assistive, adaptive, orthotic, protective, supportive, or prosthetic devices and equipment (eg, activity profiles, disability indexes, functional status questionnaires, IADL scales, observations, physical capacity tests)
- Ability to gain access to work (job/school/play), community, and leisure environments (eg, barrier identification, interviews, observations, physical capacity tests, transportation assessments)
- Safety in work (job/school/play), community, and leisure activities and environments (eg, diaries, fall scales, interviews, logs, observations, videographic assessments)

Evaluation, Diagnosis, and Prognosis (Including Plan of Care)

Physical therapists perform *evaluations* (make clinical judgments) based on the data gathered from the history, systems review, and tests and measures. In the evaluation process, physical therapists synthesize the examination data to establish the diagnosis and prognosis (including the plan of care). Factors that influence the complexity of the evaluation include the clinical findings, extent of loss of function, chronicity or severity of the problem, possibility of multisite or multisystem involvement, preexisting condition(s), potential discharge destination, social considerations, physical function, and overall health status.

A *diagnosis* is a label encompassing a cluster of signs and symptoms, syndromes, or categories. It is the result of the systematic diagnostic process, which includes integrating and evaluating the data from the examination. The diagnostic label indicates the primary dysfunction(s) toward which the therapist will direct interventions. The *prognosis* is the determination of the predicted optimal level of improvement in function and the amount of time needed to reach that level and may also include a prediction of levels of improvement that may be reached at various intervals during the course of therapy. During the prognostic process, the physical therapist develops the plan of care. The *plan of care* identifies specific interventions, proposed frequency and duration of the interventions, anticipated goals, expected outcomes, and discharge plans. The plan of care identifies realistic anticipated goals and expected outcomes, taking into consideration the expectations of the patient/client and appropriate others. These anticipated goals and expected outcomes should be measureable and time limited.

The frequency of visits and duration of the episode of care may vary from a short episode with a high intensity of intervention to a longer episode with a diminishing intensity of intervention. Frequency and duration may vary greatly among patients/clients based on a variety of factors that the physical therapist considers throughout the evaluation process, such as anatomical and physiological changes related to growth and development; caregiver consistency or expertise; chronicity or severity of the current condition; living environment; multisite or multisystem involvement; social support; potential discharge destinations; probability of prolonged impairment, functional limitation, or disability; and stability of the condition.

Prognosis

Over the course of 6 to 12 weeks, patient/client will demonstrate optimal aerobic capacity/endurance and the highest level of functioning in home, work (job/school/play), community, and leisure environments.

During the episode of care, patient/client will achieve (1) the anticipated goals and expected outcomes of the interventions that are described in the plan of care and (2) the global outcomes for patients/clients who are classified in this pattern.

Expected Range of Number of Visits Per Episode of Care

6 to 30

This range represents the lower and upper limits of the number of physical therapist visits required to achieve anticipated goals and expected outcomes. *It is anticipated that 80% of patients/clients who are classified into this pattern will achieve the anticipated goals and expected outcomes within 6 to 30 visits during a single continuous episode of care.* Frequency of visits and duration of the episode of care should be determined by the physical therapist to maximize effectiveness of care and efficiency of service delivery.

Factors That May Require New Episode of Care or That May Modify Frequency of Visits/Duration of Episode

- Accessibility and availability of resources
- Adherence to the intervention program
- Age
- Anatomical and physiological changes related to growth and development
- Caregiver consistency or expertise
- Chronicity or severity of the current condition
- Cognitive status
- Comorbitities, complications, or secondary impairments
- Concurrent medical, surgical, and therapeutic interventions
- Decline in functional independence
- Level of impairment
- Level of physical function
- Living environment
- Multisite or multisystem involvement
- Nutritional status
- Overall health status
- Potential discharge destinations
- Premorbid conditions
- Probability of prolonged impairment, functional limitation, or disability
- Psychological and socioeconomic factors
- Psychomotor abilities
- Social support
- Stability of the condition

Intervention

Intervention is the purposeful interaction of the physical therapist with the patient/client and, when appropriate, with other individuals involved in patient/client care, using various physical therapy procedures and techniques to produce changes in the condition consistent with the diagnosis and prognosis. Decisions about interventions are contingent on the timely monitoring of patient/client response and the progress made toward achieving the anticipated goals and expected outcomes.

Communication, coordination, and documentation and patient/client-related instruction are provided for all patients/clients across all settings. Procedural interventions are selected or modified based on the examination data and the evaluation, the diagnosis and the prognosis, and the anticipated goals and expected outcomes for a particular patient/client. *For clinical considerations in selecting interventions, listings of interventions, and listings of anticipated goals and expected outcomes, refer to Chapter 3.*

Coordination, Communication, and Documentation

Coordination, communication, and documentation may include:

Interventions

- Addressing required functions
  - advance directives
  - individualized family service plans (IFSPs) or individualized education plans (IEPs)
  - informed consent
  - mandatory communication and reporting (eg, patient advocacy and abuse reporting)
- Admission and discharge planning
- Case management
- Collaboration and coordination with agencies, including:
  - equipment suppliers
  - home care agencies
  - payer groups
  - schools
  - transportation agencies
- Communication across settings, including:
  - case conferences
  - documentation
- Cost-effective resource utilization
- Data collection, analysis, and reporting
  - outcome data
  - peer review findings
  - record reviews
- Documentation across settings, following APTA's *Guidelines for Physical Therapy Documentation* (Appendix 5), including:
  - changes in impairments, functional limitations, and disabilities
  - changes in interventions
  - elements of patient/client management (examination, evaluation, diagnosis, prognosis, intervention)
  - outcomes of intervention
- Interdisciplinary teamwork
  - case conferences
  - patient care rounds
  - patient/client family meetings
- Referrals to other professionals or resources

Anticipated Goals and Expected Outcomes

- Accountability for services is increased.
- Admission data and discharge planning are completed.
- Advance directives, individualized family service plans (IFSPs) or individualized education plans (IEPs), informed consent, and mandatory communication and reporting (eg, patient advocacy and abuse reporting) are obtained or completed.
- Available resources are maximally utilized.
- Care is coordinated with patient/client, family, significant others, caregivers, and other professionals.
- Case is managed throughout the episode of care.
- Collaboration and coordination occurs with agencies, including equipment suppliers, home care agencies, payer groups, schools, and transportation agencies.
- Communication enhances risk reduction and prevention.
- Communication occurs across settings through case conferences, education plans, and documentation.
- Data are collected, analyzed, and reported, including outcome data, peer review findings, and record reviews.
- Decision making is enhanced regarding health, wellness, and fitness needs.
- Decision making is enhanced regarding patient/client health and the use of health care resources by patient/client, family, significant others, and caregivers.
- Documentation occurs throughout patient/client management and across settings and follows APTA's *Guidelines for Physical Therapy Documentation* (Appendix 5).
- Interdisciplinary collaboration occurs through case conferences, patient care rounds, and patient/client family meetings.
- Patient/client, family, significant other, and caregiver understanding of anticipated goals and expected outcomes is increased.
- Placement needs are determined.
- Referrals are made to other professionals or resources whenever necessary and appropriate.
- Resources are utilized in a cost-effective way.

Patient/Client-Related Instruction

Patient/client-related instruction may include:

Interventions

- Instruction, education and training of patients/clients and caregivers regarding:
  - current condition (pathology/pathophysiology [disease, disorder, or condition], impairments, functional limitations, or disabilities)
  - enhancement of performance
  - health, wellness, and fitness programs
  - plan of care
  - risk factors for pathology/pathophysiology (disease, disorder, or condition), impairments, functional limitations, or disabilities
  - transitions across settings
  - transitions to new roles

Anticipated Goals and Expected Outcomes

- Ability to perform physical actions, tasks, or activities is improved.
- Awareness and use of community resources are improved.
- Behaviors that foster healthy habits, wellness, and prevention are acquired.
- Decision making is enhanced regarding patient/client health and the use of health care resources by patient/client, family, significant others, and caregivers.
- Disability associated with acute or chronic illnesses is reduced.
- Functional independence in activities of daily living (ADL) and instrumental activities of daily living (IADL) is increased.
- Health status is improved.
- Intensity of care is decreased.
- Level of supervision required for task performance is decreased.
- Patient/client, family, significant other, and caregiver knowledge and awareness of the diagnosis, prognosis, interventions, and anticipated goals and expected outcomes are increased.
- Patient/client knowledge of personal and environmental factors associated with the condition is increased.
- Performance levels in self-care, home management, work (job/school/play), community, or leisure actions, tasks, or activities are improved.
- Physical function is improved.
- Risk of recurrence of condition is reduced.
- Risk of secondary impairment is reduced.
- Safety of patient/client, family, significant others, and caregivers is improved.
- Self-management of symptoms is improved.
- Utilization and cost of health care services are decreased.

Procedural Interventions

Procedural interventions for this pattern may include:

Therapeutic Exercise

Interventions

- Aerobic capacity/endurance conditioning or reconditioning
  - aquatic programs
  - gait and locomotor training
  - increased workload over time
  - walking and wheelchair propulsion programs
- Balance, coordination, and agility training
  - developmental activities training
  - motor function (motor control and motor learning) training or retraining
  - neuromuscular education or reeducation
  - standardized, programmatic, complementary exercise approaches
- Body mechanics and postural stabilization
  - body mechanics training
  - postural control training
- Flexibility exercises
  - muscle lengthening
  - range of motion
  - stretching
- Gait and locomotion training
  - developmental activities training
  - gait training
  - implement and device training
  - standardized, programmatic, complementary exercise approaches
  - wheelchair training
- Relaxation
  - breathing strategies
  - movement strategies
  - relaxation techniques
  - standardized, programmatic, complementary exercise approaches
- Strength, power, and endurance training for head and neck, limb, pelvic-floor, trunk, and ventilatory muscles
  - active assistive, active, and resistive exercises (including concentric, dynamic/isotonic, isometric, and plyometric)
  - aquatic programs
  - standardized, programmatic, complementary exercise approaches

Anticipated Goals and Expected Outcomes

- Impact on pathology/pathophysiology (disease, disorder, or condition)
  - Nutrient delivery to tissue is increased.
  - Osteogenic effects of exercise are maximized.
  - Physiological response to increased oxygen demand is improved.
  - Symptoms associated with increased oxygen demand are decreased.
  - Tissue perfusion and oxygenation are enhanced.
- Impact on impairments
  - Aerobic capacity is increased.
  - Balance is improved.
  - Endurance is increased.
  - Energy expenditure per unit of work is decreased.
  - Motor function (motor control and motor learning) is improved.
  - Muscle performance (strength, power, and endurance) is increased.
  - Postural control is improved.
  - Quality and quantity of movement between and across body segments are improved.
  - Range of motion is improved.
  - Relaxation is increased.
  - Weight-bearing status is improved.
- Impact on functional limitations
  - Ability to perform physical actions, tasks, or activities related to self-care, home management, work (job/school/play), community, and leisure is improved.
  - Level of supervision required for task performance is decreased.
  - Performance of and independence in activities of daily living (ADL) and instrumental activities of daily living (IADL) with or without devices and equipment are increased.
  - Tolerance of positions and activities is increased.
- Impact on disabilities
  - Ability to assume or resume required self-care, home management, work (job/school/play), community, and leisure roles is improved.
- Risk reduction/prevention
  - Risk factors are reduced.
  - Risk of recurrence of condition is reduced.
  - Risk of secondary impairment is reduced.
  - Safety is improved.
  - Self-management of symptoms is improved.
- Impact on health, wellness, and fitness
  - Health status is improved.
  - Physical capacity is increased.
  - Physical function is improved.
- Impact on societal resources
  - Utilization of physical therapy services is optimized.
  - Utilization of physical therapy services results in efficient use of health care dollars.
- Patient/client satisfaction
  - Access, availability, and services provided are acceptable to patient/client.
  - Administrative management of practice is acceptable to patient/client.
  - Clinical proficiency of physical therapist is acceptable to patient/client.
  - Coordination of care is acceptable to patient/client.
  - Cost of health care services is decreased.
  - Intensity of care is decreased.
  - Interpersonal skills of physical therapist are acceptable to patient/client, family, and significant others.
  - Sense of well-being is improved.
  - Stressors are decreased.

Functional Training in Self-Care and Home Management (Including Activities of Daily Living [ADL] and Instrumental Activities of Daily Living [IADL])

Interventions

- ADL training
  - bathing
  - bed mobility and transfer training
  - developmental activities
- Devices and equipment use and training
  - assistive and adaptive device or equipment training during ADL and IADL
  - orthotic, protective, or supportive device or equipment training during ADL and IADL
- Functional training programs
  - simulated environments and tasks
- IADL training
  - home maintenance
  - household chores
  - shopping
  - structured play for infants and children
  - yard work
- Injury prevention or reduction
  - safety awareness training during self-care and home management

Anticipated Goals and Expected Outcomes

- Impact on pathology/pathophysiology (disease, disorder, or condition)
  - Pain is decreased.
  - Physiological response to increased oxygen demand is improved.
  - Symptoms associated with increased oxygen demand are decreased.
- Impact on impairments
  - Endurance is increased.
  - Energy expenditure per unit of work is decreased.
  - Muscle performance (strength, power, and endurance) is increased.
  - Postural control is improved.
  - Work of breathing is decreased.
- Impact on functional limitations
  - Ability to perform physical actions, tasks, or activities related to self-care and home management is increased.
  - Level of supervision required for task performance is decreased.
  - Performance of and independence in ADL and IADL with or without devices and equipment are increased.
  - Tolerance of positions and activities is increased.
- Impact on disabilities
  - Ability to assume or resume required self-care and home management roles is improved.
- Risk reduction/prevention
  - Risk factors are reduced.
  - Risk of secondary impairments is reduced.
  - Safety is improved.
  - Self-management of symptoms is improved.
- Impact on health, wellness, and fitness
  - Fitness is improved.
  - Health status is improved.
  - Physical capacity is increased.
  - Physical function is improved.
- Impact on societal resources
  - Utilization of physical therapy services is optimized.
  - Utilization of physical therapy services results in efficient use of health care dollars.
- Patient/client satisfaction
  - Access, availability, and services provided are acceptable to patient/client.
  - Administrative management of practice is acceptable to patient/client.
  - Clinical proficiency of physical therapist is acceptable to patient/client.
  - Coordination of care is acceptable to patient/client.
  - Cost of health care services is decreased.
  - Intensity of care is decreased.
  - Interpersonal skills of physical therapist are acceptable to patient/client, family, and significant others.
  - Sense of well-being is improved.
  - Stressors are decreased.

Functional Training in Work (Job/School/Play), Community, and Leisure Integration or Reintegration (Including Instrumental Activities of Daily Living [IADL], Work Hardening, and Work Conditioning)

Interventions

- Devices and equipment use and training
  - assistive and adaptive device or equipment training during IADL
  - orthotic, protective, or supportive device or equipment training during IADL
- Functional training programs
  - simulated environments and tasks
  - task adaptation
  - task training
  - work conditioning
  - work hardening
- IADL training
  - community service training involving instruments
  - school and play activities training including tools and instruments
  - work training with tools
- Injury prevention or reduction
  - injury prevention or reduction with use of devices and equipment
  - safety awareness training during work (job/school/play), community, and leisure integration and reintegration

Anticipated Goals and Expected Outcomes

- Impact on pathology/pathophysiology (disease, disorder, or condition)
  - Pain is decreased.
  - Physiological response to increased oxygen demand is improved.
  - Symptoms associated with increased oxygen demand are decreased.
- Impact on impairments
  - Endurance is increased.
  - Energy expenditure per unit of work is decreased.
  - Motor function (motor control and motor learning) is improved.
  - Muscle performance (strength, power, and endurance) is increased.
  - Postural control is improved.
  - Work of breathing is decreased.
- Impact on functional limitations
  - Ability to perform physical actions, tasks, or activities related to work (job/school/play), community, and leisure integration or reintegration is improved.
  - Level of supervision required for task performance is decreased.
  - Performance of and independence in IADL with or without devices and equipment are increased.
  - Tolerance of positions and activities is increased.
- Impact on disabilities
  - Ability to assume or resume required and work (job/school/play), community, and leisure roles is improved.
- Risk reduction/prevention
  - Risk factors are reduced.
  - Risk of secondary impairment is reduced.
  - Safety is improved.
  - Self-management of symptoms is improved.
- Impact on health, wellness, and fitness
  - Fitness is improved.
  - Health status is improved.
  - Physical capacity is increased.
  - Physical function is improved.
- Impact on societal resources
  - Utilization of physical therapy services is optimized.
  - Utilization of physical therapy services results in efficient use of health care dollars.
- Patient/client satisfaction
  - Access, availability, and services provided are acceptable to patient/client.
  - Administrative management of practice is acceptable to patient/client.
  - Clinical proficiency of physical therapist is acceptable to patient/client.
  - Coordination of care is acceptable to patient/client.
  - Cost of health care services is decreased.
  - Intensity of care is decreased.
  - Interpersonal skills of physical therapist are acceptable to patient/client, family, and significant others.
  - Sense of well-being is improved.
  - Stressors are decreased.

Prescription, Application, and, as Appropriate, Fabrication of Devices and Equipment (Assistive, Adaptive, Orthotic, Protective, Supportive, and Prosthetic)

Interventions

- Adaptive devices
  - seating systems
- Assistive devices
  - canes
  - crutches
  - power devices
  - static and dynamic splints
  - walkers
  - wheelchairs
- Orthotic devices
  - braces
  - casts
  - shoe inserts
  - splints
- Protective devices
  - braces
  - cushions
- Supportive devices
  - compression garments
  - corsets
  - elastic wraps
  - mechanical ventilators
  - neck collars
  - supplemental oxygen

Anticipated Goals and Expected Outcomes

- Impact on pathology/pathophysiology (disease, disorder, or condition)
  - Edema, lymphedema, or effusion is reduced.
  - Pain is decreased.
  - Physiological response to increased oxygen demand is improved.
  - Symptoms associated with increased oxygen demand are decreased.
- Impact on impairments
  - Balance is improved.
  - Endurance is increased.
  - Energy expenditure per unit of work is decreased.
  - Gait, locomotion, and balance are improved.
  - Joint stability is improved.
  - Motor function (motor control and motor learning) is improved.
  - Muscle performance (strength, power, and endurance) is increased.
  - Optimal joint alignment is achieved.
  - Optimal loading on a body part is achieved.
  - Postural control is improved.
  - Quality and quantity of movement between and across body segments are improved.
  - Range of motion is improved.
  - Weight-bearing status is improved.
  - Work of breathing is decreased.
- Impact on functional limitations
  - Ability to perform physical actions, tasks, or activities related to self-care, home management, work (job/school/play), community, and leisure is improved.
  - Level of supervision required for task performance is decreased.
  - Performance of and independence in activities of daily living (ADL) and instrumental activities of daily living (IADL) with or without devices and equipment are increased.
  - Tolerance of positions and activities is improved.
- Impact on disabilities
  - Ability to assume or resume required self-care, home management, work (job/school/play), community, and leisure roles is improved.
- Risk reduction/prevention
  - Pressure on body tissues is reduced.
  - Protection of body parts is increased.
  - Risk factors are reduced.
  - Risk of secondary impairment is reduced.
  - Safety is improved.
  - Self-management of symptoms is improved.
  - Stresses precipitating injury are decreased.
- Impact on health, wellness, and fitness
  - Health status is improved.
  - Physical function is improved.
- Impact on societal resources
  - Utilization of physical therapy services is optimized.
  - Utilization of physical therapy services results in efficient use of health care dollars.
- Patient/client satisfaction
  - Access, availability, and services provided are acceptable to patient/client.
  - Administrative management of practice is acceptable to patient/client.
  - Clinical proficiency of physical therapist is acceptable to patient/client.
  - Coordination of care is acceptable to patient/client.
  - Cost of health care services is decreased.
  - Intensity of care is decreased.
  - Interpersonal skills of physical therapist are acceptable to patient/client, family, and significant others.
  - Sense of well-being is improved.
  - Stressors are decreased.

Airway Clearance Techniques

Interventions

- Breathing strategies
  - paced breathing
  - pursed lip breathing
  - techniques to maximize ventilation (eg, maximum inspiratory hold, stair case breathing, manual hyperinflation)
- Positioning
  - positioning to alter work of breathing
  - positioning to maximize ventilation and perfusion

Anticipated Goals and Expected Outcomes

- Impact on pathology/pathophysiology (disease, disorder, or condition)
  - Nutrient delivery to tissue is increased.
  - Physiological response to increased oxygen demand is improved.
  - Symptoms associated with increased oxygen demand are decreased.
  - Tissue perfusion and oxygenation are enhanced.
- Impact on impairments
  - Endurance is increased.
  - Energy expenditure per unit of work is decreased.
  - Exercise tolerance is improved.
  - Muscle performance (strength, power, and endurance) is increased.
  - Ventilation and respiration/gas exchange are improved.
  - Work of breathing is decreased.
- Impact on functional limitations
  - Ability to perform physical actions, tasks, or activities related to self-care, home management, work (job/school/play), community, and leisure is improved.
  - Performance of and independence in activities of daily living (ADL) and instrumental activities of daily living (IADL) with or without devices and equipment are increased.
  - Tolerance of positions and activities is increased.
- Impact on disabilities
  - Ability to assume or resume required self-care, home management, work (job/school/play), community, and leisure roles is improved.
- Risk reduction/prevention
  - Risk factors are reduced.
  - Risk of secondary impairment is reduced.
  - Safety is improved.
  - Self-management of symptoms is improved.
- Impact on health, wellness, and fitness
  - Health status is improved.
  - Physical capacity is increased.
  - Physical function is improved.
- Impact on societal resources
  - Utilization of physical therapy services is optimized.
  - Utilization of physical therapy services results in efficient use of health care dollars.
- Patient/client satisfaction
  - Access, availability, and services provided are acceptable to patient/client.
  - Administrative management of practice is acceptable to patient/client.
  - Clinical proficiency of physical therapist is acceptable to patient/client.
  - Coordination of care is acceptable to patient/client.
  - Cost of health care services is decreased.
  - Intensity of care is decreased.
  - Interpersonal skills of physical therapist are acceptable to patient/client, family, and significant others.
  - Sense of well-being is improved.
  - Stressors are decreased.

Reexamination

Reexamination is the process of performing selected tests and measures after the initial examination to evaluate progress and to modify or redirect interventions. Reexamination may be indicated more than once during a single episode of care. It also may be performed over the course of a disease, disorder, or condition, which for some patients/clients may be over the life span. Indications for reexamination include new clinical findings or failure to respond to physical therapy interventions.

Global Outcomes for Patients/Clients in This Pattern

Throughout the entire episode of care, the physical therapist determines the anticipated goals and expected outcomes for each intervention. These anticipated goals and expected outcomes are delineated in shaded boxes that accompany the lists of interventions in each preferred practice pattern. As the patient/client reaches the termination of physical therapy services and the end of the episode of care, the physical therapist measures the global outcomes of the physical therapy services by characterizing or quantifying the impact of the physical therapy interventions in the following domains:

- Pathology/pathophysiology (disease, disorder, or condition)
- Impairments
- Functional limitations
- Disabilities
- Risk reduction/prevention
- Health, wellness, and fitness
- Societal resources
- Patient/client satisfaction

In some instances, a particular anticipated goal or expected outcome is thoroughly achieved through implementation of a single form of intervention. More commonly, however, the anticipated goals and expected outcomes are achieved as a result of the combined effects of several forms of interventions, leading to enhancement of both health status and health-related quality of life.

Criteria for Termination of Physical Therapy Services

Discharge is the process of ending physical therapy services that have been provided during a single episode of care. It occurs when the anticipated goals and expected outcomes have been achieved. Discharge does *not* occur with a *transfer* (defined as the time when a patient is moved from one site to another site within the same setting or across settings during a single episode of care). Although there may be facility-specific or payer-specific requirements for documentation regarding the conclusion of physical therapy services, *discharge occurs based on the physical therapist's analysis of the achievement of anticipated goals and expected outcomes.*

Discontinuation is the process of ending physical therapy services that have been provided during a single episode of care when (1) the patient/client, caregiver, or legal guardian declines to continue intervention; (2) the patient/client is unable to continue to progress toward outcomes because of medical or psychosocial complications or because financial/insurance resources have been expended; or (3) the physical therapist determines that the patient/client will no longer benefit from physical therapy. When physical therapy services are terminated prior to achievement of anticipated goals and expected outcomes, patient/client status and the rationale for termination are documented.

For patients/clients who require multiple episodes of care, periodic follow-up is needed over the life span to ensure safety and effective adaptation following changes in physical status, caregivers, environment, or task demands. In consultation with appropriate individuals, and in consideration of the outcomes, the physical therapist plans for discharge or discontinuation and provides for appropriate follow-up or referral.

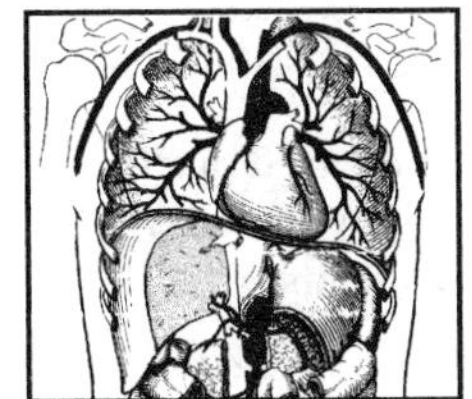

Impaired Ventilation, Respiration/Gas Exchange, and Aerobic Capacity/Endurance Associated With Airway Clearance Dysfunction

This preferred practice pattern describes the generally accepted elements of patient/client management that physical therapists provide for patients/clients who are classified in this pattern. The pattern title reflects the diagnosis made by the physical therapist. APTA emphasizes that preferred practice patterns are the boundaries within which a physical therapist may select any of a number of clinical alternatives, based on consideration of a wide variety of factors, such as individual patient/client needs; the profession's code of ethics and standards of practice; and patient/client age, culture, gender roles, race, sex, sexual orientation, and socioeconomic status.

Patient/Client Diagnostic Classification

Patients/clients will be classified into this pattern—for impaired ventilation, respiration/gas exchange, and aerobic capacity/endurance associated with airway clearance dysfunction—as a result of the physical therapist's evaluation of the examination data. The findings from the examination (history, systems review, and tests and measures) may indicate the presence or risk of pathology/pathophysiology (disease, disorder, or condition), impairments, functional limitations, or disabilities or the need for health, wellness, or fitness programs. The physical therapist integrates, synthesizes, and interprets the data to determine the diagnostic classification.

Inclusion

The following examples of examination findings may support the inclusion of patients/clients in this pattern:

Risk Factors or Consequences of Pathology/Pathophysiology (Disease, Disorder, or Condition)

- Acute lung disorders
- Acute or chronic oxygen dependency
- Bone marrow/stem cell transplants
- Cardiothoracic surgery
- Change in baseline breath sounds
- Change in baseline chest radiograph
- Chronic obstructive pulmonary disease (COPD)
- Frequent or recurring pulmonary infection
- Solid-organ transplants (eg, heart, lung, kidney)
- Tracheostomy or microtracheostomy

Impairments, Functional Limitations, or Disabilities

- Dyspnea at rest or with exertion
- Impaired airway clearance
- Impaired cough
- Impaired gas exchange
- Impaired ventilatory forces and flow
- Impaired ventilatory volumes
- Inability to perform self-care due to dyspnea
- Inability to perform work tasks due to dyspnea

Note:

Some risk factors or consequences of pathology/pathophysiology— such as *cardiac surgery with aspiration pneumonia, emphysema with acute pneumonia, and lung transplant with rejection*—may be severe and complex; *however, they do not necessarily exclude patients/clients from this pattern.* Severe and complex risk factors or consequences may require modification of the frequency of visits and duration of care. (See "Evaluation, Diagnosis, and Prognosis," page 495.)

Exclusion or Multiple-Pattern Classification

The following examples of examination findings may support exclusion from this pattern or classification into additional patterns. Depending on the level of severity or complexity of the examination findings, the physical therapist may determine that the patient/client would be more appropriately managed through (1) classification in an entirely different pattern or (2) classification in both this and another pattern.

Findings That May Require Classification in a Different Pattern

- Neonate with respiratory failure
- Respiratory failure with mechanical ventilation

Findings That May Require Classification in Additional Patterns

- Chronic obstructive pulmonary disease with diabetes
- Impairments associated with acute cerebrovascular accident with aspiration pneumonia

ICD-9-CM Codes

The listing below contains the current (as of press time) and most typical 3- and 4-digit ICD-9-CM codes related to this preferred practice pattern. Because patient/client diagnostic classification is based on impairments, functional limitations, and disabilities—not on codes—patients/clients may be classified into the pattern even though the codes listed with the pattern may not apply to those clients.

This listing is intended for general information only and should not be used for coding purposes. The codes should be confirmed by referring to the World Health Organization's *International Classification of Diseases, 9th Revision, Clinical Modification (ICD-9-CM 2001)*, Volumes 1 and 3 (Chicago, Ill: American Medical Association; 2000) or subsequent revisions or by referring to other ICD-9-CM coding manuals that contain exclusion notes and instructions regarding fifth-digit requirements.

136 Other and unspecified infectious and parasitic diseases
- **136.3** Pneumocystosis

277 Other and unspecified disorders of metabolism
- **277.0** Cystic fibrosis

482 Other bacterial pneumonia
- **482.2** Pneumonia due to Hemophilus influenzae
- **482.9** Bacterial pneumonia unspecified

491 Chronic bronchitis
- **491.8** Other chronic bronchitis
- **491.9** Unspecified chronic bronchitis

492 Emphysema
- **492.8** Other emphysema

493 Asthma

494 Bronchiectasis

496 Chronic airway obstruction, not elsewhere classified
Chronic obstructive pulmonary disease [COPD], not otherwise specified

500 Coal workers' pneumoconiosis

501 Asbestosis

502 Pneumoconiosis due to other silica or silicates

503 Pneumoconiosis due to other inorganic dust

504 Pneumonopathy due to inhalation of other dust

505 Pneumoconiosis, unspecified

507 Pneumonitis due to solids and liquids
- **507.0** Due to inhalation of food or vomitus
  Aspiration pneumonia

508 Respiratory conditions due to other and unspecified external agents
- **508.9** Respiratory conditions due to unspecified external agent

510 Empyema

511 Pleurisy

513 Abscess of lung and mediastinum
- **513.0** Abscess of lung

514 Pulmonary congestion and hypostasis

515 Postinflammatory pulmonary fibrosis

516 Other alveolar and parietoalveolar pneumonopathy
- **516.9** Unspecified alveolar and parietoalveolar pneumonopathy

518 Other diseases of lung
- **518.0** Pulmonary collapse
- **518.8** Other diseases of lung
  - **518.89** Other diseases of lung, not elsewhere classified

759 Other and unspecified congenital anomalies
- **759.3** Situs inversus

770 Other respiratory conditions of fetus and newborn
- **770.7** Chronic respiratory disease arising in the perinatal period
  Bronchopulmonary dysplasia

786 Symptoms involving respiratory system and other chest symptoms
- **786.0** Dyspnea and respiratory abnormalities
  - **786.00** Respiratory abnormality, unspecified
- **786.5** Chest pain
  - **786.52** Painful respiration

861 Injury to heart and lung
- **861.2** Lung, without mention of open wound into thorax
  - **861.21** Contusion

941 Burn of face, head, and neck

942 Burn of trunk

947 Burn of internal organs
- **947.1** Larynx, trachea, and lung
- **947.9** Unspecified site

996 Complications peculiar to certain specified procedures
- **996.0** Mechanical complication of cardiac device, implant, and graft
- **996.1** Mechanical complication of other vascular device, implant, and graft
- **996.2** Mechanical complication of nervous system device, implant, and graft
- **996.3** Mechanical complication of genitourinary device, implant, and graft
- **996.4** Mechanical complication of internal orthopedic device, implant, and graft
- **996.5** Mechanical complications of other specified prosthetic device, implant, and graft
- **996.8** Complications of transplanted organ
  - **996.85** Bone marrow

997 Complications affecting specified body system, not elsewhere classified
- **997.3** Respiratory complications

Supplemental Classification of Factors Influencing Health Status and Contact With Health Services

V42 Organ or tissue replaced by transplant

- **V42.0** Kidney
- **V42.2** Heart valve
- **V42.3** Skin
- **V42.4** Bone
- **V42.6** Lung
- **V42.7** Liver
- **V42.8** Other specified organ or tissue
    - **V42.81** Bone marrow
    - **V42.82** Peripheral stem cells
    - **V42.83** Pancreas
    - **V42.89** Other

Note:

Patients/clients who have surgical procedures involving the abdomen, chest wall, diaphragm, lung, mediastinum, thorax, and vessels of the heart also may be classified into this pattern.

Examination

Examination is a comprehensive screening and specific testing process that leads to a diagnostic classification or, when appropriate, to a referral to another practitioner. Examination is required prior to the initial intervention and is performed for all patients/clients. Through the examination, the physical therapist may identify impairments, functional limitations, disabilities, changes in physical function or overall health status, and needs related to restoration of health and to prevention, wellness, and fitness. The physical therapist synthesizes the examination findings to establish the diagnosis and the prognosis (including the plan of care). The patient/client, family, significant others, and caregivers may provide information during the examination process.

Examination has three components: the patient/client history, the systems review, and tests and measures. The *history* is a systematic gathering of past and current information (often from the patient/client) related to why the patient/client is seeking the services of the physical therapist. The *systems review* is a brief or limited examination of (1) the anatomical and physiological status of the cardiovascular/pulmonary, integumentary, musculoskeletal, and neuromuscular systems and (2) the communication ability, affect, cognition, language, and learning style of the patient/client. *Tests and measures* are the means of gathering data about the patient/client.

The selection of examination procedures and the depth of the examination vary based on patient/client age; severity of the problem; stage of recovery (acute, subacute, chronic); phase of rehabilitation (early, intermediate, late, return to activity); home, work (job/school/play), or community situation; and other relevant factors. *For clinical indications in selecting tests and measures and for listings of tests and measures, tools used to gather data, and the types of data generated by tests and measures, refer to Chapter 2.*

Patient/Client History

The history may include:

General Demographics

- Age
- Sex
- Race/ethnicity
- Primary language
- Education

Social History

- Cultural beliefs and behaviors
- Family and caregiver resources
- Social interactions, social activities, and support systems

Employment/Work (Job/School/Play)

- Current and prior work (job/school/play), community, and leisure actions, tasks, or activities

Growth and Development

- Developmental history
- Hand dominance

Living Environment

- Devices and equipment (eg, assistive, adaptive, orthotic, protective, supportive, prosthetic)
- Living environment and community characteristics
- Projected discharge destinations

General Health Status (Self-Report, Family Report, Caregiver Report)

- General health perception
- Physical function (eg, mobility, sleep patterns, restricted bed days)
- Psychological function (eg, memory, reasoning ability, depression, anxiety)
- Role function (eg, community, leisure, social, work)
- Social function (eg, social activity, social interaction, social support)

Social/Health Habits (Past and Current)

- Behavioral health risks (eg, smoking, drug abuse)
- Level of physical fitness

Family History

- Familial health risks

Medical/Surgical History

- Cardiovascular
- Endocrine/metabolic
- Gastrointestinal
- Genitourinary
- Gynecological
- Integumentary
- Musculoskeletal
- Neuromuscular
- Obstetrical
- Prior hospitalizations, surgeries, and preexisting medical and other health-related conditions
- Psychological
- Pulmonary

Current Condition(s)/Chief Complaint(s)

- Concerns that led patient/client to seek the services of a physical therapist
- Concerns or needs of patient/client who requires the services of a physical therapist
- Current therapeutic interventions
- Mechanisms of injury or disease, including date of onset and course of events
- Onset and pattern of symptoms
- Patient/client, family, significant other, and caregiver expectations and goals for the therapeutic intervention
- Patient/client, family, significant other, and caregiver perceptions of patient's/client's emotional response to the current clinical situation
- Previous occurrence of chief complaint(s)
- Prior therapeutic interventions

Functional Status and Activity Level

- Current and prior functional status in self-care and home management activities, including activities of daily living (ADL) and instrumental activities of daily living (IADL)
- Current and prior functional status in work (job/school/play), community, and leisure actions, tasks, or activities

Medications

- Medications for current condition
- Medications previously taken for current condition
- Medications for other conditions

Other Clinical Tests

- Laboratory and diagnostic tests
- Review of available records (eg, medical, education, surgical)
- Review of other clinical findings (eg, nutrition and hydration)

Systems Review

The systems review may include:

Anatomical and Physiological Status

- Cardiovascular/Pulmonary
  - Blood pressure
  - Edema
  - Heart rate
  - Respiratory rate
- Integumentary
  - Pliability (texture)
  - Presence of scar formation
  - Skin color
  - Skin integrity
- Musculoskeletal
  - Gross range of motion
  - Gross strength
  - Gross symmetry
  - Height
  - Weight
- Neuromuscular
  - Gross coordinated movements (eg, balance, gait, locomotion, transfers, transitions)
  - Motor function (motor control, motor learning)

Communication, Affect, Cognition, Language, and Learning Style

- Ability to make needs known
- Consciousness
- Expected emotional/behavioral responses
- Learning preferences (eg, education needs, learning barriers)
- Orientation (person, place, time)

Tests and Measures

Tests and measures for this pattern may include those that characterize or quantify:

Aerobic Capacity and Endurance

- Aerobic capacity during functional activities (eg, activities of daily living [ADL] scales, indexes, instrumental activities of daily living [IADL] scales, observations)
- Aerobic capacity during standardized exercise test protocols (eg, ergometry, step tests, time/distance walk/run tests, treadmill tests, wheelchair tests)
- Cardiovascular signs and symptoms in response to increased oxygen demand with exercise or activity, including pressures and flow; heart rate, rhythm, and sounds; and superficial vascular responses (eg, angina, claudication, and exertion scales; electrocardiography; observations; palpation; sphygmomanometry)
- Pulmonary signs and symptoms in response to increased oxygen demand with exercise or activity, including breath and voice sounds; cyanosis; gas exchange; respiratory pattern, rate, and rhythm; and ventilatory flow, force, and volume (eg, auscultation, dyspnea and exertion scales, gas analyses, observations, oximetry, palpation, pulmonary function tests)

Anthropometric Characteristics

- Edema (eg, girth measurement, palpation, scales, volume measurement)

Arousal, Attention, and Cognition

- Arousal and attention (eg, adaptability tests, arousal and awareness scales, indexes, profiles, questionnaires)
- Cognition, including ability to process commands (eg, developmental inventories, indexes, interviews, mental state scales, observations, questionnaires, safety checklists)
- Motivation (eg, adaptive behavior scales)
- Orientation to time, person, place, and situation (eg, attention tests, learning profiles, mental state scales)
- Recall, including memory and retention (eg, assessment scales, interviews, questionnaires)

Assistive and Adaptive Devices

- Assistive or adaptive devices and equipment use during functional activities (eg, ADL scales, functional scales, IADL scales, interviews, observations)
- Components, alignment, fit, and ability to care for assistive or adaptive devices and equipment (eg, interviews, logs, observations, pressure-sensing maps, reports)
- Remediation of impairments, functional limitations, or disabilities with use of assistive or adaptive devices and equipment (eg, activity status indexes, ADL scales, aerobic capacity tests, functional performance inventories, health assessment questionnaires, IADL scales, pain scales, play scales, videographic assessments)
- Safety during use of assistive or adaptive devices and equipment (eg, diaries, interviews, logs, observations, reports)

Circulation (Arterial, Venous, and Lymphatic)

- Cardiovascular signs, including heart rate, rhythm, and sounds; pressures and flow; and superficial vascular responses (eg, auscultation, electrocardiography, palpation, sphygmomanometry, thermography)
- Cardiovascular symptoms (eg, angina, claudication, and perceived exertion scales)
- Physiological responses to position change, including autonomic responses, central and peripheral pressures, heart rate and rhythm, respiratory rate and rhythm, ventilatory pattern (eg, auscultation, electrocardiography, observations, palpation, sphygmomanometry)

Environmental, Home, and Work (Job/School/Play) Barriers

- Current and potential barriers (eg, checklists, interviews, observations, questionnaires)
- Physical space and environment (eg, compliance standards, observations, photographic assessments, questionnaires, structural specifications, videographic assessments)

Integumentary Integrity

Associated skin

- Activities, positioning, and postures that produce or relieve trauma to the skin (eg, observations, pressure-sensing maps, scales)
- Assistive, adaptive, orthotic, protective, supportive, or prosthetic devices and equipment that may produce or relieve trauma to the skin (eg, observations, pressure-sensing maps, risk assessment scales)
- Skin characteristics, including blistering, continuity of skin color, dermatitis, hair growth, mobility, nail growth, sensation, temperature, texture, and turgor (eg, observations, palpation, photographic assessments, thermography)

Muscle Performance (Including Strength, Power, and Endurance)

- Muscle strength, power, and endurance (eg, dynamometry, manual muscle tests, muscle performance tests, physical capacity tests, technology-assisted assessments, timed activity tests)
- Muscle strength, power, and endurance during functional activities (eg, ADL scales, functional muscle tests, IADL scales, observations, videographic assessments)

Neuromotor Development and Sensory Integration

- Oral motor function, phonation, and speech production (eg, interviews, observations)

Orthotic, Protective, and Supportive Devices

- Orthotic, protective, and supportive devices and equipment use during functional activities (eg, ADL scales, functional scales, IADL scales, interviews, observations, profiles)
- Safety during use of orthotic, protective, and supportive devices and equipment (eg, diaries, fall scales, interviews, logs, observations, reports)

Pain

- Pain, soreness, and nociception (eg, angina scales, analog scales, discrimination tests, pain drawings and maps, provocation tests, verbal and pictorial descriptor tests)

Posture

- Postural alignment and position (static and dynamic), including symmetry and deviation from midline (eg, grid measurements, observations, photographic assessments, videographic assessments)
- Specific body parts (eg, angle assessments, forward-bending test, goniometry, observations, palpation, positional tests)

Range of Motion (ROM) (Including Muscle Length)

- Functional ROM (eg, observations, squat testing, toe touch tests)
- Joint active and passive movement (eg, goniometry, inclinometry, observations, photographic assessments, technology-assisted assessments, videographic assessments)
- Muscle length, soft tissue extensibility, and flexibility (eg, contracture tests, goniometry, inclinometry, ligamentous tests, linear measurement, multisegment flexibility tests, palpation)

Self-Care and Home Management (Including ADL and IADL)

- Ability to gain access to home environments (eg, barrier identification, observations, physical performance tests)
- Ability to perform self-care and home management activities with or without assistive, adaptive, orthotic, protective, supportive, or prosthetic devices and equipment (eg, ADL scales, aerobic capacity tests, IADL scales, interviews, observations, profiles)

Ventilation and Respiration/Gas Exchange

- Pulmonary signs of respiration/gas exchange, including breath sounds (eg, gas analyses, observations, oximetry)
- Pulmonary signs of ventilatory function, including airway protection; breath and voice sounds; respiratory rate, rhythm, and pattern; ventilatory flow, forces, and volumes (eg, airway clearance tests, observations, palpation, pulmonary function tests, ventilatory muscle force tests)
- Pulmonary symptoms (eg, dyspnea and perceived exertion indexes and scales)

Work (Job/School/Play), Community, and Leisure Integration or Reintegration (Including IADL)

- Ability to assume or resume work (job/school/play), community, and leisure activities with or without assistive, adaptive, orthotic, protective, supportive, or prosthetic devices and equipment (eg, activity profiles, disability indexes, functional status questionnaires, IADL scales, observations, physical capacity tests)
- Ability to gain access to work (job/school/play), community, and leisure environments (eg, barrier identification, interviews, observations, physical capacity tests, transportation assessments)
- Safety in work (job/school/play), community, and leisure activities and environments (eg, diaries, fall scales, interviews, logs, observations, videographic assessments)

Evaluation, Diagnosis, and Prognosis (Including Plan of Care)

Physical therapists perform *evaluations* (make clinical judgments) based on the data gathered from the history, systems review, and tests and measures. In the evaluation process, physical therapists synthesize the examination data to establish the diagnosis and prognosis (including the plan of care). Factors that influence the complexity of the evaluation include the clinical findings, extent of loss of function, chronicity or severity of the problem, possibility of multisite or multisystem involvement, preexisting condition(s), potential discharge destination, social considerations, physical function, and overall health status.

A *diagnosis* is a label encompassing a cluster of signs and symptoms, syndromes, or categories. It is the result of the systematic diagnostic process, which includes integrating and evaluating the data from the examination. The diagnostic label indicates the primary dysfunction(s) toward which the therapist will direct interventions. The *prognosis* is the determination of the predicted optimal level of improvement in function and the amount of time needed to reach that level and may also include a prediction of levels of improvement that may be reached at various intervals during the course of therapy. During the prognostic process, the physical therapist develops the plan of care. The *plan of care* identifies specific interventions, proposed frequency and duration of the interventions, anticipated goals, expected outcomes, and discharge plans. The plan of care identifies realistic anticipated goals and expected outcomes, taking into consideration the expectations of the patient/client and appropriate others. These anticipated goals and expected outcomes should be measureable and time limited.

The frequency of visits and duration of the episode of care may vary from a short episode with a high intensity of intervention to a longer episode with a diminishing intensity of intervention. Frequency and duration may vary greatly among patients/clients based on a variety of factors that the physical therapist considers throughout the evaluation process, such as anatomical and physiological changes related to growth and development; caregiver consistency or expertise; chronicity or severity of the current condition; living environment; multisite or multisystem involvement; social support; potential discharge destinations; probability of prolonged impairment, functional limitation, or disability; and stability of the condition.

Prognosis

Over the course of 12 to 16 weeks, patient/client will demonstrate optimal ventilation, respiration/gas exchange, and aerobic capacity/endurance and the highest level of functioning in home, work (job/school/play), community, and leisure environments, within the context of the impairments, functional limitations, and disabilities.

During the episode of care, patient/client will achieve (1) the anticipated goals and expected outcomes of the interventions that are described in the plan of care and (2) the global outcomes for patients/clients who are classified in this pattern.

Expected Range of Number of Visits Per Episode of Care

5 to 30

This range represents the lower and upper limits of the number of physical therapist visits required to achieve anticipated goals and expected outcomes. *It is anticipated that 80% of patients/clients who are classified into this pattern will achieve the anticipated goals and expected outcomes within 5 to 30 visits during a single continuous episode of care.* Frequency of visits and duration of the episode of care should be determined by the physical therapist to maximize effectiveness of care and efficiency of service delivery.

Factors That May RequireNew Episode of Care or That May Modify Frequency of Visits/ Duration of Episode

- Accessibility and availability of resources
- Adherence to the intervention program
- Age
- Anatomical and physiological changes related to growth and development
- Caregiver consistency or expertise
- Chronicity or severity of the current condition
- Cognitive status
- Comorbitities, complications, or secondary impairments
- Concurrent medical, surgical, and therapeutic interventions
- Decline in functional independence
- Level of impairment
- Level of physical function
- Living environment
- Multisite or multisystem involvement
- Nutritional status
- Overall health status
- Potential discharge destinations
- Premorbid conditions
- Probability of prolonged impairment, functional limitation, or disability
- Psychological and socioeconomic factors
- Psychomotor abilities
- Social support
- Stability of the condition

Intervention

Intervention is the purposeful interaction of the physical therapist with the patient/client and, when appropriate, with other individuals involved involved in patient/client care, using various physical therapy procedures and techniques to produce changes in the condition consistent with the diagnosis and prognosis. Decisions about interventions are contingent on the timely monitoring of patient/client response and the progress made toward achieving the anticipated goals and expected outcomes.

Communication, coordination, and documentation and patient/client-related instruction are provided for all patients/clients across all settings. Procedural interventions are selected or modified based on the examination data and the evaluation, the diagnosis and the prognosis, and the anticipated goals and expected outcomes for a particular patient/client. *For clinical considerations in selecting interventions, listings of interventions, and listings of anticipated goals and expected outcomes, refer to Chapter 3.*

Coordination, Communication, and Documentation

Coordination, communication, and documentation may include:

Interventions

- Addressing required functions
  - Advance directives
  - individualized family service plans (IFSPs) or individualized education plans (IEPs)
  - informed consent
  - mandatory communication and reporting (eg, patient advocacy and abuse reporting)
- Admission and discharge planning
- Case management
- Collaboration and coordination with agencies, including:
  - equipment suppliers
  - home care agencies
  - payer groups
  - schools
  - transportation agencies
- Communication across settings, including:
  - case conferences
  - documentation
- Cost-effective resource utilization
- Data collection, analysis, and reporting
  - outcome data
  - peer review findings
  - record reviews
- Documentation across settings, following APTA's *Guidelines for Physical Therapy Documentation* (Appendix 5), including:
  - changes in impairments, functional limitations, and disabilities
  - changes in interventions
  - elements of patient/client management (examination, evaluation, diagnosis, prognosis, intervention)
  - outcomes of intervention
- Interdisciplinary teamwork
  - case conferences
  - patient care rounds
  - patient/client family meetings
- Referrals to other professionals or resources

Anticipated Goals and Expected Outcomes

- Accountability for services is increased.
- Admission data and discharge planning are completed.
- Advance directives, individualized family service plans (IFSPs) or individualized education plans (IEPs), informed consent, and mandatory communication and reporting (eg, patient advocacy and abuse reporting) are obtained or completed.
- Available resources are maximally utilized.
- Care is coordinated with patient/client, family, significant others, caregivers, and other professionals.
- Case is managed throughout the episode of care.
- Collaboration and coordination occurs with agencies, including equipment suppliers, home care agencies, payer groups, schools, and transportation agencies.
- Communication enhances risk reduction and prevention.
- Communication occurs across settings through case conferences, and documentation.
- Data are collected, analyzed, and reported, including outcome data, peer review findings, and record reviews.
- Decision making is enhanced regarding health, wellness, and fitness needs.
- Decision making is enhanced regarding patient/client health and the use of health care resources by patient/client, family, significant others, and caregivers.
- Documentation occurs throughout patient/client management and across settings and follows APTA's *Guidelines for Physical Therapy Documentation* (Appendix 5).
- Interdisciplinary collaboration occurs through case conferences, patient care rounds, and patient/client family meetings.
- Patient/client, family, significant other, and caregiver understanding of anticipated goals and expected outcomes is increased.
- Placement needs are determined.
- Referrals are made to other professionals or resources whenever necessary and appropriate.
- Resources are utilized in a cost-effective way.

Patient/Client-Related Instruction

Patient/client-related instruction may include:

Interventions

- Instruction, education and training of patients/clients and caregivers regarding:
  - current condition (pathology/pathophysiology [disease, disorder, or condition], impairments, functional limitations, or disabilities)
  - enhancement of performance
  - health, wellness, and fitness programs
  - plan of care
  - risk factors for pathology/pathophysiology (disease, disorder, or condition), impairments, functional limitations, or disabilities
  - transitions across settings
  - transitions to new roles

Anticipated Goals and Expected Outcomes

- Ability to perform physical actions, tasks, or activities is improved.
- Awareness and use of community resources are improved.
- Behaviors that foster healthy habits, wellness, and prevention are acquired.
- Decision making is enhanced regarding patient/client health and the use of health care resources by patient/client, family, significant others, and caregivers.
- Disability associated with acute or chronic illnesses is reduced.
- Functional independence in activities of daily living (ADL) and instrumental activities of daily living (IADL) is increased.
- Health status is improved.
- Intensity of care is decreased.
- Level of supervision required for task performance is decreased.
- Patient/client, family, significant other, and caregiver knowledge and awareness of the diagnosis, prognosis, interventions, and anticipated goals and expected outcomes are increased.
- Patient/client knowledge of personal and environmental factors associated with the condition is increased.
- Performance levels in self-care, home management, work (job/school/play), community, or leisure actions, tasks, or activities are improved.
- Physical function is improved.
- Risk of recurrence of condition is reduced.
- Risk of secondary impairment is reduced.
- Safety of patient/client, family, significant others, and caregivers is improved.
- Self-management of symptoms is improved.
- Utilization and cost of health care services are decreased.

Procedural Interventions

Procedural interventions for this pattern may include:

Therapeutic Exercise

Interventions

- Aerobic capacity/endurance conditioning or reconditioning
  - aquatic programs
  - gait and locomotor training
  - increased workload over time
  - walking and wheelchair propulsion programs
- Body mechanics and postural stabilization
  - posture awareness training
  - postural control training
- Flexibility exercises
  - muscle lengthening
  - range of motion
  - stretching
- Relaxation
  - breathing strategies
  - movement strategies
  - relaxation techniques
  - standardized, programmatic, complementary exercise approaches
- Strength, power, and endurance training for head and neck, limb, pelvic-floor, trunk, and ventilatory muscles
  - active assistive, active, and resistive exercises (including concentric, dynamic/isotonic, isometric, and plyometric)
  - aquatic programs
  - standardized, programmatic, complementary exercise approaches
  - task-specific performance training

Anticipated Goals and Expected Outcomes

- Impact on pathology/pathophysiology (disease, disorder, or condition)
  - Atelectasis is decreased.
  - Nutrient delivery to tissue is increased.
  - Pain is decreased.
  - Physiological response to increased oxygen demand is improved.
  - Symptoms associated with increased oxygen demand are decreased.
  - Tissue perfusion and oxygenation are enhanced.
- Impact on impairments
  - Aerobic capacity is increased.
  - Airway clearance is improved.
  - Endurance is increased.
  - Energy expenditure per unit of work is decreased.
  - Gait, locomotion, and balance are improved.
  - Motor function (motor control and motor learning) is improved.
  - Muscle performance (strength, power, and endurance) is increased.
  - Postural control is improved.
  - Quality and quantity of movement between and across body segments are improved.
  - Range of motion is improved.
  - Relaxation is increased.
  - Ventilation and respiration/gas exchange are improved.
  - Work of breathing is decreased.
- Impact on functional limitations
  - Ability to perform physical actions, tasks, or activities related to self-care, home management, work (job/school/play), community, and leisure is improved.
  - Level of supervision required for task performance is decreased.
  - Performance of and independence in activities of daily living (ADL) and instrumental activities of daily living (IADL) with or without devices and equipment are increased.
  - Tolerance of positions and activities is increased.
- Impact on disabilities
  - Ability to assume or resume required self-care, home management, work (job/school/play), community, and leisure roles is improved.
- Risk reduction/prevention
  - Preoperative and postoperative complications are reduced.
  - Risk factors are reduced.
  - Risk of recurrence of condition is reduced.
  - Risk of secondary impairment is reduced.
  - Safety is improved.
  - Self-management of symptoms is improved.
- Impact on health, wellness, and fitness
  - Health status is improved.
  - Physical capacity is increased.
  - Physical function is improved.
- Impact on societal resources
  - Utilization of physical therapy services is optimized.
  - Utilization of physical therapy services results in efficient use of health care dollars.
- Patient/client satisfaction
  - Access, availability, and services provided are acceptable to patient/client.
  - Administrative management of practice is acceptable to patient/client.
  - Clinical proficiency of physical therapist is acceptable to patient/client.
  - Coordination of care is acceptable to patient/client.
  - Cost of health care services is decreased.
  - Intensity of care is decreased.
  - Interpersonal skills of physical therapist are acceptable to patient/client, family, and significant others.
  - Sense of well-being is improved.
  - Stressors are decreased.

Interventions Continued

Functional Training in Self-Care and Home Management (Including Activities of Daily Living [ADL] and Instrumental Activities of Daily Living [IADL])

Interventions

- ADL training
  - bed mobility and transfer training
  - developmental activities
- Devices and equipment use and training
  - assistive and adaptive device or equipment training during ADL and IADL
  - orthotic, protective, or supportive device or equipment training during ADL and IADL
  - prosthetic device or equipment training during ADL and IADL
- Functional training programs
  - simulated environments and tasks
  - task adaptation
- IADL training
  - home maintenance
  - household chores
  - shopping
  - structured play for infants and children
  - yard work
- Injury prevention or reduction
  - injury prevention education during self-care and home management
  - injury prevention or reduction with use of devices and equipment
  - safety awareness training during self-care and home management

Anticipated Goals and Expected Outcomes

- Impact on pathology/pathophysiology (disease, disorder, or condition)
  - Physiological response to increased oxygen demand is improved.
  - Symptoms associated with increased oxygen demand are decreased.
- Impact on impairments
  - Endurance is increased.
  - Energy expenditure per unit of work is decreased.
  - Muscle performance (strength, power, and endurance) is increased.
  - Work of breathing is decreased.
- Impact on functional limitations
  - Ability to perform physical actions, tasks, or activities related to self-care and home management is increased.
  - Level of supervision required for task performance is decreased.
  - Performance of and independence in ADL and IADL with or without devices and equipment are increased.
  - Tolerance of positions and activities is increased.
- Impact on disabilities
  - Ability to assume or resume required self-care and home management roles is improved.
- Risk reduction/prevention
  - Risk factors are reduced.
  - Risk of secondary impairments is reduced.
  - Safety is improved.
  - Self-management of symptoms is improved.
- Impact on health, wellness, and fitness
  - Health status is improved.
  - Physical capacity is increased.
  - Physical function is improved.
- Impact on societal resources
  - Utilization of physical therapy services is optimized.
  - Utilization of physical therapy services results in efficient use of health care dollars.
- Patient/client satisfaction
  - Access, availability, and services provided are acceptable to patient/client.
  - Administrative management of practice is acceptable to patient/client.
  - Clinical proficiency of physical therapist is acceptable to patient/client.
  - Coordination of care is acceptable to patient/client.
  - Cost of health care services is decreased.
  - Intensity of care is decreased.
  - Interpersonal skills of physical therapist are acceptable to patient/client, family, and significant others.
  - Sense of well-being is improved.
  - Stressors are decreased.

Functional Training in Work (Job/School/Play), Community, and Leisure Integration or Reintegration (Including Instrumental Activities of Daily Living [IADL], Work Hardening, and Work Conditioning)

Interventions

- Devices and equipment use and training
  - assistive and adaptive device or equipment training during IADL
  - orthotic, protective, or supportive device or equipment training during IADL
- Injury prevention or reduction
  - injury prevention education during work (job/school/play), community, and leisure integration or reintegration
  - injury prevention or reduction with use of devices and equipment
  - safety awareness training during work (job/school/play), community, and leisure integration or reintegration

Anticipated Goals and Expected Outcomes

- Impact on pathology/pathophysiology (disease, disorder, or condition)
  - Physiological response to increased oxygen demand is improved.
  - Symptoms associated with increased oxygen demand are decreased.
- Impact on impairments
  - Endurance is increased.
  - Energy expenditure per unit of work is decreased.
  - Muscle performance (strength, power, and endurance) is increased.
  - Postural control is improved.
  - Work of breathing is decreased.
- Impact on functional limitations
  - Ability to perform physical actions, tasks, or activities related to work (job/school/play), community, and leisure integration or reintegration is increased.
  - Level of supervision required for task performance is decreased.
  - Performance of and independence in IADL with or without devices and equipment are increased.
  - Tolerance of positions and activities is increased.
- Impact on disabilities
  - Ability to assume or resume required work (job/school/play), community, and leisure roles is improved.
- Risk reduction/prevention
  - Risk factors are reduced.
  - Risk of secondary impairment is reduced.
  - Safety is improved.
  - Self-management of symptoms is improved.
- Impact on health, wellness, and fitness
  - Fitness is improved.
  - Health status is improved.
  - Physical capacity is increased.
  - Physical function is improved.
- Impact on societal resources
  - Costs of work-related injury or disability are reduced.
  - Utilization of physical therapy services is optimized.
  - Utilization of physical therapy services results in efficient use of health care dollars.
- Patient/client satisfaction
  - Access, availability, and services provided are acceptable to patient/client.
  - Administrative management of practice is acceptable to patient/client.
  - Clinical proficiency of physical therapist is acceptable to patient/client.
  - Coordination of care is acceptable to patient/client.
  - Cost of health care services is decreased.
  - Intensity of care is decreased.
  - Interpersonal skills of physical therapist are acceptable to patient/client, family, and significant others.
  - Sense of well-being is improved.
  - Stressors are decreased.

Manual Therapy Techniques (Including Mobilization/Manipulation)

Interventions

- Massage
  - connective tissue massage
  - therapeutic massage
- Mobilization/manipulation
  - soft tissue
  - spinal and peripheral joints

Anticipated Goals and Expected Outcomes

- Impact on pathology/pathophysiology (disease, disorder, or condition)
  - Joint swelling, inflammation, or restriction is reduced.
  - Pain is decreased.
  - Soft tissue swelling, inflammation, or restriction is reduced.
- Impact on impairments
  - Airway clearance is improved.
  - Energy expenditure per unit of work is decreased.
  - Joint integrity and mobility are improved.
  - Muscle performance (strength, power, and endurance) is increased.
  - Postural control is improved.
  - Quality and quantity of movement between and across body segments are improved.
  - Range of motion is improved.
  - Relaxation is increased.
  - Work of breathing is decreased.
- Impact on functional limitations
  - Ability to perform movement tasks is improved.
  - Ability to perform physical actions, tasks, or activities related to self-care, home management, work (job/school/play), community, and leisure is increased.
  - Tolerance of positions and activities is increased.
- Impact on disabilities
  - Ability to assume or resume required self-care, home management, work (job/school/play), community, and leisure roles is improved.
- Risk reduction/prevention
  - Risk factors are reduced.
  - Risk of recurrence of condition is reduced.
  - Risk of secondary impairment is reduced.
  - Self-management of symptoms is improved.
- Impact on health, wellness, and fitness
  - Physical capacity is increased.
  - Physical function is improved.
- Impact on societal resources
  - Utilization of physical therapy services is optimized.
  - Utilization of physical therapy services results in efficient use of health care dollars.
- Patient/client satisfaction
  - Access, availability, and services provided are acceptable to patient/client.
  - Administrative management of practice is acceptable to patient/client.
  - Clinical proficiency of physical therapist is acceptable to patient/client.
  - Coordination of care is acceptable to patient/client.
  - Cost of health care services is decreased.
  - Intensity of care is decreased.
  - Interpersonal skills of physical therapist are acceptable to patient/client, family, and significant others.
  - Sense of well-being is improved.
  - Stressors are decreased.

Prescription, Application, and, as Appropriate, Fabrication of Devices and Equipment (Assistive, Adaptive, Orthotic, Protective, Supportive, and Prosthetic)

Interventions

- Adaptive devices
  - environmental controls
- Assistive devices
  - canes
  - crutches
  - long-handled reachers
  - percussors and vibrators
  - power devices
  - walkers
  - wheelchairs
- Orthotic devices
  - braces
- Protective devices
  - braces
  - cushions
- Supportive devices
  - compression garments
  - corsets
  - elastic wraps
  - mechanical ventilators
  - neck collars
  - supplemental oxygen

Anticipated Goals and Expected Outcomes

- Impact on pathology/pathophysiology (disease, disorder, or condition)
  - Edema, lymphedema, or effusion is reduced.
  - Joint swelling, inflammation, or restriction is reduced.
  - Pain is decreased.
  - Physiological response to increased oxygen demand is improved.
  - Soft tissue swelling, inflammation, or restriction is reduced.
  - Symptoms associated with increased oxygen demand are decreased.
- Impact on impairments
  - Balance is improved.
  - Endurance is increased.
  - Energy expenditure per unit of work is decreased.
  - Gait, locomotion, and balance are improved.
  - Integumentary integrity is improved.
  - Joint stability is improved.
  - Muscle performance (strength, power, and endurance) is increased.
  - Optimal joint alignment is achieved.
  - Optimal loading on a body part is achieved.
  - Postural control is improved.
  - Quality and quantity of movement between and across body segments are improved.
  - Range of motion is improved.
  - Ventilation and respiration/gas exchange are improved.
  - Work of breathing is decreased.
- Impact on functional limitations
  - Ability to perform physical actions, tasks, or activities related to self-care, home management, work (job/school/play), community, and leisure is improved.
  - Level of supervision required for task performance is decreased.
  - Performance of and independence in activities of daily living (ADL) and instrumental activities of daily living (IADL) with or without devices and equipment are increased.
  - Tolerance of positions and activities is improved.
- Impact on disabilities
  - Ability to assume or resume required self-care, home management, work (job/school/play), community, and leisure roles is improved.
- Risk reduction/prevention
  - Pressure on body tissues is reduced.
  - Protection of body parts is increased.
  - Risk factors are reduced.
  - Risk of secondary impairment is reduced.
  - Safety is improved.
  - Self-management of symptoms is improved.
- Impact on health, wellness, and fitness
  - Health status is improved.
  - Physical function is improved.
- Impact on societal resources
  - Utilization of physical therapy services is optimized.
  - Utilization of physical therapy services results in efficient use of health care dollars.
- Patient/client satisfaction
  - Access, availability, and services provided are acceptable to patient/client.
  - Administrative management of practice is acceptable to patient/client.
  - Clinical proficiency of physical therapist is acceptable to patient/client.
  - Coordination of care is acceptable to patient/client.
  - Cost of health care services is decreased.
  - Intensity of care is decreased.
  - Interpersonal skills of physical therapist are acceptable to patient/client, family, and significant others.
  - Sense of well-being is improved.

Airway Clearance Techniques

Interventions

- Breathing strategies
  - active cycle of breathing or forced expiratory techniques
  - assisted cough/huff techniques
  - autogenic drainage
  - paced breathing
  - pursed lip breathing
  - techniques to maximize ventilation (eg, maximum inspiratory hold, stair case breathing, manual hyperinflation)
- Manual/mechanical techniques
  - assistive devices (eg, percussors, vibrators)
  - chest percussion, vibration, and shaking
  - chest wall manipulation
  - suctioning
  - ventilatory aids
- Positioning
  - positioning to alter work of breathing
  - positioning to maximize ventilation and perfusion
  - pulmonary postural drainage

Anticipated Goals and Expected Outcomes

- Impact on pathology/pathophysiology (disease, disorder, or condition)
  - Atelectasis is decreased.
  - Tissue perfusion and oxygenation are enhanced.
- Impact on impairments
  - Airway clearance is improved.
  - Cough is improved.
  - Endurance is increased.
  - Energy expenditure per unit of work is decreased.
  - Exercise tolerance is improved.
  - Ventilation and respiration/gas exchange are improved.
  - Work of breathing is decreased.
- Impact on functional limitations
  - Ability to perform physical actions, tasks, or activities related to self-care, home management, work (job/school/play), community, and leisure is improved.
  - Performance of and independence in activities of daily living (ADL) and instrumental activities of daily living (IADL) with or without devices and equipment are increased.
  - Tolerance of positions and activities is increased.
- Impact on disabilities
  - Ability to assume or resume required self-care, home management, work (job/school/play), community, and leisure roles is improved.
- Risk reduction/prevention
  - Risk factors are reduced.
  - Risk of secondary impairment is reduced.
  - Safety is improved.
  - Self-management of symptoms is improved.
- Impact on health, wellness, and fitness
  - Health status is improved.
  - Physical capacity is increased.
  - Physical function is improved.
- Impact on societal resources
  - Utilization of physical therapy services is optimized.
  - Utilization of physical therapy services results in efficient use of health care dollars.
- Patient/client satisfaction
  - Access, availability, and services provided are acceptable to patient/client.
  - Administrative management of practice is acceptable to patient/client.
  - Clinical proficiency of physical therapist is acceptable to patient/client.
  - Coordination of care is acceptable to patient/client.
  - Cost of health care services is decreased.
  - Intensity of care is decreased.
  - Interpersonal skills of physical therapist are acceptable to patient/client, family, and significant others.
  - Sense of well-being is improved.
  - Stressors are decreased.

Reexamination

Reexamination is the process of performing selected tests and measures after the initial examination to evaluate progress and to modify or redirect interventions. Reexamination may be indicated more than once during a single episode of care. It also may be performed over the course of a disease, disorder, or condition, which for some patients/clients may be over the life span. Indications for reexamination include new clinical findings or failure to respond to physical therapy interventions.

Global Outcomes for Patients/Clients in This Pattern

Throughout the entire episode of care, the physical therapist determines the anticipated goals and expected outcomes for each intervention. These anticipated goals and expected outcomes are delineated in shaded boxes that accompany the lists of interventions in each preferred practice pattern. As the patient/client reaches the termination of physical therapy services and the end of the episode of care, the physical therapist measures the global outcomes of the physical therapy services by characterizing or quantifying the impact of the physical therapy interventions in the following domains:

- Pathology/pathophysiology (disease, disorder, or condition)
- Impairments
- Functional limitations
- Disabilities
- Risk reduction/prevention
- Health, wellness, and fitness
- Societal resources
- Patient/client satisfaction

In some instances, a particular anticipated goal or expected outcome is thoroughly achieved through implementation of a single form of intervention. More commonly, however, the anticipated goals and expected outcomes are achieved as a result of the combined effects of several forms of interventions, leading to enhancement of both health status and health-related quality of life.

Criteria for Termination of Physical Therapy Services

Discharge is the process of ending physical therapy services that have been provided during a single episode of care. It occurs when the anticipated goals and expected outcomes have been achieved. Discharge does *not* occur with a *transfer* (defined as the time when a patient is moved from one site to another site within the same setting or across settings during a single episode of care). Although there may be facility-specific or payer-specific requirements for documentation regarding the conclusion of physical therapy services, *discharge occurs based on the physical therapist's analysis of the achievement of anticipated goals and expected outcomes.*

Discontinuation is the process of ending physical therapy services that have been provided during a single episode of care when (1) the patient/client, caregiver, or legal guardian declines to continue intervention; (2) the patient/client is unable to continue to progress toward outcomes because of medical or psychosocial complications or because financial/insurance resources have been expended; or (3) the physical therapist determines that the patient/client will no longer benefit from physical therapy. When physical therapy services are terminated prior to achievement of anticipated goals and expected outcomes, patient/client status and the rationale for termination are documented.

For patients/clients who require multiple episodes of care, periodic follow-up is needed over the life span to ensure safety and effective adaptation following changes in physical status, caregivers, environment, or task demands. In consultation with appropriate individuals, and in consideration of the outcomes, the physical therapist plans for discharge or discontinuation and provides for appropriate follow-up or referral.

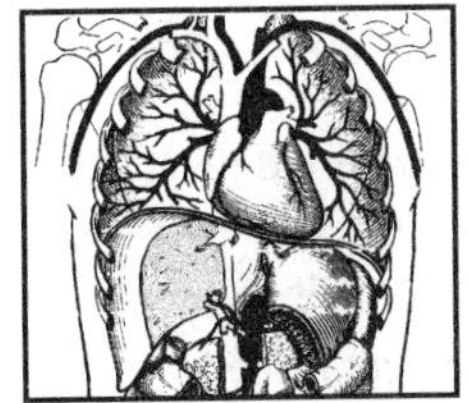

Impaired Aerobic Capacity/Endurance Associated With Cardiovascular Pump Dysfunction or Failure

This preferred practice pattern describes the generally accepted elements of patient/client management that physical therapists provide for patients/clients who are classified in this pattern. The pattern title reflects the diagnosis made by the physical therapist. APTA emphasizes that preferred practice patterns are the boundaries within which a physical therapist may select any of a number of clinical alternatives, based on consideration of a wide variety of factors, such as individual patient/client needs; the profession's code of ethics and standards of practice; and patient/client age, culture, gender roles, race, sex, sexual orientation, and socioeconomic status.

Patient/Client Diagnostic Classification

Patients/clients will be classified into this pattern—for impaired aerobic capacity/endurance associated with cardiovascular pump dysfunction or failure—as a result of the physical therapist's evaluation of the examination data. The findings from the examination (history, systems review, and tests and measures) may indicate the presence or risk of pathology/pathophysiology (disease, disorder, or condition), impairments, functional limitations, or disabilities or the need for health, wellness, or fitness programs. The physical therapist integrates, synthesizes, and interprets the data to determine the diagnostic classification.

Inclusion

The following examples of examination findings may support the inclusion of patients/clients in this pattern:

Risk Factors or Consequences of Pathology/Pathophysiology (Disease, Disorder, or Condition)

- Angioplasty or atherectomy
- Atrioventricular block
- Cardiogenic shock
- Cardiomyopathy
- Cardiothoracic surgery
- Complex ventricular arrhythmias
- Complicated myocardial infarction (failure); uncomplicated myocardial infarction (dysfunction)
- Congenital cardiac anomalies
- Coronary artery disease
- Decrease in ejection fraction (EF) on exercise testing (EF of 30-50% with dysfunction; < 30% with failure)
- Diabetes
- Exercise-induced myocardial ischemia (1-2 mm ST segment depression with dysfunction; > 2 mm ST segment with failure)
- Hypertensive heart disease
- Nonmalignant arrhythmias
- Valvular heart disease

Impairments, Functional Limitations, or Disabilities

- Abnormal heart rate response to increased oxygen demand
- Abnormal pulmonary response to increased oxygen demand
- Decreased ability or the inability to perform activities of daily living (ADL) because of symptoms
- Change in baseline breath sounds with activity
- Flat or falling blood pressure response to increased oxygen demand (failure)
- Hypertensive blood pressure response to increased oxygen demand (dysfunction)
- Impaired aerobic capacity of ≤ 5 or 6 metabolic equivalents (METS) (dysfunction) or ≤ 4 or 5 METS (failure)
- Impaired gas exchange
- Inability or decreased ability to perform work roles because of symptoms
- Presence of or increase in cardiovascular symptoms in response to increased oxygen demand

Exclusion or Multiple-Pattern Classification

The following examples of examination findings may support exclusion from this pattern or classification into additional patterns. Depending on the level of severity or complexity of the examination findings, the physical therapist may determine that the patient/client would be more appropriately managed through (1) classification in an entirely different pattern or (2) classification in both this and another pattern.

Findings That May Require Classification in a Different Pattern

- Heart failure with respiratory failure
- Neonate with cardiovascular anomaly and respiratory failure

Findings That May Require Classification in Additional Patterns

- Airway clearance impairments with pericarditis status post chest trauma

Note:

Some risk factors or consequences of pathology/pathophysiology—such as *cardiovascular pump dysfunction with multisystem impairments*—may be severe and complex; *however, they do not necessarily exclude patients/clients from this pattern.* Severe and complex risk factors or consequences may require modification of the frequency of visits and duration of care. (See "Evaluation, Diagnosis, and Prognosis," page 511.)

ICD-9-CM Codes

The listing below contains the current (as of press time) and most typical 3- and 4-digit ICD-9-CM codes related to this preferred practice pattern. Because patient/client diagnostic classification is based on impairments, functional limitations, and disabilities—not on codes—patients/clients may be classified into the pattern even though the codes listed with the pattern may not apply to those clients.

This listing is intended for general information only and should not be used for coding purposes. The codes should be confirmed by referring to the World Health Organization's *International Classification of Diseases, 9th Revision, Clinical Modification (ICD-9-CM 2001)*, Volumes 1 and 3 (Chicago, Ill: American Medical Association; 2000) or subsequent revisions or by referring to other ICD-9-CM coding manuals that contain exclusion notes and instructions regarding fifth-digit requirements.

391 Rheumatic fever with heart involvement
394 Diseases of mitral valve
395 Diseases of aortic valve
396 Diseases of mitral and aortic valves
397 Diseases of other endocardial structures
398 Other rheumatic heart disease
402 Hypertensive heart disease
403 Hypertensive renal disease
404 Hypertensive heart and renal disease
410 Acute myocardial infarction
411 Other acute and subacute forms of ischemic heart disease
412 Old myocardial infarction
413 Angina pectoris
414 Other forms of chronic ischemic heart disease
416 Chronic pulmonary heart disease
417 Other diseases of pulmonary circulation
- **417.0** Arteriovenous fistula of pulmonary vessels

422 Acute myocarditis
423 Other diseases of pericardium
- **423.2** Constrictive pericarditis

424 Other diseases of endocardium
- **424.0** Mitral valve disorders

425 Cardiomyopathy
426 Conduction disorders
427 Cardiac dysrhythmias
428 Heart failure
429 Ill-defined descriptions and complications of heart disease
- **429.0** Myocarditis, unspecified
- **429.4** Functional disturbances following cardiac surgery

440 Atherosclerosis
441 Aortic aneurysm and dissection
443 Other peripheral vascular disease
444 Arterial embolism and thrombosis
745 Bulbus cordis anomalies and anomalies of cardic septal closure
- **745.0** Common truncus
- **745.1** Transposition of great vessels
- **745.2** Tetralogy of Fallot
- **745.4** Ventricular septal defect
- **745.5** Ostium secundum type atrial septal defect

746 Other congenital anomalies of heart
747 Other congenital anonalies of circulatory system
- **747.0** Patent ductus botalli
- **747.1** Coarctation of aorta

785 Symptoms involving cardiovascular system
- **785.5** Shock without mention of trauma
  - **785.51** Cardiogenic shock

Note:

Patients/clients who have surgical procedures involving the chest wall, diaphragm, pleura, mediastinum, thorax, and vessels of the heart also may be classified into this pattern.

Examination

Examination is a comprehensive screening and specific testing process that leads to a diagnostic classification or, when appropriate, to a referral to another practitioner. Examination is required prior to the initial intervention and is performed for all patients/clients. Through the examination, the physical therapist may identify impairments, functional limitations, disabilities, changes in physical function or overall health status, and needs related to restoration of health and to prevention, wellness, and fitness. The physical therapist synthesizes the examination findings to establish the diagnosis and the prognosis (including the plan of care). The patient/client, family, significant others, and caregivers may provide information during the examination process.

Examination has three components: the patient/client history, the systems review, and tests and measures. The *history* is a systematic gathering of past and current information (often from the patient/client) related to why the patient/client is seeking the services of the physical therapist. The *systems review* is a brief or limited examination of (1) the anatomical and physiological status of the cardiovascular/pulmonary, integumentary, musculoskeletal, and neuromuscular systems and (2) the communication ability, affect, cognition, language, and learning style of the patient/client. *Tests and measures* are the means of gathering data about the patient/client.

The selection of examination procedures and the depth of the examination vary based on patient/client age; severity of the problem; stage of recovery (acute, subacute, chronic); phase of rehabilitation (early, intermediate, late, return to activity); home, work (job/school/play), or community situation; and other relevant factors. *For clinical indications in selecting tests and measures and for listings of tests and measures, tools used to gather data, and the types of data generated by tests and measures, refer to Chapter 2.*

Patient/Client History

The history may include:

General Demographics

- Age
- Sex
- Race/ethnicity
- Primary language
- Education

Social History

- Cultural beliefs and behaviors
- Family and caregiver resources
- Social interactions, social activities, and support systems

Employment/Work (Job/School/Play)

- Current and prior work (job/school/play), community, and leisure actions, tasks, or activities

Growth and Development

- Developmental history
- Hand dominance

Living Environment

- Devices and equipment (eg, assistive, adaptive, orthotic, protective, supportive, prosthetic)
- Living environment and community characteristics
- Projected discharge destinations

General Health Status (Self-Report, Family Report, Caregiver Report)

- General health perception
- Physical function (eg, mobility, sleep patterns, restricted bed days)
- Psychological function (eg, memory, reasoning ability, depression, anxiety)
- Role function (eg, community, leisure, social, work)
- Social function (eg, social activity, social interaction, social support)

Social/Health Habits (Past and Current)

- Behavioral health risks (eg, smoking, drug abuse)
- Level of physical fitness

Family History

- Familial health risks

Medical/Surgical History

- Cardiovascular
- Endocrine/metabolic
- Gastrointestinal
- Genitourinary
- Gynecological
- Integumentary
- Musculoskeletal
- Neuromuscular
- Obstetrical
- Prior hospitalizations, surgeries, and preexisting medical and other health-related conditions
- Psychological
- Pulmonary

Current Condition(s)/Chief Complaint(s)

- Concerns that led patient/client to seek the services of a physical therapist
- Concerns or needs of patient/client who requires the services of a physical therapist
- Current therapeutic interventions
- Mechanisms of injury or disease, including date of onset and course of events
- Onset and pattern of symptoms
- Patient/client, family, significant other, and caregiver expectations and goals for the therapeutic intervention
- Patient/client, family, significant other, and caregiver perceptions of patient's/client's emotional response to the current clinical situation
- Previous occurrence of chief complaint(s)
- Prior therapeutic interventions

Functional Status and Activity Level

- Current and prior functional status in self-care and home management activities, including activities of daily living (ADL) and instrumental activities of daily living (IADL)
- Current and prior functional status in work (job/school/play), community, and leisure actions, tasks, or activities

Medications

- Medications for current condition
- Medications previously taken for current condition
- Medications for other conditions

Other Clinical Tests

- Laboratory and diagnostic tests
- Review of available records (eg, medical, education, surgical)
- Review of other clinical findings (eg, nutrition and hydration)

Systems Review

The systems review may include:

Anatomical and Physiological Status

- Cardiovascular/Pulmonary
  - Blood pressure
  - Edema
  - Heart rate
  - Respiratory rate
- Integumentary
  - Pliability (texture)
  - Presence of scar formation
  - Skin color
  - Skin integrity
- Musculoskeletal
  - Gross range of motion
  - Gross strength
  - Gross symmetry
  - Height
  - Weight
- Neuromuscular
  - Gross coordinated movements (eg, balance, gait, locomotion, transfers, transitions)
  - Motor function (motor control, motor learning)

Communication, Affect, Cognition, Language, and Learning Style

- Ability to make needs known
- Consciousness
- Expected emotional/behavioral responses
- Learning preferences (eg, education needs, learning barriers)
- Orientation (person, place, time)

Tests and Measures

Tests and measures for this pattern may include those that characterize or quantify:

Aerobic Capacity and Endurance

- Aerobic capacity during functional activities (eg, activities of daily living [ADL] scales, indexes, instrumental activities of daily living [IADL] scales, observations)
- Aerobic capacity during standardized exercise test protocols (eg, ergometry, step tests, time/distance walk/run tests, treadmill tests, wheelchair tests)
- Cardiovascular signs and symptoms in response to increased oxygen demand with exercise or activity, including pressures and flow; heart rate, rhythm, and sounds; and superficial vascular responses (eg, angina, claudication, and exertion scales; electrocardiography; observations; palpation; sphygmomanometry)
- Pulmonary signs and symptoms in response to increased oxygen demand with exercise or activity, including breath and voice sounds; cyanosis; gas exchange; respiratory pattern, rate, and rhythm; and ventilatory flow, force, and volume (eg, auscultation, dyspnea and exertion scales, gas analyses, observations, oximetry, palpation, pulmonary function tests)

Anthropometric Characteristics

- Body composition (eg, body mass index, impedance measurement, skinfold thickness measurement)
- Body dimensions (eg, girth measurement, length measurement)
- Edema (eg, girth measurement, palpation, scales, volume measurement)

Arousal, Attention, and Cognition

- Arousal and attention (eg, adaptability tests, arousal and awareness scales, indexes, profiles, questionnaires)
- Cognition, including ability to process commands (eg, developmental inventories, indexes, interviews, mental state scales, observations, questionnaires, safety checklists)
- Motivation (eg, adaptive behavior scales)
- Orientation to time, person, place, and situation (eg, attention tests, learning profiles, mental state scales)
- Recall, including memory and retention (eg, assessment scales, interviews, questionnaires)

Assistive and Adaptive Devices

- Assistive or adaptive devices and equipment use during functional activities (eg, ADL scales, functional scales, IADL scales, interviews, observations)
- Components, alignment, fit, and ability to care for the assistive or adaptive devices and equipment (eg, interviews, logs, observations, pressure-sensing maps, reports)
- Remediation of impairments, functional limitations, or disabilities with use of assistive or adaptive devices and equipment (eg, activity status indexes, ADL scales, aerobic capacity tests, functional performance inventories, health assessment questionnaires, IADL scales, pain scales, play scales, videographic assessments)
- Safety during use of assistive or adaptive devices and equipment (eg, diaries, fall scales, interviews, logs, observations, reports)

Circulation (Arterial, Venous, and Lymphatic)

- Cardiovascular signs, including heart rate, rhythm, and sounds; pressures and flow; and superficial vascular responses (eg, auscultation, electrocardiography, palpation, sphygmomanometry, thermography)
- Cardiovascular symptoms (eg, angina, claudication, and perceived exertion scales)
- Physiological responses to position change, including autonomic responses, central and peripheral pressures, heart rate and rhythm, respiratory rate and rhythm, ventilatory pattern (eg, auscultation, electrocardiography, observations, palpation, sphygmomanometry)

Environmental, Home, and Work (Job/School/Play) Barriers

- Current and potential barriers (eg, checklists, interviews, observations, questionnaires)
- Physical space and environment (eg, compliance standards, observations, photographic assessments, questionnaires, structural specifications, videographic assessments)

Ergonomics and Body Mechanics

Ergonomics

- Functional capacity and performance during work actions, tasks, or activities (eg, accelerometry, dynamometry, electroneuromyography, endurance tests, force platform tests, goniometry, interviews, observations, photographic assessments, physical capacity tests, postural loading analyses, technology-assisted assessments, videographic assessments, work analyses)
- Safety in work environments (eg, hazard identification checklists, job severity indexes, lifting standards, risk assessment scales, standards for exposure limits)

Body mechanics

- Body mechanics during self-care, home management, work, community, or leisure actions, tasks, or activities (eg, ADL scales, IADL scales, observations, photographic assessments, technology-assisted assessments, videographic assessments)

Gait, Locomotion, and Balance

- Balance during functional activities with or without the use of assistive, adaptive, orthotic, protective, supportive, or prosthetic devices or equipment (eg, ADL scales, IADL scales, observations, videographic assessments)
- Gait and locomotion during functional activities with or without the use of assistive, adaptive, orthotic, protective, supportive, or prosthetic devices or equipment (eg, ADL scales, gait indexes, IADL scales, mobility skill profiles, observations, videographic assessments)
- Safety during gait, locomotion, and balance (eg, confidence scales, diaries, fall scales, functional assessment profiles, logs, reports)

Integumentary Integrity

Associated skin

- Activities, positioning, and postures that produce or relieve trauma to the skin (eg, observations, pressure-sensing maps, scales)
- Assistive, adaptive, orthotic, protective, supportive, or prosthetic devices and equipment that may produce or relieve trauma to the skin (eg, observations, pressure-sensing maps, risk assessment scales)
- Skin characteristics, including blistering, continuity of skin color, dermatitis, hair growth, mobility, nail growth, sensation, temperature, texture, and turgor (eg, observations, palpation, photographic assessments, thermography)

Wound

- Signs of infection (eg, culture results, observations, palpation)

Motor Function (Motor Control and Motor Learning)

- Dexterity, coordination, and agility (eg, coordination screens, motor impairment tests, motor proficiency tests, observations, videographic assessments)

Muscle Performance (Including Strength, Power, and Endurance)

- Muscle strength, power, and endurance (eg, dynamometry, manual muscle tests, muscle performance tests, physical capacity tests, technology-assisted assessments, timed activity tests)
- Muscle strength, power, and endurance during functional activities (eg, ADL scales, functional muscle tests, IADL scales, observations, videographic assessments)
- Muscle tension (eg, palpation)

Neuromotor Development and Sensory Integration

- Oral motor function, phonation, and speech production (eg, interviews, observations)

Orthotic, Protective, and Supportive Devices

- Components, alignment, fit, and ability to care for orthotic, protective, and supportive devices and equipment (eg, interviews, logs, observations, pressure-sensing maps, reports)
- Orthotic, protective, and supportive devices and equipment use during functional activities (eg, ADL scales, functional scales, IADL scales, interviews, observations, profiles)
- Remediation of impairments, functional limitations, or disabilities with use of orthotic, protective, and supportive devices and equipment (eg, activity status indexes, ADL scales, aerobic capacity tests, functional performance inventories, health assessment questionnaires, IADL scales, pain scales, play scales, videographic assessments)
- Safety during use of orthotic, protective, and supportive devices and equipment (eg, diaries, fall scales, interviews, logs, observations, reports)

Pain

- Pain, soreness, and nociception (eg, angina scales, analog scales, discrimination tests, pain drawings and maps, provocation tests, verbal and pictorial descriptor tests)

Posture

- Postural alignment and position (static and dynamic), including symmetry and deviation from midline (eg, grid measurement, observations, photographic assessments, technology-assisted assessments, videographic assessments)
- Specific body parts (eg, angle assessments, forward-bending test, goniometry, observations, palpation, positional tests)

Range of Motion (ROM) (Including Muscle Length)

- Functional ROM (eg, observations, squat testing, toe touch tests)
- Muscle length, soft tissue extensibility, and flexibility (eg, contracture tests, goniometry, inclinometry, ligamentous tests, linear measurement, multisegment flexibility tests, palpation)

Self-Care and Home Management (Including ADL and IADL)

- Ability to gain access to home environments (eg, barrier identification, observations, physical performance tests)
- Ability to perform self-care and home management activities with or without assistive, adaptive, orthotic, protective, supportive, or prosthetic devices and equipment (eg, ADL scales, aerobic capacity tests, IADL scales, interviews, observations, profiles)
- Safety in self-care and home management activities and environments (eg, diaries, fall scales, interviews, logs, observations, reports, videographic assessments)

Ventilation and Respiration/Gas Exchange

- Pulmonary signs of respiration/gas exchange, including breath sounds (eg, gas analyses, observations, oximetry)
- Pulmonary signs of ventilatory function, including airway protection; breath and voice sounds; respiratory rate, rhythm, and pattern; ventilatory flow, forces, and volumes (eg, airway clearance tests, observations, palpation, pulmonary function tests, ventilatory muscle force tests)
- Pulmonary symptoms (eg, dyspnea and perceived exertion indexes and scales)

Work (Job/School/Play), Community, and Leisure Integration or Reintegration (Including IADL)

- Ability to assume or resume work (job/school/play), community, and leisure activities with or without assistive, adaptive, orthotic, protective, supportive, or prosthetic devices and equipment (eg, activity profiles, disability indexes, functional status questionnaires, IADL scales, observations, physical capacity tests)
- Ability to gain access to work (job/school/play), community, and leisure environments (eg, barrier identification, interviews, observations, physical capacity tests, transportation assessments)
- Safety in work (job/school/play), community, and leisure activities and environments (eg, diaries, fall scales, interviews, logs, observations, videographic assessments)

Evaluation, Diagnosis, and Prognosis (Including Plan of Care)

Physical therapists perform *evaluations* (make clinical judgments) based on the data gathered from the history, systems review, and tests and measures. In the evaluation process, physical therapists synthesize the examination data to establish the diagnosis and prognosis (including the plan of care). Factors that influence the complexity of the evaluation include the clinical findings, extent of loss of function, chronicity or severity of the problem, possibility of multisite or multisystem involvement, preexisting condition(s), potential discharge destination, social considerations, physical function, and overall health status.

A *diagnosis* is a label encompassing a cluster of signs and symptoms, syndromes, or categories. It is the result of the systematic diagnostic process, which includes integrating and evaluating the data from the examination. The diagnostic label indicates the primary dysfunction(s) toward which the therapist will direct interventions. The *prognosis* is the determination of the predicted optimal level of improvement in function and the amount of time needed to reach that level and may also include a prediction of levels of improvement that may be reached at various intervals during the course of therapy. During the prognostic process, the physical therapist develops the plan of care. The *plan of care* identifies specific interventions, proposed frequency and duration of the interventions, anticipated goals, expected outcomes, and discharge plans. The plan of care identifies realistic anticipated goals and expected outcomes, taking into consideration the expectations of the patient/client and appropriate others. These anticipated goals and expected outcomes should be measureable and time limited.

The frequency of visits and duration of the episode of care may vary from a short episode with a high intensity of intervention to a longer episode with a diminishing intensity of intervention. Frequency and duration may vary greatly among patients/clients based on a variety of factors that the physical therapist considers throughout the evaluation process, such as anatomical and physiological changes related to growth and development; caregiver consistency or expertise; chronicity or severity of the current condition; living environment; multisite or multisystem involvement; social support; potential discharge destinations; probability of prolonged impairment, functional limitation, or disability; and stability of the condition.

Prognosis	Expected Range of Number of Visits Per Episode of Care	Factors That May Require New Episode of Care or That May Modify Frequency of Visits/ Duration of Episode
Over the course of 6 to 12 weeks, patient/ client with cardiovascular pump dysfunction will demonstrate optimal aerobic capacity/endurance and the highest level of functioning in home, work (job/ school/play), community, and leisure environments, within the context of the impairments, functional limitations, and disabilities.	3 to 30	• Accessibility and availability of resources • Adherence to the intervention program • Age • Anatomical and physiological changes related to growth and development • Caregiver consistency or expertise • Chronicity or severity of the current condition • Cognitive status
Over the course of 8 to 16 weeks, patient/client with cardiovascular pump failure will demonstrate optimal aerobic capacity/endurance and the highest level of functioning in home, work (job/ school/play), community, and leisure environments, within the context of the impairments, functional limitations, and disabilities.	14 to 44 These ranges represent the lower and upper limits of the number of physical therapist visits required to achieve anticipated goals and expected outcomes. *It is anticipated that 80% of patients/clients who are classified into this pattern will achieve the anticipated goals and expected outcomes within these ranges during a single continuous episode of care.* Frequency of visits and duration of the episode of care should be determined by the physical therapist to maximize effectiveness of care and efficiency of service delivery.	• Comorbitities, complications, or secondary impairments • Concurrent medical, surgical, and therapeutic interventions • Decline in functional independence • Level of impairment • Level of physical function • Living environment • Multisite or multisystem involvement • Nutritional status
During the episode of care, patient/client with cardiovascular pump dysfunction or failure will achieve (1) the anticipated goals and expected outcomes of the interventions that are described in the plan of care and (2) the global outcomes for patients/ clients who are classified in this pattern.		• Overall health status • Potential discharge destinations • Premorbid conditions • Probability of prolonged impairment, functional limitation, or disability • Psychological and socioeconomic factors • Psychomotor abilities • Social support • Stability of the condition

Intervention

Intervention is the purposeful interaction of the physical therapist with the patient/client and, when appropriate, with other individuals involved in patient/client care, using various physical therapy procedures and techniques to produce changes in the condition consistent with the diagnosis and prognosis. Decisions about interventions are contingent on the timely monitoring of patient/client response and the progress made toward achieving the anticipated goals and expected outcomes.

Communication, coordination, and documentation and patient/client-related instruction are provided for all patients/clients across all settings. Procedural interventions are selected or modified based on the examination data and the evaluation, the diagnosis and the prognosis, and the anticipated goals and expected outcomes for a particular patient/client. *For clinical considerations in selecting interventions, listings of interventions, and listings of anticipated goals and expected outcomes, refer to Chapter 3.*

Coordination, Communication, and Documentation

Coordination, communication, and documentation may include:

Interventions

- Addressing required functions
  - advance directives
  - individualized family service plans (IFSPs) or individualized education plans (IEPs)
  - informed consent
  - mandatory communication and reporting (eg, patient advocacy and abuse reporting)
- Admission and discharge planning
- Case management
- Collaboration and coordination with agencies, including:
  - equipment suppliers
  - home care agencies
  - payer groups
  - schools
  - transportation agencies
- Communication across settings, including:
  - case conferences
  - documentation
- Cost-effective resource utilization
- Data collection, analysis, and reporting
  - outcome data
  - peer review findings
  - record reviews
- Documentation across settings, following APTA's *Guidelines for Physical Therapy Documentation* (Appendix 5), including:
  - changes in impairments, functional limitations, and disabilities
  - changes in interventions
  - elements of patient/client management (examination, evaluation, diagnosis, prognosis, intervention)
  - outcomes of intervention
- Interdisciplinary teamwork
  - case conferences
  - patient care rounds
  - patient/client family meetings
- Referrals to other professionals or resources

Anticipated Goals and Expected Outcomes

- Accountability for services is increased.
- Admission data and discharge planning are completed.
- Advance directives, individualized family service plans (IFSPs) or individualized education plans (IEPs), informed consent, and mandatory communication and reporting (eg, patient advocacy and abuse reporting) are obtained or completed.
- Available resources are maximally utilized.
- Care is coordinated with patient/client, family, significant others, caregivers, and other professionals.
- Case is managed throughout the episode of care.
- Collaboration and coordination occurs with agencies, including equipment suppliers, home care agencies, payer groups, schools, and transportation agencies.
- Communication enhances risk reduction and prevention.
- Communication occurs across settings through case conferences, and documentation.
- Data are collected, analyzed, and reported, including outcome data, peer review findings, and record reviews.
- Decision making is enhanced regarding health, wellness, and fitness needs.
- Decision making is enhanced regarding patient/client health and the use of health care resources by patient/client, family, significant others, and caregivers.
- Documentation occurs throughout patient/client management and across settings and follows APTA's *Guidelines for Physical Therapy Documentation* (Appendix 5).
- Interdisciplinary collaboration occurs through case conferences, patient care rounds, and patient/client family meetings.
- Patient/client, family, significant other, and caregiver understanding of anticipated goals and expected outcomes is increased.
- Placement needs are determined.
- Referrals are made to other professionals or resources whenever necessary and appropriate.
- Resources are utilized in a cost-effective way.

Patient/Client-Related Instruction

Patient/client-related instruction may include:

Interventions

- Instruction, education and training of patients/clients and caregivers regarding:
  - current condition (pathology/pathophysiology [disease, disorder, or condition], impairments, functional limitations, or disabilities)
  - enhancement of performance
  - health, wellness, and fitness programs
  - plan of care
  - risk factors for pathology/pathophysiology (disease, disorder, or condition), impairments, functional limitations, or disabilities
  - transitions across settings
  - transitions to new roles

Anticipated Goals and Expected Outcomes

- Ability to perform physical actions, tasks, or activities is improved.
- Awareness and use of community resources are improved.
- Behaviors that foster healthy habits, wellness, and prevention are acquired.
- Decision making is enhanced regarding patient/client health and the use of health care resources by patient/client, family, significant others, and caregivers.
- Disability associated with acute or chronic illnesses is reduced.
- Functional independence in activities of daily living (ADL) and instrumental activities of daily living (IADL) is increased.
- Health status is improved.
- Intensity of care is decreased.
- Level of supervision required for task performance is decreased.
- Patient/client, family, significant other, and caregiver knowledge and awareness of the diagnosis, prognosis, interventions, and anticipated goals and expected outcomes are increased.
- Patient/client knowledge of personal and environmental factors associated with the condition is increased.
- Performance levels in self-care, home management, work (job/school/play), community, or leisure actions, tasks, or activities are improved.
- Physical function is improved.
- Risk of recurrence of condition is reduced.
- Risk of secondary impairment is reduced.
- Safety of patient/client, family, significant others, and caregivers is improved.
- Self-management of symptoms is improved.
- Utilization and cost of health care services are decreased.

Procedural Interventions

Procedural interventions for this pattern may include:

Therapeutic Exercise

Interventions

- Aerobic capacity/endurance conditioning or reconditioning
  - gait and locomotor training
  - increased workload over time
  - movement efficiency and energy conservation training
  - walking and wheelchair propulsion programs
- Balance, coordination, and agility training
  - developmental activities training
  - motor function (motor control and motor learning) training or retraining
  - neuromuscular education or reeducation
  - posture awareness training
  - standardized, programmatic, complementary exercise approaches
  - task-specific performance training
- Body mechanics and postural stabilization
  - body mechanics training
  - posture awareness training
- Flexibility exercises
  - muscle lengthening
  - range of motion
  - stretching
- Gait and locomotion training
  - developmental activities training
  - gait training
  - implement and device training
  - standardized, programmatic, complementary exercise approaches
  - wheelchair training
- Relaxation
  - breathing strategies
  - movement strategies
  - relaxation techniques
  - standardized, programmatic, complementary exercise approaches
- Strength, power, and endurance training for head and neck, limb, pelvic-floor, trunk, and ventilatory muscles
  - active assistive, active, and resistive exercises (including concentric, dynamic/isotonic, isometric, and plyometric)
  - standardized, programmatic, complementary exercise approaches
  - task-specific performance training

Anticipated Goals and Expected Outcomes

- Impact on pathology/pathophysiology (disease, disorder, or condition)
  - Atelectasis is decreased.
  - Joint swelling, inflammation, or restriction is reduced.
  - Nutrient delivery to tissue is increased.
  - Osteogenic effects of exercise are maximized.
  - Pain is decreased.
  - Physiological response to increased oxygen demand is improved.
  - Soft tissue swelling, inflammation, or restriction is reduced.
  - Symptoms associated with increased oxygen demand are decreased.
  - Tissue perfusion and oxygenation are enhanced.
- Impact on impairments
  - Aerobic capacity is increased.
  - Airway clearance is improved.
  - Endurance is increased.
  - Energy expenditure per unit of work is decreased.
  - Gait, locomotion, and balance are improved.
  - Integumentary integrity is improved.
  - Joint integrity and mobility are improved.
  - Motor function (motor control and motor learning) is improved.
  - Muscle performance (strength, power, and endurance) is increased.
  - Postural control is improved.
  - Range of motion is improved.
  - Relaxation is increased.
  - Work of breathing is decreased.
- Impact on functional limitations
  - Ability to perform physical actions, tasks, or activities related to self-care, home management, work (job/school/play), community, and leisure is improved.
  - Level of supervision required for task performance is decreased.
  - Performance of and independence in activities of daily living (ADL) and instrumental activities of daily living (IADL) with or without devices and equipment are increased.
  - Tolerance of positions and activities is increased.
- Impact on disabilities
  - Ability to assume or resume required self-care, home management, work (job/school/play), community, and leisure roles is improved.
- Risk reduction/prevention
  - Preoperative and postoperative complications are reduced.
  - Risk factors are reduced.
  - Risk of recurrence of condition is reduced.
  - Risk of secondary impairment is reduced.
  - Safety is improved.
  - Self-management of symptoms is improved.
- Impact on health, wellness, and fitness
  - Fitness is improved.
  - Health status is improved.
  - Physical capacity is increased.
  - Physical function is improved.
- Impact on societal resources
  - Utilization of physical therapy services is optimized.
  - Utilization of physical therapy services results in efficient use of health care dollars.
- Patient/client satisfaction
  - Access, availability, and services provided are acceptable to patient/client.
  - Administrative management of practice is acceptable to patient/client.
  - Clinical proficiency of physical therapist is acceptable to patient/client.
  - Coordination of care is acceptable to patient/client.
  - Cost of health care services is decreased.
  - Intensity of care is decreased.
  - Interpersonal skills of physical therapist are acceptable to patient/client, family, and significant others.
  - Sense of well-being is improved.
  - Stressors are decreased.

Functional Training in Self-Care and Home Management (Including Activities of Daily Living [ADL] and Instrumental Activities of Daily Living [IADL])

Interventions

- ADL training
  - bathing
  - bed mobility and transfer training
  - developmental activities
  - dressing
  - eating
  - grooming
  - toileting
- Devices and equipment use and training
  - assistive and adaptive device or equipment training during ADL and IADL
  - orthotic, protective, or supportive device or equipment training during ADL and IADL
  - prosthetic device or equipment training during ADL and IADL
- Functional training programs
  - simulated environments and tasks
  - task adaptation
- IADL training
  - caring for dependents
  - home maintenance
  - household chores
  - shopping
  - structured play for infants and children
  - yard work
- Injury prevention or reduction
  - injury prevention education during self-care and home management
  - injury prevention or reduction with use of devices and equipment
  - safety awareness training during self-care and home management

Anticipated Goals and Expected Outcomes

- Impact on pathology/pathophysiology (disease, disorder, or condition)
  - Pain is decreased.
  - Physiological response to increased oxygen demand is improved.
  - Symptoms associated with increased oxygen demand are decreased.
- Impact on impairments
  - Endurance is increased.
  - Energy expenditure per unit of work is decreased.
  - Muscle performance (strength, power, and endurance) is increased.
- Impact on functional limitations
  - Ability to perform physical actions, tasks, or activities related to self-care and home management is improved.
  - Level of supervision required for task performance is decreased.
  - Performance of and independence in ADL and IADL with or without devices and equipment are increased.
  - Tolerance of positions and activities is increased.
- Impact on disabilities
  - Ability to assume or resume required self-care and home management roles is improved.
- Risk reduction/prevention
  - Risk factors are reduced.
  - Risk of secondary impairments is reduced.
  - Safety is improved.
  - Self-management of symptoms is improved.
- Impact on health, wellness, and fitness
  - Health status is improved.
  - Physical capacity is increased.
  - Physical function is improved.
- Impact on societal resources
  - Utilization of physical therapy services is optimized.
  - Utilization of physical therapy services results in efficient use of health care dollars.
- Patient/client satisfaction
  - Access, availability, and services provided are acceptable to patient/client.
  - Administrative management of practice is acceptable to patient/client.
  - Clinical proficiency of physical therapist is acceptable to patient/client.
  - Coordination of care is acceptable to patient/client.
  - Cost of health care services is decreased.
  - Intensity of care is decreased.
  - Interpersonal skills of physical therapist are acceptable to patient/client, family, and significant others.
  - Sense of well-being is improved.
  - Stressors are decreased.

Functional Training in Work (Job/School/Play), Community, and Leisure Integration or Reintegration (Including Instrumental Activities of Daily Living [IADL], Work Hardening, and Work Conditioning)

Interventions

- Devices and equipment use and training
  - assistive and adaptive device or equipment training during IADL
  - orthotic, protective, or supportive device or equipment training during IADL
  - prosthetic device or equipment training during IADL
- Functional training programs
  - job coaching
  - simulated environments and tasks
  - task adaptation
  - task training
- IADL training
  - community service training involving instruments
  - school and play activities training including tools and instruments
  - work training with tools
- Injury prevention or reduction
  - injury prevention education during work (job/school/play), community, and leisure integration or reintegration
  - injury prevention or reduction with use of devices and equipment
  - safety awareness training during work (job/school/play), community, and leisure integration or reintegration

Anticipated Goals and Expected Outcomes

- Impact on pathology/pathophysiology (disease, disorder, or condition)
  - Pain is decreased.
  - Physiological response to increased oxygen demand is improved.
  - Symptoms associated with increased oxygen demand are decreased.
- Impact on impairments
  - Endurance is increased.
  - Energy expenditure per unit of work is decreased.
  - Muscle performance (strength, power, and endurance) is increased.
- Impact on functional limitations
  - Ability to perform physical actions, tasks, or activities related to work (job/school/play), community, and leisure integration or reintegration is improved.
  - Level of supervision required for task performance is decreased.
  - Performance of and independence in IADL with or without devices and equipment are increased.
  - Tolerance of positions and activities is increased.
- Impact on disabilities
  - Ability to assume or resume required work (job/school/play), community, and leisure roles is improved.
- Risk reduction/prevention
  - Risk factors are reduced.
  - Risk of secondary impairment is reduced.
  - Safety is improved.
  - Self-management of symptoms is improved.
- Impact on health, wellness, and fitness
  - Fitness is improved.
  - Health status is improved.
  - Physical capacity is increased.
  - Physical function is improved.
- Impact on societal resources
  - Costs of work-related injury or disability are reduced.
  - Utilization of physical therapy services is optimized.
  - Utilization of physical therapy services results in efficient use of health care dollars.
- Patient/client satisfaction
  - Access, availability, and services provided are acceptable to patient/client.
  - Administrative management of practice is acceptable to patient/client.
  - Clinical proficiency of physical therapist is acceptable to patient/client.
  - Coordination of care is acceptable to patient/client.
  - Cost of health care services is decreased.
  - Intensity of care is decreased.
  - Interpersonal skills of physical therapist are acceptable to patient/client, family, and significant others.
  - Sense of well-being is improved.
  - Stressors are decreased.

Manual Therapy Techniques (Including Mobilization/Manipulation)

Interventions

- Massage
  - connective tissue massage
  - therapeutic massage
- Mobilization/manipulation
  - soft tissue
- Passive range of motion

Anticipated Goals and Expected Outcomes

- Impact on pathology/pathophysiology (disease, disorder, or condition)
  - Edema, lymphedema, or effusion is reduced.
  - Joint swelling, inflammation, or restriction is reduced.
  - Pain is decreased.
  - Soft tissue swelling, inflammation, or restriction is reduced.
- Impact on impairments
  - Airway clearance is improved.
  - Energy expenditure per unit of work is decreased.
  - Gait, locomotion, and balance are improved.
  - Integumentary integrity is improved.
  - Joint integrity and mobility are improved.
  - Muscle performance (strength, power, and endurance) is increased.
  - Range of motion is improved.
  - Relaxation is increased.
- Impact on functional limitations
  - Ability to perform movement tasks is improved.
  - Ability to perform physical actions, tasks, or activities related to self-care, home management, work (job/school/play), community, and leisure is improved.
  - Tolerance of positions and activities is increased.
- Impact on disabilities
  - Ability to assume or resume required self-care, home management, work (job/school/play), community, and leisure roles is improved.
- Risk reduction/prevention
  - Risk factors are reduced.
  - Risk of recurrence of condition is reduced.
  - Risk of secondary impairment is reduced.
  - Self-management of symptoms is improved.
- Impact on health, wellness, and fitness
  - Physical capacity is increased.
  - Physical function is improved.
- Impact on societal resources
  - Utilization of physical therapy services is optimized.
  - Utilization of physical therapy services results in efficient use of health care dollars.
- Patient/client satisfaction
  - Access, availability, and services provided are acceptable to patient/client.
  - Administrative management of practice is acceptable to patient/client.
  - Clinical proficiency of physical therapist is acceptable to patient/client.
  - Coordination of care is acceptable to patient/client.
  - Cost of health care services is decreased.
  - Intensity of care is decreased.
  - Interpersonal skills of physical therapist are acceptable to patient/client, family, and significant others.
  - Sense of well-being is improved.
  - Stressors are decreased.

Prescription, Application, and, as Appropriate, Fabrication of Devices and Equipment (Assistive, Adaptive, Orthotic, Protective, Supportive, and Prosthetic)

Interventions

- Adaptive devices
  - environmental controls
  - hospital beds
  - raised toilet seats
  - seating systems
- Assistive devices
  - canes
  - crutches
  - long-handled reachers
  - power devices
  - static and dynamic splints
  - walkers
  - wheelchairs
- Orthotic devices
  - braces
  - shoe inserts
  - splints
- Protective devices
  - braces
  - cushions
- Supportive devices
  - compression garments
  - elastic wraps
  - mechanical ventilators
  - neck collars
  - supplemental oxygen

Anticipated Goals and Expected Outcomes

- Impact on pathology/pathophysiology (disease, disorder, or condition)
  - Edema, lymphedema, or effusion is reduced.
  - Joint swelling, inflammation, or restriction is reduced.
  - Pain is decreased.
  - Physiological response to increased oxygen demand is improved.
  - Soft tissue swelling, inflammation, or restriction is reduced.
  - Symptoms associated with increased oxygen demand are decreased.
- Impact on impairments
  - Balance is improved.
  - Endurance is increased.
  - Energy expenditure per unit of work is decreased.
  - Gait, locomotion, and balance are improved.
  - Integumentary integrity is improved.
  - Joint stability is improved.
  - Muscle performance (strength, power, and endurance) is increased.
  - Optimal joint alignment is achieved.
  - Optimal loading on a body part is achieved.
  - Work of breathing is decreased.
- Impact on functional limitations
  - Ability to perform physical actions, tasks, or activities related to self-care, home management, work (job/school/play), community, and leisure is improved.
  - Level of supervision required for task performance is decreased.
  - Performance of and independence in activities of daily living (ADL) and instrumental activities of daily living (IADL) with or without devices and equipment are increased.
  - Tolerance of positions and activities is improved.
- Impact on disabilities
  - Ability to assume or resume required self-care, home management, work (job/school/play), community, and leisure roles is improved.
- Risk reduction/prevention
  - Pressure on body tissues is reduced.
  - Protection of body parts is increased.
  - Risk factors are reduced.
  - Risk of secondary impairment is reduced.
  - Safety is improved.
  - Self-management of symptoms is improved.
- Impact on health, wellness, and fitness
  - Health status is improved.
  - Physical capacity is increased.
  - Physical function is improved.
- Impact on societal resources
  - Utilization of physical therapy services is optimized.
  - Utilization of physical therapy services results in efficient use of health care dollars.
- Patient/client satisfaction
  - Access, availability, and services provided are acceptable to patient/client.
  - Administrative management of practice is acceptable to patient/client.
  - Clinical proficiency of physical therapist is acceptable to patient/client.
  - Coordination of care is acceptable to patient/client.
  - Cost of health care services is decreased.
  - Intensity of care is decreased.
  - Interpersonal skills of physical therapist are acceptable to patient/client, family, and significant others.
  - Sense of well-being is improved.
  - Stressors are decreased.

Airway Clearance Techniques

Interventions

- Breathing strategies
  - active cycle of breathing or forced expiratory techniques
  - paced breathing
  - pursed lip breathing
  - techniques to maximize ventilation (eg, maximum inspiratory hold, stair case breathing, manual hyperinflation)
- Positioning
  - positioning to alter work of breathing
  - positioning to maximize ventilation and perfusion

Anticipated Goals and Expected Outcomes

- Impact on pathology/pathophysiology (disease, disorder, or condition)
  - Atelectasis is decreased.
  - Tissue perfusion and oxygenation are enhanced.
- Impact on impairments
  - Airway clearance is improved.
  - Cough is improved.
  - Endurance is increased.
  - Energy expenditure per unit of work is decreased.
  - Exercise tolerance is improved.
  - Ventilation and respiration/gas exchange are improved.
  - Work of breathing is decreased.
- Impact on functional limitations
  - Ability to perform physical actions, tasks, or activities related to self-care, home management, work (job/school/play), community, and leisure is improved.
  - Performance of and independence in activities of daily living (ADL) and instrumental activities of daily living (IADL) with or without devices and equipment are increased.
- Impact on disabilities
  - Ability to assume or resume required self-care, home management, work (job/school/play), community, and leisure roles is improved.
- Risk reduction/prevention
  - Risk factors are reduced.
  - Risk of secondary impairment is reduced.
  - Self-management of symptoms is improved.
- Impact on health, wellness, and fitness
  - Health status is improved.
  - Physical capacity is increased.
  - Physical function is improved.
- Impact on societal resources
  - Utilization of physical therapy services is optimized.
  - Utilization of physical therapy services results in efficient use of health care dollars.
- Patient/client satisfaction
  - Access, availability, and services provided are acceptable to patient/client.
  - Administrative management of practice is acceptable to patient/client.
  - Clinical proficiency of physical therapist is acceptable to patient/client.
  - Coordination of care is acceptable to patient/client.
  - Cost of health care services is decreased.
  - Intensity of care is decreased.
  - Interpersonal skills of physical therapist are acceptable to patient/client, family, and significant others.
  - Sense of well-being is improved.
  - Stressors are decreased.

Reexamination

Reexamination is the process of performing selected tests and measures after the initial examination to evaluate progress and to modify or redirect interventions. Reexamination may be indicated more than once during a single episode of care. It also may be performed over the course of a disease, disorder, or condition, which for some patients/clients may be over the life span. Indications for reexamination include new clinical findings or failure to respond to physical therapy interventions.

Global Outcomes for Patients/Clients in This Pattern

Throughout the entire episode of care, the physical therapist determines the anticipated goals and expected outcomes for each intervention. These anticipated goals and expected outcomes are delineated in shaded boxes that accompany the lists of interventions in each preferred practice pattern. As the patient/client reaches the termination of physical therapy services and the end of the episode of care, the physical therapist measures the global outcomes of the physical therapy services by characterizing or quantifying the impact of the physical therapy interventions in the following domains:

- Pathology/pathophysiology (disease, disorder, or condition)
- Impairments
- Functional limitations
- Disabilities
- Risk reduction/prevention
- Health, wellness, and fitness
- Societal resources
- Patient/client satisfaction

In some instances, a particular anticipated goal or expected outcome is thoroughly achieved through implementation of a single form of intervention. More commonly, however, the anticipated goals and expected outcomes are achieved as a result of the combined effects of several forms of interventions, leading to enhancement of both health status and health-related quality of life.

Criteria for Termination of Physical Therapy Services

Discharge is the process of ending physical therapy services that have been provided during a single episode of care. It occurs when the anticipated goals and expected outcomes have been achieved. Discharge does *not* occur with a *transfer* (defined as the time when a patient is moved from one site to another site within the same setting or across settings during a single episode of care). Although there may be facility-specific or payer-specific requirements for documentation regarding the conclusion of physical therapy services, *discharge occurs based on the physical therapist's analysis of the achievement of anticipated goals and expected outcomes.*

Discontinuation is the process of ending physical therapy services that have been provided during a single episode of care when (1) the patient/client, caregiver, or legal guardian declines to continue intervention; (2) the patient/client is unable to continue to progress toward outcomes because of medical or psychosocial complications or because financial/insurance resources have been expended; or (3) the physical therapist determines that the patient/client will no longer benefit from physical therapy. When physical therapy services are terminated prior to achievement of anticipated goals and expected outcomes, patient/client status and the rationale for termination are documented.

For patients/clients who require multiple episodes of care, periodic follow-up is needed over the life span to ensure safety and effective adaptation following changes in physical status, caregivers, environment, or task demands. In consultation with appropriate individuals, and in consideration of the outcomes, the physical therapist plans for discharge or discontinuation and provides for appropriate follow-up or referral.

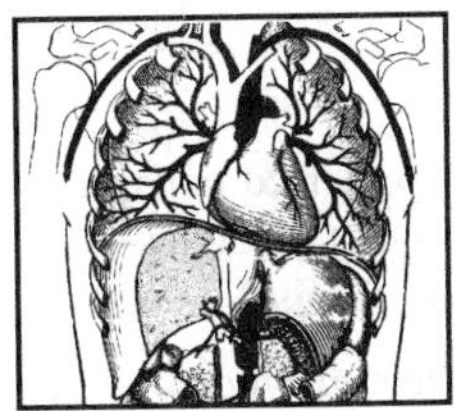

Impaired Ventilation and Respiration/ Gas Exchange Associated With Ventilatory Pump Dysfunction or Failure

This preferred practice pattern describes the generally accepted elements of patient/client management that physical therapists provide for patients/clients who are classified in this pattern. The pattern title reflects the diagnosis made by the physical therapist. APTA emphasizes that preferred practice patterns are the boundaries within which a physical therapist may select any of a number of clinical alternatives, based on consideration of a wide variety of factors, such as individual patient/client needs; the profession's code of ethics and standards of practice; and patient/client age, culture, gender roles, race, sex, sexual orientation, and socioeconomic status.

Patient/Client Diagnostic Classification

Patients/clients will be classified into this pattern—for impaired ventilation and respiration/gas exchange associated with ventilatory pump dysfunction or failure—as a result of the physical therapist's evaluation of the examination data. The findings from the examination (history, systems review, and tests and measures) may indicate the presence or risk of pathology/pathophysiology (disease, disorder, or condition), impairments, functional limitations, or disabilities or the need for health, wellness, or fitness programs. The physical therapist integrates, synthesizes, and interprets the data to determine the diagnostic classification.

Inclusion

The following examples of examination findings may support the inclusion of patients/clients in this pattern:

Risk Factors or Consequences of Pathology/Pathophysiology (Disease, Disorder, or Condition)

- Elevated diaphragm and volume loss on chest radiograph
- Neuromuscular disorders
- Partial or complete diaphragmatic paralysis
- Poliomyelitis
- Pulmonary fibrosis
- Restrictive lung disease
- Severe kyphoscoliosis
- Spinal/cerebral neoplasm
- Spinal cord injury

Impairments, Functional Limitations, or Disabilities

- Abnormal or adventitious breath sounds
- Abnormal increased respiratory rate and decreased tidal volume at rest
- Airway clearance dysfunction secondary to ventilatory pump impairment
- Decreased to severely impaired strength and endurance of ventilatory muscles
- Dyspnea with self-care
- Dyspnea with work tasks
- Dyssynchronous or paradoxical breathing at rest or with activity
- Progressive decrease in arterial oxygen and increase in carbon dioxide off ventilator
- Ventilatory pump impairment requiring assistive ventilatory support to maintain gas exchange

Note:

Some risk factors or consequences of pathology/pathophysiology—such as *spinal cord injury with joint contracture*—may be severe and complex; *however, they do not necessarily exclude patients/clients from this pattern.* Severe and complex risk factors or consequences may require modification of the frequency of visits and duration of care. (See "Evaluation, Diagnosis, and Prognosis," page 527.)

Exclusion or Multiple-Pattern Classification

The following examples of examination findings may support exclusion from this pattern or classification into additional patterns. Depending on the level of severity or complexity of the examination findings, the physical therapist may determine that the patient/client would be more appropriately managed through (1) classification in an entirely different pattern or (2) classification in both this and another pattern.

Findings That May Require Classification in a Different Pattern

- Impairments associated with acute pneumonia
- Impairments associated with acute respiratory failure
- Impairments associated with primary airway clearance disorders

Findings That May Require Classification in Additional Patterns

- Cardiothoracic surgery
- Decubitus ulcer

ICD-9-CM Codes

The listing below contains the current (as of press time) and most typical 3- and 4-digit ICD-9-CM codes related to this preferred practice pattern. Because patient/client diagnostic classification is based on impairments, functional limitations, and disabilities—not on codes—patients/clients may be classified into the pattern even though the codes listed with the pattern may not apply to those clients.

This listing is intended for general information only and should not be used for coding purposes. The codes should be confirmed by referring to the World Health Organization's *International Classification of Diseases, 9th Revision, Clinical Modification (ICD-9-CM 2001)*, Volumes 1 and 3 (Chicago, Ill: American Medical Association; 2000) or subsequent revisions or by referring to other ICD-9-CM coding manuals that contain exclusion notes and instructions regarding fifth-digit requirements.

045 Acute poliomyelitis

192 Malignant neoplasm of other and unspecified parts of nervous system

- **192.2** Spinal cord
  - Cauda equina

237 Neoplasm of uncertain behavior of endocrine glands and nervous system

- **237.5** Brain and spinal cord

239 Neoplasms of unspecified nature

- **239.9** Site unspecified

277 Other and unspecified disorders of metabolism

- **277.0** Cystic fibrosis

332 Parkinson's disease

333 Other extrapyramidal disease and abnormal movement disorders

- **333.4** Huntington's chorea

334 Spinocerebellar disease

- **334.2** Primary cerebellar degeneration

335 Anterior horn cell disease

- **335.2** Motor neuron disease
  - **335.20** Amyotrophic lateral sclerosis

340 Multiple sclerosis

343 Infantile cerebral palsy

344 Other paralytic syndromes

- **344.0** Quadriplegia and quadriparesis

348 Other conditions of brain

- **348.1** Anoxic brain damage

357 Inflammatory and toxic neuropathy

- **357.0** Acute infective polyneuritis
  - Guillain-Barré syndrome

359 Muscular dystrophies and other myopathies

- **359.1** Hereditary progressive muscular dystrophy

430 Subarachnoid hemorrhage

431 Intracerebral hemorrhage

432 Other and unspecified intracranial hemorrhage

434 Occlusion of cerebral arteries

- **434.1** Cerebral embolism

492 Emphysema

- **492.8** Other emphysema

493 Asthma

505 Pneumoconiosis, unspecified

515 Postinflammatory pulmonary fibrosis

518 Other diseases of lung

519 Other diseases of respiratory system

- **519.4** Disorders of diaphragm

737 Curvature of spine

- **737.3** Kyphoscoliosis and scoliosis

786 Symptoms involving respiratory system and other chest symptoms

- **786.0** Dyspnea and respiratory abnormalities
- **786.9** Other symptoms involving respiratory system and chest

852 Subarachnoid, subdural, and extradural hemorrhage, following injury

853 Other and unspecified intracranial hemorrhage following injury

854 Intracranial injury of other and unspecified nature

941 Burn of face, head, and neck

942 Burn of trunk

946 Burns of multiple specified sites

947 Burn of internal organs

948 Burns classified according to extent of body surface involved

949 Burn, unspecified

977 Poisoning by other and unspecified drugs and medicinal substances

- **977.9** Unspecified drug or medicinal substance

Note:

Patients/clients who have nonsurgical procedures such as intubation, irrigation, and other continuous mechanical ventilation also may be classified into this pattern.

Examination

Examination is a comprehensive screening and specific testing process that leads to a diagnostic classification or, when appropriate, to a referral to another practitioner. Examination is required prior to the initial intervention and is performed for all patients/clients. Through the examination, the physical therapist may identify impairments, functional limitations, disabilities, changes in physical function or overall health status, and needs related to restoration of health and to prevention, wellness, and fitness. The physical therapist synthesizes the examination findings to establish the diagnosis and the prognosis (including the plan of care). The patient/client, family, significant others, and caregivers may provide information during the examination process.

Examination has three components: the patient/client history, the systems review, and tests and measures. The *history* is a systematic gathering of past and current information (often from the patient/client) related to why the patient/client is seeking the services of the physical therapist. The *systems review* is a brief or limited examination of (1) the anatomical and physiological status of the cardiovascular/pulmonary, integumentary, musculoskeletal, and neuromuscular systems and (2) the communication ability, affect, cognition, language, and learning style of the patient/client. *Tests and measures* are the means of gathering data about the patient/client.

The selection of examination procedures and the depth of the examination vary based on patient/client age; severity of the problem; stage of recovery (acute, subacute, chronic); phase of rehabilitation (early, intermediate, late, return to activity); home, work (job/school/play), or community situation; and other relevant factors. *For clinical indications in selecting tests and measures and for listings of tests and measures, tools used to gather data, and the types of data generated by tests and measures, refer to Chapter 2.*

Patient/Client History

The history may include:

General Demographics

- Age
- Sex
- Race/ethnicity
- Primary language
- Education

Social History

- Cultural beliefs and behaviors
- Family and caregiver resources
- Social interactions, social activities, and support systems

Employment/Work (Job/School/Play)

- Current and prior work (job/school/play), community, and leisure actions, tasks, or activities

Growth and Development

- Developmental history
- Hand dominance

Living Environment

- Devices and equipment (eg, assistive, adaptive, orthotic, protective, supportive, prosthetic)
- Living environment and community characteristics
- Projected discharge destinations

General Health Status (Self-Report, Family Report, Caregiver Report)

- General health perception
- Physical function (eg, mobility, sleep patterns, restricted bed days)
- Psychological function (eg, memory, reasoning ability, depression, anxiety)
- Role function (eg, community, leisure, social, work)
- Social function (eg, social activity, social interaction, social support)

Social/Health Habits (Past and Current)

- Behavioral health risks (eg, smoking, drug abuse)
- Level of physical fitness

Family History

- Familial health risks

Medical/Surgical History

- Cardiovascular
- Endocrine/metabolic
- Gastrointestinal
- Genitourinary
- Gynecological
- Integumentary
- Musculoskeletal
- Neuromuscular
- Obstetrical
- Prior hospitalizations, surgeries, and preexisting medical and other health-related conditions
- Psychological
- Pulmonary

Current Condition(s)/Chief Complaint(s)

- Concerns that led patient/client to seek the services of a physical therapist
- Concerns or needs of patient/client who requires the services of a physical therapist
- Current therapeutic interventions
- Mechanisms of injury or disease, including date of onset and course of events
- Onset and pattern of symptoms
- Patient/client, family, significant other, and caregiver expectations and goals for the therapeutic intervention
- Patient/client, family, significant other, and caregiver perceptions of patient's/client's emotional response to the current clinical situation
- Previous occurrence of chief complaint(s)
- Prior therapeutic interventions

Functional Status and Activity Level

- Current and prior functional status in self-care and home management activities, including activities of daily living (ADL) and instrumental activities of daily living (IADL)
- Current and prior functional status in work (job/school/play), community, and leisure actions, tasks, or activities

Medications

- Medications for current condition
- Medications previously taken for current condition
- Medications for other conditions

Other Clinical Tests

- Laboratory and diagnostic tests
- Review of available records (eg, medical, education, surgical)
- Review of other clinical findings (eg, nutrition and hydration)

Systems Review

The systems review may include:

Anatomical and Physiological Status

- Cardiovascular/Pulmonary
  - Blood pressure
  - Edema
  - Heart rate
  - Respiratory rate
- Integumentary
  - Pliability (texture)
  - Presence of scar formation
  - Skin color
  - Skin integrity
- Musculoskeletal
  - Gross range of motion
  - Gross strength
  - Gross symmetry
  - Height
  - Weight
- Neuromuscular
  - Gross coordinated movements (eg, balance, gait, locomotion, transfers, transitions)
  - Motor function (motor control, motor learning)

Communication, Affect, Cognition, Language, and Learning Style

- Ability to make needs known
- Consciousness
- Expected emotional/behavioral responses
- Learning preferences (eg, education needs, learning barriers)
- Orientation (person, place, time)

Tests and Measures

Tests and measures for this pattern may include those that characterize or quantify:

Aerobic Capacity and Endurance

- Aerobic capacity during functional activities (eg, activities of daily living [ADL] scales, indexes, instrumental activities of daily living [IADL] scales, observations)
- Aerobic capacity during standardized exercise test protocols (eg, ergometry, step tests, time/distance walk/run tests, treadmill tests, wheelchair tests)
- Cardiovascular signs and symptoms in response to increased oxygen demand with exercise or activity, including pressures and flow; heart rate, rhythm, and sounds; and superficial vascular responses (eg, angina, claudication, and exertion scales; electrocardiography; observations; palpation; sphygmomanometry)
- Pulmonary signs and symptoms in response to increased oxygen demand with exercise or activity, including breath and voice sounds; cyanosis; gas exchange; respiratory pattern, rate, and rhythm; and ventilatory flow, force, and volume (eg, auscultation, dyspnea and exertion scales, gas analyses, observations, oximetry, palpation, pulmonary function tests)

Anthropometric Characteristics

- Body dimensions (eg, girth measurement, length measurement)
- Edema (eg, girth measurement, palpation, scales, volume measurement)

Arousal, Attention, and Cognition

- Arousal and attention (eg, adaptability tests, arousal and awareness scales, indexes, profiles, questionnaires)
- Cognition, including ability to process commands (eg, developmental inventories, indexes, interviews, mental state scales, observations, questionnaires, safety checklists)
- Motivation (eg, adaptive behavior scales)
- Orientation to time, person, place, and situation (eg, attention tests, learning profiles, mental state scales)
- Recall, including memory and retention (eg, assessment scales, interviews, questionnaires)

Assistive and Adaptive Devices

- Assistive or adaptive devices and equipment use during functional activities (eg, ADL scales, functional scales, IADL scales, interviews, observations)
- Components, alignment, fit, and ability to care for assistive or adaptive devices and equipment (eg, interviews, logs, observations, reports)
- Remediation of impairments, functional limitations, or disabilities with use of assistive or adaptive devices and equipment (eg, activity status indexes, ADL scales, aerobic capacity tests, functional performance inventories, health assessment questionnaires, IADL scales, pain scales, play scales, videographic assessments)
- Safety during use of assistive or adaptive devices and equipment (eg, diaries, fall scales, interviews, logs, observations, reports)

Circulation (Arterial, Venous, and Lymphatic)

- Cardiovascular signs, including heart rate, rhythm, and sounds; pressures and flow; and superficial vascular responses (eg, auscultation, electrocardiography, girth measurement, observations, palpation, sphygmomanometry, thermography)
- Cardiovascular symptoms (eg, angina, claudication, and perceived exertion scales)
- Physiological responses to position change, including autonomic responses, central and peripheral pressures, heart rate and rhythm, respiratory rate and rhythm, ventilatory pattern (eg, auscultation, electrocardiography, observations, palpation, sphygmomanometry)

Cranial Nerve Integrity

- Motor distribution of the cranial nerves (eg, dynamometry, muscle tests, observations)
- Response to stimuli, including auditory, gustatory, olfactory, pharyngeal, vestibular, and visual (eg, observations, provocation tests)

Environmental, Home, and Work (Job/School/Play) Barriers

- Current and potential barriers (eg, checklists, interviews, observations, questionnaires)
- Physical space and environment (eg, compliance standards, observations, photographic assessments, questionnaires, structural specifications, videographic assessments)

Ergonomics and Body Mechanics

Ergonomics

- Functional capacity and performance during work actions, tasks, or activities (eg, accelerometry, dynamometry, electroneuromyography, endurance tests, force platform tests, goniometry, interviews, observations, photographic assessments, physical capacity tests, postural loading analyses, technology-assisted assessments, videographic assessments, work analyses)
- Safety in work environments (eg, hazard identification checklists, job severity indexes, lifting standards, risk assessment scales, standards for exposure limits)

Gait, Locomotion, and Balance

- Balance during functional activities with or without the use of assistive, adaptive, orthotic, protective, supportive, or prosthetic devices or equipment (eg, ADL scales, IADL scales, observations, videographic assessments)
- Balance (dynamic and static) with or without the use of assistive, adaptive, orthotic, protective, supportive, or prosthetic devices or equipment (eg, balance scales, dizziness inventories, dynamic posturography, fall scales, motor impairment tests, observations, photographic assessments, postural control tests)
- Gait and locomotion during functional activities with or without the use of assistive, adaptive, orthotic, protective, supportive, or prosthetic devices or equipment (eg, ADL scales, gait indexes, IADL scales, mobility skill profiles, observations, videographic assessments)
- Safety during gait, locomotion, and balance (eg, confidence scales, diaries, fall scales, functional assessment profiles, logs, reports)

Integumentary Integrity

Associated skin

- Activities, positioning, and postures that produce or relieve trauma to the skin (eg, observations, pressure-sensing maps, scales)
- Assistive, adaptive, orthotic, protective, supportive, or prosthetic devices and equipment that may produce or relieve trauma to the skin (eg, observations, pressure-sensing maps, risk assessment scales)
- Skin characteristics, including blistering, continuity of skin color, dermatitis, hair growth, mobility, nail growth, sensation, temperature, texture, and turgor (eg, observations, palpation, photographic assessments, thermography)

Wound

- Signs of infection (eg, cultures, observations, palpation)
- Wound scar tissue characteristics, including banding, pliability, sensation, and texture (eg, observations, scar-rating scales)

Joint Integrity and Mobility

- Joint play movements, including end feel (all joints of the axial and appendicular skeletal system) (eg, palpation)

Muscle Performance (Including Strength, Power, and Endurance)

- Electrophysiological integrity (eg, electroneuromyography)
- Muscle strength, power, and endurance (eg, dynamometry, manual muscle tests, muscle performance tests, physical capacity tests, technology-assisted assessments, timed activity tests)
- Muscle strength, power, and endurance during functional activities (eg, ADL scales, functional muscle tests, IADL scales, observations, videographic assessments)

Neuromotor Development and Sensory Integration

- Oral motor function, phonation, and speech production (eg, interviews, observations)

Orthotic, Protective, and Supportive Devices

- Components, alignment, fit, and ability to care for orthotic, protective, and supportive devices and equipment (eg, interviews, logs, observations, pressure-sensing maps, reports)
- Orthotic, protective, and supportive devices and equipment use during functional activities (eg, ADL scales, functional scales, IADL scales, interviews, observations, profiles)
- Remediation of impairments, functional limitations, or disabilities with use of orthotic, protective, and supportive devices and equipment (eg, activity status indexes, ADL scales, aerobic capacity tests, functional performance inventories, health assessment questionnaires, IADL scales, pain scales, play scales, videographic assessments)
- Safety during use of orthotic, protective, and supportive devices and equipment (eg, diaries, fall scales, interviews, logs, observations, reports)

Pain

- Pain, soreness, and nociception (eg, angina scales, analog scales, discrimination tests, pain drawings and maps, provocation tests, verbal and pictorial descriptor tests)

Posture

- Postural alignment and position (static and dynamic), including symmetry and deviation from midline (eg, grid measurement, observations, photographic assessments, technology-assisted assessments, videographic assessments)
- Specific body parts (eg, angle assessments, forward-bending test, goniometry, observations, palpation, positional tests)

Range of Motion (ROM) (Including Muscle Length)

- Functional ROM (eg, observations)
- Joint active and passive movement (eg, goniometry, inclinometry, observations, photographic assessments, technology-assisted assessments, videographic assessments)
- Muscle length, soft tissue extensibility, and flexibility (eg, contracture tests, goniometry, inclinometry, ligamentous tests, linear measurement, multisegment flexibility tests, palpation)

Reflex Integrity

- Deep reflexes (eg, myotatic reflex scale, observations, reflex tests)
- Electrophysiological integrity (eg, electroneuromyography)
- Superficial reflexes and reactions (eg, observations, provocation tests)

Self-Care and Home Management (Including ADL and IADL)

- Ability to gain access to home environments (eg, barrier identification, observations, physical performance tests)
- Ability to perform self-care and home management activities with or without assistive, adaptive, orthotic, protective, supportive, or prosthetic devices and equipment (eg,ADL scales, aerobic capacity tests, IADL scales, interviews, observations, profiles)
- Safety in self-care and home management activities and environments (eg, diaries, fall scales, interviews, logs, observations, reports, videographic assessments)

Sensory Integrity

- Electrophysiological integrity (eg,electroneuromyography)

Ventilation and Respiration/Gas Exchange

- Pulmonary signs of respiration/gas exchange, including breath sounds (eg, gas analyses, observations, oximetry)
- Pulmonary signs of ventilatory function, including airway protection; breath and voice sounds; respiratory rate, rhythm, and pattern; ventilatory flow, forces, and volumes (eg, airway clearance tests, observations, palpation, pulmonary function tests, ventilatory muscle force tests)
- Pulmonary symptoms (eg, dyspnea and perceived exertion indexes and scales)

Work (Job/School/Play), Community, and Leisure Integration or Reintegration (Including Instrumental Activities of Daily Living [IADL])

- Ability to assume or resume work (job/school/play), community, and leisure activities with or without assistive, adaptive, orthotic, protective, supportive, or prosthetic devices and equipment (eg, activity profiles, disability indexes, functional status questionnaires, IADL scales, observations, physical capacity tests)
- Ability to gain access to work (job/school/play), community, and leisure environments (eg, barrier identification, interviews, observations, physical capacity tests, transportation assessments)
- Safety in work (job/school/play), community, and leisure activities and environments (eg, diaries, fall scales, interviews, logs, observations, videographic assessments)

Evaluation, Diagnosis, and Prognosis (Including Plan of Care)

Physical therapists perform *evaluations* (make clinical judgments) based on the data gathered from the history, systems review, and tests and measures. In the evaluation process, physical therapists synthesize the examination data to establish the diagnosis and prognosis (including the plan of care). Factors that influence the complexity of the evaluation include the clinical findings, extent of loss of function, chronicity or severity of the problem, possibility of multisite or multisystem involvement, preexisting condition(s), potential discharge destination, social considerations, physical function, and overall health status.

A *diagnosis* is a label encompassing a cluster of signs and symptoms, syndromes, or categories. It is the result of the systematic diagnostic process, which includes integrating and evaluating the data from the examination. The diagnostic label indicates the primary dysfunction(s) toward which the therapist will direct interventions. The *prognosis* is the determination of the predicted optimal level of improvement in function and the amount of time needed to reach that level and may also include a prediction of levels of improvement that may be reached at various intervals during the course of therapy. During the prognostic process, the physical therapist develops the plan of care. The *plan of care* identifies specific interventions, proposed frequency and duration of the interventions, anticipated goals, expected outcomes, and discharge plans. The plan of care identifies realistic anticipated goals and expected outcomes, taking into consideration the expectations of the patient/client and appropriate others. These anticipated goals and expected outcomes should be measureable and time limited.

The frequency of visits and duration of the episode of care may vary from a short episode with a high intensity of intervention to a longer episode with a diminishing intensity of intervention. Frequency and duration may vary greatly among patients/clients based on a variety of factors that the physical therapist considers throughout the evaluation process, such as anatomical and physiological changes related to growth and development; caregiver consistency or expertise; chronicity or severity of the current condition; living environment; multisite or multisystem involvement; social support; potential discharge destinations; probability of prolonged impairment, functional limitation, or disability; and stability of the condition.

Prognosis	Expected Range of Number of Visits Per Episode of Care	Factors That May Require New Episode of Care or That May Modify Frequency of Visits/ Duration of Episode
Over the course of 3 to 6 weeks, patient/client with ventilatory pump dysfunction or reversible ventilatory pump failure will demonstrate optimal independence with ventilation and respiration/gas exchange and the highest level of functioning in home, work (job/school/play), community, and leisure environments, within the context of the impairments, functional limitations, and disabilities.	**5 to 20**	• Accessibility and availability of resources • Adherence to the intervention program • Age • Anatomical and physiological changes related to growth and development • Caregiver consistency or expertise • Chronicity or severity of the current condition • Cognitive status • Comorbitities, complications, or secondary impairments • Concurrent medical, surgical, and therapeutic interventions • Decline in functional independence • Level of impairment • Level of physical function • Living environment • Multisite or multisystem involvement • Nutritional status • Overall health status • Potential discharge destinations • Premorbid conditions • Probability of prolonged impairment, functional limitation, or disability • Psychological and socioeconomic factors • Psychomotor abilities • Social support • Stability of the condition
Over the course of 8 to10 weeks, patient/client with prolonged, severe, or chronic ventilatory pump failure will demonstrate optimal independence with ventilation and respiration/gas exchange and the highest level of functioning in home, work (job/school/play), community, and leisure environments, within the context of the impairments, functional limitations, and disabilities.	**20 to 60** These ranges represent the lower and upper limits of the number of physical therapist visits required to achieve anticipated goals and expected outcomes. *It is anticipated that 80% of patients/clients who are classified into this pattern will achieve the anticipated goals and expected outcomes within these ranges during a single continuous episode of care.* Frequency of visits and duration of the episode of care should be determined by the physical therapist to maximize effectiveness of care and efficiency of service delivery.	
During the episode of care, patient/client with ventilatory pump dysfunction, with reversible ventilatory pump failure, or with prolonged, severe, or chronic ventilatory pump failure will achieve (1) the anticipated goals and expected outcomes of the interventions that are described in the plan of care and (2) the global outcomes for patients/ clients who are classified in this pattern.		

Intervention

Intervention is the purposeful interaction of the physical therapist with the patient/client and, when appropriate, with other individuals involved in patient/client care, using various physical therapy procedures and techniques to produce changes in the condition consistent with the diagnosis and prognosis. Decisions about interventions are contingent on the timely monitoring of patient/client response and the progress made toward achieving the anticipated goals and expected outcomes.

Communication, coordination, and documentation and patient/client-related instruction are provided for all patients/clients across all settings. Procedural interventions are selected or modified based on the examination data and the evaluation, the diagnosis and the prognosis, and the anticipated goals and expected outcomes for a particular patient/client. *For clinical considerations in selecting interventions, listings of interventions, and listings of anticipated goals and expected outcomes, refer to Chapter 3.*

Coordination, Communication, and Documentation

Coordination, communication, and documentation may include:

Interventions

- Addressing required functions
  - advance directives
  - individualized family service plans (IFSPs) or individualized education plans (IEPs)
  - informed consent
  - mandatory communication and reporting (eg, patient advocacy and abuse reporting)
- Admission and discharge planning
- Case management
- Collaboration and coordination with agencies, including:
  - equipment suppliers
  - home care agencies
  - payer groups
  - schools
  - transportation agencies
- Communication across settings, including:
  - case conferences
  - documentation
- Cost-effective resource utilization
- Data collection, analysis, and reporting
  - outcome data
  - peer review findings
  - record reviews
- Documentation across settings, following APTA's *Guidelines for Physical Therapy Documentation* (Appendix 5), including:
  - changes in impairments, functional limitations, and disabilities
  - changes in interventions
  - elements of patient/client management (examination, evaluation, diagnosis, prognosis, intervention)
  - outcomes of intervention
- Interdisciplinary teamwork
  - case conferences
  - patient care rounds
  - patient/client family meetings
- Referrals to other professionals or resources

Anticipated Goals and Expected Outcomes

- Accountability for services is increased.
- Admission data and discharge planning are completed.
- Advance directives, individualized family service plans (IFSPs) or individualized education plans (IEPs), informed consent, and mandatory communication and reporting (eg, patient advocacy and abuse reporting) are obtained or completed.
- Available resources are maximally utilized.
- Care is coordinated with patient/client, family, significant others, caregivers, and other professionals.
- Case is managed throughout the episode of care.
- Collaboration and coordination occurs with agencies, including equipment suppliers, home care agencies, payer groups, schools, and transportation agencies.
- Communication enhances risk reduction and prevention.
- Communication occurs across settings through case conferences, and documentation.
- Data are collected, analyzed, and reported, including outcome data, peer review findings, and record reviews.
- Decision making is enhanced regarding health, wellness, and fitness needs.
- Decision making is enhanced regarding patient/client health and the use of health care resources by patient/client, family, significant others, and caregivers.
- Documentation occurs throughout patient/client management and across settings and follows APTA's *Guidelines for Physical Therapy Documentation* (Appendix 5).
- Interdisciplinary collaboration occurs through case conferences, patient care rounds, and patient/client family meetings.
- Patient/client, family, significant other, and caregiver understanding of anticipated goals and expected outcomes is increased.
- Placement needs are determined.
- Referrals are made to other professionals or resources whenever necessary and appropriate.
- Resources are utilized in a cost-effective way.

Patient/Client-Related Instruction

Patient/client-related instruction may include:

Interventions

- Instruction, education and training of patients/clients and caregivers regarding:
  - current condition (pathology/pathophysiology [disease, disorder, or condition], impairments, functional limitations, or disabilities)
  - enhancement of performance
  - health, wellness, and fitness programs
  - plan of care
  - risk factors for pathology/pathophysiology (disease, disorder, or condition), impairments, functional limitations, or disabilities
  - transitions across settings
  - transitions to new roles

Anticipated Goals and Expected Outcomes

- Ability to perform physical actions, tasks, or activities is improved.
- Awareness and use of community resources are improved.
- Behaviors that foster healthy habits, wellness, and prevention are acquired.
- Decision making is enhanced regarding patient/client health and the use of health care resources by patient/client, family, significant others, and caregivers.
- Disability associated with acute or chronic illnesses is reduced.
- Functional independence in activities of daily living (ADL) and instrumental activities of daily living (IADL) is increased.
- Health status is improved.
- Intensity of care is decreased.
- Level of supervision required for task performance is decreased.
- Patient/client, family, significant other, and caregiver knowledge and awareness of the diagnosis, prognosis, interventions, and anticipated goals and expected outcomes are increased.
- Patient/client knowledge of personal and environmental factors associated with the condition is increased.
- Performance levels in self-care, home management, work (job/school/play), community, or leisure actions, tasks, or activities are improved.
- Physical function is improved.
- Risk of recurrence of condition is reduced.
- Risk of secondary impairment is reduced.
- Safety of patient/client, family, significant others, and caregivers is improved.
- Self-management of symptoms is improved.
- Utilization and cost of health care services are decreased.

Procedural Interventions

Procedural interventions for this pattern may include:

Therapeutic Exercise

Interventions

- Aerobic capacity/endurance conditioning or reconditioning
  - gait and locomotor training
  - increased workload over time
  - movement efficiency and energy conservation training
  - walking and wheelchair propulsion programs
- Balance, coordination, and agility training
  - developmental activities training
  - motor function (motor control and motor learning) training or retraining
  - neuromuscular education or reeducation
  - posture awareness training
  - task-specific performance training
- Body mechanics and postural stabilization
  - body mechanics training
  - postural control training
  - postural stabilization activities
  - posture awareness training
- Flexibility exercises
  - muscle lengthening
  - range of motion
  - stretching
- Gait and locomotion training
  - developmental activities training
  - gait training
  - implement and device training
  - perceptual training
  - standardized, programmatic, complementary exercise approaches
  - wheelchair training
- Relaxation
  - breathing strategies
  - movement strategies
  - relaxation techniques
  - standardized, programmatic, complementary exercise approaches
- Strength, power, and endurance training for head, neck, limb, pelvic-floor, trunk, and ventilatory muscles
  - active assistive, active, and resistive exercises (including concentric, dynamic/isotonic, isometric, and plyometric)
  - task-specific performance training

Anticipated Goals and Expected Outcomes

- Impact on pathology/pathophysiology (disease, disorder, or condition)
  - Atelectasis is decreased.
  - Joint swelling, inflammation, or restriction is reduced.
  - Nutrient delivery to tissue is increased.
  - Osteogenic effects of exercise are maximized.
  - Pain is decreased.
  - Physiological response to increased oxygen demand is improved.
  - Soft tissue swelling, inflammation, or restriction is reduced.
  - Symptoms associated with increased oxygen demand are decreased.
  - Tissue perfusion and oxygenation are enhanced.
- Impact on impairments
  - Aerobic capacity is increased.
  - Airway clearance is improved.
  - Balance is improved.
  - Endurance is increased.
  - Energy expenditure per unit of work is decreased.
  - Gait, locomotion, and balance are improved.
  - Integumentary integrity is improved.
  - Joint integrity and mobility are improved.
  - Motor function (motor control and motor learning) is improved.
  - Muscle performance (strength, power, and endurance) is increased.
  - Postural control is improved.
  - Quality and quantity of movement between and across body segments are improved.
  - Range of motion is improved.
  - Relaxation is increased.
  - Sensory awareness is increased.
  - Ventilation and respiration/gas exchange are improved.
  - Weight-bearing status is improved.
  - Work of breathing is decreased.
- Impact on functional limitations
  - Ability to perform physical actions, tasks, or activities related to self-care, home management, work (job/school/play), community, and leisure is improved.
  - Level of supervision required for task performance is decreased.
  - Performance of and independence in activities of daily living (ADL) and instrumental activities of daily living (IADL) with or without devices and equipment are increased.
  - Tolerance of positions and activities is increased.
- Impact on disabilities
  - Ability to assume or resume required self-care, home management, work (job/school/play), community, and leisure roles is improved.
- Risk reduction/prevention
  - Risk factors are reduced.
  - Risk of secondary impairment is reduced.
  - Safety is improved.
  - Self-management of symptoms is improved.
- Impact on health, wellness, and fitness
  - Fitness is improved.
  - Health status is improved.
  - Physical capacity is increased.
  - Physical function is improved.
- Impact on societal resources
  - Utilization of physical therapy services is optimized.
  - Utilization of physical therapy services results in efficient use of health care dollars.
- Patient/client satisfaction
  - Access, availability, and services provided are acceptable to patient/client.
  - Administrative management of practice is acceptable to patient/client.
  - Clinical proficiency of physical therapist is acceptable to patient/client.
  - Coordination of care is acceptable to patient/client.
  - Cost of health care services is decreased.
  - Intensity of care is decreased.
  - Interpersonal skills of physical therapist are acceptable to patient/client, family, and significant others.
  - Sense of well-being is improved.
  - Stressors are decreased.

Functional Training in Self-Care and Home Management (Including Activities of Daily Living [ADL] and Instrumental Activities of Daily Living [IADL])

Interventions

- ADL training
  - bathing
  - bed mobility and transfer training
  - developmental activities
  - dressing
  - eating
  - grooming
  - toileting
- Devices and equipment use and training
  - assistive and adaptive device or equipment training during ADL and IADL
  - orthotic, protective, or supportive device or equipment training during ADL and IADL
  - prosthetic device or equipment training during ADL and IADL
- Functional training programs
  - simulated environments and tasks
  - task adaptation
- IADL training
  - caring for dependents
  - home maintenance
  - shopping
  - structured play for infants and children
- Injury prevention or reduction
  - injury prevention education during self-care and home management
  - injury prevention or reduction with use of devices and equipment
  - safety awareness training during self-care and home management

Anticipated Goals and Expected Outcomes

- Impact on pathology/pathophysiology (disease/disorder/condition)
  - Pain is decreased.
  - Physiological response to increased oxygen demand is improved.
  - Symptoms associated with increased oxygen demand are decreased.
- Impact on impairments
  - Balance is improved.
  - Endurance is increased.
  - Energy expenditure per unit of work is decreased.
  - Motor function (motor control and motor learning) is improved.
  - Muscle performance (strength, power, and endurance) is increased.
  - Postural control is improved.
  - Sensory awareness is increased.
  - Weight-bearing status is improved.
  - Work of breathing is decreased.
- Impact on functional limitations
  - Ability to perform physical actions, tasks, or activities related to self-care and home management is improved.
  - Level of supervision required for task performance is decreased.
  - Performance of and independence in ADL and IADL with or without devices and equipment are increased.
  - Tolerance of positions and activities is increased.
- Impact on disabilities
  - Ability to assume or resume required self-care and home management roles is improved.
- Risk reduction/prevention
  - Risk factors are reduced.
  - Risk of secondary impairments is reduced.
  - Safety is improved.
  - Self-management of symptoms is improved.
- Impact on health, wellness, and fitness
  - Health status is improved.
  - Physical capacity is increased.
  - Physical function is improved.
- Impact on societal resources
  - Utilization of physical therapy services results in efficient use of health care dollars.
  - Utilization of physical therapy services is optimized.
- Patient/client satisfaction
  - Access, availability, and services provided are acceptable to patient/client.
  - Administrative management of practice is acceptable to patient/client.
  - Clinical proficiency of physical therapist is acceptable to patient/client.
  - Coordination of care is acceptable to patient/client.
  - Cost of health care services is decreased.
  - Intensity of care is decreased.
  - Interpersonal skills of physical therapist are acceptable to patient/client, family, and significant others.
  - Sense of well-being is improved.
  - Stressors are decreased.

Functional Training in Work (Job/School/Play), Community, and Leisure Integration or Reintegration (Including Instrumental Activities of Daily Living [IADL], Work Hardening, and Work Conditioning)

Interventions

- Devices and equipment use and training
  - assistive and adaptive device or equipment training during IADL
  - orthotic, protective, or supportive device or equipment training during IADL
  - prosthetic device or equipment training during IADL
- Functional training programs
  - job coaching
  - simulated environments and tasks
  - task adaptation
  - task training
- IADL training
  - community service training involving instruments
  - school and play activities training including tools and instruments
  - work training with tools
- Injury prevention or reduction
  - injury prevention education during work (job/school/play), community, and leisure integration
  - injury prevention or reduction with use of devices and equipment
  - safety awareness training during work (job/school/play), community, and leisure integration

Anticipated Goals and Expected Outcomes

- Impact on pathology/pathophysiology (disease, disorder, or condition)
  - Pain is decreased.
  - Physiological response to increased oxygen demand is improved.
  - Symptoms associated with increased oxygen demand are decreased.
- Impact on impairments
  - Balance is improved.
  - Endurance is increased.
  - Energy expenditure per unit of work is decreased.
  - Motor function (motor control and motor learning) is improved.
  - Muscle performance (strength, power, and endurance) is increased.
  - Postural control is improved.
  - Sensory awareness is increased.
  - Weight-bearing status is improved.
  - Work of breathing is decreased.
- Impact on functional limitations
  - Ability to perform physical actions, tasks, or activities related to work (job/school/play), community, and leisure integration or reintegration is improved.
  - Level of supervision required for task performance is decreased.
  - Performance of and independence in IADL with or without devices and equipment are increased.
  - Tolerance of positions and activities is increased.
- Impact on disabilities
  - Ability to assume or resume required work (job/school/play), community, and leisure roles is improved.
- Risk reduction/prevention
  - Risk factors are reduced.
  - Risk of secondary impairment is reduced.
  - Safety is improved.
  - Self-management of symptoms is improved.
- Impact on health, wellness, and fitness
  - Fitness is improved.
  - Health status is improved.
  - Physical capacity is increased.
  - Physical function is improved.
- Impact on societal resources
  - Costs of work-related injury or disability are reduced.
  - Utilization of physical therapy services is optimized.
  - Utilization of physical therapy services results in efficient use of health care dollars.
- Patient/client satisfaction
  - Access, availability, and services provided are acceptable to patient/client.
  - Administrative management of practice is acceptable to patient/client.
  - Clinical proficiency of physical therapist is acceptable to patient/client.
  - Coordination of care is acceptable to patient/client.
  - Cost of health care services is decreased.
  - Intensity of care is decreased.
  - Interpersonal skills of physical therapist are acceptable to patient/client, family, and significant others.
  - Sense of well-being is improved.
  - Stressors are decreased.

Manual Therapy Techniques (Including Mobilization/Manipulation)

Interventions

- Massage
  - connective tissue massage
  - therapeutic massage
- Mobilization/manipulation
  - soft tissue
  - spinal and peripheral joints
- Passive range of motion

Anticipated Goals and Expected Outcomes

- Impact on pathology/pathophysiology (disease, disorder, or condition)
  - Edema, lymphedema, or effusion is reduced.
  - Joint swelling, inflammation, or restriction is reduced.
  - Pain is decreased.
  - Soft tissue swelling, inflammation, or restriction is reduced.
- Impact on impairments
  - Airway clearance is improved.
  - Balance is improved.
  - Energy expenditure per unit of work is decreased.
  - Gait, locomotion, and balance are improved.
  - Integumentary integrity is improved.
  - Joint integrity and mobility are improved.
  - Muscle performance (strength, power, and endurance) is increased.
  - Postural control is improved.
  - Quality and quantity of movement between and across body segments are improved.
  - Range of motion is improved.
  - Relaxation is increased.
  - Sensory awareness is increased.
  - Weight-bearing status is improved.
  - Work of breathing is decreased.
- Impact on functional limitations
  - Ability to perform movement tasks is improved.
  - Ability to perform physical actions, tasks, or activities related to self-care, home management, work (job/school/play), community, and leisure is improved.
  - Tolerance of positions and activities is increased.
- Impact on disabilities
  - Ability to assume or resume required self-care, home management, work (job/school/play), community, and leisure roles is improved.
- Risk reduction/prevention
  - Risk factors are reduced.
  - Risk of recurrence of condition is reduced.
  - Risk of secondary impairment is reduced.
  - Self-management of symptoms is improved.
- Impact on health, wellness, and fitness
  - Physical capacity is increased.
  - Physical function is improved.
- Impact on societal resources
  - Utilization of physical therapy services is optimized.
  - Utilization of physical therapy services results in efficient use of health care dollars.
- Patient/client satisfaction
  - Access, availability, and services provided are acceptable to patient/client.
  - Administrative management of practice is acceptable to patient/client.
  - Clinical proficiency of physical therapist is acceptable to patient/client.
  - Coordination of care is acceptable to patient/client.
  - Cost of health care services is decreased.
  - Intensity of care is decreased.
  - Interpersonal skills of physical therapist are acceptable to patient/client, family, and significant others.
  - Sense of well-being is improved.
  - Stressors are decreased.

Prescription, Application, and, as Appropriate, Fabrication of Devices and Equipment (Assistive, Adaptive, Orthotic, Protective, Supportive, and Prosthetic)

Interventions

- Adaptive devices
  - environmental controls
  - hospital beds
  - raised toilet seats
  - seating systems
- Assistive devices
  - canes
  - crutches
  - long-handled reachers
  - percussors and vibrators
  - power devices
  - static and dynamic splints
  - walkers
  - wheelchairs
- Orthotic devices
  - braces
  - casts
  - shoe inserts
  - splints
- Prosthetic devices (lower-extremity and upper-extremity)
- Protective devices
  - cushions
- Supportive devices
  - compression garments
  - mechanical ventilators
  - supplemental oxygen

Anticipated Goals and Expected Outcomes

- Impact on pathology/pathophysiology (disease, disorder, or condition)
  - Edema, lymphedema, or effusion is reduced.
  - Joint swelling, inflammation, or restriction is reduced.
  - Pain is decreased.
  - Physiological response to increased oxygen demand is improved.
  - Soft tissue swelling, inflammation, or restriction is reduced.
  - Symptoms associated with increased oxygen demand are decreased.
- Impact on impairments
  - Balance is improved.
  - Endurance is increased.
  - Energy expenditure per unit of work is decreased.
  - Gait, locomotion, and balance are improved.
  - Integumentary integrity is improved.
  - Joint stability is improved.
  - Motor function (motor control and motor learning) is improved.
  - Muscle performance (strength, power, and endurance) is increased.
  - Optimal joint alignment is achieved.
  - Optimal loading on a body part is achieved.
  - Postural control is improved.
  - Quality and quantity of movement between and across body segments are improved.
  - Range of motion is improved.
  - Ventilation and respiratory/gas exchange are improved.
  - Weight-bearing status is improved.
  - Work of breathing is decreased.
- Impact on functional limitations
  - Ability to perform physical actions, tasks, or activities related to self-care, home management, work (job/school/play), community, and leisure is improved.
  - Level of supervision required for task performance is decreased.
  - Performance of and independence in activities of daily living (ADL) and instrumental activities of daily living (IADL) with or without devices and equipment are increased.
  - Tolerance of positions and activities is improved.
- Impact on disabilities
  - Ability to assume or resume required self-care, home management, work (job/school/play), community, and leisure roles is improved.
- Risk reduction/prevention
  - Pressure on body tissues is reduced.
  - Protection of body parts is increased.
  - Risk factors are reduced.
  - Risk of secondary impairment is reduced.
  - Safety is improved.
  - Self-management of symptoms is improved.
- Impact on health, wellness, and fitness
  - Health status is improved.
  - Physical capacity is increased.
  - Physical function is improved.
- Impact on societal resources
  - Utilization of physical therapy services is optimized.
  - Utilization of physical therapy services results in efficient use of health care dollars.
- Patient/client satisfaction
  - Access, availability, and services provided are acceptable to patient/client.
  - Administrative management of practice is acceptable to patient/client.
  - Clinical proficiency of physical therapist is acceptable to patient/client.
  - Coordination of care is acceptable to patient/client.
  - Cost of health care services is decreased.
  - Intensity of care is decreased.
  - Interpersonal skills of physical therapist are acceptable to patient/client, family, and significant others.
  - Sense of well-being is improved.
  - Stressors are decreased.

Airway Clearance Techniques

Interventions

- Breathing strategies
  - active cycle of breathing or forced expiratory techniques
  - assisted cough/huff techniques
  - autogenic drainage
  - paced breathing
  - pursed lip breathing
  - techniques to maximize ventilation (eg, maximum inspiratory hold, stair case breathing, manual hyperinflation)
- Manual/mechanical techniques
  - assistive devices
  - chest percussion, vibration, and shaking
  - chest wall manipulation
  - suctioning
  - ventilatory aids
- Positioning
  - positioning to alter work of breathing
  - positioning to maximize ventilation and perfusion
  - pulmonary postural drainage

Anticipated Goals and Expected Outcomes

- Impact on pathology/pathophysiology (disease, disorder, or condition)
  - Atelectasis is decreased.
  - Tissue perfusion and oxygenation are enhanced.
- Impact on impairments
  - Airway clearance is improved.
  - Cough is improved.
  - Endurance is increased.
  - Energy expenditure per unit of work is decreased.
  - Exercise tolerance is improved.
  - Ventilation and respiration/gas exchange are improved.
  - Work of breathing is decreased.
- Impact on functional limitations
  - Ability to perform physical actions, tasks, or activities related to self-care, home management, work (job/school/play), community, and leisure is improved.
  - Performance of and independence in activities of daily living (ADL) and instrumental activities of daily living (IADL) with or without devices and equipment are increased.
  - Tolerance of positions and activities is increased.
- Impact on disabilities
  - Ability to assume or resume required self-care, home management, work (job/school/play), community, and leisure roles is improved.
- Risk reduction/prevention
  - Risk factors are reduced.
  - Risk of secondary impairment is reduced.
  - Self-management of symptoms is improved.
- Impact on health, wellness, and fitness
  - Health status is improved.
  - Physical capacity is increased.
  - Physical function is improved.
- Impact on societal resources
  - Utilization of physical therapy services is optimized.
  - Utilization of physical therapy services results in efficient use of health care dollars.
- Patient/client satisfaction
  - Access, availability, and services provided are acceptable to patient/client.
  - Administrative management of practice is acceptable to patient/client.
  - Clinical proficiency of physical therapist is acceptable to patient/client.
  - Coordination of care is acceptable to patient/client.
  - Cost of health care services is decreased.
  - Intensity of care is decreased.
  - Interpersonal skills of physical therapist are acceptable to patient/client, family, and significant others.
  - Sense of well-being is improved.
  - Stressors are decreased.

Electrotherapeutic Modalities

Interventions

- Biofeedback
- Electrical stimulation
  - electrical muscle stimulation (EMS)
  - functional electrical stimulation (FES)
  - neuromuscular electrical stimulation (NMES)
  - transcutaneous electrical nerve stimulation (TENS)

Anticipated Goals and Expected Outcomes

- Impact on pathology/pathophysiology (disease, disorder, or condition)
  - Nutrient delivery to tissue is increased.
  - Pain is decreased.
  - Tissue perfusion and oxygenation are enhanced.
- Impact on impairments
  - Motor function (motor control and motor learning) is improved.
  - Muscle performance (strength, power, and endurance) is increased.
  - Postural control is improved.
  - Quality and quantity of movement between and across body segments are improved.
  - Relaxation is increased.
  - Sensory awareness is increased.
  - Work of breathing is decreased.
- Impact on functional limitations
  - Ability to perform physical actions, tasks, or activities related to self-care, home management, work (job/school/play), community, and leisure is improved.
  - Level of supervision required for task performance is decreased.
  - Performance of and independence in activities of daily living (ADL) and instrumental activities of daily living (IADL) with or without devices and equipment are increased.
  - Tolerance of positions and activities is increased.
- Impact on disabilities
  - Ability to assume or resume required self-care, home management, work (job/school/play), community, and leisure roles is improved.
- Risk reduction/prevention
  - Complications of immobility are reduced.
  - Risk factors are reduced.
  - Risk of recurrence of condition is reduced.
  - Risk of secondary impairment is reduced.
  - Self-management of symptoms is improved.
- Impact on health, wellness, and fitness
  - Physical capacity is increased.
  - Physical function is improved.
- Impact on societal resources
  - Utilization of physical therapy services is optimized.
  - Utilization of physical therapy services results in efficient use of health care dollars.
- Patient/client satisfaction
  - Access, availability, and services provided are acceptable to patient/client.
  - Administrative management of practice is acceptable to patient/client.
  - Clinical proficiency of physical therapist is acceptable to patient/client.
  - Coordination of care is acceptable to patient/client.
  - Interpersonal skills of physical therapist are acceptable to patient/client, family, and significant others.
  - Sense of well-being is improved.
  - Stressors are decreased.

Reexamination

Reexamination is the process of performing selected tests and measures after the initial examination to evaluate progress and to modify or redirect interventions. Reexamination may be indicated more than once during a single episode of care. It also may be performed over the course of a disease, disorder, or condition, which for some patients/clients may be over the life span. Indications for reexamination include new clinical findings or failure to respond to physical therapy interventions.

Global Outcomes for Patients/Clients in This Pattern

Throughout the entire episode of care, the physical therapist determines the anticipated goals and expected outcomes for each intervention. These anticipated goals and expected outcomes are delineated in shaded boxes that accompany the lists of interventions in each preferred practice pattern. As the patient/client reaches the termination of physical therapy services and the end of the episode of care, the physical therapist measures the global outcomes of the physical therapy services by characterizing or quantifying the impact of the physical therapy interventions in the following domains:

- Pathology/pathophysiology (disease, disorder, or condition)
- Impairments
- Functional limitations
- Disabilities
- Risk reduction/prevention
- Health, wellness, and fitness
- Societal resources
- Patient/client satisfaction

In some instances, a particular anticipated goal or expected outcome is thoroughly achieved through implementation of a single form of intervention. More commonly, however, the anticipated goals and expected outcomes are achieved as a result of the combined effects of several forms of interventions, leading to enhancement of both health status and health-related quality of life.

Criteria for Termination of Physical Therapy Services

Discharge is the process of ending physical therapy services that have been provided during a single episode of care. It occurs when the anticipated goals and expected outcomes have been achieved. Discharge does *not* occur with a *transfer* (defined as the time when a patient is moved from one site to another site within the same setting or across settings during a single episode of care). Although there may be facility-specific or payer-specific requirements for documentation regarding the conclusion of physical therapy services, ***discharge occurs based on the physical therapist's analysis of the achievement of anticipated goals and expected outcomes.***

Discontinuation is the process of ending physical therapy services that have been provided during a single episode of care when (1) the patient/client, caregiver, or legal guardian declines to continue intervention; (2) the patient/client is unable to continue to progress toward outcomes because of medical or psychosocial complications or because financial/insurance resources have been expended; or (3) the physical therapist determines that the patient/client will no longer benefit from physical therapy. When physical therapy services are terminated prior to achievement of anticipated goals and expected outcomes, patient/client status and the rationale for termination are documented.

For patients/clients who require multiple episodes of care, periodic follow-up is needed over the life span to ensure safety and effective adaptation following changes in physical status, caregivers, environment, or task demands. In consultation with appropriate individuals, and in consideration of the outcomes, the physical therapist plans for discharge or discontinuation and provides for appropriate follow-up or referral.

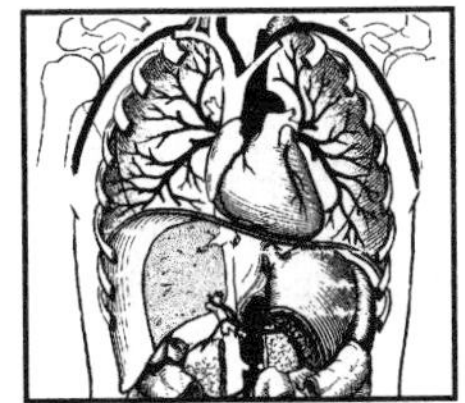

Impaired Ventilation and Respiration/ Gas Exchange Associated With Respiratory Failure

This preferred practice pattern describes the generally accepted elements of patient/client management that physical therapists provide for patients/clients who are classified in this pattern. The pattern title reflects the diagnosis made by the physical therapist. APTA emphasizes that preferred practice patterns are the boundaries within which a physical therapist may select any of a number of clinical alternatives, based on consideration of a wide variety of factors, such as individual patient/client needs; the profession's code of ethics and standards of practice; and patient/client age, culture, gender roles, race, sex, sexual orientation, and socioeconomic status.

Patient/Client Diagnostic Classification

Patients/clients will be classified into this pattern—for impaired ventilation and respiration/gas exchange associated with respiratory failure—as a result of the physical therapist's evaluation of the examination data. The findings from the examination (history, systems review, and tests and measures) may indicate the presence or risk of pathology/pathophysiology (disease, disorder, or condition), impairments, functional limitations, or disabilities or the need for health, wellness, or fitness programs. The physical therapist integrates, synthesizes, and interprets the data to determine the diagnostic classification.

Inclusion

The following examples of examination findings may support the inclusion of patients/clients in this pattern:

Risk Factors or Consequences of Pathology/Pathophysiology (Disease, Disorder, or Condition)

- Abnormal chest radiograph
- Acute neuromuscular dysfunction
- Adult respiratory distress syndrome
- Abnormal alveolar to arterial oxygen tension differences
- Asthma
- Cardiothoracic surgery
- Chronic obstructive pulmonary disease (COPD)
- Inability to maintain adequate oxygen tension with supplemental oxygen
- Multisystem failure
- Pneumonia
- Pre- and post-lung transplant or rejection
- Rapid rise in arterial carbon dioxide at rest or with activity
- Sepsis
- Thoracic or multisystem trauma

Impairments, Functional Limitations, or Disabilities

- Abnormal or adventitious breath sounds
- Abnormal vital capacity
- Airway clearance dysfunction
- Dyspnea at rest
- Dyssynchronous or paradoxical breathing pattern
- Impaired gas exchange
- Significantly increased respiratory rate at rest (>35)

Note:

Some risk factors or consequences of pathology/pathophysiology—such as *respiratory failure with sepsis*—may be severe and complex; *however, they do not necessarily exclude patients/clients from this pattern.* Severe and complex risk factors or consequences may require modification of the frequency of visits and duration of care. (See "Evaluation, Diagnosis, and Prognosis," page 545.)

Exclusion or Multiple-Pattern Classification

The following examples of examination findings may support exclusion from this pattern or classification into additional patterns. Depending on the level of severity or complexity of the examination findings, the physical therapist may determine that the patient/client would be more appropriately managed through (1) classification in an entirely different pattern or (2) classification in both this and another pattern.

Findings That May Require Classification in a Different Pattern

- Age of less than 4 months
- Impairments associated with cardiovascular pump failure
- Impairments associated with chronic ventilatory pump failure

Findings That May Require Classification in Additional Patterns

- Multisite fracture
- Multitrauma with open wounds

ICD-9-CM Codes

The listing below contains the current (as of press time) and most typical 3- and 4-digit ICD-9-CM codes related to this preferred practice pattern. Because patient/client diagnostic classification is based on impairments, functional limitations, and disabilities—not on codes—patients/clients may be classified into the pattern even though the codes listed with the pattern may not apply to those clients.

This listing is intended for general information only and should not be used for coding purposes. The codes should be confirmed by referring to the World Health Organization's *International Classification of Diseases, 9th Revision, Clinical Modification (ICD-9-CM 2001)*, Volumes 1 and 3 (Chicago, Ill: American Medical Association; 2000) or subsequent revisions or by referring to other ICD-9-CM coding manuals that contain exclusion notes and instructions regarding fifth-digit requirements.

136 Other and unspecified infectious and parasitic diseases
- **136.3** Pneumocystosis

277 Other and unspecified disorders of metabolism
- **277.0** Cystic fibrosis

286 Coagulation defects
- **286.6** Defribrination syndrome
  Diffuse or disseminated intravascular coagulation [DIC syndrome]

348 Other conditions of brain
- **348.1** Anoxic brain damage

415 Acute pulmonary heart disease
- **415.1** Pulmonary embolism and infarction

480 Viral pneumonia

481 Pneumococcal pneumonia [Streptococcus pneumoniae pneumonia]

482 Other bacterial pneumonia

483 Pneumonia due to other specified organism

484 Pneumonia in infectious diseases classified elsewhere

485 Bronchopneumonia, organism unspecified

486 Pneumonia, organism unspecified

491 Chronic bronchitis

492 Emphysema
- **492.8** Other emphysema
  Emphysema (lung or pulmonary), not otherwise specified

493 Asthma

494 Bronchiectasis

495 Extrinsic allergic alveolitis
- **495.7** "Ventilation" pneumonitis

496 Chronic airway obstruction, not elsewhere classified
  Chronic obstructive pulmonary disease [COPD], not otherwise specified

507 Pneumonitis due to solids and liquids
- **507.0** Due to inhalation of food or vomitus
  Aspiration pneumonia

511 Pleurisy
- **511.8** Other specified forms of effusion, except tuberculous
  Hemothorax

512 Pneumothorax
- **512.8** Other spontaneous pneumothorax

513 Abscess of lung and mediastinum

514 Pulmonary congestion and hypostasis
  Pulmonary edema, not otherwise specified

516 Other alveolar and parietoalveolar pneumonopathy
- **516.9** Unspecified alveolar and parietoalveolar pneumonopathy

517 Lung involvement in conditions classified elsewhere

518 Other diseases of lung
- **518.0** Pulmonary collapse
- **518.5** Pulmonary insufficiency following trauma and surgery
  Adult respiratory distress syndrome
- **518.8** Other diseases of lung
  - **518.81** Acute respiratory failure
  - **518.82** Other pulmonary insufficiency, not elsewhere classified
    Acute respiratory distress

519 Other diseases of respiratory system
- **519.4** Disorders of diaphragm

786 Symptoms involving respiratory system and other chest symptoms

852 Subarachnoid, subdural, and extradural hemorrhage, following injury

853 Other and unspecified intracranial hemorrhage following injury

854 Intracranial injury of other and unspecified nature

861 Injury to heart and lung
- **861.2** Lung, without mention of open wound into thorax
  - **861.21** Contusion

959 Injury, other and unspecified

996 Complications peculiar to certain specified procedures
- **996.0** Mechanical complication of cardiac device, implant, and graft
- **996.1** Mechanical complication of other vascular device, implant, and graft
- **996.2** Mechanical complication of nervous system device, implant, and graft
- **996.3** Mechanical complication of genitourinary device, implant, and graft
- **996.4** Mechanical complication of internal orthopedic device, implant, and graft
- **996.5** Mechanical complications of other specified prosthetic device, implant, and graft
- **996.8** Complications of transplanted organ
  - **996.85** Bone marrow

997 Complications affecting specified body system, not elsewhere classified
- **997.3** Respiratory complications

Supplemental Classification of Factors Influencing Health Status and Contact With Health Services

V42 Organ or tissue replaced by transplant

- **V42.0** Kidney
- **V42.1** Heart
- **V42.4** Bone
- **V42.6** Lung
- **V42.7** Liver
- **V42.8** Other specified organ or tissue
  - **V42.81** Bone marrow

Note:

Patients/clients who have surgical procedures involving the abdomen, chest wall, diaphragm, lung, pleura, mediastinum, thorax, and vessels of the heart and patients/clients who have nonsurgical procedures such as intubation, irrigation, and other continuous mechanical ventilation also may be classified into this pattern.

Examination

Examination is a comprehensive screening and specific testing process that leads to a diagnostic classification or, when appropriate, to a referral to another practitioner. Examination is required prior to the initial intervention and is performed for all patients/clients. Through the examination, the physical therapist may identify impairments, functional limitations, disabilities, changes in physical function or overall health status, and needs related to restoration of health and to prevention, wellness, and fitness. The physical therapist synthesizes the examination findings to establish the diagnosis and the prognosis (including the plan of care). The patient/client, family, significant others, and caregivers may provide information during the examination process.

Examination has three components: the patient/client history, the systems review, and tests and measures. The *history* is a systematic gathering of past and current information (often from the patient/client) related to why the patient/client is seeking the services of the physical therapist. The *systems review* is a brief or limited examination of (1) the anatomical and physiological status of the cardiovascular/pulmonary, integumentary, musculoskeletal, and neuromuscular systems and (2) the communication ability, affect, cognition, language, and learning style of the patient/client. *Tests and measures* are the means of gathering data about the patient/client.

The selection of examination procedures and the depth of the examination vary based on patient/client age; severity of the problem; stage of recovery (acute, subacute, chronic); phase of rehabilitation (early, intermediate, late, return to activity); home, work (job/school/play), or community situation; and other relevant factors. *For clinical indications in selecting tests and measures and for listings of tests and measures, tools used to gather data, and the types of data generated by tests and measures, refer to Chapter 2.*

Patient/Client History

The history may include:

General Demographics
- Age
- Sex
- Race/ethnicity
- Primary language
- Education

Social History
- Cultural beliefs and behaviors
- Family and caregiver resources
- Social interactions, social activities, and support systems

Employment/Work (Job/School/Play)
- Current and prior work (job/school/play), community, and leisure actions, tasks, or activities

Growth and Development
- Developmental history
- Hand dominance

Living Environment
- Devices and equipment (eg, assistive, adaptive, orthotic, protective, supportive, prosthetic)
- Living environment and community characteristics
- Projected discharge destinations

General Health Status (Self-Report, Family Report, Caregiver Report)
- General health perception
- Physical function (eg, mobility, sleep patterns, restricted bed days)
- Psychological function (eg, memory, reasoning ability, depression, anxiety)
- Role function (eg, community, leisure, social, work)
- Social function (eg, social activity, social interaction, social support)

Social/Health Habits (Past and Current)
- Behavioral health risks (eg, smoking, drug abuse)
- Level of physical fitness

Family History
- Familial health risks

Medical/Surgical History
- Cardiovascular
- Endocrine/metabolic
- Gastrointestinal
- Genitourinary
- Gynecological
- Integumentary
- Musculoskeletal
- Neuromuscular
- Obstetrical
- Prior hospitalizations, surgeries, and preexisting medical and other health-related conditions
- Psychological
- Pulmonary

Current Condition(s)/Chief Complaint(s)
- Concerns that led patient/client to seek the services of a physical therapist
- Concerns or needs of patient/client who requires the services of a physical therapist
- Current therapeutic interventions
- Mechanisms of injury or disease, including date of onset and course of events
- Onset and pattern of symptoms
- Patient/client, family, significant other, and caregiver expectations and goals for the therapeutic intervention
- Patient/client, family, significant other, and caregiver perceptions of patient's/client's emotional response to the current clinical situation
- Previous occurrence of chief complaint(s)
- Prior therapeutic interventions

Functional Status and Activity Level
- Current and prior functional status in self-care and home management activities, including activities of daily living (ADL) and instrumental activities of daily living (IADL)
- Current and prior functional status in work (job/school/play), community, and leisure actions, tasks, or activities

Medications
- Medications for current condition
- Medications previously taken for current condition
- Medications for other conditions

Other Clinical Tests
- Laboratory and diagnostic tests
- Review of available records (eg, medical, education, surgical)
- Review of other clinical findings (eg, nutrition and hydration)

Systems Review

The systems review may include:

Anatomical and Physiological Status

- Cardiovascular/Pulmonary
  - Blood pressure
  - Edema
  - Heart rate
  - Respiratory rate
- Integumentary
  - Pliability (texture)
  - Presence of scar formation
  - Skin color
  - Skin integrity
- Musculoskeletal
  - Gross range of motion
  - Gross strength
  - Gross symmetry
  - Height
  - Weight
- Neuromuscular
  - Gross coordinated movements (eg, balance, gait, locomotion, transfers, transitions)
  - Motor function (motor control, motor learning)

Communication, Affect, Cognition, Language, and Learning Style

- Ability to make needs known
- Consciousness
- Expected emotional/behavioral responses
- Learning preferences (eg, education needs, learning barriers)
- Orientation (person, place, time)

Tests and Measures

Tests and measures for this pattern may include those that characterize or quantify:

Aerobic Capacity and Endurance

- Cardiovascular signs and symptoms in response to increased oxygen demand with exercise or activity, including pressures and flow; heart rate, rhythm, and sounds; and superficial vascular responses (eg, angina, claudication, and exertion scales; electrocardiography; observations; palpation; sphygmomanometry)
- Pulmonary signs and symptoms in response to increased oxygen demand with exercise or activity, including breath and voice sounds; cyanosis; gas exchange; respiratory pattern, rate, and rhythm; and ventilatory flow, force, and volume (eg, auscultation, dyspnea and exertion scales, gas analyses, observations, oximetry, palpation, pulmonary function tests)

Anthropometric Characteristics

- Body composition (eg, body mass index, impedance measurement, skinfold thickness measurement)
- Edema (eg, girth measurement, palpation, scales, volume measurement)

Arousal, Attention, and Cognition

- Arousal and attention (eg, adaptability tests, arousal and awareness scales, indexes, profiles, questionnaires)
- Cognition, including ability to process commands (eg, developmental inventories, indexes, interviews, mental state scales, observations, questionnaires, safety checklists)
- Motivation (eg, adaptive behavior scales)
- Orientation to time, person, place, and situation (eg, attention tests, learning profiles, mental state scales)
- Recall, including memory and retention (eg, assessment scales, interviews, questionnaires)

Assistive and Adaptive Devices

- Assistive or adaptive devices and equipment use during functional activities (eg, ADL scales, functional scales, interviews, observations)
- Remediation of impairments, functional limitations, or disabilities with use of assistive or adaptive devices and equipment (eg, activity status indexes, ADL scales, aerobic capacity tests, functional performance inventories, health assessment questionnaires, IADL scales, pain scales, play scales, videographic assessments)
- Safety during use of assistive or adaptive devices and equipment (eg, fall scales, interviews, logs, observations, reports)

Circulation (Arterial, Venous, and Lymphatic)

- Cardiovascular signs, including heart rate, rhythm, and sounds; pressures and flow; and superficial vascular responses (eg, auscultation, electrocardiography, girth measurement, palpation, sphygmomanometry, thermography)
- Cardiovascular symptoms (eg, angina, claudication, and perceived exertion scales)
- Physiological responses to position change, including autonomic responses, central and peripheral pressures, heart rate and rhythm, respiratory rate and rhythm, ventilatory pattern (eg, auscultation, electrocardiography, observations, palpation, sphygmomanometry)

Cranial and Peripheral Nerve Integrity

- Motor distribution of the peripheral nerves (eg, dynamometry, muscle tests, observations, thoracic outlet tests)
- Response to stimuli, including auditory, gustatory, olfactory, pharyngeal, vestibular, and visual (eg, observations, provocation tests)
- Sensory distribution of the peripheral nerves (eg, discrimination tests; tactile tests, including coarse and light touch, cold and heat, pain, pressure, and vibration; thoracic outlet tests)

Gait, Locomotion, and Balance

- Balance during functional activities with or without the use of assistive, adaptive, orthotic, protective, supportive, or prosthetic devices or equipment (eg, ADL scales, IADL scales, observations, videographic assessments)
- Balance (dynamic and static) with or without the use of assistive, adaptive, orthotic, protective, supportive, or prosthetic devices or equipment (eg, balance scales, dizziness inventories, dynamic posturography, fall scales, motor impairment tests, observations, photographic assessments, postural control tests)
- Gait and locomotion during functional activities with or without the use of assistive, adaptive, orthotic, protective, supportive, or prosthetic devices or equipment (eg, ADL scales, gait indexes, IADL scales, mobility skill profiles, observations, videographic assessments)
- Safety during gait, locomotion, and balance (eg, confidence scales, diaries, fall scales, functional assessment profiles, logs, reports)

Integumentary Integrity

Associated skin

- Activities, positioning, and postures that produce or relieve trauma to the skin (eg, observations, pressure-sensing maps, scales)
- Assistive, adaptive, orthotic, protective, supportive, or prosthetic devices and equipment that may produce or relieve trauma to the skin (eg, observations, pressure-sensing maps, risk assessment scales)
- Skin characteristics, including blistering, continuity of skin color, dermatitis, hair growth, mobility, nail growth, sensation, temperature, texture, and turgor (eg, observations, palpation, photographic assessments, thermography)

Motor Function (Motor Control and Motor Learning)

- Initiation, modification, and control of movement patterns and voluntary postures (eg, activity indexes, developmental scales, gross motor function profiles, motor scales, movement assessment batteries, neuromotor tests, observations, physical performance tests, postural challenge tests, videographic assessments)

Muscle Performance (Including Strength, Power, and Endurance)

- Muscle strength, power, and endurance during functional activities (eg, ADL scales, functional muscle tests, IADL scales, observations, videographic assessments)
- Muscle tension (eg, palpation)

Orthotic, Protective, and Supportive Devices

- Components, alignment, fit, and ability to care for orthotic, protective, and supportive devices and equipment (eg, interviews, logs, observations, pressure-sensing maps, reports)
- Orthotic, protective, and supportive devices and equipment use during functional activities (eg, ADL scales, functional scales, IADL scales, interviews, observations, profiles)
- Remediation of impairments, functional limitations, or disabilities with use of orthotic, protective, and supportive devices and equipment (eg, activity status indexes, ADL scales, aerobic capacity tests, functional performance inventories, health assessment questionnaires, IADL scales, pain scales, play scales, videographic assessments)
- Safety during use of orthotic, protective, and supportive devices and equipment (eg, fall scales, interviews, logs, observations, reports)

Pain

- Pain, soreness, and nociception (eg, angina scales, analog scales, discrimination tests, pain drawings and maps, provocation tests, verbal and pictorial descriptor tests)
- Pain in specific body parts (eg, pain indexes, pain questionnaires, structural provocation tests)

Posture

- Postural alignment and position (static and dynamic), including symmetry and deviation from midline (eg, grid measurements, observations, photographic assessments, technology-assisted assessments, videographic assessments)
- Specific body parts (eg, angle assessments, forward-bending test, goniometry, observations, palpation, positional tests)

Range of Motion (ROM) (Including Muscle Length)

- Functional ROM (eg, observations)
- Joint active and passive movement (eg, goniometry, inclinometry, observations, photographic assessments, videographic assessments)
- Muscle length, soft tissue extensibility, and flexibility (eg, contracture tests, goniometry, inclinometry, ligamentous tests, linear measurement, multisegment flexibility tests, palpation)

Reflex Integrity

- Deep reflexes (eg, myotatic reflex scale, observations, reflex tests)
- Resistance to passive stretch (eg, tone scales)
- Superficial reflexes and reactions (eg, observations, provocation tests)

Self-Care and Home Management (Including ADL and IADL)

- Ability to gain access to home environments (eg, barrier identification, observations, physical performance tests)
- Ability to perform self-care and home management activities with or without assistive, adaptive, orthotic, protective, supportive, or prosthetic devices and equipment (eg, ADL scales, aerobic capacity tests, IADL scales, interviews, observations, profiles)
- Safety in self-care and home management activities and environments (eg, diaries, fall scales, interviews, logs, observations, reports, videographic assessments)

Sensory Integrity

- Combined/cortical sensations (eg, stereognosis tests, tactile discrimination tests)
- Deep sensations (eg, kinesthesiometry, observations, photographic assessments, vibration tests)

Ventilation and Respiration/Gas Exchange

- Pulmonary signs of respiration/gas exchange, including breath sounds (eg, gas analyses, observations, oximetry)
- Pulmonary signs of ventilatory function, including airway protection; breath and voice sounds; respiratory rate, rhythm, and pattern; ventilatory flow, forces, and volumes (eg, airway clearance tests, observations, palpation, pulmonary function tests, ventilatory muscle force tests)
- Pulmonary symptoms (eg, dyspnea and perceived exertion indexes and scales)

Work (Job/School/Play), Community, and Leisure Integration or Reintegration (Including IADL)

- Ability to assume or resume work (job/school/play), community, and leisure activities with or without assistive, adaptive, orthotic, protective, supportive, or prosthetic devices and equipment (eg, activity profiles, disability indexes, functional status questionnaires, IADL scales, observations, physical capacity tests)
- Ability to gain access to work (job/school/play), community, and leisure environments (eg, barrier identification, interviews, observations, physical capacity tests, transportation assessments)
- Safety in work (job/school/play), community, and leisure activities and environments (eg, diaries, fall scales, interviews, logs, observations, videographic assessments)

Evaluation, Diagnosis, and Prognosis (Including Plan of Care)

Physical therapists perform *evaluations* (make clinical judgments) based on the data gathered from the history, systems review, and tests and measures. In the evaluation process, physical therapists synthesize the examination data to establish the diagnosis and prognosis (including the plan of care). Factors that influence the complexity of the evaluation include the clinical findings, extent of loss of function, chronicity or severity of the problem, possibility of multisite or multisystem involvement, preexisting condition(s), potential discharge destination, social considerations, physical function, and overall health status.

A *diagnosis* is a label encompassing a cluster of signs and symptoms, syndromes, or categories. It is the result of the systematic diagnostic process, which includes integrating and evaluating the data from the examination. The diagnostic label indicates the primary dysfunction(s) toward which the therapist will direct interventions. The *prognosis* is the determination of the predicted optimal level of improvement in function and the amount of time needed to reach that level and may also include a prediction of levels of improvement that may be reached at various intervals during the course of therapy. During the prognostic process, the physical therapist develops the plan of care. The *plan of care* identifies specific interventions, proposed frequency and duration of the interventions, anticipated goals, expected outcomes, and discharge plans. The plan of care identifies realistic anticipated goals and expected outcomes, taking into consideration the expectations of the patient/client and appropriate others. These anticipated goals and expected outcomes should be measureable and time limited.

The frequency of visits and duration of the episode of care may vary from a short episode with a high intensity of intervention to a longer episode with a diminishing intensity of intervention. Frequency and duration may vary greatly among patients/clients based on a variety of factors that the physical therapist considers throughout the evaluation process, such as anatomical and physiological changes related to growth and development; caregiver consistency or expertise; chronicity or severity of the current condition; living environment; multisite or multisystem involvement; social support; potential discharge destinations; probability of prolonged impairment, functional limitation, or disability; and stability of the condition.

Prognosis	Expected Range of Number of Visits Per Episode of Care
Over the course of 72 hours, patient/client with acute reversible respiratory failure will demonstrate optimal independence with ventilation and respiration/gas exchange and the highest level of functioning in home, work (job/school/play), community, and leisure environments.	**3 to 9**
Over the course of 3 weeks, patient/client with prolonged respiratory failure will demonstrate optimal independence with ventilation and respiration/gas exchange and the highest level of functioning in home, work (job/school/play), community, and leisure environments.	**10 to 25**
Over the course of 4 to 6 weeks, patient/client with severe or chronic respiratory failure will demonstrate optimal independence with ventilation and respiration/gas exchange and the highest level of functioning in home, work (job/school/play), community, and leisure environments.	**20 to 45**

During the episode of care, patient/client with acute reversible respiratory failure, prolonged respiratory failure, or severe or chronic respiratory failure will achieve (1) the anticipated goals and expected outcomes of the interventions that are described in the plan of care and (2) the global outcomes for patients/clients who are classified in this pattern.

These ranges represent the lower and upper limits of the number of physical therapist visits required to achieve anticipated goals and expected outcomes. *It is anticipated that 80% of patients/clients who are classified into this pattern will achieve the anticipated goals and expected outcomes within these ranges during a single continuous episode of care.* Frequency of visits and duration of the episode of care should be determined by the physical therapist to maximize effectiveness of care and efficiency of service delivery.

Factors That May Require New Episode of Care or That May Modify Frequency of Visits/Duration of Episode

- Accessibility and availability of resources
- Adherence to the intervention program
- Age
- Anatomical and physiological changes related to growth and development
- Caregiver consistency or expertise
- Chronicity or severity of the current condition
- Cognitive status
- Comorbitities, complications, or secondary impairments
- Concurrent medical, surgical, and therapeutic interventions
- Decline in functional independence
- Level of impairment
- Level of physical function
- Living environment
- Multisite or multisystem involvement
- Nutritional status
- Overall health status
- Potential discharge destinations
- Premorbid conditions
- Probability of prolonged impairment, functional limitation, or disability
- Psychological and socioeconomic factors
- Psychomotor abilities
- Social support
- Stability of the condition

Intervention

Intervention is the purposeful interaction of the physical therapist with the patient/client and, when appropriate, with other individuals involved in patient/client care, using various physical therapy procedures and techniques to produce changes in the condition consistent with the diagnosis and prognosis. Decisions about interventions are contingent on the timely monitoring of patient/client response and the progress made toward achieving the anticipated goals and expected outcomes.

Communication, coordination, and documentation and patient/client-related instruction are provided for all patients/clients across all settings. Procedural interventions are selected or modified based on the examination data and the evaluation, the diagnosis and the prognosis, and the anticipated goals and expected outcomes for a particular patient/client. *For clinical considerations in selecting interventions, listings of interventions, and listings of anticipated goals and expected outcomes, refer to Chapter 3.*

Coordination, Communication, and Documentation

Coordination, communication, and documentation may include:

Interventions

- Addressing required functions
  - advance directives
  - informed consent
  - mandatory communication and reporting (eg, patient advocacy and abuse reporting)
- Admission and discharge planning
- Case management
- Collaboration and coordination with agencies, including:
  - equipment suppliers
  - home care agencies
  - payer groups
  - transportation agencies
- Communication across settings, including:
  - case conferences
  - documentation
- Cost-effective resource utilization
- Data collection, analysis, and reporting
  - outcome data
  - peer review findings
  - record reviews
- Documentation across settings, following APTA's *Guidelines for Physical Therapy Documentation* (Appendix 5), including:
  - changes in impairments, functional limitations, and disabilities
  - changes in interventions
  - elements of patient/client management (examination, evaluation, diagnosis, prognosis, intervention)
  - outcomes of intervention
- Interdisciplinary teamwork
  - case conferences
  - patient care rounds
  - patient/client family meetings
- Referrals to other professionals or resources

Anticipated Goals and Expected Outcomes

- Accountability for services is increased.
- Admission data and discharge planning are completed.
- Advance directives, informed consent, and mandatory communication and reporting (eg, patient advocacy and abuse reporting) are obtained or completed.
- Available resources are maximally utilized.
- Care is coordinated with patient/client, family, significant others, caregivers, and other professionals.
- Case is managed throughout the episode of care.
- Collaboration and coordination occurs with agencies, including equipment suppliers, home care agencies, payer groups, and transportation agencies.
- Communication enhances risk reduction and prevention.
- Communication occurs across settings through case conferences and documentation.
- Data are collected, analyzed, and reported, including outcome data, peer review findings, and record reviews.
- Decision making is enhanced regarding health, wellness, and fitness needs.
- Decision making is enhanced regarding patient/client health and the use of health care resources by patient/client, family, significant others, and caregivers.
- Documentation occurs throughout patient/client management and across settings and follows APTA's *Guidelines for Physical Therapy Documentation* (Appendix 5).
- Interdisciplinary collaboration occurs through case conferences, patient care rounds, and patient/client family meetings.
- Patient/client, family, significant other, and caregiver understanding of anticipated goals and expected outcomes is increased.
- Placement needs are determined.
- Referrals are made to other professionals or resources whenever necessary and appropriate.
- Resources are utilized in a cost-effective way.

Patient/Client-Related Instruction

Patient/client-related instruction may include:

Interventions

- Instruction, education and training of patients/clients and caregivers regarding:
  - current condition (pathology/pathophysiology [disease, disorder, or condition], impairments, functional limitations, or disabilities)
  - enhancement of performance
  - health, wellness, and fitness programs
  - plan of care
  - risk factors for pathology/pathophysiology (disease, disorder, or condition), impairments, functional limitations, or disabilities
  - transitions across settings
  - transitions to new roles

Anticipated Goals and Expected Outcomes

- Ability to perform physical actions, tasks, or activities is improved.
- Awareness and use of community resources are improved.
- Behaviors that foster healthy habits, wellness, and prevention are acquired.
- Decision making is enhanced regarding patient/client health and the use of health care resources by patient/client, family, significant others, and caregivers.
- Disability associated with acute or chronic illnesses is reduced.
- Functional independence in activities of daily living (ADL) and instrumental activities of daily living (IADL) is increased.
- Health status is improved.
- Intensity of care is decreased.
- Level of supervision required for task performance is decreased.
- Patient/client, family, significant other, and caregiver knowledge and awareness of the diagnosis, prognosis, interventions, and anticipated goals and expected outcomes are increased.
- Patient/client knowledge of personal and environmental factors associated with the condition is increased.
- Performance levels in self-care, home management, work (job/school/play), community, or leisure actions, tasks, or activities are improved.
- Physical function is improved.
- Risk of recurrence of condition is reduced.
- Risk of secondary impairment is reduced.
- Safety of patient/client, family, significant others, and caregivers is improved.
- Self-management of symptoms is improved.
- Utilization and cost of health care services are decreased.

Direct Interventions

Direct interventions for this pattern may include, in order of preferred usage:

Therapeutic Exercise

Interventions

- Aerobic capacity/endurance conditioning or reconditioning
  - gait and locomotor training
  - increased workload over time
  - movement efficiency and energy conservation training
  - walking and wheelchair propulsion programs
- Balance, coordination, and agility training
  - neuromuscular education or reeducation
  - posture awareness training
- Body mechanics and postural stabilization
  - body mechanics training
  - postural control training
  - posture awareness training
- Flexibility exercises
  - muscle lengthening
  - range of motion
  - stretching
- Relaxation
  - breathing strategies
  - movement strategies
  - relaxation techniques
  - standardized, programmatic, complementary exercise approaches
- Strength, power, and endurance training for head, neck, limb, pelvic-floor, trunk, and ventilatory muscles
  - active assistive, active, and resistive exercises (including concentric, dynamic/isotonic, isometric, and plyometric)
  - task-specific performance training

Anticipated Goals and Expected Outcomes

- Impact on pathology/pathophysiology (disease, disorder, or condition)
  - Atelectasis is decreased.
  - Joint swelling, inflammation, or restriction is reduced.
  - Nutrient delivery to tissue is increased.
  - Osteogenic effects of exercise are maximized.
  - Pain is decreased.
  - Physiological response to increased oxygen demand is improved.
  - Soft tissue swelling, inflammation, or restriction is reduced.
  - Symptoms associated with increased oxygen demand are decreased.
  - Tissue perfusion and oxygenation are enhanced.
  - Ventilation and respiration/gas exchange are improved.
- Impact on impairments
  - Aerobic capacity is increased.
  - Airway clearance is improved.
  - Balance is improved.
  - Endurance is increased.
  - Energy expenditure per unit of work is decreased.
  - Gait, locomotion, and balance are improved.
  - Integumentary integrity is improved.
  - Joint integrity and mobility are improved.
  - Motor function (motor control and motor learning) is improved.
  - Muscle performance (strength, power, and endurance) is increased.
  - Postural control is improved.
  - Quality and quantity of movement between and across body segments are improved.
  - Range of motion is improved.
  - Relaxation is increased.
  - Sensory awareness is increased.
  - Weight-bearing status is improved.
  - Work of breathing is decreased.
- Impact on functional limitations
  - Ability to perform physical actions, tasks, or activities related to self-care, home management, work (job/school/play), community, and leisure is improved.
  - Level of supervision required for task performance is decreased.
  - Performance of and independence in activities of daily living (ADL) and instrumental activities of daily living (IADL) with or without devices and equipment are increased.
  - Tolerance of positions and activities is increased.
- Impact on disabilities
  - Ability to assume or resume required self-care, home management, work (job/school/play), community, and leisure roles is improved.
- Risk reduction/prevention
  - Preoperative and postoperative complications are reduced.
  - Risk factors are reduced.
  - Risk of secondary impairment is reduced.
  - Safety is improved.
  - Self-management of symptoms is improved.
- Impact on health, wellness, and fitness
  - Fitness is improved.
  - Health status is improved.
  - Physical capacity is increased.
  - Physical function is improved.
- Impact on societal resources
  - Utilization of physical therapy services is optimized.
  - Utilization of physical therapy services results in efficient use of health care dollars.
- Patient/client satisfaction
  - Access, availability, and services provided are acceptable to patient/client.
  - Administrative management of practice is acceptable to patient/client.
  - Clinical proficiency of physical therapist is acceptable to patient/client.
  - Coordination of care is acceptable to patient/client.
  - Cost of health care services is decreased.
  - Intensity of care is decreased.
  - Interpersonal skills of physical therapist are acceptable to patient/client, family, and significant others.
  - Sense of well-being is improved.
  - Stressors are decreased.

Functional Training in Self-Care and Home Management (Including Activities of Daily Living [ADL] and Instrumental Activities of Daily Living [IADL])

Interventions

- ADL training
  - bathing
  - bed mobility and transfer training
  - developmental activities
  - dressing
  - eating
  - grooming
  - toileting
- Devices and equipment use and training
  - assistive and adaptive device or equipment training during ADL and IADL
  - orthotic, protective, or supportive device or equipment training during ADL and IADL
  - prosthetic device or equipment training during ADL and IADL
- IADL training
  - home maintenance
  - household chores
- Injury prevention or reduction
  - injury prevention education during self-care and home management
  - injury prevention or reduction with use of devices and equipment
  - safety awareness training during self-care and home management

Anticipated Goals and Expected Outcomes

- Impact on pathology/pathophysiology (disease, disorder, or condition)
  - Pain is decreased.
  - Physiological response to increased oxygen demand is improved.
  - Symptoms associated with increased oxygen demand are decreased.
- Impact on impairments
  - Balance is improved.
  - Endurance is increased.
  - Energy expenditure per unit of work is decreased.
  - Motor function (motor control and motor learning) is improved.
  - Muscle performance (strength, power, and endurance) is increased.
  - Postural control is improved.
  - Sensory awareness is increased.
  - Weight-bearing status is improved.
- Impact on functional limitations
  - Ability to perform physical actions, tasks, or activities related to self-care and home management is improved.
  - Level of supervision required for task performance is decreased.
  - Performance of and independence in ADL and IADL with or without devices and equipment are increased.
  - Tolerance of positions and activities is increased.
- Impact on disabilities
  - Ability to assume or resume required self-care and home management roles is improved.
- Risk reduction/prevention
  - Risk factors are reduced.
  - Risk of secondary impairments is reduced.
  - Safety is improved.
  - Self-management of symptoms is improved.
- Impact on health, wellness, and fitness
  - Health status is improved.
  - Physical capacity is increased.
  - Physical function is improved.
- Impact on societal resources
  - Utilization of physical therapy services is optimized.
  - Utilization of physical therapy services results in efficient use of health care dollars.
- Patient/client satisfaction
  - Access, availability, and services provided are acceptable to patient/client.
  - Administrative management of practice is acceptable to patient/client.
  - Clinical proficiency of physical therapist is acceptable to patient/client.
  - Coordination of care is acceptable to patient/client.
  - Cost of health care services is decreased.
  - Intensity of care is decreased.
  - Interpersonal skills of physical therapist are acceptable to patient/client, family, and significant others.
  - Sense of well-being is improved.
  - Stressors are decreased.

Manual Therapy Techniques (Including Mobilization/Manipulation)

Interventions

- Massage
  - connective tissue massage
  - therapeutic massage
- Mobilization/manipulation
  - soft tissue
- Passive range of motion

Anticipated Goals and Expected Outcomes

- Impact on pathology/pathophysiology (disease, disorder, or condition)
  - Edema, lymphedema, or effusion is reduced.
  - Joint swelling, inflammation, or restriction is reduced.
  - Pain is decreased.
  - Soft tissue swelling, inflammation, or restriction is reduced.
- Impact on impairments
  - Airway clearance is improved.
  - Balance is improved.
  - Energy expenditure per unit of work is decreased.
  - Gait, locomotion, and balance are improved.
  - Integumentary integrity is improved.
  - Joint integrity and mobility are improved.
  - Muscle performance (strength, power, and endurance) is increased.
  - Postural control is improved.
  - Quality and quantity of movement between and across body segments are improved.
  - Range of motion is improved.
  - Relaxation is increased.
  - Sensory awareness is increased.
  - Weight-bearing status is improved.
  - Work of breathing is decreased.
- Impact on functional limitations
  - Ability to perform movement tasks is improved.
  - Ability to perform physical actions, tasks, or activities related to self-care, home management, work (job/school/play), community, and leisure is improved.
  - Tolerance of positions and activities is increased.
- Impact on disabilities
  - Ability to assume or resume required self-care, home management, work (job/school/play), community, and leisure roles is improved.
- Risk reduction/prevention
  - Risk factors are reduced.
  - Risk of secondary impairment is reduced.
  - Self-management of symptoms is improved.
- Impact on health, wellness, and fitness
  - Physical capacity is increased.
  - Physical function is improved.
- Impact on societal resources
  - Utilization of physical therapy services is optimized.
  - Utilization of physical therapy services results in efficient use of health care dollars.
- Patient/client satisfaction
  - Access, availability, and services provided are acceptable to patient/client.
  - Administrative management of practice is acceptable to patient/client.
  - Clinical proficiency of physical therapist is acceptable to patient/client.
  - Coordination of care is acceptable to patient/client.
  - Cost of health care services is decreased.
  - Intensity of care is decreased.
  - Interpersonal skills of physical therapist are acceptable to patient/client, family, and significant others.
  - Sense of well-being is improved.
  - Stressors are decreased.

Prescription, Application, and, as Appropriate, Fabrication of Devices and Equipment (Assistive, Adaptive, Orthotic, Protective, Supportive, and Prosthetic)

Interventions

- Adaptive devices
  - environmental controls
  - hospital beds
  - raised toilet seats
  - seating systems
- Assistive devices
  - canes
  - crutches
  - long-handled reachers
  - percussors and vibrators
  - power devices
  - static and dynamic splints
  - walkers
  - wheelchairs
- Orthotic devices
  - braces
  - casts
  - shoe inserts
  - splints
- Protective devices
  - braces
  - cushions
- Supportive devices
  - compression garments
  - elastic wrap
  - mechanical ventilators
  - neck collars
  - supplemental oxygen

Anticipated Goals and Expected Outcomes

- Impact on pathology/pathophysiology (disease, disorder, or condition)
  - Edema, lymphedema, or effusion is reduced.
  - Joint swelling, inflammation, or restriction is reduced.
  - Pain is decreased.
  - Physiological response to increased oxygen demand is improved.
  - Soft tissue swelling, inflammation, or restriction is reduced.
  - Symptoms associated with increased oxygen demand are decreased.
- Impact on impairments
  - Balance is improved.
  - Endurance is increased.
  - Energy expenditure per unit of work is decreased.
  - Gait, locomotion, and balance are improved.
  - Integumentary integrity is improved.
  - Joint stability is improved.
  - Motor function (motor control and motor learning) is improved.
  - Muscle performance (strength, power, and endurance) is increased.
  - Optimal joint alignment is achieved.
  - Optimal loading on a body part is achieved.
  - Postural control is improved.
  - Quality and quantity of movement between and across body segments are improved.
  - Range of motion is improved.
  - Weight-bearing status is improved.
  - Work of breathing is decreased.
- Impact on functional limitations
  - Ability to perform physical actions, tasks, or activities related to self-care, home management, work (job/school/play), community, and leisure is improved.
  - Level of supervision required for task performance is decreased.
  - Performance of and independence in activities of daily living (ADL) and instrumental activities of daily living (IADL) with or without devices and equipment are increased.
  - Tolerance of positions and activities is improved.
- Impact on disabilities
  - Ability to assume or resume required self-care, home management, work (job/school/play), community, and leisure roles is improved.
- Risk reduction/prevention
  - Pressure on body tissues is reduced.
  - Protection of body parts is increased.
  - Risk factors are reduced.
  - Risk of secondary impairment is reduced.
  - Safety is improved.
  - Self-management of symptoms is improved.
- Impact on health, wellness, and fitness
  - Health status is improved.
  - Physical capacity is increased.
  - Physical function is improved.
- Impact on societal resources
  - Utilization of physical therapy services is optimized.
  - Utilization of physical therapy services results in efficient use of health care dollars.
- Patient/client satisfaction
  - Access, availability, and services provided are acceptable to patient/client.
  - Administrative management of practice is acceptable to patient/client.
  - Clinical proficiency of physical therapist is acceptable to patient/client.
  - Coordination of care is acceptable to patient/client.
  - Cost of health care services is decreased.
  - Intensity of care is decreased.
  - Interpersonal skills of physical therapist are acceptable to patient/client, family, and significant others.
  - Sense of well-being is improved.
  - Stressors are decreased.

Airway Clearance Techniques

Interventions

- Breathing strategies
  - active cycle of breathing or forced expiratory techniques
  - assisted cough/huff techniques
  - autogenic drainage
  - paced breathing
  - pursed lip breathing
  - techniques to maximize ventilation (eg, maximum inspiratory hold, stair case breathing, manual hyperinflation)
- Manual/mechanical techniques
  - assistive devices
  - chest percussion, vibration, and shaking
  - chest wall manipulation
  - suctioning
  - ventilatory aids
- Positioning
  - positioning to alter work of breathing
  - positioning to maximize ventilation and perfusion
  - pulmonary postural drainage

Anticipated Goals and Expected Outcomes

- Impact on pathology/pathophysiology (disease, disorder, or condition)
  - Atelectasis is decreased.
  - Tissue perfusion and oxygenation are enhanced.
- Impact on impairments
  - Airway clearance is improved.
  - Cough is improved.
  - Endurance is increased.
  - Energy expenditure per unit of work is decreased.
  - Exercise tolerance is improved.
  - Ventilation and respiration/gas exchange are improved.
  - Work of breathing is decreased.
- Impact on functional limitations
  - Ability to perform physical actions, tasks, or activities related to self-care, home management, work (job/school/play), community, and leisure is improved.
  - Performance of and independence in activities of daily living (ADL) and instrumental activities of daily living (IADL) with or without devices and equipment are increased.
  - Tolerance of positions and activities is increased.
- Impact on disabilities
  - Ability to assume or resume required self-care, home management, work (job/school/play), community, and leisure roles is improved.
- Risk reduction/prevention
  - Risk factors are reduced.
  - Risk of secondary impairment is reduced.
  - Self-management of symptoms is improved.
- Impact on health, wellness, and fitness
  - Health status is improved.
  - Physical capacity is increased.
  - Physical function is improved.
- Impact on societal resources
  - Utilization of physical therapy services is optimized.
  - Utilization of physical therapy services results in efficient use of health care dollars.
- Patient/client satisfaction
  - Access, availability, and services provided are acceptable to patient/client.
  - Administrative management of practice is acceptable to patient/client.
  - Clinical proficiency of physical therapist is acceptable to patient/client.
  - Coordination of care is acceptable to patient/client.
  - Cost of health care services is decreased.
  - Intensity of care is decreased.
  - Interpersonal skills of physical therapist are acceptable to patient/client, family, and significant others.
  - Sense of well-being is improved.
  - Stressors are decreased.

Reexamination

Reexamination is the process of performing selected tests and measures after the initial examination to evaluate progress and to modify or redirect interventions. Reexamination may be indicated more than once during a single episode of care. It also may be performed over the course of a disease, disorder, or condition, which for some patients/clients may be over the life span. Indications for reexamination include new clinical findings or failure to respond to physical therapy interventions.

Global Outcomes for Patients/Clients in This Pattern

Throughout the entire episode of care, the physical therapist determines the anticipated goals and expected outcomes for each intervention. These anticipated goals and expected outcomes are delineated in shaded boxes that accompany the lists of interventions in each preferred practice pattern. As the patient/client reaches the termination of physical therapy services and the end of the episode of care, the physical therapist measures the global outcomes of the physical therapy services by characterizing or quantifying the impact of the physical therapy interventions in the following domains:

- Pathology/pathophysiology (disease, disorder, or condition)
- Impairments
- Functional limitations
- Disabilities
- Risk reduction/prevention
- Health, wellness, and fitness
- Societal resources
- Patient/client satisfaction

In some instances, a particular anticipated goal or expected outcome is thoroughly achieved through implementation of a single form of intervention. More commonly, however, the anticipated goals and expected outcomes are achieved as a result of the combined effects of several forms of interventions, leading to enhancement of both health status and health-related quality of life.

Criteria for Termination of Physical Therapy Services

Discharge is the process of ending physical therapy services that have been provided during a single episode of care. It occurs when the anticipated goals and expected outcomes have been achieved. Discharge does *not* occur with a *transfer* (defined as the time when a patient is moved from one site to another site within the same setting or across settings during a single episode of care). Although there may be facility-specific or payer-specific requirements for documentation regarding the conclusion of physical therapy services, *discharge occurs based on the physical therapist's analysis of the achievement of anticipated goals and expected outcomes.*

Discontinuation is the process of ending physical therapy services that have been provided during a single episode of care when (1) the patient/client, caregiver, or legal guardian declines to continue intervention; (2) the patient/client is unable to continue to progress toward outcomes because of medical or psychosocial complications or because financial/insurance resources have been expended; or (3) the physical therapist determines that the patient/client will no longer benefit from physical therapy. When physical therapy services are terminated prior to achievement of anticipated goals and expected outcomes, patient/client status and the rationale for termination are documented.

For patients/clients who require multiple episodes of care, periodic follow-up is needed over the life span to ensure safety and effective adaptation following changes in physical status, caregivers, environment, or task demands. In consultation with appropriate individuals, and in consideration of the outcomes, the physical therapist plans for discharge or discontinuation and provides for appropriate follow-up or referral.

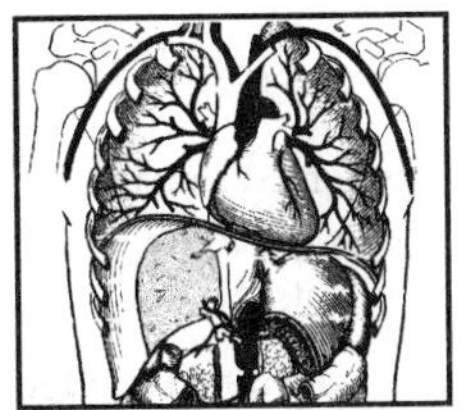

Impaired Ventilation, Respiration/ Gas Exchange, and Aerobic Capacity/ Endurance Associated With Respiratory Failure in the Neonate

This preferred practice pattern describes the generally accepted elements of patient/client management that physical therapists provide for patients/clients who are classified in this pattern. The pattern title reflects the diagnosis made by the physical therapist. APTA emphasizes that preferred practice patterns are the boundaries within which a physical therapist may select any of a number of clinical alternatives, based on consideration of a wide variety of factors, such as individual patient/client needs; the profession's code of ethics and standards of practice; and patient/client age, culture, gender roles, race, sex, sexual orientation, and socioeconomic status.

Patient/Client Diagnostic Classification

Patients/clients will be classified into this pattern—for impaired ventilation, respiration/gas exchange, and aerobic capacity/endurance associated with respiratory failure in the neonate—as a result of the physical therapist's evaluation of the examination data. The findings from the examination (history, systems review, and tests and measures) may indicate the presence or risk of pathology/pathophysiology (disease, disorder, or condition), impairments, functional limitations, or disabilities or the need for health, wellness, or fitness programs. The physical therapist integrates, synthesizes, and interprets the data to determine the diagnostic classification.

Inclusion

The following examples of examination findings may support the inclusion of patients/clients in this pattern:

Risk Factors or Consequences of Pathology/Pathophysiology (Disease, Disorder, or Condition)

- Abdominal thoracic surgeries
- Apnea and bradycardia
- Bronchopulmonary dysphasia
- Congenital anomalies
- Hyaline membranes disease
- Meconium aspiration syndrome
- Neurovascular disorders
- Pneumonia
- Rapid desaturation with movement or crying

Impairments, Functional Limitations, or Disabilities

- Abnormal pulmonary responses to activity
- Impaired airway clearance
- Impaired cough
- Impaired gas exchange
- Intercostal or subcostal retraction on inspiration
- Paradoxical or abnormal breathing pattern at rest or with activity
- Physiological intolerance of routine care

Note:

Some risk factors or consequences of pathology/pathophysiology—such as *bronchopulmonary dysphasia*—may be severe and complex; *however, they do not necessarily exclude patients/clients from this pattern.* Severe and complex risk factors or consequences may require modification of the frequency of visits and duration of care. (See "Evaluation, Diagnosis, and Prognosis," page 560.)

Exclusion or Multiple-Pattern Classification

The following examples of examination findings may support exclusion from this pattern or classification into additional patterns. Depending on the level of severity or complexity of the examination findings, the physical therapist may determine that the patient/client would be more appropriately managed through (1) classification in an entirely different pattern or (2) classification in both this and another pattern.

Findings That May Require Classification in a Different Pattern

- Age of greater than 4 months
- Neonate with central nervous system disorder without respiratory failure

Findings That May Require Classification in Additional Patterns

- Neonate with an intracranial bleed and respiratory failure

ICD-9-CM Codes

The listing below contains the current (as of press time) and most typical 3- and 4-digit ICD-9-CM codes related to this preferred practice pattern. Because patient/client diagnostic classification is based on impairments, functional limitations, and disabilities—not on codes—patients/clients may be classified into the pattern even though the codes listed with the pattern may not apply to those clients.

This listing is intended for general information only and should not be used for coding purposes. The codes should be confirmed by referring to the World Health Organization's *International Classification of Diseases, 9th Revision, Clinical Modification (ICD-9-CM 2001)*, Volumes 1 and 3 (Chicago, Ill: American Medical Association; 2000) or subsequent revisions or by referring to other ICD-9-CM coding manuals that contain exclusion notes and instructions regarding fifth-digit requirements.

508 Respiratory conditions due to other and unspecified external agents
- **508.9** Respiratory conditions due to unspecified external agent

514 Pulmonary congestion and hypostasis

516 Other alveolar and parietoalveolar pneumonopathy
- **516.9** Unspecified alveolar and parietoalveolar pneumonopathy

518 Other diseases of lung
- **518.0** Pulmonary collapse
- **518.8** Other diseases of lung
  - **518.89** Other diseases of lung, not elsewhere classified

553 Other hernia of abdominal cavity without mention of obstruction or gangrene
- **553.3** Diaphragmatic hernia

748 Congenital anomalies of respiratory system
- **748.3** Other anomalies of larynx, trachea, and bronchus
- **748.5** Agenesis, hypoplasia, and dysplasia of lung
- **748.6** Other anomalies of lung

750 Other congenital anomalies of upper alimentary tract
- **750.3** Tracheoesophageal fistula, esophageal atresia and stenosis

765 Disorders relating to short gestation and unspecified low birth weight
- **765.0** Extreme immaturity
- **765.1** Other preterm infants

767 Birth trauma
- **767.7** Other cranial and peripheral nerve injuries
  Phrenic nerve paralysis

769 Respiratory distress syndrome
Hyaline membrane disease (pulmonary)

770 Other respiratory conditions of fetus and newborn
- **770.1** Meconium aspiration syndrome
- **770.6** Transitory tachypnea of newborn
- **770.7** Chronic respiratory disease arising in the perinatal period
  Bronchopulmonary dysplasia

786 Symptoms involving respiratory system and other chest symptoms
- **786.0** Dyspnea and respiratory abnormalities
  - **786.00** Respiratory abnormality, unspecified

Examination

Examination is a comprehensive screening and specific testing process that leads to a diagnostic classification or, when appropriate, to a referral to another practitioner. Examination is required prior to the initial intervention and is performed for all patients/clients. Through the examination, the physical therapist may identify impairments, functional limitations, disabilities, changes in physical function or overall health status, and needs related to restoration of health and to prevention, wellness, and fitness. The physical therapist synthesizes the examination findings to establish the diagnosis and the prognosis (including the plan of care). The patient/client, family, significant others, and caregivers may provide information during the examination process.

Examination has three components: the patient/client history, the systems review, and tests and measures. The *history* is a systematic gathering of past and current information (often from the patient/client) related to why the patient/client is seeking the services of the physical therapist. The *systems review* is a brief or limited examination of (1) the anatomical and physiological status of the cardiovascular/pulmonary, integumentary, musculoskeletal, and neuromuscular systems and (2) the communication ability, affect, cognition, language, and learning style of the patient/client. *Tests and measures* are the means of gathering data about the patient/client.

The selection of examination procedures and the depth of the examination vary based on patient/client age; severity of the problem; stage of recovery (acute, subacute, chronic); phase of rehabilitation (early, intermediate, late, return to activity); home, work (job/school/play), or community situation; and other relevant factors. *For clinical indications in selecting tests and measures and for listings of tests and measures, tools used to gather data, and the types of data generated by tests and measures, refer to Chapter 2.*

Patient/Client History

The history may include:

General Demographics

- Age
- Sex
- Race/ethnicity
- Primary language
- Education

Social History

- Cultural beliefs and behaviors
- Family and caregiver resources
- Social interactions, social activities, and support systems

Employment/Work (Job/School/Play)

- Current and prior work (job/school/play), community, and leisure actions, tasks, or activities

Growth and Development

- Developmental history
- Hand dominance

Living Environment

- Devices and equipment (eg, assistive, adaptive, orthotic, protective, supportive, prosthetic)
- Living environment and community characteristics
- Projected discharge destinations

General Health Status (Self-Report, Family Report, Caregiver Report)

- General health perception
- Physical function (eg, mobility, sleep patterns, restricted bed days)
- Psychological function (eg, memory, reasoning ability, depression, anxiety)
- Role function (eg, community, leisure, social, work)
- Social function (eg, social activity, social interaction, social support)

Social/Health Habits (Past and Current)

- Behavioral health risks (eg, smoking, drug abuse)
- Level of physical fitness

Family History

- Familial health risks

Medical/Surgical History

- Cardiovascular
- Endocrine/metabolic
- Gastrointestinal
- Genitourinary
- Gynecological
- Integumentary
- Musculoskeletal
- Neuromuscular
- Obstetrical
- Prior hospitalizations, surgeries, and preexisting medical and other health-related conditions
- Psychological
- Pulmonary

Current Condition(s)/Chief Complaint(s)

- Concerns that led patient/client to seek the services of a physical therapist
- Concerns or needs of patient/client who requires the services of a physical therapist
- Current therapeutic interventions
- Mechanisms of injury or disease, including date of onset and course of events
- Onset and pattern of symptoms
- Patient/client, family, significant other, and caregiver expectations and goals for the therapeutic intervention
- Patient/client, family, significant other, and caregiver perceptions of patient's/client's emotional response to the current clinical situation
- Previous occurrence of chief complaint(s)
- Prior therapeutic interventions

Functional Status and Activity Level

- Current and prior functional status in self-care and home management activities, including activities of daily living (ADL) and instrumental activities of daily living (IADL)
- Current and prior functional status in work (job/school/play), community, and leisure actions, tasks, or activities

Medications

- Medications for current condition
- Medications previously taken for current condition
- Medications for other conditions

Other Clinical Tests

- Laboratory and diagnostic tests
- Review of available records (eg, medical, education, surgical)
- Review of other clinical findings (eg, nutrition and hydration)

Systems Review

The systems review may include:

Anatomical and Physiological Status

- Cardiovascular/Pulmonary
  - Blood pressure
  - Edema
  - Heart rate
  - Respiratory rate
- Integumentary
  - Pliability (texture)
  - Presence of scar formation
  - Skin color
  - Skin integrity
- Musculoskeletal
  - Gross range of motion
  - Gross strength
  - Gross symmetry
  - Height
  - Weight
- Neuromuscular
  - Gross coordinated movements (eg, balance, gait, locomotion, transfers, transitions)
  - Motor function (motor control, motor learning)

Communication, Affect, Cognition, Language, and Learning Style

- Ability to make needs known
- Consciousness

Tests and Measures

Tests and measures for this pattern may include those that characterize or quantify:

Aerobic Capacity and Endurance

- Cardiovascular signs and symptoms in response to increased oxygen demand with exercise or activity, including pressures and flow; heart rate, rhythm, and sounds; and superficial vascular responses (eg, electrocardiography, observations, palpation, sphygmomanometry)
- Pulmonary signs and symptoms in response to increased oxygen demand with exercise or activity, including breath and voice sounds; cyanosis; gas exchange; respiratory pattern, rate, and rhythm; and ventilatory flow, force, and volume (eg, auscultation, dyspnea and exertion scales, gas analyses, observations, oximetry, palpation, pulmonary function tests)

Anthropometric Characteristics

- Body dimensions (eg, girth measurement, length measurement)
- Edema (eg, girth measurement, palpation, scales, volume measurement)

Arousal, Attention, and Cognition

- Arousal and attention (eg, adaptability tests, arousal and awareness scales, indexes, profiles, questionnaires)

Circulation (Arterial, Venous, and Lymphatic)

- Cardiovascular signs, including heart rate, rhythm, and sounds; pressures and flow; and superficial vascular responses (eg, auscultation, electrocardiography, palpation, sphygmomanometry, thermography)
- Physiological responses to position change, including autonomic responses, central and peripheral pressures, heart rate and rhythm, respiratory rate and rhythm, ventilatory pattern (eg, auscultation, electrocardiography, observations, palpation, sphygmomanometry)

Cranial and Peripheral Nerve Integrity

- Motor distribution of the cranial nerves (eg, observations)
- Motor distribution of the peripheral nerves (eg, observations)
- Response to stimuli, including auditory, gustatory, olfactory, pharyngeal, vestibular, and visual (eg, observations, provocation tests)
- Sensory distribution of the cranial nerves (eg, tactile tests, including coarse and light touch, cold and heat, pain, pressure, and vibration)
- Sensory distribution of the peripheral nerves (eg, tactile tests, including coarse and light touch, cold and heat, pain, pressure, and vibration, thoracic outlet tests)

Integumentary Integrity

Associated skin

- Activities, positioning, and postures that produce or relieve trauma to the skin (eg, observations)
- Skin characteristics, including blistering, continuity of skin color, dermatitis, hair growth, mobility, nail growth, sensation, temperature, texture, and turgor (eg, observations, palpation, photographic assessments, thermography)

Motor Function (Motor Control and Motor Learning)

- Initiation, modification, and control of movement patterns and voluntary postures (eg, activity indexes, developmental scales, gross motor function profiles, motor scales, movement assessment batteries, neuromotor tests, observations, physical performance tests, postural challenge tests, videographic assessments)

Muscle Performance (Including Strength, Power, and Endurance)

- Muscle strength, power, and endurance during functional activities (eg, ADL scales, functional muscle tests, IADL scales)

Neuromotor Development and Sensory Integration

- Acquisition and evolution of motor skills, including age-appropriate development (eg, activity indexes, developmental inventories and questionnaires, infant and toddler motor assessments, learning profiles, motor function tests, motor proficiency assessments, neuromotor assessments, reflex tests, screens, videographic assessments)
- Oral motor function, phonation, and speech production (eg, interviews, observations)
- Sensorimotor integration, including postural, equilibrium, and righting reactions (eg, behavioral assessment scales, motor and processing skill tests, observations, postural challenge tests, reflex tests, sensory profiles)

Orthotic, Protective, and Supportive Devices

- Components, alignment, fit, and ability to care for orthotic, protective, and supportive devices and equipment (eg, interviews, logs, observations, reports)
- Orthotic, protective, and supportive devices and equipment use during functional activities (eg, activities of daily living [ADL] scales, functional scales, interviews, observations, profiles)
- Remediation of impairments, functional limitations, or disabilities with use of orthotic, protective, and supportive devices and equipment (eg, activity status indexes, ADL scales, pain scales)
- Safety during use of orthotic, protective, and supportive devices and equipment (eg, reports, observations)

Pain

- Pain, soreness, and nociception (eg, provocation tests)

Posture

- Postural alignment and position (static and dynamic), including symmetry and deviation from midline (eg, grid measurement, observations, photographic assessments, videographic assessments)
- Specific body parts (eg, angle assessments, forward-bending test, goniometry, observations, palpation, positional tests)

Range of Motion (ROM) (Including Muscle Length)

- Functional ROM (eg, observations)

Reflex Integrity

- Deep reflexes (eg, myotatic reflex scale, observations, reflex tests)
- Postural reflexes and reactions, including righting, equilibrium, and protective reactions (eg, observations, postural challenge tests, reflex profiles, videographic assessments)
- Primitive reflexes and reactions, including developmental (eg, reflex profiles, screening tests)
- Resistance to passive stretch (eg, tone scales)
- Superficial reflexes and reactions (eg, observations, provocation tests)

Ventilation and Respiration/Gas Exchange

- Pulmonary signs of respiration/gas exchange, including breath sounds (eg, gas analyses, observations, oximetry)
- Pulmonary signs of ventilatory function, including airway protection; breath and voice sounds; respiratory rate, rhythm, and pattern; ventilatory flow, forces, and volumes (eg, airway clearance tests, observations, palpation, pulmonary function tests, ventilatory muscle force tests)

Evaluation, Diagnosis, and Prognosis (Including Plan of Care)

Physical therapists perform *evaluations* (make clinical judgments) based on the data gathered from the history, systems review, and tests and measures. In the evaluation process, physical therapists synthesize the examination data to establish the diagnosis and prognosis (including the plan of care). Factors that influence the complexity of the evaluation include the clinical findings, extent of loss of function, chronicity or severity of the problem, possibility of multisite or multisystem involvement, preexisting condition(s), potential discharge destination, social considerations, physical function, and overall health status.

A *diagnosis* is a label encompassing a cluster of signs and symptoms, syndromes, or categories. It is the result of the systematic diagnostic process, which includes integrating and evaluating the data from the examination. The diagnostic label indicates the primary dysfunction(s) toward which the therapist will direct interventions. The *prognosis* is the determination of the predicted optimal level of improvement in function and the amount of time needed to reach that level and may also include a prediction of levels of improvement that may be reached at various intervals during the course of therapy. During the prognostic process, the physical therapist develops the plan of care. The *plan of care* identifies specific interventions, proposed frequency and duration of the interventions, anticipated goals, expected outcomes, and discharge plans. The plan of care identifies realistic anticipated goals and expected outcomes, taking into consideration the expectations of the patient/client and appropriate others. These anticipated goals and expected outcomes should be measureable and time limited.

The frequency of visits and duration of the episode of care may vary from a short episode with a high intensity of intervention to a longer episode with a diminishing intensity of intervention. Frequency and duration may vary greatly among patients/clients based on a variety of factors that the physical therapist considers throughout the evaluation process, such as anatomical and physiological changes related to growth and development; caregiver consistency or expertise; chronicity or severity of the current condition; living environment; multisite or multisystem involvement; social support; potential discharge destinations; probability of prolonged impairment, functional limitation, or disability; and stability of the condition.

Prognosis

Over the course of 6 to 12 months, patient/client will demonstrate optimal ventilation, respiration/gas exchange, and aerobic capacity/endurance and the highest level of age-appropriate functioning.

During the episode of care, patient/client will achieve (1) the anticipated goals and expected outcomes of the interventions that are described in the plan of care and (2) the global outcomes for patients/clients who are classified in this pattern.

Expected Range of Number of Visits Per Episode of Care

16 to 84

This range represents the lower and upper limits of the number of physical therapist visits required to achieve anticipated goals and expected outcomes. *It is anticipated that 80% of patients/clients who are classified into this pattern will achieve the anticipated goals and expected outcomes within 16 to 84 visits during a single continuous episode of care.* Frequency of visits and duration of the episode of care should be determined by the physical therapist to maximize effectiveness of care and efficiency of service delivery.

Factors That May Require New Episode of Care or That May Modify Frequency of Visits/Duration of Episode

- Accessibility and availability of resources
- Adherence to the intervention program
- Age
- Anatomical and physiological changes related to growth and development
- Caregiver consistency or expertise
- Chronicity or severity of the current condition
- Cognitive status
- Comorbitities, complications, or secondary impairments
- Concurrent medical, surgical, and therapeutic interventions
- Decline in functional independence
- Level of impairment
- Level of physical function
- Living environment
- Multisite or multisystem involvement
- Nutritional status
- Overall health status
- Potential discharge destinations
- Premorbid conditions
- Probability of prolonged impairment, functional limitation, or disability
- Psychological and socioeconomic factors
- Psychomotor abilities
- Social support
- Stability of the condition

Intervention

Intervention is the purposeful interaction of the physical therapist with the patient/client and, when appropriate, with other individuals involved in patient/client care, using various physical therapy procedures and techniques to produce changes in the condition consistent with the diagnosis and prognosis. Decisions about interventions are contingent on the timely monitoring of patient/client response and the progress made toward achieving the anticipated goals and expected outcomes.

Communication, coordination, and documentation and patient/client-related instruction are provided for all patients/clients across all settings. Procedural interventions are selected or modified based on the examination data and the evaluation, the diagnosis and the prognosis, and the anticipated goals and expected outcomes for a particular patient/client. *For clinical considerations in selecting interventions, listings of interventions, and listings of anticipated goals and expected outcomes, refer to Chapter 3.*

Coordination, Communication, and Documentation

Coordination, communication, and documentation may include:

Interventions

- Addressing required functions
  - advance directives
  - individualized family service plans (IFSPs)
  - informed parent/guardian consent
  - mandatory communication and reporting (eg, patient advocacy and abuse reporting)
- Admission and discharge planning
- Case management
- Collaboration and coordination with agencies, including:
  - equipment suppliers
  - home care agencies
  - payer groups
  - transportation agencies
- Communication across settings, including:
  - case conferences
  - documentation
- Cost-effective resource utilization
- Data collection, analysis, and reporting
  - outcome data
  - peer review findings
  - record reviews
- Documentation across settings, following APTA's *Guidelines for Physical Therapy Documentation* (Appendix 5), including:
  - changes in impairments, functional limitations, and disabilities
  - changes in interventions
  - elements of patient/client management (examination, evaluation, diagnosis, prognosis, intervention)
  - outcomes of intervention
- Interdisciplinary teamwork
  - case conferences
  - patient care rounds
  - patient/client family meetings
- Referrals to other professionals or resources

Anticipated Goals and Expected Outcomes

- Accountability for services is increased.
- Admission data and discharge planning are completed.
- Advance directives, individualized family service plans (IFSPs), informed consent, and mandatory communication and reporting (eg, patient/client advocacy and abuse reporting) are obtained or completed.
- Available resources are maximally utilized.
- Care is coordinated with family, significant others, caregivers, and other professionals.
- Case is managed throughout the episode of care.
- Collaboration and coordination occurs with agencies, including equipment suppliers, home care agencies, payer groups, schools, and transportation agencies.
- Communication enhances risk reduction and prevention.
- Communication occurs across settings through case conferences and documentation.
- Data are collected, analyzed, and reported, including outcome data, peer review findings, and record reviews.
- Decision making is enhanced regarding patient/client health and the use of health care resources by family, significant others, and caregivers.
- Documentation occurs throughout patient/client management and across settings and follows APTA's *Guidelines for Physical Therapy Documentation* (Appendix 5).
- Interdisciplinary collaboration occurs through case conferences, patient care rounds, and patient/client family meetings.
- Family, significant other, and caregiver understanding of anticipated goals and expected outcomes is increased.
- Placement needs are determined.
- Referrals are made to other professionals or resources whenever necessary and appropriate.
- Resources are utilized in a cost-effective way.

Patient/Client-Related Instruction

Patient/client-related instruction may include:

Interventions

- Instruction, education and training of caregivers regarding:
  - current condition (pathology/pathophysiology [disease, disorder, or condition], impairments, functional limitations, or disabilities)
  - plan of care
  - risk factors for pathology/pathophysiology (disease, disorder, or condition), impairments, functional limitations, or disabilities
  - transitions across settings

Anticipated Goals and Expected Outcomes

- Ability to perform physical actions, tasks, or activities is improved.
- Awareness and use of community resources by family or caregivers are improved.
- Decision making is enhanced regarding patient/client health and the use of health care resources by family, significant others, and caregivers.
- Disability associated with acute or chronic illnesses is reduced.
- Family, significant other, and caregiver knowledge and awareness of the diagnosis, prognosis, interventions, and anticipated goals and expected outcomes are increased.
- Health status is improved.
- Intensity of care is decreased.
- Level of supervision required for task performance by family or caregiver is decreased.
- Physical function is improved.
- Risk of recurrence of condition is reduced.
- Risk of secondary impairment is reduced.
- Safety of patient/client, family, significant others, and caregivers is improved.
- Utilization and cost of health care services are decreased.

Procedural Interventions

Procedural interventions for this pattern may include:

Therapeutic Exercise

Interventions

- Flexibility exercises
  - muscle lengthening
  - range of motion
  - stretching
- Neuromotor development training
  - developmental activities training
  - motor training
  - movement patterns
  - neuromuscular education or reeducation

Anticipated Goals and Expected Outcomes

- Impact on pathology/pathophysiology (disease, disorder, or condition)
  - Atelectasis is decreased.
  - Nutrient delivery to tissue is increased.
  - Physiological response to increased oxygen demand is improved.
  - Symptoms associated with increased oxygen demand are decreased.
  - Tissue perfusion and oxygenation are enhanced.
- Impact on impairments
  - Airway clearance is improved.
  - Endurance is increased.
  - Energy expenditure per unit of work is decreased.
  - Muscle performance (strength, power, and endurance) is increased.
  - Quality and quantity of movement between and across body segments are improved.
  - Ventilation and respiration/gas exchange are improved.
  - Work of breathing is decreased.
- Impact on functional limitations
  - Ability to perform age-appropriate physical actions, tasks, or activities is improved.
  - Tolerance of positions and activities is increased.
- Impact on disabilities
  - Ability to assume required age-appropriate roles is improved.
- Risk reduction/prevention
  - Preoperative and postoperative complications are reduced.
  - Risk factors are reduced.
  - Risk of secondary impairment is reduced.
  - Safety is improved.
- Impact on health, wellness, and fitness
  - Health status is improved.
  - Physical function is improved.
- Impact on societal resources
  - Utilization of physical therapy services is optimized.
  - Utilization of physical therapy services results in efficient use of health care dollars.
- Patient/client satisfaction
  - Access, availability, and services provided are acceptable to caregiver.
  - Administrative management of practice is acceptable to caregiver.
  - Caregiver's sense of well-being is improved.
  - Caregiver's stressors are decreased.
  - Clinical proficiency of physical therapist is acceptable to caregiver.
  - Coordination of care is acceptable to caregiver.
  - Cost of health care services is decreased.
  - Intensity of care is decreased.
  - Interpersonal skills of physical therapist are acceptable to caregiver.

Functional Training in Self-Care and Home Management (Including Activities of Daily Living [ADL] and Instrumental Activities of Daily Living [IADL])

Interventions

- ADL training for caregivers
  - developmental activities
  - feeding
- Devices and equipment use and training for caregivers
  - assistive and adaptive device or equipment training during ADL
  - orthotic, protective, or supportive device or equipment training during ADL
- Injury prevention or reduction
  - injury prevention education for caregivers during ADL
  - safety awareness training for caregivers during ADL

Anticipated Goals and Expected Outcomes

- Impact on pathology/pathophysiology (disease, disorder, or condition)
  - Physiological response to increased oxygen demand is improved.
  - Symptoms associated with increased oxygen demand are decreased.
- Impact on impairments
  - Endurance is increased.
  - Energy expenditure per unit of work is decreased.
  - Muscle performance (strength, power, and endurance) is increased.
  - Work of breathing is decreased.
- Impact on functional limitations
  - Ability to perform age-appropriate physical actions, tasks, or activities is improved.
  - Tolerance of positions and activities is increased.
- Impact on disabilities
  - Ability to assume age-appropriate roles is improved.
- Risk reduction/prevention
  - Risk factors are reduced.
  - Risk of secondary impairments is reduced.
- Impact on health, wellness, and fitness
  - Health status is improved.
  - Physical function is improved.
- Impact on societal resources
  - Utilization of physical therapy services is optimized.
  - Utilization of physical therapy services results in efficient use of health care dollars.
- Patient/client satisfaction
  - Access, availability, and services provided are acceptable to caregiver.
  - Administrative management of practice is acceptable to caregiver.
  - Caregiver's sense of well-being is improved.
  - Caregiver's stressors are decreased.
  - Clinical proficiency of physical therapist is acceptable to caregiver.
  - Coordination of care is acceptable to caregiver.
  - Cost of health care services is decreased.
  - Intensity of care is decreased.
  - Interpersonal skills of physical therapist are acceptable to caregiver.

Manual Therapy Techniques (Including Mobilization/Manipulation)

Interventions

- Massage
  - connective tissue massage
  - therapeutic massage
- Mobilization/manipulation
  - soft tissue
- Passive range of motion

Anticipated Goals and Expected Outcomes

- Impact on pathology/pathophysiology (disease, disorder, or condition)
  - Soft tissue swelling, inflammation, or restriction is reduced.
- Impact on impairments
  - Joint integrity and mobility are improved.
- Impact on functional limitations
  - Ability to perform age-appropriate physical actions, tasks, or activities is improved.
  - Tolerance of positions and activities is increased.
- Impact on disabilities
  - Ability to assume age-appropriate roles is improved.
- Risk reduction/prevention
  - Risk of secondary impairment is reduced.
- Impact on health, wellness, and fitness
  - Physical function is improved.
- Impact on societal resources
  - Utilization of physical therapy services is optimized.
  - Utilization of physical therapy services results in efficient use of health care dollars.
- Patient/client satisfaction
  - Access, availability, and services provided are acceptable to caregiver.
  - Administrative management of practice is acceptable to caregiver.
  - Caregiver's sense of well-being is improved.
  - Caregiver's stressors are decreased.
  - Clinical proficiency of physical therapist is acceptable to caregiver.
  - Coordination of care is acceptable to caregiver.
  - Cost of health care services is decreased.
  - Intensity of care is decreased.
  - Interpersonal skills of physical therapist are acceptable to caregiver.

Prescription, Application, and, as Appropriate, Fabrication of Devices and Equipment (Assistive, Adaptive, Orthotic, Protective, Supportive, and Prosthetic)

Interventions

- Assistive devices
  - percussors and vibrators
- Orthotic devices
  - braces
  - casts
  - splints
- Protective devices
  - braces
  - cushions
- Supportive devices
  - mechanical ventilators
  - supplemental oxygen

Anticipated Goals and Expected Outcomes

- Impact on pathology/pathophysiology (disease, disorder, or condition)
  - Edema, lymphedema, or effusion is reduced.
  - Physiological response to increased oxygen demand is improved.
- Impact on impairments
  - Endurance is increased.
  - Energy expenditure per unit of work is decreased.
  - Work of breathing is decreased.
- Impact on functional limitations
  - Ability to perform age-appropriate physical actions, tasks, or activities is improved.
  - Tolerance of positions and activities is improved.
- Impact on disabilities
  - Ability to assume age-appropriate roles is improved.
- Risk reduction/prevention
  - Pressure on body tissues is reduced.
  - Protection of body parts is increased.
  - Risk factors are reduced.
  - Risk of secondary impairment is reduced.
  - Safety is improved.
- Impact on health, wellness, and fitness
  - Physical function is improved.
- Impact on societal resources
  - Utilization of physical therapy services is optimized.
  - Utilization of physical therapy services results in efficient use of health care dollars.
- Patient/client satisfaction
  - Access, availability, and services provided are acceptable to caregiver.
  - Administrative management of practice is acceptable to caregiver.
  - Caregiver's sense of well-being is improved.
  - Caregiver's stressors are decreased.
  - Clinical proficiency of physical therapist is acceptable to caregiver.
  - Coordination of care is acceptable to caregiver.
  - Cost of health care services is decreased.
  - Intensity of care is decreased.
  - Interpersonal skills of physical therapist are acceptable to caregiver.

Procedural Interventions

Airway Clearance Techniques

Interventions

- Manual/mechanical techniques
  - assistive devices
  - chest percussion, vibration, and shaking
  - suctioning
  - ventilatory aids
- Positioning
  - positioning to alter work of breathing
  - positioning to maximize ventilation and perfusion
  - pulmonary postural drainage

Anticipated Goals and Expected Outcomes

- Impact on pathology/pathophysiology (disease, disorder, or condition)
  - Atelectasis is decreased.
  - Tissue perfusion and oxygenation are enhanced.
- Impact on impairments
  - Airway clearance is improved.
  - Cough is improved.
  - Endurance is increased.
  - Energy expenditure per unit of work is decreased.
  - Ventilation and respiration/gas exchange are improved.
  - Work of breathing is decreased.
- Impact on functional limitations
  - Ability to perform age-appropriate physical actions, tasks, or activities is improved.
  - Tolerance of positions and activities is increased.
- Impact on disabilities
  - Ability to assume age-appropriate roles is improved.
- Risk reduction/prevention
  - Risk of secondary impairment is reduced.
- Impact on health, wellness, and fitness
  - Physical function is improved.
- Impact on societal resources
  - Utilization of physical therapy services is optimized.
  - Utilization of physical therapy services results in efficient use of health care dollars.
- Patient/client satisfaction
  - Access, availability, and services provided are acceptable to caregiver.
  - Administrative management of practice is acceptable to caregiver.
  - Caregiver's sense of well-being is improved.
  - Caregiver's stressors are decreased.
  - Clinical proficiency of physical therapist is acceptable to caregiver.
  - Coordination of care is acceptable to caregiver.
  - Cost of health care services is decreased.
  - Intensity of care is decreased.
  - Interpersonal skills of physical therapist are acceptable to caregiver.

Reexamination

Reexamination is the process of performing selected tests and measures after the initial examination to evaluate progress and to modify or redirect interventions. Reexamination may be indicated more than once during a single episode of care. It also may be performed over the course of a disease, disorder, or condition, which for some patients/clients may be over the life span. Indications for reexamination include new clinical findings or failure to respond to physical therapy interventions.

Global Outcomes for Patients/Clients in This Pattern

Throughout the entire episode of care, the physical therapist determines the anticipated goals and expected outcomes for each intervention. These anticipated goals and expected outcomes are delineated in shaded boxes that accompany the lists of interventions in each preferred practice pattern. As the patient/client reaches the termination of physical therapy services and the end of the episode of care, the physical therapist measures the global outcomes of the physical therapy services by characterizing or quantifying the impact of the physical therapy interventions in the following domains:

- Pathology/pathophysiology (disease, disorder, or condition)
- Impairments
- Functional limitations
- Disabilities
- Risk reduction/prevention
- Health, wellness, and fitness
- Societal resources
- Patient/client satisfaction

In some instances, a particular anticipated goal or expected outcome is thoroughly achieved through implementation of a single form of intervention. More commonly, however, the anticipated goals and expected outcomes are achieved as a result of the combined effects of several forms of interventions, leading to enhancement of both health status and health-related quality of life.

Criteria for Termination of Physical Therapy Services

Discharge is the process of ending physical therapy services that have been provided during a single episode of care. It occurs when the anticipated goals and expected outcomes have been achieved. Discharge does *not* occur with a *transfer* (defined as the time when a patient is moved from one site to another site within the same setting or across settings during a single episode of care). Although there may be facility-specific or payer-specific requirements for documentation regarding the conclusion of physical therapy services, *discharge occurs based on the physical therapist's analysis of the achievement of anticipated goals and expected outcomes.*

Discontinuation is the process of ending physical therapy services that have been provided during a single episode of care when (1) the patient/client, caregiver, or legal guardian declines to continue intervention; (2) the patient/client is unable to continue to progress toward outcomes because of medical or psychosocial complications or because financial/insurance resources have been expended; or (3) the physical therapist determines that the patient/client will no longer benefit from physical therapy. When physical therapy services are terminated prior to achievement of anticipated goals and expected outcomes, patient/client status and the rationale for termination are documented.

For patients/clients who require multiple episodes of care, periodic follow-up is needed over the life span to ensure safety and effective adaptation following changes in physical status, caregivers, environment, or task demands. In consultation with appropriate individuals, and in consideration of the outcomes, the physical therapist plans for discharge or discontinuation and provides for appropriate follow-up or referral.

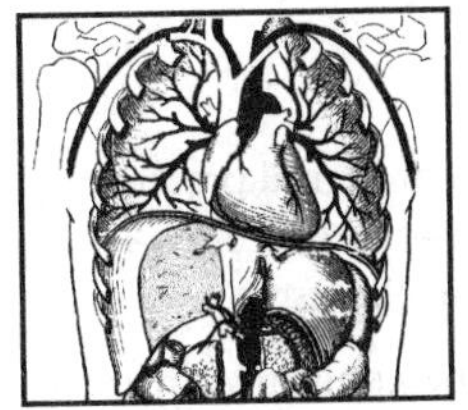

Impaired Circulation and Anthropometric Dimensions Associated With Lymphatic System Disorders

This preferred practice pattern describes the generally accepted elements of patient/client management that physical therapists provide for patients/clients who are classified in this pattern. The pattern title reflects the diagnosis made by the physical therapist. APTA emphasizes that preferred practice patterns are the boundaries within which a physical therapist may select any of a number of clinical alternatives, based on consideration of a wide variety of factors, such as individual patient/client needs; the profession's code of ethics and standards of practice; and patient/client age, culture, gender roles, race, sex, sexual orientation, and socioeconomic status.

Patient/Client Diagnostic Classification

Patients/clients will be classified into this pattern—for impaired circulation and anthropometric dimensions associated with lymphatic system disorders—as a result of the physical therapist's evaluation of the examination data. The findings from the examination (history, systems review, and tests and measures) may indicate the presence or risk of pathology/pathophysiology (disease, disorder, or condition), impairments, functional limitations, or disabilities or the need for health, wellness, or fitness programs. The physical therapist integrates, synthesizes, and interprets the data to determine the diagnostic classification.

Inclusion

The following examples of examination findings may support the inclusion of patients/clients in this pattern:

Risk Factors or Consequences of Pathology/Pathophysiology (Disease, Disorder, or Condition)

- Acquired immune deficiency syndrome
- Cellulitis
- Filariasis
- Infection/sepsis
- Lymphedema
- Post-radiation
- Reconstructive surgery
- Reflex sympathetic dystrophy
- Status post lymph node dissection
- Trauma

Impairments, Functional Limitations, or Disabilities

- Decreased participation in social activities as a result of perceived body image
- Difficulty dressing
- Edema
- Impaired skin integrity
- Pain

Note:

Some risk factors or consequences of pathology/pathophysiology—such as *deep vein thrombosis, lymphangiosarcoma*, and *lymphangitis*—may be severe and complex; *however, they do not necessarily exclude patients/clients from this pattern.* Severe and complex risk factors or consequences may require modification of the frequency of visits and duration of care. (See "Evaluation, Diagnosis, and Prognosis," page 575.)

Exclusion or Multiple-Pattern Classification

The following examples of examination findings may support exclusion from this pattern or classification into additional patterns. Depending on the level of severity or complexity of the examination findings, the physical therapist may determine that the patient/client would be more appropriately managed through (1) classification in an entirely different pattern or (2) classification in both this and another pattern.

Findings That May Require Classification in a Different Pattern

- Impairments associated with congestive heart failure

Findings That May Require Classification in Additional Patterns

- Dependent edema with cellulitis

ICD-9-CM Codes

The listing below contains the current (as of press time) and most typical 3- and 4-digit ICD-9-CM codes related to this preferred practice pattern. Because patient/client diagnostic classification is based on impairments, functional limitations, and disabilities—not on codes—patients/clients may be classified into the pattern even though the codes listed with the pattern may not apply to those clients.

This listing is intended for general information only and should not be used for coding purposes. The codes should be confirmed by referring to the World Health Organization's *International Classification of Diseases, 9th Revision, Clinical Modification (ICD-9-CM 2001)*, Volumes 1 and 3 (Chicago, Ill: American Medical Association; 2000) or subsequent revisions or by referring to other ICD-9-CM coding manuals that contain exclusion notes and instructions regarding fifth-digit requirements.

038 Septicemia
- **038.9** Unspecified septicemia

040 Other bacterial diseases
- **040.0** Gas gangrene
  - Malignant edema

125 Filarial infection and dracontiasis
- **125.9** Unspecified filariasis

176 Kaposi's sarcoma
- **176.5** Lymph nodes

457 Noninfectious disorders of lymphatic channels
- **457.0** Postmastectomy lymphedema syndrome
- **457.1** Other lymphedema
- **457.8** Other noninfectious disorders of lymphatic channels
- **457.9** Unspecified noninfectious disorder of lymphatic channels

646 Other complications of pregnancy, not elsewhere classified
- **646.1** Edema or excessive weight gain in pregnancy, without mention of hypertension

682 Other cellulitis and abscess
- **682.3** Upper arm and forearm
- **682.4** Hand, except fingers and thumb
- **682.6** Leg, except foot
- **682.7** Foot, except toes
- **682.9** Unspecified site
  - Abscess not otherwise specified
  - Cellulitis not otherwise specified
  - Lymphangitis, acute not otherwise specified

683 Acute lymphadenitis

757 Congenital anomalies of the integument
- **757.0** Hereditary edema of legs

782 Symptoms involving skin and other integumentary tissue
- **782.3** Edema
- **782.8** Changes in skin texture

995 Certain adverse effects not elsewhere classified
- **995.1** Angioneurotic edema

Examination

Examination is a comprehensive screening and specific testing process that leads to a diagnostic classification or, when appropriate, to a referral to another practitioner. Examination is required prior to the initial intervention and is performed for all patients/clients. Through the examination, the physical therapist may identify impairments, functional limitations, disabilities, changes in physical function or overall health status, and needs related to restoration of health and to prevention, wellness, and fitness. The physical therapist synthesizes the examination findings to establish the diagnosis and the prognosis (including the plan of care). The patient/client, family, significant others, and caregivers may provide information during the examination process.

Examination has three components: the patient/client history, the systems review, and tests and measures. The *history* is a systematic gathering of past and current information (often from the patient/client) related to why the patient/client is seeking the services of the physical therapist. The *systems review* is a brief or limited examination of (1) the anatomical and physiological status of the cardiovascular/pulmonary, integumentary, musculoskeletal, and neuromuscular systems and (2) the communication ability, affect, cognition, language, and learning style of the patient/client. *Tests and measures* are the means of gathering data about the patient/client.

The selection of examination procedures and the depth of the examination vary based on patient/client age; severity of the problem; stage of recovery (acute, subacute, chronic); phase of rehabilitation (early, intermediate, late, return to activity); home, work (job/school/play), or community situation; and other relevant factors. *For clinical indications in selecting tests and measures and for listings of tests and measures, tools used to gather data, and the types of data generated by tests and measures, refer to Chapter 2.*

Patient/Client History

The history may include:

General Demographics

- Age
- Sex
- Race/ethnicity
- Primary language
- Education

Social History

- Cultural beliefs and behaviors
- Family and caregiver resources
- Social interactions, social activities, and support systems

Employment/Work (Job/School/Play)

- Current and prior work (job/school/play), community, and leisure actions, tasks, or activities

Growth and Development

- Developmental history
- Hand dominance

Living Environment

- Devices and equipment (eg, assistive, adaptive, orthotic, protective, supportive, prosthetic)
- Living environment and community characteristics
- Projected discharge destinations

General Health Status (Self-Report, Family Report, Caregiver Report)

- General health perception
- Physical function (eg, mobility, sleep patterns, restricted bed days)
- Psychological function (eg, memory, reasoning ability, depression, anxiety)
- Role function (eg, community, leisure, social, work)
- Social function (eg, social activity, social interaction, social support)

Social/Health Habits (Past and Current)

- Behavioral health risks (eg, smoking, drug abuse)
- Level of physical fitness

Family History

- Familial health risks

Medical/Surgical History

- Cardiovascular
- Endocrine/metabolic
- Gastrointestinal
- Genitourinary
- Gynecological
- Integumentary
- Musculoskeletal
- Neuromuscular
- Obstetrical
- Prior hospitalizations, surgeries, and preexisting medical and other health-related conditions
- Psychological
- Pulmonary

Current Condition(s)/Chief Complaint(s)

- Concerns that led patient/client to seek the services of a physical therapist
- Concerns or needs of patient/client who requires the services of a physical therapist
- Current therapeutic interventions
- Mechanisms of injury or disease, including date of onset and course of events
- Onset and pattern of symptoms
- Patient/client, family, significant other, and caregiver expectations and goals for the therapeutic intervention
- Patient/client, family, significant other, and caregiver perceptions of patient's/client's emotional response to the current clinical situation
- Previous occurrence of chief complaint(s)
- Prior therapeutic interventions

Functional Status and Activity Level

- Current and prior functional status in self-care and home management activities, including activities of daily living (ADL) and instrumental activities of daily living (IADL)
- Current and prior functional status in work (job/school/play), community, and leisure actions, tasks, or activities

Medications

- Medications for current condition
- Medications previously taken for current condition
- Medications for other conditions

Other Clinical Tests

- Laboratory and diagnostic tests
- Review of available records (eg, medical, education, surgical)
- Review of other clinical findings (eg, nutrition and hydration)

Systems Review

The systems review may include:

Anatomical and Physiological Status

- Cardiovascular/Pulmonary
  - Blood pressure
  - Edema
  - Heart rate
  - Respiratory rate
- Integumentary
  - Pliability (texture)
  - Presence of scar formation
  - Skin color
  - Skin integrity
- Musculoskeletal
  - Gross range of motion
  - Gross strength
  - Gross symmetry
  - Height
  - Weight
- Neuromuscular
  - Gross coordinated movements (eg, balance, gait, locomotion, transfers, transitions)
  - Motor function (motor control, motor learning)

Communication, Affect, Cognition, Language, and Learning Style

- Ability to make needs known
- Consciousness
- Expected emotional/behavioral responses
- Learning preferences (eg, education needs, learning barriers)
- Orientation (person, place, time)

Tests and Measures

Tests and measures for this pattern may include those that characterize or quantify:

Aerobic Capacity and Endurance

- Cardiovascular signs and symptoms in response to increased oxygen demand with exercise or activity, including pressures and flow; heart rate, rhythm, and sounds; and superficial vascular responses (eg, claudication and exertion scales; observations; palpation; sphygmomanometry)
- Pulmonary signs and symptoms in response to increased oxygen demand with exercise or activity, including breath and voice sounds; cyanosis; gas exchange; respiratory pattern, rate, and rhythm; and ventilatory flow, force, and volume (eg, auscultation, dyspnea and exertion scales, observations, oximetry, palpation)

Anthropometric Characteristics

- Body composition (eg, body mass index, impedance measurement, skinfold thickness measurement)
- Body dimensions (eg, girth measurement, length measurement)
- Edema (eg, girth measurement, palpation, scales, volume measurement)

Arousal, Attention, and Cognition

- Cognition, including ability to process commands (eg, developmental inventories, indexes, interviews, mental state scales, observations, questionnaires, safety checklists)
- Motivation (eg, adaptive behavior scales)
- Recall, including memory and retention (eg, assessment scales, interviews, questionnaires)

Assistive and Adaptive Devices

- Assistive or adaptive devices and equipment use during functional activities (eg, activities of daily living [ADL] scales, functional scales, instrumental activities of daily living [IADL] scales, interviews, observations)
- Components, alignment, fit, and ability to care for assistive or adaptive devices and equipment (eg, interviews, logs, observations, pressure-sensing maps, reports)
- Remediation of impairments, functional limitations, or disabilities with use of assistive or adaptive devices and equipment (eg, activity status indexes, ADL scales, aerobic capacity tests, functional performance inventories, health assessment questionnaires, IADL scales, pain scales, play scales, videographic assessments)
- Safety during use of assistive or adaptive devices and equipment (eg, diaries, fall scales, interviews, logs, observations, reports)

Circulation (Arterial, Venous, and Lymphatic)

- Cardiovascular signs, including heart rate, rhythm, and sounds; pressures and flow; and superficial vascular responses (eg, auscultation, girth measurement, palpation, sphygmomanometry, thermography)
- Cardiovascular symptoms (eg, angina, claudication, and perceived exertion scales)
- Physiological responses to position change, including autonomic responses, central and peripheral pressures, heart rate and rhythm, respiratory rate and rhythm, ventilatory pattern (eg, auscultation, electrocardiography, observations, palpation, sphygmomanometry)

Cranial and Peripheral Nerve Integrity

- Motor distribution of the peripheral nerves (eg, dynamometry, muscle tests, observations, thoracic outlet tests)
- Sensory distribution of the peripheral nerves (eg, discrimination tests; tactile tests, including coarse and light touch, cold and heat, pain, pressure, and vibration; thoracic outlet tests)

Environmental, Home, and Work (Job/School/Play) Barriers

- Current and potential barriers (eg, checklists, interviews, observations, questionnaires)

Ergonomics and Body Mechanics

Ergonomics

- Dexterity and coordination during work (job/school/play) (eg, hand function tests, impairment rating scales, manipulative ability tests)
- Functional capacity and performance during work actions, tasks, or activities (eg, accelerometry, dynamometry, electroneuromyography, endurance tests, force platform tests, goniometry, interviews, observations, photographic assessments, physical capacity tests, postural loading analyses, technology-assisted assessments, videographic assessments, work analyses)
- Safety in work environments (eg, hazard identification checklists, job severity indexes, lifting standards, risk assessment scales, standards for exposure limits)
- Specific work conditions or activities (eg, handling checklists, job simulations, lifting models, preemployment screenings, task analysis checklists, workstation checklists)
- Tools, devices, equipment, and workstations related to work actions, tasks, or activities (eg, observations, tool analysis checklists, vibration assessments)

Body mechanics

- Body mechanics during self-care, home management, work, community, or leisure actions, tasks, or activities (eg, ADL scales, IADL scales, observations, photographic assessments, technology-assisted assessments, videographic assessments)

Gait, Locomotion, and Balance

- Balance during functional activities with or without the use of assistive, adaptive, orthotic, protective, supportive, or prosthetic devices or equipment (eg, ADL scales, IADL scales, observations, videographic assessments)
- Balance (dynamic and static) with or without the use of assistive, adaptive, orthotic, protective, supportive, or prosthetic devices or equipment (eg, balance scales, dizziness inventories, dynamic posturography, fall scales, motor impairment tests, observations, photographic assessments, postural control tests)
- Gait and locomotion during functional activities with or without the use of assistive, adaptive, orthotic, protective, supportive, or prosthetic devices or equipment (eg, ADL scales, gait indexes, IADL scales, mobility skill profiles, observations, videographic assessments)
- Gait and locomotion with or without the use of assistive, adaptive, orthotic, protective, supportive, or prosthetic devices or equipment (eg, dynamometry, electroneuromyography, footprint analyses, gait indexes, mobility skill profiles, observations, photographic assessments, technology-assisted assessments, videographic assessments, weight-bearing scales, wheelchair mobility tests)
- Safety during gait, locomotion, and balance (eg, confidence scales, diaries, fall scales, functional assessment profiles, logs, reports)

Integumentary Integrity

Associated skin

- Activities, positioning, and postures that produce or relieve trauma to the skin (eg, observations, pressure-sensing maps, scales)
- Assistive, adaptive, orthotic, protective, supportive, or prosthetic devices and equipment that may produce or relieve trauma to the skin (eg, observations, pressure-sensing maps, risk assessment scales)
- Skin characteristics, including blistering, continuity of skin color, dermatitis, hair growth, mobility, nail growth, sensation, temperature, texture, and turgor (eg, observations, palpation, photographic assessments, thermography)

Wound

- Activities, positioning, and postures that aggravate the wound or scar or that produce or relieve trauma (eg, observations, pressure-sensing maps)
- Burn (body charting, planimetry)
- Signs of infection (eg, cultures, observations, palpation)
- Wound characteristics, including bleeding, contraction, depth, drainage, exposed anatomical structures, location, odor, pigment, shape, size, staging and progression, tunneling, and undermining (eg, digital and grid measurement, grading of sores and ulcers, observations, palpation, photographic assessments, wound tracing)
- Wound scar tissue characteristics, including banding, pliability, sensation, and texture (eg, observations, scar-rating scales)

Muscle Performance (Including Strength, Power, and Endurance)

- Muscle strength, power, and endurance (eg, dynamometry, manual muscle tests, muscle performance tests, physical capacity tests, technology-assisted assessments, timed activity tests)
- Muscle strength, power, and endurance during functional activities (eg, ADL scales, functional muscle tests, IADL scales, observations, videographic assessments)
- Muscle tension (eg, palpation)

Orthotic, Protective, and Supportive Devices

- Components, alignment, fit, and ability to care for orthotic, protective, and supportive devices and equipment (eg, interviews, logs, observations, pressure-sensing maps, reports)
- Orthotic, protective, and supportive devices and equipment use during functional activities (eg, ADL scales, functional scales, IADL scales, interviews, observations, profiles)
- Remediation of impairments, functional limitations, or disabilities with use of orthotic, protective, and supportive devices and equipment (eg, activity status indexes, ADL scales, aerobic capacity tests, functional performance inventories, health assessment questionnaires, IADL scales, pain scales, play scales, videographic assessments)
- Safety during use of orthotic, protective, and supportive devices and equipment (eg, diaries, fall scales, interviews, logs, observations, reports)

Pain

- Pain, soreness, and nociception (eg, angina scales, analog scales, discrimination tests, pain drawings and maps, provocation tests, verbal and pictorial descriptor tests)
- Pain in specific body parts (eg, pain indexes, pain questionnaires, structural provocation tests)

Posture

- Postural alignment and position (static and dynamic), including symmetry and deviation from midline (eg, grid measurement, observations, photographic assessments, technology-assisted assessments, videographic assessments)
- Specific body parts (eg, angle assessments, forward-bending test, goniometry, observations, palpation, positional tests)

Range of Motion (ROM) (Including Muscle Length)

- Functional ROM (eg, observations, squat testing, toe touch tests)
- Joint active and passive movement (eg, goniometry, inclinometry, observations, photographic assessments, technology-assisted assessments, videographic assessments)
- Muscle length, soft tissue extensibility, and flexibility (eg, contracture tests, goniometry, inclinometry, ligamentous tests, linear measurement, multisegment flexibility tests, palpation)

Reflex Integrity

- Deep reflexes (eg, myotatic reflex scale, observations, reflex tests)
- Superficial reflexes and reactions (eg, observations, provocation tests)

Self-Care and Home Management (Including ADL and IADL)

- Ability to gain access to home environments (eg, barrier identification, observations, physical performance tests)
- Ability to perform self-care and home management activities with or without assistive, adaptive, orthotic, protective, supportive, or prosthetic devices and equipment (eg, ADL scales, aerobic capacity tests, IADL scales, interviews, observations, profiles)
- Safety in self-care and home management activities and environments (eg, diaries, fall scales, interviews, logs, observations, reports, videographic assessments)

Sensory Integrity

- Combined/cortical sensations (eg, stereognosis tests, tactile discrimination tests)
- Deep sensations (eg, kinesthesiometry, observations, photographic assessments, vibration tests)
- Electrophysiological integrity (eg, electroneuromyography)

Ventilation and Respiration/Gas Exchange

- Pulmonary signs of respiration/gas exchange, including breath sounds (eg, gas analyses, observations, oximetry)
- Pulmonary symptoms (eg, dyspnea and perceived exertion indexes and scales)

Work (Job/School/Play), Community, and Leisure Integration or Reintegration (Including IADL)

- Ability to assume or resume work (job/school/play), community, and leisure activities with or without assistive, adaptive, orthotic, protective, supportive, or prosthetic devices and equipment (eg, activity profiles, disability indexes, functional status questionnaires, IADL scales, observations, physical capacity tests)
- Ability to gain access to work (job/school/play), community, and leisure environments (eg, barrier identification, interviews, observations, physical capacity tests, transportation assessments)
- Safety in work (job/school/play), community, and leisure activities and environments (eg, diaries, fall scales, interviews, logs, observations, videographic assessments)

Evaluation, Diagnosis, and Prognosis (Including Plan of Care)

Physical therapists perform *evaluations* (make clinical judgments) based on the data gathered from the history, systems review, and tests and measures. In the evaluation process, physical therapists synthesize the examination data to establish the diagnosis and prognosis (including the plan of care). Factors that influence the complexity of the evaluation include the clinical findings, extent of loss of function, chronicity or severity of the problem, possibility of multisite or multisystem involvement, preexisting condition(s), potential discharge destination, social considerations, physical function, and overall health status.

A *diagnosis* is a label encompassing a cluster of signs and symptoms, syndromes, or categories. It is the result of the systematic diagnostic process, which includes integrating and evaluating the data from the examination. The diagnostic label indicates the primary dysfunction(s) toward which the therapist will direct interventions. The *prognosis* is the determination of the predicted optimal level of improvement in function and the amount of time needed to reach that level and may also include a prediction of levels of improvement that may be reached at various intervals during the course of therapy. During the prognostic process, the physical therapist develops the plan of care. The *plan of care* identifies specific interventions, proposed frequency and duration of the interventions, anticipated goals, expected outcomes, and discharge plans. The plan of care identifies realistic anticipated goals and expected outcomes, taking into consideration the expectations of the patient/client and appropriate others. These anticipated goals and expected outcomes should be measureable and time limited.

The frequency of visits and duration of the episode of care may vary from a short episode with a high intensity of intervention to a longer episode with a diminishing intensity of intervention. Frequency and duration may vary greatly among patients/clients based on a variety of factors that the physical therapist considers throughout the evaluation process, such as anatomical and physiological changes related to growth and development; caregiver consistency or expertise; chronicity or severity of the current condition; living environment; multisite or multisystem involvement; social support; potential discharge destinations; probability of prolonged impairment, functional limitation, or disability; and stability of the condition.

Prognosis	Expected Range of Number of Visits Per Episode of Care
Over the course of 1 to 8 weeks, patient/client with *mild lymphedema (less than 3-cm differential between affected limb and unaffected limb)* will demonstrate optimal circulation and anthropometric dimensions and the highest level of functioning in home, work (job/school/play), community, and leisure environments, within the context of the impairments, functional limitations, and disabilities.	**5 to 10**
Over the course of 1 to 8 weeks, patient/client with *moderate lymphedema (3- to 5-cm differential between affected limb and unaffected limb)* will demonstrate optimal circulation and anthropometric dimensions and the highest level of functioning in home, work (job/school/play), community, and leisure environments, within the context of the impairments, functional limitations, and disabilities.	**8 to 16**
Over the course of 1 to 8 weeks, patient/client with *severe lymphedema (5-plus-cm differential between affected limb and unaffected limb)* will demonstrate optimal circulation and anthropometric dimensions and the highest level of functioning in home, work (job/school/ play), community, and leisure environments, within the context of the impairments, functional limitations, and disabilities.	**14 to 24**

During the episode of care, patient/client with lymphedema will achieve (1) the anticipated goals and expected outcomes of the interventions that are described in the plan of care and (2) the global outcomes for patients/ clients who are classified in this pattern.

These ranges represent the lower and upper limits of the number of physical therapist visits required to achieve the anticipated goals and expected outcomes. ***It is anticipated that 80% of patients/clients who are classified into this pattern will achieve the anticipated goals and expected outcomes within these ranges during a single continuous episode of care.*** Frequency of visits and duration of the episode of care should be determined by the physical therapist to maximize effectiveness of care and efficiency of service delivery.

Factors That May Require New Episode of Care or That May Modify Frequency of Visits/ Duration of Episode

- Accessibility and availability of resources
- Adherence to the intervention program
- Age
- Anatomical and physiological changes related to growth and development
- Caregiver consistency or expertise
- Chronicity or severity of the current condition
- Cognitive status
- Comorbitities, complications, or secondary impairments
- Concurrent medical, surgical, and therapeutic interventions
- Decline in functional independence
- Level of impairment
- Level of physical function
- Living environment
- Multisite or multisystem involvement
- Nutritional status
- Overall health status
- Potential discharge destinations
- Premorbid conditions
- Probability of prolonged impairment, functional limitation, or disability
- Psychological and socioeconomic factors
- Psychomotor abilities
- Social support
- Stability of the condition

Note:

Patients/clients may require multiple episodes of care for lymphatic management over the lifetime.

Intervention

Intervention is the purposeful interaction of the physical therapist with the patient/client and, when appropriate, with other individuals involved in patient/client care, using various physical therapy procedures and techniques to produce changes in the condition consistent with the diagnosis and prognosis. Decisions about interventions are contingent on the timely monitoring of patient/client response and the progress made toward achieving the anticipated goals and expected outcomes.

Communication, coordination, and documentation and patient/client-related instruction are provided for all patients/clients across all settings. Procedural interventions are selected or modified based on the examination data and the evaluation, the diagnosis and the prognosis, and the anticipated goals and expected outcomes for a particular patient/client. *For clinical considerations in selecting interventions, listings of interventions, and listings of anticipated goals and expected outcomes, refer to Chapter 3.*

Coordination, Communication, and Documentation

Coordination, communication, and documentation may include:

Interventions

- Addressing required functions
  - advance directives
  - individualized family service plans (IFSPs) or individualized education plans (IEPs)
  - informed consent
  - mandatory communication and reporting (eg, patient advocacy and abuse reporting)
- Admission and discharge planning
- Case management
- Collaboration and coordination with agencies, including:
  - equipment suppliers
  - home care agencies
  - payer groups
  - schools
  - transportation agencies
- Communication across settings, including:
  - case conferences
  - documentation
- Cost-effective resource utilization
- Data collection, analysis, and reporting
  - outcome data
  - peer review findings
  - record reviews
- Documentation across settings, following APTA's *Guidelines for Physical Therapy Documentation* (Appendix 5), including:
  - changes in impairments, functional limitations, and disabilities
  - changes in interventions
  - elements of patient/client management (examination, evaluation, diagnosis, prognosis, intervention)
  - outcomes of intervention
- Interdisciplinary teamwork
  - case conferences
  - patient care rounds
  - patient/client family meetings
- Referrals to other professionals or resources

Anticipated Goals and Expected Outcomes

- Accountability for services is increased.
- Admission data and discharge planning are completed.
- Advance directives, individualized family service plans (IFSPs) or individualized education plans (IEPs), informed consent, and mandatory communication and reporting (eg, patient advocacy and abuse reporting) are obtained or completed.
- Available resources are maximally utilized.
- Care is coordinated with patient/client, family, significant others, caregivers, and other professionals.
- Case is managed throughout the episode of care.
- Collaboration and coordination occurs with agencies, including equipment suppliers, home care agencies, payer groups, schools, and transportation agencies.
- Communication enhances risk reduction and prevention.
- Communication occurs across settings through case conferences, and documentation.
- Data are collected, analyzed, and reported, including outcome data, peer review findings, and record reviews.
- Decision making is enhanced regarding health, wellness, and fitness needs.
- Decision making is enhanced regarding patient/client health and the use of health care resources by patient/client, family, significant others, and caregivers.
- Documentation occurs throughout patient/client management and across settings and follows APTA's *Guidelines for Physical Therapy Documentation* (Appendix 5).
- Interdisciplinary collaboration occurs through case conferences, patient care rounds, and patient/client family meetings.
- Patient/client, family, significant other, and caregiver understanding of anticipated goals and expected outcomes is increased.
- Placement needs are determined.
- Referrals are made to other professionals or resources whenever necessary and appropriate.
- Resources are utilized in a cost-effective way.

Patient/Client-Related Instruction

Patient/client-related instruction may include:

Interventions

- Instruction, education and training of patients/clients and caregivers regarding:
  - current condition (pathology/pathophysiology [disease, disorder, or condition], impairments, functional limitations, or disabilities)
  - enhancement of performance
  - health, wellness, and fitness programs
  - plan of care
  - risk factors for pathology/pathophysiology (disease, disorder, or condition), impairments, functional limitations, or disabilities
  - transitions across settings
  - transitions to new roles

Anticipated Goals and Expected Outcomes

- Ability to perform physical actions, tasks, or activities is improved.
- Awareness and use of community resources are improved.
- Behaviors that foster healthy habits, wellness, and prevention are acquired.
- Decision making is enhanced regarding patient/client health and the use of health care resources by patient/client, family, significant others, and caregivers.
- Disability associated with acute or chronic illnesses is reduced.
- Functional independence in activities of daily living (ADL) and instrumental activities of daily living (IADL) is increased.
- Health status is improved.
- Intensity of care is decreased.
- Level of supervision required for task performance is decreased.
- Patient/client, family, significant other, and caregiver knowledge and awareness of the diagnosis, prognosis, interventions, and anticipated goals and expected outcomes are increased.
- Patient/client knowledge of personal and environmental factors associated with the condition is increased.
- Performance levels in self-care, home management, work (job/school/play), community, or leisure actions, tasks, or activities are improved.
- Physical function is improved.
- Risk of recurrence of condition is reduced.
- Risk of secondary impairment is reduced.
- Safety of patient/client, family, significant others, and caregivers is improved.
- Self-management of symptoms is improved.
- Utilization and cost of health care services are decreased.

Procedural Interventions

Procedural interventions for this pattern may include:

Therapeutic Exercise

Interventions

- Aerobic capacity/endurance conditioning or reconditioning
  - aquatic programs
  - gait and locomotor training
  - increased workload over time
  - walking and wheelchair propulsion programs
- Balance, coordination, and agility training
  - developmental activities training
  - motor function (motor control and motor learning) training or retraining
  - neuromuscular education or reeducation
  - perceptual training
  - posture awareness training
  - standardized, programmatic, complementary exercise approaches
  - sensory training and retraining
  - task-specific performance training
- Body mechanics and postural stabilization
  - body mechanics training
  - postural control training
  - postural stabilization activities
  - posture awareness training
- Flexibility exercises
  - muscle lengthening
  - range of motion
  - stretching
- Gait and locomotion training
  - developmental activities training
  - gait training
  - implement and device training
  - perceptual training
    standardized, programmatic, complementary exercise approaches
  - wheelchair training
- Relaxation
  - breathing strategies
  - movement strategies
  - relaxation techniques
    standardized, programmatic, complementary exercise approaches
- Strength, power, and endurance training for head, neck, limb, pelvic-floor, trunk, and ventilatory muscles
  - active assistive, active, and resistive exercises (including concentric, dynamic/isotonic, isometric, and plyometric)
  - aquatic programs
  - standardized, programmatic, complementary exercise approaches
  - task-specific performance training

Anticipated Goals and Expected Outcomes

- Impact on pathology/pathophysiology (disease, disorder, or condition)
  - Joint swelling, inflammation, or restriction is reduced.
  - Nutrient delivery to tissue is increased.
  - Osteogenic effects of exercise are maximized.
  - Pain is decreased.
  - Physiological response to increased oxygen demand is improved.
  - Soft tissue swelling, inflammation, or restriction is reduced.
  - Tissue perfusion and oxygenation are enhanced.
- Impact on impairments
  - Aerobic capacity is increased.
  - Balance is improved.
  - Endurance is increased.
  - Energy expenditure per unit of work is decreased.
  - Gait, locomotion, and balance are improved.
  - Integumentary integrity is improved.
  - Joint integrity and mobility are improved.
  - Motor function (motor control and motor learning) is improved.
  - Muscle performance (strength, power, and endurance) is increased.
  - Postural control is improved.
  - Quality and quantity of movement between and across body segments are improved.
  - Range of motion is improved.
  - Relaxation is increased.
  - Sensory awareness is increased.
  - Weight-bearing status is improved.
- Impact on functional limitations
  - Ability to perform physical actions, tasks, or activities related to self-care, home management, work (job/school/play), community, and leisure is improved.
  - Level of supervision required for task performance is decreased.
  - Performance of and independence in activities of daily living (ADL) and instrumental activities of daily living (IADL) with or without devices and equipment are increased.
  - Tolerance of positions and activities is increased.
- Impact on disabilities
  - Ability to assume or resume required self-care, home management, work (job/school/play), community, and leisure roles is improved.
- Risk reduction/prevention
  - Preoperative and postoperative complications are reduced.
  - Risk factors are reduced.
  - Risk of recurrence of condition is reduced.
  - Risk of secondary impairment is reduced.
  - Safety is improved.
  - Self-management of symptoms is improved.
- Impact on health, wellness, and fitness
  - Fitness is improved.
  - Health status is improved.
  - Physical capacity is increased.
  - Physical function is improved.
- Impact on societal resources
  - Utilization of physical therapy services is optimized.
  - Utilization of physical therapy services results in efficient use of health care dollars.
- Patient/client satisfaction
  - Access, availability, and services provided are acceptable to patient/client.
  - Administrative management of practice is acceptable to patient/client.
  - Clinical proficiency of physical therapist is acceptable to patient/client.
  - Coordination of care is acceptable to patient/client.
  - Cost of health care services is decreased.
  - Intensity of care is decreased.
  - Interpersonal skills of physical therapist are acceptable to patient/client, family, and significant others.
  - Sense of well-being is improved.
  - Stressors are decreased.

Functional Training in Self-Care and Home Management (Including Activities of Daily Living [ADL] and Instrumental Activities of Daily Living [IADL])

Interventions

- ADL training
  - bathing
  - bed mobility and transfer training
  - developmental activities
  - dressing
  - eating
  - grooming
  - toileting
- Devices and equipment use and training
  - assistive and adaptive device or equipment training during ADL and IADL
  - orthotic, protective, or supportive device or equipment training during ADL and IADL
  - prosthetic device or equipment training during ADL and IADL
- Functional training programs
  - simulated environments and tasks
  - task adaptation
- IADL training
  - caring for dependents
  - home maintenance
  - household chores
  - shopping
  - structured play for infants and children
  - yard work
- Injury prevention or reduction
  - injury prevention education during self-care and home management
  - injury prevention or reduction with use of devices and equipment
  - safety awareness training during self-care and home management

Anticipated Goals and Expected Outcomes

- Impact on pathology/pathophysiology (disease, disorder, or condition)
  - Pain is decreased.
  - Physiological response to increased oxygen demand is improved.
- Impact on impairments
  - Balance is improved.
  - Endurance is increased.
  - Energy expenditure per unit of work is decreased.
  - Motor function (motor control and motor learning) is improved.
  - Muscle performance (strength, power, and endurance) is increased.
  - Postural control is improved.
  - Sensory awareness is increased.
  - Weight-bearing status is improved.
- Impact on functional limitations
  - Ability to perform physical actions, tasks, or activities related to self-care and home management is improved.
  - Level of supervision required for task performance is decreased.
  - Performance of and independence in ADL and IADL with or without devices and equipment are increased.
  - Tolerance of positions and activities is increased.
- Impact on disabilities
  - Ability to assume or resume required self-care and home management roles is improved.
- Risk reduction/prevention
  - Risk factors are reduced.
  - Risk of secondary impairments is reduced.
  - Safety is improved.
  - Self-management of symptoms is improved.
- Impact on health, wellness, and fitness
  - Health status is improved.
  - Physical capacity is increased.
  - Physical function is improved.
- Impact on societal resources
  - Utilization of physical therapy services is optimized.
  - Utilization of physical therapy services results in efficient use of health care dollars.
- Patient/client satisfaction
  - Access, availability, and services provided are acceptable to patient/client.
  - Administrative management of practice is acceptable to patient/client.
  - Clinical proficiency of physical therapist is acceptable to patient/client.
  - Coordination of care is acceptable to patient/client.
  - Cost of health care services is decreased.
  - Intensity of care is decreased.
  - Interpersonal skills of physical therapist are acceptable to patient/client, family, and significant others.
  - Sense of well-being is improved.
  - Stressors are decreased.

Functional Training in Work (Job/School/Play), Community, and Leisure Integration or Reintegration (Including Instrumental Activities of Daily Living [IADL], Work Hardening, and Work Conditioning)

Interventions

- Devices and equipment use and training
  - assistive and adaptive device or equipment training during IADL
  - orthotic, protective, or supportive device or equipment training during IADL
  - prosthetic device or equipment training during IADL
- IADL training
  - community service training involving instruments
  - school and play activities training including tools and instruments
  - work training with tools
- Injury prevention or reduction
  - injury prevention education during work (job/school/play), community, and leisure integration or reintegration
  - injury prevention or reduction with use of devices and equipment
  - safety awareness training during work (job/school/play), community, and leisure integration or reintegration

Anticipated Goals and Expected Outcomes

- Impact on pathology/pathophysiology (disease, disorder, or condition)
  - Pain is decreased.
  - Physiological response to increased oxygen demand is improved.
- Impact on impairments
  - Balance is improved.
  - Endurance is increased.
  - Energy expenditure per unit of work is decreased.
  - Motor function (motor control and motor learning) is improved.
  - Muscle performance (strength, power, and endurance) is increased.
  - Postural control is improved.
  - Sensory awareness is increased.
  - Weight-bearing status is improved.
- Impact on functional limitations
  - Ability to perform physical actions, tasks, or activities related to work (job/school/play), community, and leisure integration or reintegration is improved.
  - Level of supervision required for task performance is decreased.
  - Performance of and independence in IADL with or without devices and equipment are increased.
  - Tolerance of positions and activities is increased.
- Impact on disabilities
  - Ability to assume or resume required work (job/school/play), community, and leisure roles is improved.
- Risk reduction/prevention
  - Risk factors are reduced.
  - Risk of secondary impairment is reduced.
  - Safety is improved.
  - Self-management of symptoms is improved.
- Impact on health, wellness, and fitness
  - Fitness is improved.
  - Health status is improved.
  - Physical capacity is increased.
  - Physical function is improved.
- Impact on societal resources
  - Costs of work-related injury or disability are reduced.
  - Utilization of physical therapy services is optimized.
  - Utilization of physical therapy services results in efficient use of health care dollars.
- Patient/client satisfaction
  - Access, availability, and services provided are acceptable to patient/client.
  - Administrative management of practice is acceptable to patient/client.
  - Clinical proficiency of physical therapist is acceptable to patient/client.
  - Coordination of care is acceptable to patient/client.
  - Cost of health care services is decreased.
  - Intensity of care is decreased.
  - Interpersonal skills of physical therapist are acceptable to patient/client, family, and significant others.
  - Sense of well-being is improved.
  - Stressors are decreased.

Manual Therapy Techniques (Including Mobilization/Manipulation)

Interventions

- Manual lymphatic drainage
- Massage
  - connective tissue massage
  - therapeutic massage
- Mobilization/manipulation
  - soft tissue
- Passive range of motion

Anticipated Goals and Expected Outcomes

- Impact on pathology/pathophysiology (disease, disorder, or condition)
  - Edema, lymphedema, or effusion is reduced.
  - Joint swelling, inflammation, or restriction is reduced.
  - Pain is decreased.
  - Soft tissue swelling, inflammation, or restriction is reduced.
- Impact on impairments
  - Balance is improved.
  - Energy expenditure per unit of work is decreased.
  - Gait, locomotion, and balance are improved.
  - Integumentary integrity is improved.
  - Joint integrity and mobility are improved.
  - Muscle performance (strength, power, and endurance) is increased.
  - Postural control is improved.
  - Quality and quantity of movement between and across body segments are improved.
  - Range of motion is improved.
  - Relaxation is increased.
  - Sensory awareness is increased.
  - Weight-bearing status is improved.
- Impact on functional limitations
  - Ability to perform movement tasks is improved.
  - Ability to perform physical actions, tasks, or activities related to self-care, home management, work (job/school/play), community, and leisure is improved.
  - Tolerance of positions and activities is increased.
- Impact on disabilities
  - Ability to assume or resume required self-care, home management, work (job/school/play), community, and leisure roles is improved.
- Risk reduction/prevention
  - Risk factors are reduced.
  - Risk of recurrence of condition is reduced.
  - Risk of secondary impairment is reduced.
  - Self-management of symptoms is improved.
- Impact on health, wellness, and fitness
  - Physical capacity is increased.
  - Physical function is improved.
- Impact on societal resources
  - Utilization of physical therapy services is optimized.
  - Utilization of physical therapy services results in efficient use of health care dollars.
- Patient/client satisfaction
  - Access, availability, and services provided are acceptable to patient/client.
  - Administrative management of practice is acceptable to patient/client.
  - Clinical proficiency of physical therapist is acceptable to patient/client.
  - Coordination of care is acceptable to patient/client.
  - Cost of health care services is decreased.
  - Intensity of care is decreased.
  - Interpersonal skills of physical therapist are acceptable to patient/client, family, and significant others.
  - Sense of well-being is improved.
  - Stressors are decreased.

Prescription, Application, and, as Appropriate, Fabrication of Devices and Equipment (Assistive, Adaptive, Orthotic, Protective, Supportive, and Prosthetic)

Interventions

- Adaptive devices
  - environmental controls
  - hospital beds
  - raised toilet seats
  - seating systems
- Assistive devices
  - canes
  - crutches
  - long-handled reachers
  - power devices
  - static and dynamic splints
  - walkers
  - wheelchairs
- Orthotic devices
  - braces
  - casts
  - shoe inserts
  - splints
- Prosthetic devices (lower-extremity and upper-extremity)
- Protective devices
  - braces
  - cushions
  - protective taping
- Supportive devices
  - compression garments
  - corsets
  - elastic wraps
  - neck collars
  - slings
  - supportive taping

Anticipated Goals and Expected Outcomes

- Impact on pathology/pathophysiology (disease, disorder, or condition)
  - Edema, lymphedema, or effusion is reduced.
  - Joint swelling, inflammation, or restriction is reduced.
  - Pain is decreased.
  - Physiological response to increased oxygen demand is improved.
  - Soft tissue swelling, inflammation, or restriction is reduced.
- Impact on impairments
  - Balance is improved.
  - Endurance is increased.
  - Energy expenditure per unit of work is decreased.
  - Gait, locomotion, and balance are improved.
  - Integumentary integrity is improved.
  - Joint stability is improved.
  - Motor function (motor control and motor learning) is improved.
  - Muscle performance (strength, power, and endurance) is increased.
  - Optimal joint alignment is achieved.
  - Optimal loading on a body part is achieved.
  - Postural control is improved.
  - Quality and quantity of movement between and across body segments are improved.
  - Range of motion is improved.
  - Weight-bearing status is improved.
- Impact on functional limitations
  - Ability to perform physical actions, tasks, or activities related to self-care, home management, work (job/school/play), community, and leisure is improved.
  - Level of supervision required for task performance is decreased.
  - Performance of and independence in activities of daily living (ADL) and instrumental activities of daily living (IADL) with or without devices and equipment are increased.
  - Tolerance of positions and activities is improved.
- Impact on disabilities
  - Ability to assume or resume required self-care, home management, work (job/school/play), community, and leisure roles is improved.
- Risk reduction/prevention
  - Pressure on body tissues is reduced.
  - Protection of body parts is increased.
  - Risk factors are reduced.
  - Risk of secondary impairment is reduced.
  - Safety is improved.
  - Self-management of symptoms is improved.
- Impact on health, wellness, and fitness
  - Health status is improved.
  - Physical capacity is increased.
  - Physical function is improved.
- Impact on societal resources
  - Utilization of physical therapy services is optimized.
  - Utilization of physical therapy services results in efficient use of health care dollars.
- Patient/client satisfaction
  - Access, availability, and services provided are acceptable to patient/client.
  - Administrative management of practice is acceptable to patient/client.
  - Clinical proficiency of physical therapist is acceptable to patient/client.
  - Coordination of care is acceptable to patient/client.
  - Cost of health care services is decreased.
  - Intensity of care is decreased.
  - Interpersonal skills of physical therapist are acceptable to patient/client, family, and significant others.
  - Sense of well-being is improved.
  - Stressors are decreased.

Electrotherapeutic Modalities

Interventions

- Electrical stimulation
  - electrical muscle stimulation (EMS)
  - transcutaneous electrical nerve stimulation (TENS)

Anticipated Goals and Expected Outcomes

- Impact on pathology/pathophysiology (disease, disorder, or condition)
  - Edema, lymphedema, or effusion is reduced.
  - Joint swelling, inflammation, or restriction is reduced.
  - Nutrient delivery to tissue is increased.
  - Osteogenic effects of exercise are maximized.
  - Pain is decreased.
  - Soft tissue or wound healing is enhanced.
  - Soft tissue swelling, inflammation, or restriction is reduced.
  - Tissue perfusion and oxygenation are enhanced.
- Impact on impairments
  - Integumentary integrity is improved.
  - Motor function (motor control and motor learning) is improved.
  - Muscle performance (strength, power, and endurance) is increased.
  - Postural control is improved.
  - Quality and quantity of movement between and across body segments are improved.
  - Range of motion is improved.
  - Relaxation is increased.
  - Sensory awareness is increased.
- Impact on functional limitations
  - Ability to perform physical actions, tasks, or activities related to self-care, home management, work (job/school/play), community, and leisure is improved.
  - Level of supervision required for task performance is decreased.
  - Performance of and independence in activities of daily living (ADL) and instrumental activities of daily living (IADL) with or without devices and equipment are increased.
  - Tolerance of positions and activities is increased.
- Impact on disabilities
  - Ability to assume or resume required self-care, home management, work (job/school/play), community, and leisure roles is improved.
- Risk reduction/prevention
  - Complications of immobility are reduced.
  - Preoperative and postoperative complications are reduced.
  - Risk factors are reduced.
  - Risk of recurrence of condition is reduced.
  - Risk of secondary impairment is reduced.
  - Self-management of symptoms is improved.
- Impact on health, wellness, and fitness
  - Physical capacity is increased.
  - Physical function is improved.
- Impact on societal resources
  - Utilization of physical therapy services is optimized.
  - Utilization of physical therapy services results in efficient use of health care dollars.
- Patient/client satisfaction
  - Access, availability, and services provided are acceptable to patient/client.
  - Administrative management of practice is acceptable to patient/client.
  - Clinical proficiency of physical therapist is acceptable to patient/client.
  - Coordination of care is acceptable to patient/client.
  - Interpersonal skills of physical therapist are acceptable to patient/client, family, and significant others.
  - Sense of well-being is improved.
  - Stressors are reduced.

Physical Agents and Mechanical Modalities

Interventions

Physical agents may include:

- Cryotherapy
  - cold packs
  - ice massage
- Hydrotherapy
  - contrast bath
  - pools
  - whirlpool tanks
- Sound agents
  - phonophoresis
  - ultrasound
- Thermotherapy
  - dry heat
  - hot packs

Mechanical modalities may include:

- Compression therapies
  - compression bandaging
  - compression garments
  - vasopneumatic compression devices
- Mechanical motion devices
  - continuous passive motion (CPM)

Anticipated Goals and Expected Outcomes

- Impact on pathology/pathophysiology (disease, disorder, or condition)
  - Edema, lymphedema, or effusion is reduced.
  - Joint swelling, inflammation, or restriction is reduced.
  - Nutrient delivery to tissue is increased.
  - Pain is decreased.
  - Soft tissue swelling, inflammation, or restriction is reduced.
  - Tissue perfusion and oxygenation are enhanced.
- Impact on impairments
  - Integumentary integrity is improved.
  - Muscle performance (strength, power, and endurance) is increased.
  - Range of motion is improved.
  - Weight-bearing status is improved.
- Impact on functional limitations
  - Ability to perform physical actions, tasks, or activities related to self-care, home management, work (job/school/play), community, and leisure is improved.
  - Performance of and independence in activities of daily living (ADL) and instrumental activities of daily living (IADL) with or without devices and equipment are increased.
  - Tolerance of positions and activities is increased.
- Impact on disabilities
  - Ability to assume or resume required self-care, home management, work (job/school/play), community, and leisure roles is improved.
- Risk reduction/prevention
  - Complications of soft tissue and circulatory disorders are decreased.
  - Risk of secondary impairment is reduced.
  - Self-management of symptoms is improved.
  - Stresses precipitating injury are decreased.
- Impact on health, wellness, and fitness
  - Physical function is improved.
- Impact on societal resources
  - Utilization of physical therapy services is optimized.
- Patient/client satisfaction
  - Access, availability, and services provided are acceptable to patient/client.
  - Administrative management of practice is acceptable to patient/client.
  - Clinical proficiency of physical therapist is acceptable to patient/client.
  - Coordination of care is acceptable to patient/client.
  - Interpersonal skills of physical therapist are acceptable to patient/client, family, and significant others.
  - Sense of well-being is improved.
  - Stressors are decreased.

Reexamination

Reexamination is the process of performing selected tests and measures after the initial examination to evaluate progress and to modify or redirect interventions. Reexamination may be indicated more than once during a single episode of care. It also may be performed over the course of a disease, disorder, or condition, which for some patients/clients may be over the life span. Indications for reexamination include new clinical findings or failure to respond to physical therapy interventions.

Global Outcomes for Patients/Clients in This Pattern

Throughout the entire episode of care, the physical therapist determines the anticipated goals and expected outcomes for each intervention. These anticipated goals and expected outcomes are delineated in shaded boxes that accompany the lists of interventions in each preferred practice pattern. As the patient/client reaches the termination of physical therapy services and the end of the episode of care, the physical therapist measures the global outcomes of the physical therapy services by characterizing or quantifying the impact of the physical therapy interventions in the following domains:

- Pathology/pathophysiology (disease, disorder, or condition)
- Impairments
- Functional limitations
- Disabilities
- Risk reduction/prevention
- Health, wellness, and fitness
- Societal resources
- Patient/client satisfaction

In some instances, a particular anticipated goal or expected outcome is thoroughly achieved through implementation of a single form of intervention. More commonly, however, the anticipated goals and expected outcomes are achieved as a result of the combined effects of several forms of interventions, leading to enhancement of both health status and health-related quality of life.

Criteria for Termination of Physical Therapy Services

Discharge is the process of ending physical therapy services that have been provided during a single episode of care. It occurs when the anticipated goals and expected outcomes have been achieved. Discharge does *not* occur with a *transfer* (defined as the time when a patient is moved from one site to another site within the same setting or across settings during a single episode of care). Although there may be facility-specific or payer-specific requirements for documentation regarding the conclusion of physical therapy services, *discharge occurs based on the physical therapist's analysis of the achievement of anticipated goals and expected outcomes.*

Discontinuation is the process of ending physical therapy services that have been provided during a single episode of care when (1) the patient/client, caregiver, or legal guardian declines to continue intervention; (2) the patient/client is unable to continue to progress toward outcomes because of medical or psychosocial complications or because financial/insurance resources have been expended; or (3) the physical therapist determines that the patient/client will no longer benefit from physical therapy. When physical therapy services are terminated prior to achievement of anticipated goals and expected outcomes, patient/client status and the rationale for termination are documented.

For patients/clients who require multiple episodes of care, periodic follow-up is needed over the life span to ensure safety and effective adaptation following changes in physical status, caregivers, environment, or task demands. In consultation with appropriate individuals, and in consideration of the outcomes, the physical therapist plans for discharge or discontinuation and provides for appropriate follow-up or referral.

CHAPTER 7

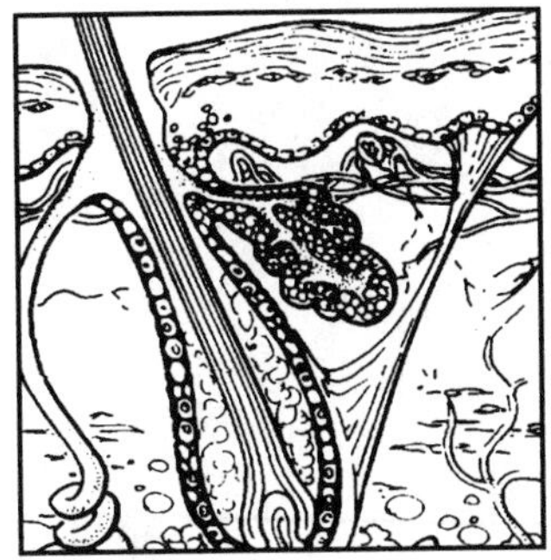

Preferred Physical Therapist Practice Patterns: Integumentary

Preferred Physical Therapist Practice Patterns describe the five elements of patient/client management that are provided by physical therapists: examination (history, systems review, and tests and measures), evaluation, diagnosis, prognosis (including plan of care), and intervention (with anticipated goals and expected outcomes). Each pattern also addresses reexamination, global outcomes, and criteria for termination of physical therapy services. Examples of ICD-9-CM codes are included.

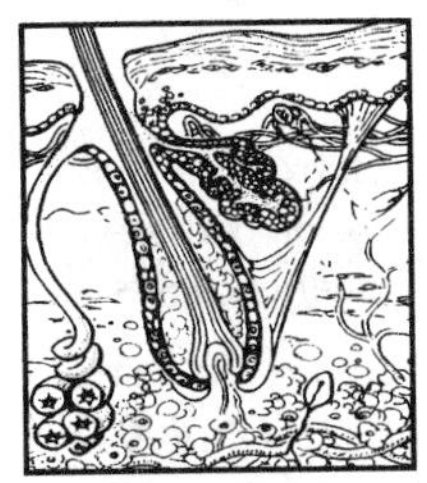

Primary Prevention/Risk Reduction for Integumentary Disorders

This preferred practice pattern describes the generally accepted elements of patient/client management that physical therapists provide for patients/clients who are classified in this pattern. The pattern title reflects the diagnosis made by the physical therapist. APTA emphasizes that preferred practice patterns are the boundaries within which a physical therapist may select any of a number of clinical alternatives, based on consideration of a wide variety of factors, such as individual patient/client needs; the profession's code of ethics and standards of practice; and patient/client age, culture, gender roles, race, sex, sexual orientation, and socioeconomic status.

Patient/Client Diagnostic Classification

Patients/clients will be classified in this primary prevention/risk reduction pattern as a result of the physical therapist's evaluation of the examination data. The findings from the examination (history, systems review, and tests and measures) may indicate the need for a prevention/risk reduction program. The physical therapist integrates, synthesizes, and interprets the data to determine inclusion in this diagnostic category.

Inclusion

The following examples of examination findings may support the inclusion of patients/clients in this pattern:

Risk Factors or Consequences of Pathology/Pathophysiology (Disease, Disorder, or Condition)

- Amputation
- Congestive heart failure
- Diabetes
- Malnutrition
- Neuromuscular dysfunction
- Obesity
- Peripheral nerve involvement
- Polyneuropathy
- Prior scar
- Spinal cord involvement
- Surgery
- Vascular disease

Impairments, Functional Limitations, or Disabilities

- Decreased level of activity
- Decreased sensation
- Edema
- Inflammation
- Ischemia
- Pain

Note:

Prevention and risk reduction are inherent in all diagnostic patterns. Patients/clients included in this pattern are in need of primary prevention/risk reduction only.

ICD-9-CM Codes

The listing below contains the current (as of press time) and most typical 3- and 4-digit ICD-9-CM codes related to this preferred practice pattern. Because patient/client diagnostic classification is based on impairments, functional limitations, and disabilities—not on codes—patients/clients may be classified into the pattern even though the codes listed with the pattern may not apply to those patients/clients.

This listing is intended for general information only and should not be used for coding purposes. The codes should be confirmed by referring to the World Health Organization's *International Classification of Diseases, 9th Revision, Clinical Modification (ICD-9-CM 2001)*, Volumes 1 and 3 (Chicago, Ill: American Medical Association; 2000) or subsequent revisions or by referring to other ICD-9-CM coding manuals that contain exclusion notes and instructions regarding fifth-digit requirements.

250 Diabetes mellitus

263 Other and unspecified protein-calorie malnutrition
- **263.0** Malnutrition of moderate degree
- **263.1** Malnutrition of mild degree

277 Other and unspecified disorders of metabolism
- **277.6** Other deficiencies of circulating enzymes
  Hereditary angioedema

278 Obesity and other hyperalimentation
- **278.0** Obesity

320 Bacterial meningitis

322 Meningitis of unspecified cause
- **322.9** Meningitis, unspecified

323 Encephalitis, myelitis, and encephalomyelitis

331 Other cerebral degenerations
- **331.7** Cerebral degeneration in diseases classified elsewhere*
- **331.9** Cerebral degeneration, unspecified

332 Parkinson's disease

333 Other extrapyramidal disease and abnormal movement disorders
- **333.2** Myoclonus

334 Spinocerebellar disease
- **334.0** Friedreich's ataxia
- **334.1** Hereditary spastic paraplegia
- **334.2** Primary cerebellar degeneration
- **334.9** Spinocerebellar disease, unspecified

335 Anterior horn cell disease

336 Other diseases of spinal cord
- **336.0** Syringomyelia and syringobulbia
- **336.1** Vascular myelopathies
- **336.9** Unspecified disease of spinal cord

337 Disorders of the autonomic nervous system

340 Multiple sclerosis

341 Other demyelinating diseases of central nervous system

342 Hemiplegia and hemiparesis

343 Infantile cerebral palsy

344 Other paralytic syndromes
- **344.0** Quadriplegia and quadriparesis
- **344.1** Paraplegia
- **344.3** Monoplegia of lower limb

353 Nerve root and plexus disorders
- **353.9** Unspecified nerve root and plexus disorder

357 Inflammatory and toxic neuropathy
- **357.2** Polyneuropathy in diabetes*
- **357.3** Polyneuropathy in malignant disease*
- **357.4** Polyneuropathy in other diseases classified elsewhere*
- **357.6** Polyneuropathy due to drugs

428 Heart failure
- **428.0** Congestive heart failure

435 Transient cerebral ischemia
- **435.1** Vertebral artery syndrome
- **435.8** Other specified transient cerebral ischemias

440 Atherosclerosis

443 Other peripheral vascular disease
- **443.0** Raynaud's syndrome
- **443.1** Thromboangiitis obliterans [Buerger's disease]
- **443.9** Peripheral vascular disease, unspecified

454 Varicose veins of lower extremities

457 Noninfectious disorders of lymphatic channels
- **457.0** Postmastectomy lymphedema syndrome
- **457.1** Other lymphedema

459 Other disorders of circulatory system
- **459.1** Postphlebitic syndrome
- **459.8** Other specified disorders of circulatory system
  - **459.81** Venous (peripheral) insufficiency, unspecified
- **459.9** Unspecified circulatory system disorder

581 Nephrotic syndrome
- **581.9** Nephrotic syndrome with unspecified pathological lesion in kidney
  Nephritis with edema, not otherwise specified

593 Other disorders of kidney and ureter
- **593.8** Other specified disorders of kidney and ureter
  - **593.81** Vascular disorders of kidney

686 Other local infections of skin and subcutaneous tissue
- **686.9** Unspecified local infection of skin and subcutaneous tissue

701 Other hypertrophic and atrophic conditions of skin
- **701.4** Keloid scar
  Hypertrophic scar

709 Other disorders of skin and subcutaneous tissue
- **709.2** Scar conditions and fibrosis of skin

* Not a primary diagnosis

716 Other and unspecified arthropathies

- **716.6** Unspecified monoarthritis

719 Other and unspecified disorders of joint

- **719.4** Pain in joint

728 Disorders of muscle, ligament, and fascia

- **728.9** Unspecified disorder of muscle, ligament, and fascia

729 Other disorders of soft tissues

- **729.5** Pain in limb

757 Congenital anomalies of the integument

- **757.0** Hereditary edema of legs

782 Symptoms involving skin and other integumentary tissue

- **782.0** Disturbance of skin sensation
- **782.3** Edema

895 Traumatic amputation of toe(s) (complete) (partial)

- **895.0** Without mention of complication

896 Traumatic amputation of foot (complete) (partial)

- **896.2** Bilateral, without mention of complication

897 Traumatic amputation of leg(s) (complete) (partial)

- **897.0** Unilateral, below knee, without mention of complication
- **897.2** Unilateral, at or above knee, without mention of complication
- **897.4** Unilateral, level not specified, without mention of complication
- **897.6** Bilateral [any level], without mention of complication

995 Certain adverse effects not elsewhere classified

- **995.1** Angioneurotic edema

Examination

Examination is a comprehensive screening and specific testing process that leads to a diagnostic classification or, when appropriate, to a referral to another practitioner. Examination is required prior to the initial intervention and is performed for all patients/clients. Through the examination, the physical therapist may identify impairments, functional limitations, disabilities, changes in physical function or overall health status, and needs related to restoration of health and to prevention, wellness, and fitness. The physical therapist synthesizes the examination findings to establish the diagnosis and the prognosis (including the plan of care). The patient/client, family, significant others, and caregivers may provide information during the examination process.

Examination has three components: the patient/client history, the systems review, and tests and measures. The *history* is a systematic gathering of past and current information (often from the patient/client) related to why the patient/client is seeking the services of the physical therapist. The *systems review* is a brief or limited examination of (1) the anatomical and physiological status of the cardiovascular/pulmonary, integumentary, musculoskeletal, and neuromuscular systems and (2) the communication ability, affect, cognition, language, and learning style of the patient/client. *Tests and measures* are the means of gathering data about the patient/client.

The selection of examination procedures and the depth of the examination vary based on patient/client age; severity of the problem; stage of recovery (acute, subacute, chronic); phase of rehabilitation (early, intermediate, late, return to activity); home, work (job/school/play), or community situation; and other relevant factors. *For clinical indications in selecting tests and measures and for listings of tests and measures, tools used to gather data, and the types of data generated by tests and measures, refer to Chapter 2.*

Patient/Client History

The history may include:

General Demographics

- Age
- Sex
- Race/ethnicity
- Primary language
- Education

Social History

- Cultural beliefs and behaviors
- Family and caregiver resources
- Social interactions, social activities, and support systems

Employment/Work (Job/School/Play)

- Current and prior work (job/school/play), community, and leisure actions, tasks, or activities

Growth and Development

- Developmental history
- Hand dominance

Living Environment

- Devices and equipment (eg, assistive, adaptive, orthotic, protective, supportive, prosthetic)
- Living environment and community characteristics
- Projected discharge destinations

General Health Status (Self-Report, Family Report, Caregiver Report)

- General health perception
- Physical function (eg, mobility, sleep patterns, restricted bed days)
- Psychological function (eg, memory, reasoning ability, depression, anxiety)
- Role function (eg, community, leisure, social, work)
- Social function (eg, social activity, social interaction, social support)

Social/Health Habits (Past and Current)

- Behavioral health risks (eg, smoking, drug abuse)
- Level of physical fitness

Family History

- Familial health risks

Medical/Surgical History

- Cardiovascular
- Endocrine/metabolic
- Gastrointestinal
- Genitourinary
- Gynecological
- Integumentary
- Musculoskeletal
- Neuromuscular
- Obstetrical
- Prior hospitalizations, surgeries, and preexisting medical and other health-related conditions
- Psychological
- Pulmonary

Current Condition(s)/Chief Complaint(s)

- Concerns that led patient/client to seek the services of a physical therapist
- Concerns or needs of patient/client who requires the services of a physical therapist
- Current therapeutic interventions
- Mechanisms of injury or disease, including date of onset and course of events
- Onset and pattern of symptoms
- Patient/client, family, significant other, and caregiver expectations and goals for the therapeutic intervention
- Patient/client, family, significant other, and caregiver perceptions of patient's/client's emotional response to the current clinical situation
- Previous occurrence of chief complaint(s)
- Prior therapeutic interventions

Functional Status and Activity Level

- Current and prior functional status in self-care and home management activities, including activities of daily living (ADL) and instrumental activities of daily living (IADL)
- Current and prior functional status in work (job/school/play), community, and leisure actions, tasks, or activities

Medications

- Medications for current condition
- Medications previously taken for current condition
- Medications for other conditions

Other Clinical Tests

- Laboratory and diagnostic tests
- Review of available records (eg, medical, education, surgical)
- Review of other clinical findings (eg, nutrition and hydration)

Systems Review

The systems review may include:

Anatomical and Physiological Status

- Cardiovascular/Pulmonary
  - Blood pressure
  - Edema
  - Heart rate
  - Respiratory rate
- Integumentary
  - Pliability (texture)
  - Presence of scar formation
  - Skin color
  - Skin integrity
- Musculoskeletal
  - Gross range of motion
  - Gross strength
  - Gross symmetry
  - Height
  - Weight
- Neuromuscular
  - Gross coordinated movements (eg, balance, gait, locomotion, transfers, transitions)
  - Motor function (motor control, motor learning)

Communication, Affect, Cognition, Language, and Learning Style

- Ability to make needs known
- Consciousness
- Expected emotional/behavioral responses
- Learning preferences (eg, education needs, learning barriers)
- Orientation (person, place, time)

Tests and Measures

Tests and measures for this pattern may include those that characterize or quantify:

Anthropometric Characteristics

- Body composition (eg, body mass index, impedance measurement, skinfold thickness measurement)
- Body dimensions (eg, girth measurement, length measurement)
- Edema (eg, girth measurement, palpation, scales, volume measurement)

Arousal, Attention, and Cognition

- Motivation (eg, adaptive behavior scales)

Circulation (Arterial, Venous, and Lymphatic)

- Cardiovascular signs, including heart rate, rhythm, and sounds; pressures and flow; and superficial vascular responses (eg, auscultation, electrocardiography, girth measurement, observations, palpation, sphygmomanometry, thermography)
- Cardiovascular symptoms (eg, angina, claudication, and perceived exertion scales)

Cranial and Peripheral Nerve Integrity

- Motor distribution of the peripheral nerves (eg, dynamometry, muscle tests, observations, thoracic outlet tests)
- Sensory distribution of the peripheral nerves (eg, discrimination tests; tactile tests, including coarse and light touch, cold and heat, pain, pressure, and vibration; thoracic outlet tests)

Integumentary Integrity

Associated skin

- Activities, positioning, and postures that produce or relieve trauma to the skin (eg, observations, pressure-sensing maps, scales)
- Assistive, adaptive, orthotic, protective, supportive, or prosthetic devices and equipment that may produce or relieve trauma to the skin (eg, observations, pressure-sensing maps, risk assessment scales)
- Skin characteristics, including blistering, continuity of skin color, dermatitis, hair growth, mobility, nail growth, sensation, temperature, texture, and turgor (eg, observations, palpation, photographic assessments, thermography)

Muscle Performance (Including Strength, Power, and Endurance)

- Muscle strength, power, and endurance during functional activities (eg, ADL scales, functional muscle tests, IADL scales, observations, videographic assessments)

Orthotic, Protective, and Supportive Devices

- Components, alignment, fit, and ability to care for orthotic, protective, and supportive devices and equipment (eg, interviews, logs, observations, pressure-sensing maps, reports)
- Safety during use of orthotic, protective, and supportive devices and equipment (eg, diaries, fall scales, interviews, logs, observations, reports)

Posture

- Postural alignment and position (static and dynamic), including symmetry and deviation from midline (eg, grid measurement, observations, photographic assessments, technology-assisted assessments, videographic assessments)
- Specific body parts (eg, angle assessments, forward-bending test, goniometry, observations, palpation, positional tests)

Prosthetic Requirements

- Components, alignment, fit, and ability to care for the prosthetic device (eg, interviews, logs, observations, pressure-sensing maps, reports)
- Safety during use of the prosthetic device (eg, diaries, fall scales, interviews, logs, observations, reports)

Sensory Integrity

- Deep sensations (eg, kinesthesiometry, observations, photographic assessments, vibration tests)

Evaluation, Diagnosis, and Prognosis (Including Plan of Care)

Physical therapists perform *evaluations* (make clinical judgments) based on the data gathered from the history, systems review, and tests and measures. In the evaluation process, physical therapists synthesize the examination data to establish the diagnosis and prognosis (including the plan of care). Factors that influence the complexity of the evaluation include the clinical findings, extent of loss of function, chronicity or severity of the problem, possibility of multisite or multisystem involvement, preexisting condition(s), potential discharge destination, social considerations, physical function, and overall health status.

A *diagnosis* is a label encompassing a cluster of signs and symptoms, syndromes, or categories. It is the result of the systematic diagnostic process, which includes integrating and evaluating the data from the examination. The diagnostic label indicates the primary dysfunction(s) toward which the therapist will direct interventions. The *prognosis* is the determination of the predicted optimal level of improvement in function and the amount of time needed to reach that level and may also include a prediction of levels of improvement that may be reached at various intervals during the course of therapy. During the prognostic process, the physical therapist develops the plan of care. The *plan of care* identifies specific interventions, proposed frequency and duration of the interventions, anticipated goals, expected outcomes, and discharge plans. The plan of care identifies realistic anticipated goals and expected outcomes, taking into consideration the expectations of the patient/client and appropriate others. These anticipated goals and expected outcomes should be measureable and time limited.

The frequency of visits and duration of the episode of care may vary from a short episode with a high intensity of intervention to a longer episode with a diminishing intensity of intervention. Frequency and duration may vary greatly among patients/clients based on a variety of factors that the physical therapist considers throughout the evaluation process, such as anatomical and physiological changes related to growth and development; caregiver consistency or expertise; chronicity or severity of the current condition; living environment; multisite or multisystem involvement; social support; potential discharge destinations; probability of prolonged impairment, functional limitation, or disability; and stability of the condition.

Prognosis

Patient/client will reduce the risk of integumentary disorders through therapeutic exercise, functional training, and lifestyle modification.

Expected Range of Number of Visits Per Episode of Care

1 to 6

This range represents the lower and upper limits of the number of physical therapist visits required to achieve anticipated goals and expected outcomes. *It is anticipated that 80% of patients/clients who are classified into this pattern will achieve the anticipated goals and expected outcomes within 1 to 6 visits during a single continuous episode of care.* Frequency of visits and duration of the episode of care should be determined by the physical therapist to maximize effectiveness of care and efficiency of service delivery.

Factors That May Modify Frequency of Visits

- Accessibility and availability of resources
- Adherence to the intervention program
- Age
- Anatomical and physiological changes related to growth and development
- Caregiver consistency or expertise
- Chronicity or severity of the current condition
- Cognitive status
- Comorbitities, complications, or secondary impairments
- Concurrent medical, surgical, and therapeutic interventions
- Decline in functional independence
- Level of impairment
- Level of physical function
- Living environment
- Multisite or multisystem involvement
- Nutritional status
- Overall health status
- Potential discharge destinations
- Premorbid conditions
- Probability of prolonged impairment, functional limitation, or disability
- Psychological and socioeconomic factors
- Psychomotor abilities
- Social support
- Stability of the condition

Intervention

Intervention is the purposeful interaction of the physical therapist with the patient/client and, when appropriate, with other individuals involved with the patient/client, using various physical therapy procedures and techniques to produce changes in the condition consistent with the diagnosis and prognosis. Decisions about interventions are contingent on the timely monitoring of patient/client response and the progress made toward achieving the anticipated goals and expected outcomes.

Communication, coordination, and documentation and patient/client-related instruction are provided for all patients/clients across all settings. Procedural interventions are selected or modified based on the examination data and the evaluation, the diagnosis and the prognosis, and the anticipated goals and expected outcomes for a particular patient/client. *For clinical considerations in selecting interventions, listings of interventions, and listings of anticipated goals and expected outcomes, refer to Chapter 3.*

Coordination, Communication, and Documentation

Coordination, communication, and documentation for primary prevention/risk reduction may include:

Interventions

- Addressing required functions
  - individualized family service plans (IFSPs) or individualized education plans (IEPs)
  - informed consent
  - mandatory communication and reporting (eg, patient/client advocacy and abuse reporting)
- Collaboration and coordination with agencies, including:
  - equipment suppliers
  - home care agencies
  - payer groups
  - schools
  - transportation agencies
- Communication, including:
  - education plans
  - documentation
- Data collection, analysis and reporting
  - outcome data
  - peer review findings
  - record reviews
- Documentation
  - elements of patient/client management (examination, evaluation, diagnosis, prognosis, intervention)
  - outcomes of intervention
- Referrals to other professionals or resources

Anticipated Goals and Expected Outcomes

- Accountability for services is increased.
- Individualized family service plans (IFSPs) or individualized education plans (IEPs), informed consent, and mandatory communication and reporting (eg, patient/client advocacy and abuse reporting) are obtained or completed.
- Available resources are maximally utilized.
- Collaboration and coordination occurs with agencies, including equipment suppliers, home care agencies, payer groups, schools, and transportation agencies.
- Communication occurs through education plans and documentation.
- Data are collected, analyzed, and reported, including outcome data, peer review findings, and record reviews.
- Decision making is enhanced regarding patient/client health and the use of health care resources by patient/client, family, significant others, and caregivers.
- Documentation occurs throughout patient/client management and follows APTA's *Guidelines for Physical Therapy Documentation* (Appendix 5).
- Patient/client, family, significant other, and caregiver understanding of anticipated goals and expected outcomes is increased.
- Referrals are made to other professionals or resources whenever necessary and appropriate.
- Resources are utilized in a cost-effective way.

Patient/Client-Related Instruction

Patient/client-related instruction may include:

Interventions

- Instruction, education, and training of patients/clients and caregivers regarding:
  - enhancement of performance
  - health, wellness, and fitness programs
  - plan for intervention
  - risk factors for pathology/pathophysiology (disease, disorder, or condition), impairments, functional limitations, or disabilities

Anticipated Goals and Expected Outcomes

- Ability to perform physical actions, tasks, or activities is improved.
- Awareness and use of community resources are improved.
- Behaviors that foster healthy habits, wellness, and prevention are acquired.
- Decision making is enhanced regarding patient/client health and the use of health care resources by patient/client, family, significant others, and caregivers.
- Health status is improved.
- Performance levels in self-care, home management, work (job/school/play), community, or leisure actions, tasks, or activities are improved.
- Patient/client, family, significant other, and caregiver knowledge and awareness of the diagnosis, prognosis, interventions, and anticipated goals and expected outcomes are increased.
- Patient/client knowledge of personal and environmental factors associated with the condition is increased.
- Physical function is improved.
- Risk of recurrence of condition is reduced.
- Safety of patient/client, family, significant others, and caregivers is improved.
- Utilization and cost of health care services are decreased.

Procedural Interventions

Procedural interventions for this pattern may include:

Therapeutic Exercise

Interventions

- Aerobic capacity/endurance conditioning or reconditioning
  - walking and wheelchair propulsion programs
- Balance, coordination, and agility training
  - developmental activities training
  - motor function (motor control and motor learning) training or retraining
  - neuromuscular education or reeducation
  - posture awareness training
  - standardized, programmatic, complementary exercise approaches
  - task-specific performance training
- Body mechanics and postural stabilization
  - body mechanics training
  - postural control training
  - postural stabilization activities
  - posture awareness training
- Strength, power, and endurance training for head, neck, limb, pelvic-floor, trunk, and ventilatory muscles
  - active assistive, active, and resistive exercises (including concentric, dynamic/isotonic, eccentric, isokinetic, isometric, and plyometric)
  - standardized, programmatic, complementary exercise approaches
  - task-specific performance training

Anticipated Goals and Expected Outcomes

- Impact on pathology/pathophysiology (disease, disorder, or condition)
  - Nutrient delivery to tissue is increased.
  - Osteogenic effects of exercise are maximized.
  - Physiological response to increased oxygen demand is improved.
  - Tissue perfusion and oxygenation are enhanced.
- Impact on impairments
  - Balance is improved.
  - Endurance is increased.
  - Energy expenditure per unit of work is decreased.
  - Integumentary integrity is improved.
  - Joint integrity and mobility are improved.
  - Muscle performance (strength, power, and endurance) is increased.
  - Postural control is improved.
  - Quality and quantity of movement between and across body segments are improved.
  - Range of motion is improved.
  - Sensory awareness is increased.
  - Weight-bearing status is improved.
- Impact on functional limitations
  - Ability to perform physical actions, tasks, or activities related to self-care, home management, work (job/school/play), community, and leisure is improved.
  - Level of supervision required for task performance is decreased.
  - Performance of and independence in activities of daily living (ADL) and instrumental activities of daily living (IADL) with or without devices and equipment are increased.
  - Tolerance of positions and activities is increased.
- Impact on disabilities
  - Ability to assume or resume required self-care, home management, work (job/school/play), community, and leisure roles is improved.
- Risk reduction/prevention
  - Risk factors are reduced.
  - Risk of secondary impairment is reduced.
  - Safety is improved.
  - Self-management of symptoms is improved.
- Impact on health, wellness, and fitness
  - Fitness is improved.
  - Health status is improved.
  - Physical capacity is increased.
  - Physical function is improved.
- Impact on societal resources
  - Utilization of physical therapy services is optimized.
  - Utilization of physical therapy services results in efficient use of health care dollars.
- Patient/client satisfaction
  - Access, availability, and services provided are acceptable to patient/client.
  - Administrative management of practice is acceptable to patient/client.
  - Clinical proficiency of physical therapist is acceptable to patient/client.
  - Coordination of care is acceptable to patient/client.
  - Cost of health care services is decreased.
  - Interpersonal skills of physical therapist are acceptable to patient/client, family, and significant others.
  - Sense of well-being is improved.
  - Stressors are decreased.

Functional Training in Self-Care and Home Management (Including Activities of Daily Living [ADL] and Instrumental Activities of Daily Living [IADL])

Interventions

- Injury prevention or reduction
  - injury prevention education during self-care and home management
  - injury prevention or reduction with use of devices and equipment
  - safety awareness training during self-care and home management

Anticipated Goals and Expected Outcomes

- Impact on pathology/pathophysiology (disease, disorder, or condition)
  - Physiological response to increased oxygen demand is improved.
- Impact on impairments
  - Weight-bearing status is improved.
- Impact on functional limitations
  - Ability to perform physical actions, tasks, or activities related to self-care and home management is improved.
  - Level of supervision required for task performance is decreased.
  - Performance of and independence in ADL and IADL with or without devices and equipment are increased.
  - Tolerance of positions and activities is increased.
- Impact on disabilities
  - Ability to assume or resume required self-care, home management, work (job/school/play), community, and leisure roles is improved.
- Risk reduction/prevention
  - Risk factors are reduced.
  - Risk of secondary impairments is reduced.
  - Safety is improved.
- Impact on health, wellness, and fitness
  - Health status is improved.
  - Physical function is improved.
- Impact on societal resources
  - Utilization of physical therapy services is optimized.
  - Utilization of physical therapy services results in efficient use of health care dollars.
- Patient/client satisfaction
  - Access, availability, and services provided are acceptable to patient/client.
  - Administrative management of practice is acceptable to patient/client.
  - Clinical proficiency of physical therapist is acceptable to patient/client.
  - Coordination of care is acceptable to patient/client.
  - Cost of health care services is decreased.
  - Interpersonal skills of physical therapist are acceptable to patient/client, family, and significant others.
  - Sense of well-being is improved.
  - Stressors are decreased.

Functional Training in Work (Job/School/Play), Community, and Leisure Integration or Reintegration (Including Instrumental Activities of Daily Living [IADL], Work Hardening, and Work Conditioning)

Interventions

- Injury prevention or reduction
  - injury prevention education during work (job/school/play), community, and leisure integration or reintegration
  - injury prevention or reduction with use of devices and equipment
  - safety awareness training during work (job/school/play), community, and leisure integration or reintegration

Anticipated Goals and Expected Outcomes

- Impact on pathology/pathophysiology (disease, disorder, or condition)
  - Physiological response to increased oxygen demand is improved.
- Impact on impairments
  - Weight-bearing status is improved.
- Impact on functional limitations
  - Ability to perform physical actions, tasks, or activities related to work (job/school/play), community, and leisure integration or reintegration is improved.
  - Level of supervision required for task performance is decreased.
  - Performance of and independence in IADL with or without devices and equipment are increased.
  - Tolerance of positions and activities is increased.
- Impact on disabilities
  - Ability to assume or resume required self-care, home management, work (job/school/play), community, and leisure roles is improved.
- Risk reduction/prevention
  - Risk factors are reduced.
  - Risk of secondary impairment is reduced.
  - Safety is improved.
- Impact on health, wellness, and fitness
  - Health status is improved.
  - Physical function is improved.
- Impact on societal resources
  - Costs of work-related injury or disability are reduced.
  - Utilization of physical therapy services is optimized.
  - Utilization of physical therapy services results in efficient use of health care dollars.
- Patient/client satisfaction
  - Access, availability, and services provided are acceptable to patient/client.
  - Administrative management of practice is acceptable to patient/client.
  - Clinical proficiency of physical therapist is acceptable to patient/client.
  - Coordination of care is acceptable to patient/client.
  - Cost of health care services is decreased.
  - Interpersonal skills of physical therapist are acceptable to patient/client, family, and significant others.
  - Sense of well-being is improved.
  - Stressors are decreased.

Procedural Interventions continued

Prescription, Application, and, as Appropriate, Fabrication of Devices and Equipment (Assistive, Adaptive, Orthotic, Protective, Supportive, and Prosthetic)

Interventions

- Adaptive devices
  - seating systems
- Assistive devices
  - canes
  - crutches
  - power devices
  - static and dynamic splints
  - walkers
  - wheelchairs
- Orthotic devices
  - braces
  - shoe inserts
  - splints
- Prosthetic devices (lower-extremity and upper-extremity)
- Protective devices
  - braces
  - cushions
  - protective taping
- Supportive devices
  - compression garments
  - elastic wraps
  - slings
  - supportive taping

Anticipated Goals and Expected Outcomes

- Impact on pathology/pathophysiology (disease, disorder, or condition)
  - Pain is decreased.
- Impact on impairments
  - Integumentary integrity is improved.
  - Joint stability is improved.
  - Optimal joint alignment is achieved.
  - Optimal loading on a body part is achieved.
  - Weight-bearing status is improved.
- Impact on functional limitations
  - Ability to perform physical actions, tasks, or activities related to self-care, home management, work (job/school/play), community, and leisure is improved.
  - Level of supervision required for task performance is decreased.
  - Performance of and independence in activities in daily living (ADL) and instrumental activities of daily living (IADL) with or without devices and equipment are increased.
  - Tolerance of positions and activities is improved.
- Impact on disabilities
  - Ability to assume or resume required self-care, home management, work (job/school/play), community, and leisure roles is improved.
- Risk reduction/prevention
  - Pressure on body tissues is reduced.
  - Protection of body parts is increased.
  - Risk factors are reduced.
  - Risk of secondary impairment is reduced.
  - Safety is improved.
  - Self-management of symptoms is improved.
- Impact on health, wellness, and fitness
  - Health status is improved.
  - Physical function is improved.
- Impact on societal resources
  - Utilization of physical therapy services is optimized.
  - Utilization of physical therapy services results in efficient use of health care dollars.
- Patient/client satisfaction
  - Access, availability, and services provided are acceptable to patient/client.
  - Administrative management of practice is acceptable to patient/client.
  - Clinical proficiency of physical therapist is acceptable to patient/client.
  - Coordination is acceptable to patient/client.
  - Cost of health care services is decreased.
  - Interpersonal skills of physical therapist are acceptable to patient/client, family, and significant others.
  - Sense of well-being is improved.
  - Stressors are decreased.

Reexamination

Reexamination is the process of performing selected tests and measures after the initial examination to evaluate progress and to modify or redirect interventions. Reexamination may be indicated more than once during a single episode of care. It also may be performed over the course of a disease, disorder, or condition, which for some patients/clients may be over the life span. Indications for reexamination include new clinical findings or failure to respond to physical therapy interventions.

Global Outcomes for Patients/Clients in This Pattern

Throughout the entire episode of care, the physical therapist determines the anticipated goals and expected outcomes for each intervention. These anticipated goals and expected outcomes are delineated in shaded boxes that accompany the lists of interventions in each preferred practice pattern. As the patient/client reaches the termination of physical therapy services and the end of the episode of care, the physical therapist measures the global outcomes of the physical therapy services by characterizing or quantifying the impact of the physical therapy interventions in the following domains:

- Pathology/pathophysiology (disease, disorder, or condition)
- Impairments
- Functional limitations
- Disabilities
- Risk reduction/prevention
- Health, wellness, and fitness
- Societal resources
- Patient/client satisfaction

In some instances, a particular anticipated goal or expected outcome is thoroughly achieved through implementation of a single form of intervention. More commonly, however, the anticipated goals and expected outcomes are achieved as a result of the combined effects of several forms of interventions, leading to enhancement of both health status and health-related quality of life.

Criteria for Termination of Physical Therapy Services

Discharge is the process of ending physical therapy services that have been provided during a single episode of care. It occurs when the anticipated goals and expected outcomes have been achieved. Discharge does *not* occur with a *transfer* (defined as the time when a patient is moved from one site to another site within the same setting or across settings during a single episode of care). Although there may be facility-specific or payer-specific requirements for documentation regarding the conclusion of physical therapy services, *discharge occurs based on the physical therapist's analysis of the achievement of anticipated goals and expected outcomes.*

Discontinuation is the process of ending physical therapy services that have been provided during a single episode of care when (1) the patient/client, caregiver, or legal guardian declines to continue intervention; (2) the patient/client is unable to continue to progress toward outcomes because of medical or psychosocial complications or because financial/insurance resources have been expended; or (3) the physical therapist determines that the patient/client will no longer benefit from physical therapy. When physical therapy services are terminated prior to achievement of anticipated goals and expected outcomes, patient/client status and the rationale for termination are documented.

For patients/clients who require multiple episodes of care, periodic follow-up is needed over the life span to ensure safety and effective adaptation following changes in physical status, caregivers, environment, or task demands. In consultation with appropriate individuals, and in consideration of the outcomes, the physical therapist plans for discharge or discontinuation and provides for appropriate follow-up or referral.

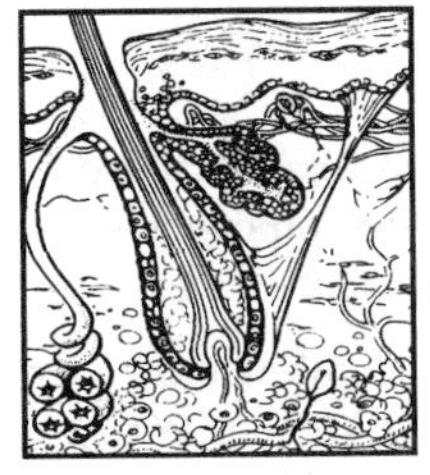

Impaired Integumentary Integrity Associated With Superficial Skin Involvement

This preferred practice pattern describes the generally accepted elements of patient/client management that physical therapists provide for patients/clients who are classified in this pattern. The pattern title reflects the diagnosis made by the physical therapist. APTA emphasizes that preferred practice patterns are the boundaries within which a physical therapist may select any of a number of clinical alternatives, based on consideration of a wide variety of factors, such as individual patient/client needs; the profession's code of ethics and standards of practice; and patient/client age, culture, gender roles, race, sex, sexual orientation, and socioeconomic status.

Patient/Client Diagnostic Classification

Patients/clients will be classified into this pattern—for impaired integumentary integrity associated with superficial skin involvement—as a result of the physical therapist's evaluation of the examination data. The findings from the examination (history, systems review, and tests and measures) may indicate the presence or risk of pathology/pathophysiology (disease, disorder, or condition), impairments, functional limitations, or disabilities or the need for health, wellness, or fitness programs. The physical therapist integrates, synthesizes, and interprets the data to determine the diagnostic classification.

Inclusion

The following examples of examination findings may support the inclusion of patients/clients in this pattern:

Risk Factors or Consequences of Pathology/Pathophysiology (Disease, Disorder, or Condition)

- Amputation
- Burns (superficial/first degree)
- Cellulitis
- Contusion
- Dermopathy
- Dermatitis
- Malnutrition
- Neuropathic ulcers (grade 0)
- Pressure ulcers (stage 2)
- Vascular disease
  - Arterial
  - Diabetic
  - Venous

Impairments, Functional Limitations, or Disabilities

- Edema
- Impaired sensation
- Impairments associated with abnormal fluid distribution
- Impaired skin
- Ischemia

Note:

Some risk factors or consequences of pathology/pathophysiology— such as *contusion with dermatitis*—may be severe and complex; *however, they do not necessarily exclude patients/ clients from this pattern.* Severe and complex risk factors or consequences may require modification of the frequency of visits and duration of care. (See "Evaluation, Diagnosis, and Prognosis," page 606.)

Exclusion or Multiple-Pattern Classification

The following examples of examination findings may support exclusion from this pattern or classification into additional patterns. Depending on the level of severity or complexity of the examination findings, the physical therapist may determine that the patient/client would be more appropriately managed through (1) classification in an entirely different pattern or (2) classification in both this and another pattern.

Findings That May Require Classification in a Different Pattern

- Frostbite
- Recent amputation

Findings That May Require Classification in Additional Patterns

- Superficial burn with inhalation injury

ICD-9-CM Codes

The listing below contains the current (as of press time) and most typical 3- and 4-digit ICD-9-CM codes related to this preferred practice pattern. Because patient/client diagnostic classification is based on impairments, functional limitations, and disabilities—not on codes—patients/clients may be classified into the pattern even though the codes listed with the pattern may not apply to those clients.

This listing is intended for general information only and should not be used for coding purposes. The codes should be confirmed by referring to the World Health Organization's *International Classification of Diseases, 9th Revision, Clinical Modification (ICD-9-CM 2001)*, Volumes 1 and 3 (Chicago, Ill: American Medical Association; 2000) or subsequent revisions or by referring to other ICD-9-CM coding manuals that contain exclusion notes and instructions regarding fifth-digit requirements.

176 Kaposi's sarcoma
- **176.0** Skin

250 Diabetes mellitus

263 Other and unspecified protein-calorie malnutrition

269 Other nutritional deficiencies

337 Disorders of the autonomic nervous system
- **337.2** Reflex sympathetic dystrophy

344 Other paralytic syndromes
- **344.0** Quadriplegia and quadriparesis
- **344.1** Paraplegia

443 Other peripheral vascular disease

454 Varicose veins of lower extremities
- **454.1** With inflammation

459 Other disorders of circulatory system

681 Cellulitis and abscess of finger and toe

682 Other cellulitis and abscess

690 Erythematosquamous dermatosis

691 Atopic dermatitis and related conditions

692 Contact dermatitis and other eczema
- **692.7** Due to solar radiation
  - **692.71** Sunburn

700 Corns and callosities

707 Chronic ulcer of skin
- **707.0** Decubitus ulcer
- **707.1** Ulcer of lower limbs, except decubitus

731 Osteitis deformans and osteopathies associated with other disorders classified elsewhere
- **731.8** Other bone involvement in diseases classified elsewhere*

782 Symptoms involving skin and other integumentary tissue
- **782.2** Localized superficial swelling, mass, or lump
- **782.7** Spontaneous ecchymoses
- **782.8** Changes in skin texture

920 Contusion of face, scalp, and neck except eye(s)

922 Contusion of trunk
- **922.0** Breast
- **922.1** Chest wall
- **922.2** Abdominal wall
- **922.3** Back
- **922.8** Multiple sites of trunk

923 Contusion of upper limb
- **923.0** Shoulder and upper arm
- **923.1** Elbow and forearm
- **923.2** Wrist and hand(s), except finger(s) alone
- **923.3** Finger
- **923.8** Multiple sites of upper limb

924 Contusion of lower limb and of other and unspecified sites
- **924.0** Hip and thigh
- **924.1** Knee and lower leg
- **924.2** Ankle and foot, excluding toe(s)
- **924.3** Toe
- **924.4** Multiple sites of lower limb

942 Burn of trunk
- **942.1** Erythema [first degree]

943 Burn of upper limb, except wrist and hand
- **943.1** Erythema [first degree]

944 Burn of wrist(s) and hand(s)
- **944.1** Erythema [first degree]

945 Burn of lower limb(s)
- **945.1** Erythema [first degree]

946 Burns of multiple specified sites
- **946.1** Erythema [first degree]

948 Burns classified according to extent of body surface involved

949 Burn, unspecified
- **949.1** Erythema [first degree]

997 Complications affecting specified body system, not elsewhere classified
- **997.6** Amputation stump complication

* Not a primary diagnosis

Examination

Examination is a comprehensive screening and specific testing process that leads to a diagnostic classification or, when appropriate, to a referral to another practitioner. Examination is required prior to the initial intervention and is performed for all patients/clients. Through the examination, the physical therapist may identify impairments, functional limitations, disabilities, changes in physical function or overall health status, and needs related to restoration of health and to prevention, wellness, and fitness. The physical therapist synthesizes the examination findings to establish the diagnosis and the prognosis (including the plan of care). The patient/client, family, significant others, and caregivers may provide information during the examination process.

Examination has three components: the patient/client history, the systems review, and tests and measures. The *history* is a systematic gathering of past and current information (often from the patient/client) related to why the patient/client is seeking the services of the physical therapist. The *systems review* is a brief or limited examination of (1) the anatomical and physiological status of the cardiovascular/pulmonary, integumentary, musculoskeletal, and neuromuscular systems and (2) the communication ability, affect, cognition, language, and learning style of the patient/client. *Tests and measures* are the means of gathering data about the patient/client.

The selection of examination procedures and the depth of the examination vary based on patient/client age; severity of the problem; stage of recovery (acute, subacute, chronic); phase of rehabilitation (early, intermediate, late, return to activity); home, work (job/school/play), or community situation; and other relevant factors. *For clinical indications in selecting tests and measures and for listings of tests and measures, tools used to gather data, and the types of data generated by tests and measures, refer to Chapter 2.*

Patient/Client History

The history may include:

General Demographics
- Age
- Sex
- Race/ethnicity
- Primary language
- Education

Social History
- Cultural beliefs and behaviors
- Family and caregiver resources
- Social interactions, social activities, and support systems

Employment/Work (Job/School/Play)
- Current and prior work (job/school/play), community, and leisure actions, tasks, or activities

Growth and Development
- Developmental history
- Hand dominance

Living Environment
- Devices and equipment (eg, assistive, adaptive, orthotic, protective, supportive, prosthetic)
- Living environment and community characteristics
- Projected discharge destinations

General Health Status (Self-Report, Family Report, Caregiver Report)
- General health perception
- Physical function (eg, mobility, sleep patterns, restricted bed days)
- Psychological function (eg, memory, reasoning ability, depression, anxiety)
- Role function (eg, community, leisure, social, work)
- Social function (eg, social activity, social interaction, social support)

Social/Health Habits (Past and Current)
- Behavioral health risks (eg, smoking, drug abuse)
- Level of physical fitness

Family History
- Familial health risks

Medical/Surgical History
- Cardiovascular
- Endocrine/metabolic
- Gastrointestinal
- Genitourinary
- Gynecological
- Integumentary
- Musculoskeletal
- Neuromuscular
- Obstetrical
- Prior hospitalizations, surgeries, and preexisting medical and other health-related conditions
- Psychological
- Pulmonary

Current Condition(s)/Chief Complaint(s)
- Concerns that led patient/client to seek the services of a physical therapist
- Concerns or needs of patient/client who requires the services of a physical therapist
- Current therapeutic interventions
- Mechanisms of injury or disease, including date of onset and course of events
- Onset and pattern of symptoms
- Patient/client, family, significant other, and caregiver expectations and goals for the therapeutic intervention
- Patient/client, family, significant other, and caregiver perceptions of patient's/client's emotional response to the current clinical situation
- Previous occurrence of chief complaint(s)
- Prior therapeutic interventions

Functional Status and Activity Level
- Current and prior functional status in self-care and home management activities, including activities of daily living (ADL) and instrumental activities of daily living (IADL)
- Current and prior functional status in work (job/school/play), community, and leisure actions, tasks, or activities

Medications
- Medications for current condition
- Medications previously taken for current condition
- Medications for other conditions

Other Clinical Tests
- Laboratory and diagnostic tests
- Review of available records (eg, medical, education, surgical)
- Review of other clinical findings (eg, nutrition and hydration)

Systems Review

The systems review may include:

Anatomical and Physiological Status

- Cardiovascular/Pulmonary
  - Blood pressure
  - Edema
  - Heart rate
  - Respiratory rate
- Integumentary
  - Pliability (texture)
  - Presence of scar formation
  - Skin color
  - Skin integrity
- Musculoskeletal
  - Gross range of motion
  - Gross strength
  - Gross symmetry
  - Height
  - Weight
- Neuromuscular
  - Gross coordinated movements (eg, balance, gait, locomotion, transfers, transitions)
  - Motor function (motor control, motor learning)

Communication, Affect, Cognition, Language, and Learning Style

- Ability to make needs known
- Consciousness
- Expected emotional/behavioral responses
- Learning preferences (eg, education needs, learning barriers)
- Orientation (person, place, time)

Tests and Measures

Tests and measures for this pattern may include those that characterize or quantify:

Anthropometric Characteristics

- Body composition (eg, body mass index, impedance measurement, skinfold thickness measurement)
- Edema (eg, girth measurement, palpation, scales, volume measurement)

Circulation (Arterial, Venous, and Lymphatic)

- Cardiovascular signs, including heart rate, rhythm, and sounds; pressures and flow; and superficial vascular responses (eg, auscultation, electrocardiography, girth measurement, observations, palpation, sphygmomanometry, thermography)
- Cardiovascular symptoms (eg, angina, claudication, and perceived exertion scales)

Cranial and Peripheral Nerve Integrity

- Sensory distribution of the cranial nerves (eg, discrimination tests; tactile tests, including coarse and light touch, cold and heat, pain, pressure, and vibration)
- Sensory distribution of the peripheral nerves (eg, discrimination tests; tactile tests, including coarse and light touch, cold and heat, pain, pressure, and vibration; thoracic outlet tests)

Gait, Locomotion, and Balance

- Safety during gait, locomotion, and balance (eg, confidence scales, diaries, fall scales, functional assessment profiles, logs, reports)

Integumentary Integrity

Associated skin

- Activities, positioning, and postures that produce or relieve trauma to the skin (eg, observations, pressure-sensing maps, scales)
- Assistive, adaptive, orthotic, protective, supportive, or prosthetic devices and equipment that may produce or relieve trauma to the skin (eg, observations, pressure-sensing maps, risk assessment scales)
- Skin characteristics, including blistering, continuity of skin color, dermatitis, hair growth, mobility, nail growth, sensation, temperature, texture, and turgor (eg, observations, palpation, photographic assessments, thermography)

Wound

- Activities, positioning, and postures that aggravate the wound or scar or that produce or relieve trauma (eg, observations, pressure-sensing maps)
- Burn (eg, body charting, planimetry)
- Signs of infection (eg, cultures, observations, palpation)
- Wound characteristics, including bleeding, contraction, depth, drainage, exposed anatomical structures, location, odor, pigment, shape, size, staging and progression, tunneling, and undermining (eg, digital and grid measurement, grading of sores and ulcers, observations, palpation, photographic assessments, wound tracing)
- Wound scar tissue characteristics, including banding, pliability, sensation, and texture (eg, observations, scar-rating scales)

Muscle Performance (Including Strength, Power, and Endurance)

- Muscle strength, power, and endurance during functional activities (eg, ADL scales, functional muscle tests, IADL scales, observations, videographic assessments)

Orthotic, Protective, and Supportive Devices

- Components, alignment, fit, and ability to care for orthotic, protective, and supportive devices and equipment (eg, interviews, logs, observations, pressure-sensing maps, reports)
- Orthotic, protective, and supportive devices and equipment use during functional activities (eg, ADL scales, functional scales, IADL scales, interviews, observations, profiles)
- Remediation of impairments, functional limitations, or disabilities with use of orthotic, protective, and supportive devices and equipment (eg, activity status indexes, ADL scales, aerobic capacity tests, functional performance inventories, health assessment questionnaires, IADL scales, pain scales, play scales, videographic assessments)
- Safety during use of orthotic, protective, and supportive devices and equipment (eg, diaries, fall scales, interviews, logs, observations, reports)

Pain

- Pain, soreness, and nociception (eg, analog scales, discrimination tests, pain drawings and maps, provocation tests, verbal and pictorial descriptor tests)
- Pain in specific body parts (eg, pain indexes, pain questionnaires, structural provocation tests)

Prosthetic Requirements

- Components, alignment, fit, and ability to care for the prosthetic device (eg, interviews, logs, observations, pressure-sensing maps, reports)
- Safety during use of the prosthetic device (eg, diaries, fall scales, interviews, logs, observations, reports)

Range of Motion (ROM) (Including Muscle Length)

- Muscle length, soft tissue extensibility, and flexibility (eg, contracture tests, goniometry, inclinometry, ligamentous tests, linear measurement, multisegment flexibility tests, palpation)

Self-Care and Home Management (Including ADL and IADL)

- Safety in self-care and home management activities and environments (eg, diaries, fall scales, interviews, logs, observations, reports, videographic assessments)

Sensory Integrity

- Deep sensations (eg, kinesthesiometry, observations, photographic assessments, vibration tests)

Evaluation, Diagnosis, and Prognosis (Including Plan of Care)

Physical therapists perform *evaluations* (make clinical judgments) based on the data gathered from the history, systems review, and tests and measures. In the evaluation process, physical therapists synthesize the examination data to establish the diagnosis and prognosis (including the plan of care). Factors that influence the complexity of the evaluation include the clinical findings, extent of loss of function, chronicity or severity of the problem, possibility of multisite or multisystem involvement, preexisting condition(s), potential discharge destination, social considerations, physical function, and overall health status.

A *diagnosis* is a label encompassing a cluster of signs and symptoms, syndromes, or categories. It is the result of the systematic diagnostic process, which includes integrating and evaluating the data from the examination. The diagnostic label indicates the primary dysfunction(s) toward which the therapist will direct interventions. The *prognosis* is the determination of the predicted optimal level of improvement in function and the amount of time needed to reach that level and may also include a prediction of levels of improvement that may be reached at various intervals during the course of therapy. During the prognostic process, the physical therapist develops the plan of care. The *plan of care* identifies specific interventions, proposed frequency and duration of the interventions, anticipated goals, expected outcomes, and discharge plans. The plan of care identifies realistic anticipated goals and expected outcomes, taking into consideration the expectations of the patient/client and appropriate others. These anticipated goals and expected outcomes should be measureable and time limited.

The frequency of visits and duration of the episode of care may vary from a short episode with a high intensity of intervention to a longer episode with a diminishing intensity of intervention. Frequency and duration may vary greatly among patients/clients based on a variety of factors that the physical therapist considers throughout the evaluation process, such as anatomical and physiological changes related to growth and development; caregiver consistency or expertise; chronicity or severity of the current condition; living environment; multisite or multisystem involvement; social support; potential discharge destinations; probability of prolonged impairment, functional limitation, or disability; and stability of the condition.

Prognosis

Over the course of 2 weeks, patient/client will demonstrate optimal integumentary integrity and the highest level of functioning in home, work (job/school/play), community, and leisure environments.

During the episode of care, patient/client will achieve (1) the anticipated goals and expected outcomes of the interventions that are described in the plan of care and (2) the global outcomes for patients/clients who are classified in this pattern.

Expected Range of Number of Visits Per Episode of Care

1 to 6

This range represents the lower and upper limits of the number of physical therapist visits required to achieve anticipated goals and expected outcomes. *It is anticipated that 80% of patients/clients who are classified into this pattern will achieve the anticipated goals and expected outcomes within 1 to 6 visits during a single continuous episode of care.* Frequency of visits and duration of the episode of care should be determined by the physical therapist to maximize effectiveness of care and efficiency of service delivery.

Factors That May Require New Episode of Care or That May Modify Frequency of Visits/Duration of Episode

- Accessibility and availability of resources
- Adherence to the intervention program
- Age
- Anatomical and physiological changes related to growth and development
- Caregiver consistency or expertise
- Chronicity or severity of the current condition
- Cognitive status
- Comorbitities, complications, or secondary impairments
- Concurrent medical, surgical, and therapeutic interventions
- Decline in functional independence
- Level of impairment
- Level of physical function
- Living environment
- Multisite or multisystem involvement
- Nutritional status
- Overall health status
- Potential discharge destinations
- Premorbid conditions
- Probability of prolonged impairment, functional limitation, or disability
- Psychological and socioeconomic factors
- Psychomotor abilities
- Social support
- Stability of the condition

Intervention

Intervention is the purposeful interaction of the physical therapist with the patient/client and, when appropriate, with other individuals involved in patient/client care, using various physical therapy procedures and techniques to produce changes in the condition consistent with the diagnosis and prognosis. Decisions about interventions are contingent on the timely monitoring of patient/client response and the progress made toward achieving the anticipated goals and expected outcomes.

Communication, coordination, and documentation and patient/client-related instruction are provided for all patients/clients across all settings. Procedural interventions are selected or modified based on the examination data and the evaluation, the diagnosis and the prognosis, and the anticipated goals and expected outcomes for a particular patient/client. *For clinical considerations in selecting interventions, listings of interventions, and listings of anticipated goals and expected outcomes, refer to Chapter 3.*

Coordination, Communication, and Documentation

Coordination, communication, and documentation may include:

Interventions

- Addressing required functions
  - advance directives
  - individualized family service plans (IFSPs) or individualized education plans (IEPs)
  - informed consent
  - mandatory communication and reporting (eg, patient advocacy and abuse reporting)
- Admission and discharge planning
- Case management
- Collaboration and coordination with agencies, including:
  - equipment suppliers
  - home care agencies
  - payer groups
  - schools
  - transportation agencies
- Communication across settings, including:
  - case conferences
  - documentation
  - education plans
- Cost-effective resource utilization
- Data collection, analysis, and reporting
  - outcome data
  - peer review findings
  - record reviews
- Documentation across settings, following *APTA's Guidelines for Physical Therapy Documentation* (Appendix 5), including:
  - changes in impairments, functional limitations, and disabilities
  - changes in interventions
  - elements of patient/client management (examination, evaluation, diagnosis, prognosis, intervention)
  - outcomes of intervention
- Interdisciplinary teamwork
  - case conferences
  - patient care rounds
  - patient/client family meetings
- Referrals to other professionals or resources

Anticipated Goals and Expected Outcomes

- Accountability for services is increased.
- Admission data and discharge planning are completed.
- Advance directives, individualized family service plans (IFSPs) or individualized education plans (IEPs), informed consent, and mandatory communication and reporting (eg, patient advocacy and abuse reporting) are obtained or completed.
- Available resources are maximally utilized.
- Care is coordinated with patient/client, family, significant others, caregivers, and other professionals.
- Case is managed throughout the episode of care.
- Collaboration and coordination occurs with agencies, including equipment suppliers, home care agencies, payer groups, schools, and transportation agencies.
- Communication enhances risk reduction and prevention.
- Communication occurs across settings through case conferences, education plans, and documentation.
- Data are collected, analyzed, and reported, including outcome data, peer review findings, and record reviews.
- Decision making is enhanced regarding health, wellness, and fitness needs.
- Decision making is enhanced regarding patient/client health and the use of health care resources by patient/client, family, significant others, and caregivers.
- Documentation occurs throughout patient/client management and across settings and follows APTA's *Guidelines for Physical Therapy Documentation* (Appendix 5).
- Interdisciplinary collaboration occurs through case conferences, patient care rounds, and patient/client family meetings.
- Patient/client, family, significant other, and caregiver understanding of anticipated goals and expected outcomes is increased.
- Placement needs are determined.
- Referrals are made to other professionals or resources whenever necessary and appropriate.
- Resources are utilized in a cost-effective way.

Patient/Client-Related Instruction

Patient/client-related instruction may include:

Interventions

- Instruction, education and training of patients/clients and caregivers regarding:
  - current condition (pathology/pathophysiology [disease, disorder, or condition], impairments, functional limitations, or disabilities)
  - enhancement of performance
  - health, wellness, and fitness programs
  - plan of care
  - risk factors for pathology/pathophysiology (disease, disorder, or condition), impairments, functional limitations, or disabilities
  - transitions across settings
  - transitions to new roles

Anticipated Goals and Expected Outcomes

- Ability to perform physical actions, tasks, or activities is improved.
- Awareness and use of community resources are improved.
- Behaviors that foster healthy habits, wellness, and prevention are acquired.
- Decision making is enhanced regarding patient/client health and the use of health care resources by patient/client, family, significant others, and caregivers.
- Disability associated with acute or chronic illnesses is reduced.
- Functional independence in activities of daily living (ADL) and instrumental activities of daily living (IADL) is increased.
- Health status is improved.
- Intensity of care is decreased.
- Level of supervision required for task performance is decreased.
- Patient/client, family, significant other, and caregiver knowledge and awareness of the diagnosis, prognosis, interventions, and anticipated goals and expected outcomes are increased.
- Patient/client knowledge of personal and environmental factors associated with the condition is increased.
- Performance levels in self-care, home management, work (job/school/play), community, or leisure actions, tasks, or activities are improved.
- Physical function is improved.
- Risk of recurrence of condition is reduced.
- Risk of secondary impairment is reduced.
- Safety of patient/client, family, significant others, and caregivers is improved.
- Self-management of symptoms is improved.
- Utilization and cost of health care services are decreased.

Procedural Interventions

Procedural interventions for this pattern may include:

Therapeutic Exercise

Interventions

- Aerobic capacity/endurance conditioning or reconditioning
  - aquatic programs
  - gait and locomotor training
  - walking and wheelchair propulsion programs
- Body mechanics and postural stabilization
  - posture awareness training
- Flexibility exercises
  - muscle lengthening
  - range of motion
  - stretching
- Strength, power, and endurance training for head, neck, limb, pelvic-floor, trunk, and ventilatory muscles
  - active assistive, active, and resistive exercises (including concentric, dynamic/isotonic, eccentric, isokinetic, isometric, and plyometric)
  - task-specific performance training

Anticipated Goals and Expected Outcomes

- Impact on pathology/pathophysiology (disease, disorder, or condition)
  - Joint swelling, inflammation, or restriction is reduced.
  - Nutrient delivery to tissue is increased.
  - Pain is decreased.
  - Physiological response to increased oxygen demand is improved.
  - Soft tissue swelling, inflammation, or restriction is reduced.
  - Tissue perfusion and oxygenation are enhanced.
- Impact on impairments
  - Integumentary integrity is improved.
  - Joint integrity and mobility are improved.
  - Muscle performance (strength, power, and endurance) is increased.
  - Postural control is improved.
  - Range of motion is improved.
  - Sensory awareness is increased.
  - Weight-bearing status is improved.
- Impact on functional limitations
  - Ability to perform physical actions, tasks, or activities related to self-care, home management, work (job/school/play), community, and leisure is improved.
  - Level of supervision required for task performance is decreased.
  - Performance of and independence in activities of daily living (ADL) and instrumental activities of daily living (IADL) with or without devices and equipment are increased.
  - Tolerance of positions and activities is increased.
- Impact on disabilities
  - Ability to assume or resume required self-care, home management, work (job/school/play), community, and leisure roles is improved.
- Risk reduction/prevention
  - Risk factors are reduced.
  - Risk of recurrence of condition is reduced.
  - Risk of secondary impairment is reduced.
  - Safety is improved.
  - Self-management of symptoms is improved.
- Impact on health, wellness, and fitness
  - Health status is improved.
  - Physical capacity is increased.
  - Physical function is improved.
- Impact on societal resources
  - Utilization of physical therapy services is optimized.
  - Utilization of physical therapy services results in efficient use of health care dollars.
- Patient/client satisfaction
  - Access, availability, and services provided are acceptable to patient/client.
  - Administrative management of practice is acceptable to patient/client.
  - Clinical proficiency of physical therapist is acceptable to patient/client.
  - Coordination of care is acceptable to patient/client.
  - Cost of health care services is decreased.
  - Intensity of care is decreased.
  - Interpersonal skills of physical therapist are acceptable to patient/client, family, and significant others.
  - Sense of well-being is improved.
  - Stressors are decreased.

Functional Training in Self-Care and Home Management (Including Activities of Daily Living [ADL] and Instrumental Activities of Daily Living [IADL])

Interventions

- Injury prevention or reduction
  - injury prevention education during self-care and home management
  - injury prevention or reduction with use of devices and equipment
  - safety awareness training during self-care and home management

Anticipated Goals and Expected Outcomes

- Impact on pathology/pathophysiology (disease/disorder/condition)
  - Pain is decreased.
- Impact on impairments
  - Sensory awareness is increased.
  - Weight-bearing status is improved.
- Impact on functional limitations
  - Ability to perform physical actions, tasks, or activities related to self-care and home management is improved.
  - Level of supervision required for task performance is decreased.
  - Performance of and independence in ADL and IADL with or without devices and equipment are increased.
  - Tolerance of positions and activities is increased.
- Impact on disabilities
  - Ability to assume or resume required self-care and home management roles is improved.
- Risk reduction/prevention
  - Risk factors are reduced.
  - Risk of secondary impairments is reduced.
  - Safety is improved.
  - Self-management of symptoms is improved.
- Impact on health, wellness, and fitness
  - Health status is improved.
  - Physical function is improved.
- Impact on societal resources
  - Utilization of physical therapy services is optimized.
  - Utilization of physical therapy services results in efficient use of health care dollars.
- Patient/client satisfaction
  - Access, availability, and services provided are acceptable to patient/client.
  - Administrative management of practice is acceptable to patient/client.
  - Clinical proficiency of physical therapist is acceptable to patient/client.
  - Coordination of care is acceptable to patient/client.
  - Cost of health care services is decreased.
  - Intensity of care is decreased.
  - Interpersonal skills of physical therapist are acceptable to patient/client, family, and significant others.
  - Sense of well-being is improved.
  - Stressors are decreased.

Functional Training in Work (Job/School/Play), Community, and Leisure Integration or Reintegration (Including Instrumental Activities of Daily Living [IADL], Work Hardening, and Work Conditioning)

Interventions

- Injury prevention or reduction
  - injury prevention education during work (job/school/play), community, and leisure integration or reintegration
  - injury prevention or reduction with use of devices and equipment
  - safety awareness training during work (job/school/play), community, and leisure integration or reintegration

Anticipated Goals and Expected Outcomes

- Impact on pathology/pathophysiology (disease, disorder, or condition)
  - Pain is decreased.
- Impact on impairments
  - Sensory awareness is increased.
  - Weight-bearing status is improved.
- Impact on functional limitations
  - Ability to perform physical actions, tasks, or activities related to work (job/school/play), community, and leisure integration or reintegration is improved.
  - Level of supervision required for task performance is decreased.
  - Performance of and independence in IADL with or without devices and equipment are increased.
  - Tolerance of positions and activities is increased.
- Impact on disabilities
  - Ability to assume or resume required work (job/school/play), community, and leisure roles is improved.
- Risk reduction/prevention
  - Risk factors are reduced.
  - Risk of secondary impairment is reduced.
  - Safety is improved.
  - Self-management of symptoms is improved.
- Impact on health, wellness, and fitness
  - Health status is improved.
  - Physical function is improved.
- Impact on societal resources
  - Costs of work-related injury or disability are reduced.
  - Utilization of physical therapy services is optimized.
  - Utilization of physical therapy services results in efficient use of health care dollars.
- Patient/client satisfaction
  - Access, availability, and services provided are acceptable to patient/client.
  - Administrative management of practice is acceptable to patient/client.
  - Clinical proficiency of physical therapist is acceptable to patient/client.
  - Coordination of care is acceptable to patient/client.
  - Cost of health care services is decreased.
  - Intensity of care is decreased.
  - Interpersonal skills of physical therapist are acceptable to patient/client, family, and significant others.
  - Sense of well being is improved.
  - Stressors are decreased.

Manual Therapy Techniques (Including Mobilization/Manipulation)

Interventions

- Manual lymphatic drainage
- Massage
  - therapeutic massage

Anticipated Goals and Expected Outcomes

- Impact on pathology/pathophysiology (disease, disorder, or condition)
  - Edema, lymphedema, or effusion is reduced.
  - Joint swelling, inflammation, or restriction is reduced.
  - Pain is decreased.
  - Soft tissue swelling, inflammation, or restriction is reduced.
- Impact on impairments
  - Integumentary integrity is improved.
  - Relaxation is increased.
  - Sensory awareness is increased.
- Impact on functional limitations
  - Ability to perform movement tasks is improved.
  - Ability to perform physical actions, tasks, or activities related to self-care, home management, work (job/school/play), community, and leisure is improved.
  - Tolerance of positions and activities is increased.
- Impact on disabilities
  - Ability to assume or resume required self-care, home management, work (job/school/play), community, and leisure roles is improved.
- Risk reduction/prevention
  - Risk factors are reduced.
  - Risk of recurrence of condition is reduced.
  - Risk of secondary impairment is reduced.
  - Self-management of symptoms is improved.
- Impact on health, wellness, and fitness
  - Physical function is improved.
- Impact on societal resources
  - Utilization of physical therapy services is optimized.
  - Utilization of physical therapy services results in efficient use of health care dollars.
- Patient/client satisfaction
  - Access, availability, and services provided are acceptable to patient/client.
  - Administrative management of practice is acceptable to patient/client.
  - Clinical proficiency of physical therapist is acceptable to patient/client.
  - Coordination of care is acceptable to patient/client.
  - Cost of health care services is decreased.
  - Intensity of care is decreased.
  - Interpersonal skills of physical therapist are acceptable to patient/client, family, and significant others.
  - Sense of well-being is improved.
  - Stressors are decreased.

Prescription, Application, and, as Appropriate, Fabrication of Devices and Equipment (Assistive, Adaptive, Orthotic, Protective, Supportive, and Prosthetic)

Interventions

- Adaptive devices
  - hospital beds
  - seating systems
- Assistive devices
  - canes
  - crutches
  - long-handled reachers
  - power devices
  - static and dynamic splints
  - walkers
  - wheelchairs
- Orthotic devices
  - braces
  - casts
  - shoe inserts
  - splints
- Prosthetic devices (lower-extremity and upper-extremity)
- Protective devices
  - braces
  - cushions
  - protective taping
- Supportive devices
  - compression garments
  - elastic wraps
  - slings
  - supportive taping

Anticipated Goals and Expected Outcomes

- Impact on pathology/pathophysiology (disease, disorder, or condition)
  - Edema, lymphedema, or effusion is reduced.
  - Joint swelling, inflammation, or restriction is reduced.
  - Pain is decreased.
  - Soft tissue swelling, inflammation, or restriction is reduced.
- Impact on impairments
  - Balance is improved.
  - Energy expenditure per unit of work is decreased.
  - Gait, locomotion, and balance are improved.
  - Integumentary integrity is improved.
  - Optimal joint alignment is achieved.
  - Optimal loading on a body part is achieved.
  - Quality and quantity of movement between and across body segments are improved.
  - Weight-bearing status is improved.
- Impact on functional limitations
  - Ability to perform physical actions, tasks, or activities related to self-care, home management, work (job/school/play), community, and leisure is improved.
  - Level of supervision required for task performance is decreased.
  - Performance of and independence in activities of daily living (ADL) and instrumental activities of daily living (IADL) with or without devices and equipment are increased.
  - Tolerance of positions and activities is increased.
- Impact on disabilities
  - Ability to assume or resume required self-care, home management, work (job/school/play), community, and leisure roles is improved.
- Risk reduction/prevention
  - Pressure on body tissues is reduced.
  - Protection of body parts is increased.
  - Risk factors are reduced.
  - Risk of secondary impairment is reduced.
  - Safety is improved.
  - Self-management of symptoms is improved.
- Impact on health, wellness, and fitness
  - Health status is improved.
  - Physical function is improved.
- Impact on societal resources
  - Utilization of physical therapy services is optimized.
  - Utilization of physical therapy services results in efficient use of health care dollars.
- Patient/client satisfaction
  - Access, availability, and services provided are acceptable to patient/client.
  - Administrative management of practice is acceptable to patient/client.
  - Clinical proficiency of physical therapist is acceptable to patient/client.
  - Coordination of care is acceptable to patient/client.
  - Cost of health care services is decreased.
  - Intensity of care is decreased.
  - Interpersonal skills of physical therapist are acceptable to patient/client, family, and significant others.
  - Sense of well-being is improved.
  - Stressors are decreased.

Integumentary Repair and Protection Techniques

Interventions

- Dressings
  - wound coverings
- Topical agents
  - cleansers
  - creams
  - moisturizers
  - ointments
  - sealants

Anticipated Goals and Expected Outcomes

- Impact on pathology/pathophysiology (disease, disorder, or condition)
  - Debridement of nonviable tissue is achieved.
  - Pain is decreased.
  - Tissue perfusion and oxygenation are enhanced.
  - Soft tissue and wound healing is enhanced.
  - Wound size is reduced.
- Impact on impairments
  - Integumentary integrity is improved.
  - Weight-bearing status is improved.
- Impact on functional limitations
  - Ability to perform physical actions, tasks, or activities related to self-care, home management, work (job/ school/play), community, and leisure is improved.
  - Level of supervision required for task performance is decreased.
  - Performance of and independence in activities of daily living (ADL) and instrumental activities of daily living (IADL) with or without devices and equipment are increased.
  - Tolerance of positions and activities is increased.
- Impact on disabilities
  - Ability to assume or resume required self-care, home management, work (job/school/play), community, and leisure roles is improved.
- Risk reduction/prevention
  - Risk factors are reduced.
  - Risk of secondary impairment is reduced.
  - Self-management of symptoms is improved.
- Impact on health, wellness, and fitness
  - Health status is improved.
  - Physical function is improved.
- Impact on societal resources
  - Utilization of physical therapy services is optimized.
  - Utilization of physical therapy services results in efficient use of health care dollars.
- Patient/client satisfaction
  - Access, availability, and services provided are acceptable to patient/client.
  - Administrative management of practice is acceptable to patient/client.
  - Clinical proficiency of physical therapist is acceptable to patient/client.
  - Coordination of care is acceptable to patient/client.
  - Cost of health care services is decreased.
  - Intensity of care is decreased.
  - Interpersonal skills of physical therapist are acceptable to patient/client, family, and significant others.
  - Sense of well-being is improved.
  - Stressors are decreased.

Electrotherapeutic Modalities

Interventions

- Electrical stimulation
  - electrical muscle stimulation (EMS)
  - high voltage pulsed current (HVPC)
  - transcutaneous electrical nerve stimulation (TENS)

Anticipated Goals and Expected Outcomes

- Impact on pathology/pathophysiology (disease, disorder, or condition)
  - Edema, lymphedema, or effusion is reduced.
  - Joint swelling, inflammation, or restriction is reduced.
  - Nutrient delivery to tissue is increased.
  - Pain is decreased.
  - Soft tissue and wound healing is enhanced.
  - Soft tissue swelling, inflammation, or restriction is reduced.
  - Tissue perfusion and oxygenation are enhanced.
- Impact on impairments
  - Integumentary integrity is improved.
  - Sensory awareness is increased.
- Impact on functional limitations
  - Ability to perform physical actions, tasks, or activities related to self-care, home management, work (job/school/play), community, and leisure is increased.
  - Level of supervision required for task performance is decreased.
  - Performance of and independence in activities of daily living (ADL) and instrumental activities of daily living (IADL) with or without devices and equipment are increased.
  - Tolerance of positions and activities is increased.
- Impact on disabilities
  - Ability to assume or resume required self-care, home management, work (job/school/play), community, and leisure roles is improved.
- Risk reduction/prevention
  - Complications of immobility are reduced.
  - Risk factors are reduced.
  - Risk of secondary impairment is reduced.
  - Self-management of symptoms is improved.
- Impact on health, wellness, and fitness
  - Physical function is improved.
- Impact on societal resources
  - Utilization of physical therapy services is optimized.
  - Utilization of physical therapy services results in efficient use of health care dollars.
- Patient/client satisfaction
  - Access, availability, and services provided are acceptable to patient/client.
  - Administrative management of practice is acceptable to patient/client.
  - Clinical proficiency of physical therapist is acceptable to patient/client.
  - Coordination of care is acceptable to patient/client.
  - Interpersonal skills of physical therapist are acceptable to patient/client, family, and significant others.
  - Sense of well-being is improved.
  - Stressors are decreased.

Physical Agents and Mechanical Modalities

Interventions

Physical agents may include:

- Hydrotherapy
  - whirlpool tanks
- Light agents
  - ultraviolet
- Sound agents
  - phonophoresis
  - ultrasound

Mechanical modalities may include:

- Compression therapies
  - compression bandaging
  - compression garments

Anticipated Goals and Expected Outcomes

- Impact on pathology/pathophysiology (disease, disorder, or condition)
  - Debridement of nonviable tissue is achieved.
  - Edema, lymphedema, or effusion is reduced.
  - Joint swelling, inflammation, or restriction is reduced.
  - Nutrient delivery to tissue is increased.
  - Pain is decreased.
  - Soft tissue swelling, inflammation, or restriction is reduced.
  - Tissue perfusion and oxygenation are enhanced.
- Impact on impairments
  - Integumentary integrity is improved.
  - Range of motion is improved.
  - Weight-bearing status is improved.
- Impact on functional limitations
  - Ability to perform physical actions, tasks, or activities related to self-care, home management, work (job/school/play), community, and leisure is improved.
  - Performance of and independence in activities of daily living (ADL) and instrumental activities of daily living (IADL) with or without devices and equipment are increased.
  - Tolerance of positions and activities is increased.
- Impact on disabilities
  - Ability to assume or resume required self-care, home management, work (job/school/play), community, and leisure roles is improved.
- Risk reduction/prevention
  - Complications of soft tissue and circulatory disorders are decreased.
  - Risk of secondary impairment is reduced.
  - Self-management of symptoms is improved.
  - Stresses precipitating injury are decreased.
- Impact on health, wellness, and fitness
  - Physical function is improved.
- Impact on societal resources
  - Utilization of physical therapy services is optimized.
- Patient/client satisfaction
  - Access, availability, and services provided are acceptable to patient/client.
  - Administrative management of practice is acceptable to patient/client.
  - Clinical proficiency of physical therapist is acceptable to patient/client.
  - Coordination of care is acceptable to patient/client.
  - Interpersonal skills of physical therapist are acceptable to patient/client, family, and significant others.
  - Sense of well-being is improved.
  - Stressors are decreased.

Reexamination

Reexamination is the process of performing selected tests and measures after the initial examination to evaluate progress and to modify or redirect interventions. Reexamination may be indicated more than once during a single episode of care. It also may be performed over the course of a disease, disorder, or condition, which for some patients/clients may be over the life span. Indications for reexamination include new clinical findings or failure to respond to physical therapy interventions.

Global Outcomes for Patients/Clients in This Pattern

Throughout the entire episode of care, the physical therapist determines the anticipated goals and expected outcomes for each intervention. These anticipated goals and expected outcomes are delineated in shaded boxes that accompany the lists of interventions in each preferred practice pattern. As the patient/client reaches the termination of physical therapy services and the end of the episode of care, the physical therapist measures the global outcomes of the physical therapy services by characterizing or quantifying the impact of the physical therapy interventions in the following domains:

- Pathology/pathophysiology (disease, disorder, or condition)
- Impairments
- Functional limitations
- Disabilities
- Risk reduction/prevention
- Health, wellness, and fitness
- Societal resources
- Patient/client satisfaction

In some instances, a particular anticipated goal or expected outcome is thoroughly achieved through implementation of a single form of intervention. More commonly, however, the anticipated goals and expected outcomes are achieved as a result of the combined effects of several forms of interventions, leading to enhancement of both health status and health-related quality of life.

Criteria for Termination of Physical Therapy Services

Discharge is the process of ending physical therapy services that have been provided during a single episode of care. It occurs when the anticipated goals and expected outcomes have been achieved. Discharge does *not* occur with a *transfer* (defined as the time when a patient is moved from one site to another site within the same setting or across settings during a single episode of care). Although there may be facility-specific or payer-specific requirements for documentation regarding the conclusion of physical therapy services, *discharge occurs based on the physical therapist's analysis of the achievement of anticipated goals and expected outcomes.*

Discontinuation is the process of ending physical therapy services that have been provided during a single episode of care when (1) the patient/client, caregiver, or legal guardian declines to continue intervention; (2) the patient/client is unable to continue to progress toward outcomes because of medical or psychosocial complications or because financial/insurance resources have been expended; or (3) the physical therapist determines that the patient/client will no longer benefit from physical therapy. When physical therapy services are terminated prior to achievement of anticipated goals and expected outcomes, patient/client status and the rationale for termination are documented.

For patients/clients who require multiple episodes of care, periodic follow-up is needed over the life span to ensure safety and effective adaptation following changes in physical status, caregivers, environment, or task demands. In consultation with appropriate individuals, and in consideration of the outcomes, the physical therapist plans for discharge or discontinuation and provides for appropriate follow-up or referral.

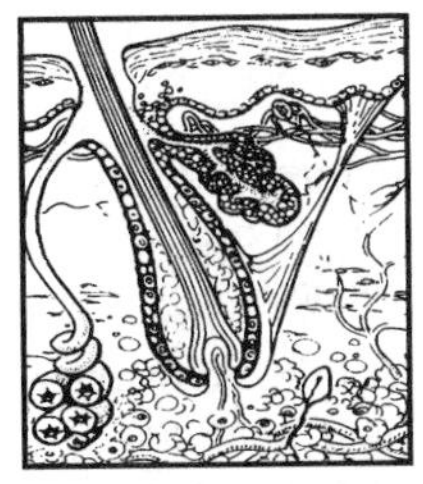

Impaired Integumentary Integrity Associated With Partial-Thickness Skin Involvement and Scar Formation

This preferred practice pattern describes the generally accepted elements of patient/client management that physical therapists provide for patients/clients who are classified in this pattern. The pattern title reflects the diagnosis made by the physical therapist. APTA emphasizes that preferred practice patterns are the boundaries within which a physical therapist may select any of a number of clinical alternatives, based on consideration of a wide variety of factors, such as individual patient/client needs; the profession's code of ethics and standards of practice; and patient/client age, culture, gender roles, race, sex, sexual orientation, and socioeconomic status.

Patient/Client Diagnostic Classification

Patients/clients will be classified into this pattern—for impaired integumentary integrity associated with partial-thickness skin involvement and scar formation—as a result of the physical therapist's evaluation of the examination data. The findings from the examination (history, systems review, and tests and measures) may indicate the presence or risk of pathology/pathophysiology (disease, disorder, or condition), impairments, functional limitations, or disabilities or the need for health, wellness, or fitness programs. The physical therapist integrates, synthesizes, and interprets the data to determine the diagnostic classification.

Inclusion

The following examples of examination findings may support the inclusion of patients/clients in this pattern:

Risk Factors or Consequences of Pathology/Pathophysiology (Disease, Disorder, or Condition)

- Amputation
- Burns (partial thickness/ second degree)
- Dermatologic disorders
- Epidermolysis bullosa
- Hematoma
- Immature scar
- Malnutrition
- Neoplasms (including Kaposi's sarcoma)
- Neuropathic ulcers (grade 1)
- Pressure ulcers (stage 2)
- Prior scar
- Status post spinal cord injury
- Surgical wounds
- Toxic epidermal necrolysis
- Traumatic injury
- Vascular ulcers
  - Arterial
  - Diabetic
  - Venous

Impairments, Functional Limitations, or Disabilities

- Impairments associated with abnormal fluid distribution
- Impaired sensation
- Impaired skin
- Muscle weakness

Note:

Some risk factors or consequences of pathology/ pathophysiology— such as *infection*—may be severe and complex; *however, they do not necessarily exclude patients/clients from this pattern.* Severe and complex risk factors or consequences may require modification of the frequency of visits and duration of care. (See "Evaluation, Diagnosis, and Prognosis," page 625.)

Exclusion or Multiple-Pattern Classification

The following examples of examination findings may support exclusion from this pattern or classification into additional patterns. Depending on the level of severity or complexity of the examination findings, the physical therapist may determine that the patient/client would be more appropriately managed through (1) classification in an entirely different pattern or (2) classification in both this and another pattern.

Findings That May Require Classification in a Different Pattern

- Electricity-related injuries
- Frostbite
- Multiple fractures
- Recent amputation

Findings That May Require Classification in Additional Patterns

- Spinal cord injury

ICD-9-CM Codes

The listing below contains the current (as of press time) and most typical 3- and 4-digit ICD-9-CM codes related to this preferred practice pattern. Because patient/client diagnostic classification is based on impairments, functional limitations, and disabilities—not on codes—patients/clients may be classified into the pattern even though the codes listed with the pattern may not apply to those clients.

This listing is intended for general information only and should not be used for coding purposes. The codes should be confirmed by referring to the World Health Organization's *International Classification of Diseases, 9th Revision, Clinical Modification (ICD-9-CM 2001)*, Volumes 1 and 3 (Chicago, Ill: American Medical Association; 2000) or subsequent revisions or by referring to other ICD-9-CM coding manuals that contain exclusion notes and instructions regarding fifth-digit requirements.

017 Tuberculosis of other organs
- **017.0** Skin and subcutaneous cellular tissue

031 Diseases due to other mycobacteria
- **031.1** Cutaneous

176 Kaposi's sarcoma
- **176.0** Skin

216 Benign neoplasm of skin
- **216.5** Skin of trunk, except scrotum
- **216.6** Skin of upper limb, including shoulder
- **216.7** Skin of lower limb, including hip

232 Carcinoma in situ of skin
- **232.5** Skin of trunk, except scrotum
- **232.6** Skin of upper limb, including shoulder
- **232.7** Skin of lower limb, including hip

239 Neoplasms of unspecified nature
- **239.2** Bone, soft tissue, and skin

263 Other and unspecified protein-calorie malnutrition

269 Other nutritional deficiencies

344 Other paralytic syndromes
- **344.0** Quadriplegia and quadriparesis
- **344.1** Paraplegia

443 Other peripheral vascular disease

454 Varicose veins of lower extremities
- **454.0** With ulcer
- **454.2** With ulcer and inflammation

459 Other disorders of circulatory system

682 Other cellulitis and abscess

686 Other local infections of skin and subcutaneous tissue

694 Bullous dermatoses
- **694.5** Pemphigoid

695 Erythematous conditions
- **695.1** Erythema multiforme
  Toxic epidermal necrolysis
- **695.4** Lupus erythematosus

696 Psoriasis and similar disorders
- **696.1** Other psoriasis

701 Other hypertrophic and atrophic conditions of skin
- **701.0** Circumscribed scleroderma
- **701.3** Striae atrophicae
  Atrophy blanche (of Milian)
- **701.4** Keloid scar

707 Chronic ulcer of skin
- **707.0** Decubitus ulcer
- **707.1** Ulcer of lower limbs, except decubitus
- **707.8** Chronic ulcer of other specified sites

709 Other disorders of skin and subcutaneous tissue
- **709.2** Scar conditions and fibrosis of skin
- **709.3** Degenerative skin disorders

757 Congenital anomalies of the integument

911 Superficial injury of trunk
- **911.0** Abrasion or friction burn without mention of infection
- **911.1** Abrasion or friction burn, infected
- **911.2** Blister without mention of infection
- **911.3** Blister, infected

912 Superficial injury of shoulder and upper arm
- **912.0** Abrasion or friction burn without mention of infection
- **912.1** Abrasion or friction burn, infected
- **912.2** Blister without mention of infection
- **912.3** Blister, infected

913 Superficial injury of elbow, forearm, and wrist
- **913.0** Abrasion or friction burn without mention of infection
- **913.1** Abrasion or friction burn, infected
- **913.2** Blister without mention of infection
- **913.3** Blister, infected

914 Superficial injury of hand(s), except finger(s) alone
- **914.0** Abrasion or friction burn without mention of infection
- **914.1** Abrasion or friction burn, infected
- **914.2** Blister without mention of infection
- **914.3** Blister, infected

915 Superficial injury of finger(s)
- **915.0** Abrasion or friction burn without mention of infection
- **915.1** Abrasion or friction burn, infected
- **915.2** Blister without mention of infection
- **915.3** Blister, infected

916 Superficial injury of hip, thigh, leg, and ankle
- **916.0** Abrasion or friction burn without mention of infection
- **916.1** Abrasion or friction burn, infected
- **916.2** Blister without mention of infection
- **916.3** Blister, infected

917 Superficial injury of foot and toe(s)
- **917.0** Abrasion or friction burn without mention of infection
- **917.1** Abrasion or friction burn, infected
- **917.2** Blister without mention of infection
- **917.3** Blister, infected

942 Burn of trunk
- **942.2** Blisters, epidermal loss [second degree]

943 Burn of upper limb, except wrist and hand
- **943.2** Blisters, epidermal loss [second degree]

944 Burn of wrist(s) and hand(s)
- **944.2** Blisters, epidermal loss [second degree]

945 Burn of lower limb(s)
- **945.2** Blisters, epidermal loss [second degree]

946 Burns of multiple specified sites
- **946.2** Blisters, epidermal loss [second degree]

948 Burns classified according to extent of body surface involved

949 Burn, unspecified
- **949.2** Blisters, epidermal loss [second degree]

997 Complications affecting specified body system, not elsewhere classified
- **997.6** Amputation stump complication

Examination

Examination is a comprehensive screening and specific testing process that leads to a diagnostic classification or, when appropriate, to a referral to another practitioner. Examination is required prior to the initial intervention and is performed for all patients/clients. Through the examination, the physical therapist may identify impairments, functional limitations, disabilities, changes in physical function or overall health status, and needs related to restoration of health and to prevention, wellness, and fitness. The physical therapist synthesizes the examination findings to establish the diagnosis and the prognosis (including the plan of care). The patient/client, family, significant others, and caregivers may provide information during the examination process.

Examination has three components: the patient/client history, the systems review, and tests and measures. The *history* is a systematic gathering of past and current information (often from the patient/client) related to why the patient/client is seeking the services of the physical therapist. The *systems review* is a brief or limited examination of (1) the anatomical and physiological status of the cardiovascular/pulmonary, integumentary, musculoskeletal, and neuromuscular systems and (2) the communication ability, affect, cognition, language, and learning style of the patient/client. *Tests and measures* are the means of gathering data about the patient/client.

The selection of examination procedures and the depth of the examination vary based on patient/client age; severity of the problem; stage of recovery (acute, subacute, chronic); phase of rehabilitation (early, intermediate, late, return to activity); home, work (job/school/play), or community situation; and other relevant factors. *For clinical indications in selecting tests and measures and for listings of tests and measures, tools used to gather data, and the types of data generated by tests and measures, refer to Chapter 2.*

Patient/Client History

The history may include:

General Demographics

- Age
- Sex
- Race/ethnicity
- Primary language
- Education

Social History

- Cultural beliefs and behaviors
- Family and caregiver resources
- Social interactions, social activities, and support systems

Employment/Work (Job/School/Play)

- Current and prior work (job/school/play), community, and leisure actions, tasks, or activities

Growth and Development

- Developmental history
- Hand dominance

Living Environment

- Devices and equipment (eg, assistive, adaptive, orthotic, protective, supportive, prosthetic)
- Living environment and community characteristics
- Projected discharge destinations

General Health Status (Self-Report, Family Report, Caregiver Report)

- General health perception
- Physical function (eg, mobility, sleep patterns, restricted bed days)
- Psychological function (eg, memory, reasoning ability, depression, anxiety)
- Role function (eg, community, leisure, social, work)
- Social function (eg, social activity, social interaction, social support)

Social/Health Habits (Past and Current)

- Behavioral health risks (eg, smoking, drug abuse)
- Level of physical fitness

Family History

- Familial health risks

Medical/Surgical History

- Cardiovascular
- Endocrine/metabolic
- Gastrointestinal
- Genitourinary
- Gynecological
- Integumentary
- Musculoskeletal
- Neuromuscular
- Obstetrical
- Prior hospitalizations, surgeries, and preexisting medical and other health-related conditions
- Psychological
- Pulmonary

Current Condition(s)/Chief Complaint(s)

- Concerns that led patient/client to seek the services of a physical therapist
- Concerns or needs of patient/client who requires the services of a physical therapist
- Current therapeutic interventions
- Mechanisms of injury or disease, including date of onset and course of events
- Onset and pattern of symptoms
- Patient/client, family, significant other, and caregiver expectations and goals for the therapeutic intervention
- Patient/client, family, significant other, and caregiver perceptions of patient's/client's emotional response to the current clinical situation
- Previous occurrence of chief complaint(s)
- Prior therapeutic interventions

Functional Status and Activity Level

- Current and prior functional status in self-care and home management activities, including activities of daily living (ADL) and instrumental activities of daily living (IADL)
- Current and prior functional status in work (job/school/play), community, and leisure actions, tasks, or activities

Medications

- Medications for current condition
- Medications previously taken for current condition
- Medications for other conditions

Other Clinical Tests

- Laboratory and diagnostic tests
- Review of available records (eg, medical, education, surgical)
- Review of other clinical findings (eg, nutrition and hydration)

Systems Review

The systems review may include:

Anatomical and Physiological Status

- Cardiovascular/Pulmonary
  - Blood pressure
  - Edema
  - Heart rate
  - Respiratory rate
- Integumentary
  - Pliability (texture)
  - Presence of scar formation
  - Skin color
  - Skin integrity
- Musculoskeletal
  - Gross range of motion
  - Gross strength
  - Gross symmetry
  - Height
  - Weight
- Neuromuscular
  - Gross coordinated movements (eg, balance, gait, locomotion, transfers, transitions)
  - Motor function (motor control, motor learning)

Communication, Affect, Cognition, Language, and Learning Style

- Ability to make needs known
- Consciousness
- Expected emotional/behavioral responses
- Learning preferences (eg, education needs, learning barriers)
- Orientation (person, place, time)

Tests and Measures

Tests and measures for this pattern may include those that characterize or quantify:

Anthropometric Characteristics

- Body composition (eg, body mass index, impedance measurement, skinfold thickness measurement)
- Edema (eg, girth measurement, palpation, scales, volume measurement)

Assistive and Adaptive Devices

- Safety during use of assistive or adaptive devices and equipment (eg, diaries, fall scales, interviews, logs, observations, reports)

Circulation (Arterial, Venous, and Lymphatic)

- Cardiovascular signs, including heart rate, rhythm, and sounds; pressures and flow; and superficial vascular responses (eg, auscultation, electrocardiography, girth measurement, observations, palpation, sphygmomanometry, thermography)
- Cardiovascular symptoms (eg, angina, claudication, and perceived exertion scales)

Cranial and Peripheral Nerve Integrity

- Sensory distribution of the cranial nerves (eg, discrimination tests; tactile tests, including coarse and light touch, cold and heat, pain, pressure, and vibration)
- Sensory distribution of the peripheral nerves (eg, discrimination tests; tactile tests, including coarse and light touch, cold and heat, pain, pressure, and vibration; thoracic outlet tests)

Gait, Locomotion, and Balance

- Gait and locomotion during functional activities with or without the use of assistive, adaptive, orthotic, protective, supportive, or prosthetic devices or equipment (eg, ADL scales, gait indexes, IADL scales, mobility skill profiles, observations, videographic assessments)
- Gait and locomotion with or without the use of assistive, adaptive, orthotic, protective, supportive, or prosthetic devices or equipment (eg, dynamometry, electroneuromyography, footprint analyses, gait indexes, mobility skill profiles, observations, photographic assessments, technology-assisted assessments, videographic assessments, weight-bearing scales, wheelchair mobility tests)
- Safety during gait, locomotion, and balance (eg, confidence scales, diaries, fall scales, functional assessment profiles, logs, reports)

Integumentary Integrity

Associated skin

- Activities, positioning, and postures that produce or relieve trauma to the skin (eg, observations, pressure-sensing maps, scales)
- Assistive, adaptive, orthotic, protective, supportive, or prosthetic devices and equipment that may produce or relieve trauma to the skin (eg, observations, pressure-sensing maps, risk assessment scales)
- Skin characteristics, including blistering, continuity of skin color, dermatitis, hair growth, mobility, nail growth, sensation, temperature, texture, and turgor (eg, observations, palpation, photographic assessments, thermography)

Tests and Measures

Tests and measures for this pattern may include those that characterize or quantify:

Wound

- Activities, positioning, and postures that aggravate the wound or scar or that produce or relieve trauma (eg, observations, pressure-sensing maps)
- Burn (eg, body charts, planimetry)
- Signs of infection (eg, cultures, observations, palpation)
- Wound characteristics, including bleeding, contraction, depth, drainage, exposed anatomical structures, location, odor, pigment, shape, size, staging and progression, tunneling, and undermining (eg, digital and grid measurement, grading of sores and ulcers, observations, palpation, photographic assessments, wound tracing)
- Wound scar tissue characteristics, including banding, pliability, sensation, and texture (eg, observations, scar-rating scales)

Muscle Performance (Including Strength, Power, and Endurance)

- Muscle strength, power, and endurance during functional activities (eg, ADL scales, functional muscle tests, IADL scales, observations, videographic assessments)
- Muscle tension (eg, palpation)

Orthotic, Protective, and Supportive Devices

- Components, alignment, fit, and ability to care for orthotic, protective, and supportive devices and equipment (eg, interviews, logs, observations, pressure-sensing maps, reports)
- Orthotic, protective, and supportive devices and equipment use during functional activities (eg, ADL scales, functional scales, IADL scales, interviews, observations, profiles)
- Remediation of impairments, functional limitations, or disabilities with use of orthotic, protective, and supportive devices and equipment (eg, activity status indexes, ADL scales, aerobic capacity tests, functional performance inventories, health assessment questionnaires, IADL scales, pain scales, play scales, videographic assessments)
- Safety during use of orthotic, protective, and supportive devices and equipment (eg, diaries, fall scales, interviews, logs, observations, reports)

Pain

- Pain, soreness, and nociception (eg, angina scales, analog scales, discrimination tests, pain drawings and maps, provocation tests, verbal and pictorial descriptor tests)
- Pain in specific body parts (eg, pain indexes, pain questionnaires, structural provocation tests)

Prosthetic Requirements

- Components, alignment, fit, and ability to care for the prosthetic device (eg, interviews, logs, observations, pressure-sensing maps, reports)
- Safety during use of the prosthetic device (eg, diaries, fall scales, interviews, logs, observations, reports)

Range of Motion (ROM) (Including Muscle Length)

- Functional ROM (eg, observations, squat testing, toe touch tests)
- Joint active and passive movement (eg, goniometry, inclinometry, observations, photographic assessments, technology-assisted assessments, videographic assessments)
- Muscle length, soft tissue extensibility, and flexibility (eg, contracture tests, goniometry, inclinometry, ligamentous tests, linear measurement, multisegment flexibility tests, palpation)

Self-Care and Home Management (Including ADL and IADL)

- Safety in self-care and home management activities and environments (eg, diaries, fall scales, interviews, logs, observations, reports, videographic assessments)

Sensory Integrity

- Deep sensations (eg, kinesthesiometry, observations, photographic assessments, vibration tests)

Work (Job/School/Play), Community, and Leisure Integration or Reintegration (Including IADL)

- Safety in work (job/school/play), community, and leisure activities and environments (eg, diaries, fall scales, interviews, logs, observations, videographic assessments)

Evaluation, Diagnosis, and Prognosis (Including Plan of Care)

Physical therapists perform *evaluations* (make clinical judgments) based on the data gathered from the history, systems review, and tests and measures. In the evaluation process, physical therapists synthesize the examination data to establish the diagnosis and prognosis (including the plan of care). Factors that influence the complexity of the evaluation include the clinical findings, extent of loss of function, chronicity or severity of the problem, possibility of multisite or multisystem involvement, preexisting condition(s), potential discharge destination, social considerations, physical function, and overall health status.

A *diagnosis* is a label encompassing a cluster of signs and symptoms, syndromes, or categories. It is the result of the systematic diagnostic process, which includes integrating and evaluating the data from the examination.The diagnostic label indicates the primary dysfunction(s) toward which the therapist will direct interventions. The *prognosis* is the determination of the predicted optimal level of improvement in function and the amount of time needed to reach that level and may also include a prediction of levels of improvement that may be reached at various intervals during the course of therapy. During the prognostic process, the physical therapist develops the plan of care. The *plan of care* identifies specific interventions, proposed frequency and duration of the interventions, anticipated goals, expected outcomes, and discharge plans. The plan of care identifies realistic anticipated goals and expected outcomes, taking into consideration the expectations of the patient/client and appropriate others.These anticipated goals and expected outcomes should be measureable and time limited.

The frequency of visits and duration of the episode of care may vary from a short episode with a high intensity of intervention to a longer episode with a diminishing intensity of intervention. Frequency and duration may vary greatly among patients/clients based on a variety of factors that the physical therapist considers throughout the evaluation process, such as anatomical and physiological changes related to growth and development; caregiver consistency or expertise; chronicity or severity of the current condition; living environment; multisite or multisystem involvement; social support; potential discharge destinations; probability of prolonged impairment, functional limitation, or disability; and stability of the condition.

Prognosis

Over the course of 4 weeks, patient/client will demonstrate optimal integumentary integrity and the highest level of functioning in home, work (job/school/play), community, and leisure environments.

During the episode of care, patient/client will achieve (1) the anticipated goals and expected outcomes of the interventions that are described in the plan of care and (2) the global outcomes for patients/clients who are classified in this pattern.

Expected Range of Number of Visits Per Episode of Care

4 to 30

This range represents the lower and upper limits of the number of physical therapist visits required to achieve anticipated goals and expected outcomes. *It is anticipated that 80% of patients/clients who are classified into this pattern will achieve the anticipated goals and expected outcomes within 4 to 30 visits during a single continuous episode of care.* Frequency of visits and duration of the episode of care should be determined by the physical therapist to maximize effectiveness of care and efficiency of service delivery.

Factors That May Require New Episode of Care or That May Modify Frequency of Visits/Duration of Episode

- Accessibility and availability of resources
- Adherence to the intervention program
- Age
- Anatomical and physiological changes related to growth and development
- Caregiver consistency or expertise
- Chronicity or severity of the current condition
- Cognitive status
- Comorbitities, complications, or secondary impairments
- Concurrent medical, surgical, and therapeutic interventions
- Decline in functional independence
- Level of impairment
- Level of physical function
- Living environment
- Multisite or multisystem involvement
- Nutritional status
- Overall health status
- Potential discharge destinations
- Premorbid conditions
- Probability of prolonged impairment, functional limitation, or disability
- Psychological and socioeconomic factors
- Psychomotor abilities
- Social support
- Stability of the condition

Intervention

Intervention is the purposeful interaction of the physical therapist with the patient/client and, when appropriate, with other individuals involved in patient/client care, using various physical therapy procedures and techniques to produce changes in the condition consistent with the diagnosis and prognosis. Decisions about interventions are contingent on the timely monitoring of patient/client response and the progress made toward achieving the anticipated goals and expected outcomes.

Communication, coordination, and documentation and patient/client-related instruction are provided for all patients/clients across all settings. Procedural interventions are selected or modified based on the examination data and the evaluation, the diagnosis and the prognosis, and the anticipated goals and expected outcomes for a particular patient/client. *For clinical considerations in selecting interventions, listings of interventions, and listings of anticipated goals and expected outcomes, refer to Chapter 3.*

Coordination, Communication, and Documentation

Coordination, communication, and documentation may include:

Interventions

- Addressing required functions
  - advance directives
  - individualized family service plans (IFSPs) or individualized education plans (IEPs)
  - informed consent
  - mandatory communication and reporting (eg, patient advocacy and abuse reporting)
- Admission and discharge planning
- Case management
- Collaboration and coordination with agencies, including:
  - equipment suppliers
  - home care agencies
  - payer groups
  - schools
  - transportation agencies
- Communication across settings, including:
  - case conferences
  - documentation
  - education plans
- Cost-effective resource utilization
- Data collection, analysis, and reporting
  - outcome data
  - peer review findings
  - record reviews
- Documentation across settings, following APTA's *Guidelines for Physical Therapy Documentation* (Appendix 5), including:
  - changes in impairments, functional limitations, and disabilities
  - changes in interventions
  - elements of patient/client management (examination, evaluation, diagnosis, prognosis, intervention)
  - outcomes of intervention
- Interdisciplinary teamwork
  - case conferences
  - patient care rounds
  - patient/client family meetings
- Referrals to other professionals or resources

Anticipated Goals and Expected Outcomes

- Accountability for services is increased.
- Admission data and discharge planning are completed.
- Advance directives, individualized family service plans (IFSPs) or individualized education plans (IEPs), informed consent, and mandatory communication and reporting (eg, patient advocacy and abuse reporting) are obtained or completed.
- Available resources are maximally utilized.
- Care is coordinated with patient/client, family, significant others, caregivers, and other professionals.
- Case is managed throughout the episode of care.
- Collaboration and coordination occurs with agencies, including equipment suppliers, home care agencies, payer groups, schools, and transportation agencies.
- Communication enhances risk reduction and prevention.
- Communication occurs across settings through case conferences, education plans, and documentation.
- Data are collected, analyzed, and reported, including outcome data, peer review findings, and record reviews.
- Decision making is enhanced regarding health, wellness, and fitness needs.
- Decision making is enhanced regarding patient/client health and the use of health care resources by patient/client, family, significant others, and caregivers.
- Documentation occurs throughout patient/client management and across settings and follows APTA's *Guidelines for Physical Therapy Documentation* (Appendix 5).
- Interdisciplinary collaboration occurs through case conferences, patient care rounds, and patient/client family meetings.
- Patient/client, family, significant other, and caregiver understanding of anticipated goals and expected outcomes is increased.
- Placement needs are determined.
- Referrals are made to other professionals or resources whenever necessary and appropriate.
- Resources are utilized in a cost-effective way.

Patient/Client-Related Instruction

Patient/client-related instruction may include:

Interventions

- Instruction, education and training of patients/clients and caregivers regarding:
  - current condition (pathology/pathophysiology [disease, disorder, or condition], impairments, functional limitations, or disabilities)
  - enhancement of performance
  - health, wellness, and fitness programs
  - plan of care
  - risk factors for pathology/pathophysiology (disease, disorder, or condition), impairments, functional limitations, or disabilities
  - transitions across settings
  - transitions to new roles

Anticipated Goals and Expected Outcomes

- Ability to perform physical actions, tasks, or activities is improved.
- Awareness and use of community resources are improved.
- Behaviors that foster healthy habits, wellness, and prevention are acquired.
- Decision making is enhanced regarding patient/client health and the use of health care resources by patient/client, family, significant others, and caregivers.
- Disability associated with acute or chronic illnesses is reduced.
- Functional independence in activities of daily living (ADL) and instrumental activities of daily living (IADL) is increased.
- Health status is improved.
- Intensity of care is decreased.
- Level of supervision required for task performance is decreased.
- Patient/client, family, significant other, and caregiver knowledge and awareness of the diagnosis, prognosis, interventions, and anticipated goals and expected outcomes are increased.
- Patient/client knowledge of personal and environmental factors associated with the condition is increased.
- Performance levels in self-care, home management, work (job/school/play), community, or leisure actions, tasks, or activities are improved.
- Physical function is improved.
- Risk of recurrence of condition is reduced.
- Risk of secondary impairment is reduced.
- Safety of patient/client, family, significant others, and caregivers is improved.
- Self-management of symptoms is improved.
- Utilization and cost of health care services are decreased.

Procedural Interventions

Procedural interventions for this pattern may include:

Therapeutic Exercise

Interventions

- Balance, coordination, and agility training
  - perceptual training
  - posture awareness training
  - sensory training or retraining
  - task-specific performance training
- Body mechanics and postural stabilization
  - posture awareness training
- Flexibility exercises
  - muscle lengthening
  - range of motion
  - stretching
- Gait and locomotion training
  - perceptual training
  - standardized, programmatic, complementary exercise approaches
- Strength, power, and endurance training for head, neck, limb, pelvic-floor, trunk, and ventilatory muscles
  - active assistive, active, and resistive exercises (including concentric, dynamic/isotonic, eccentric, isokinetic, isometric, and plyometric)
  - task-specific performance training

Anticipated Goals and Expected Outcomes

- Impact on pathology/pathophysiology (disease, disorder, or condition)
  - Joint swelling, inflammation, or restriction is reduced.
  - Nutrient delivery to tissue is increased.
  - Pain is decreased.
  - Soft tissue swelling, inflammation, or restriction is reduced.
  - Tissue perfusion and oxygenation are enhanced.
- Impact on impairments
  - Balance is improved.
  - Gait, locomotion, and balance are improved.
  - Integumentary integrity is improved.
  - Joint integrity and mobility are improved.
  - Muscle performance (strength, power, and endurance) is increased.
  - Postural control is improved.
  - Range of motion is improved.
  - Sensory awareness is increased.
  - Weight-bearing status is improved.
- Impact on functional limitations
  - Ability to perform physical actions, tasks, or activities related to self-care, home management, work (job/school/play), community, and leisure is improved.
  - Level of supervision required for task performance is decreased.
  - Performance of and independence in activities of daily living (ADL) and instrumental activities of daily living (IADL) with or without devices and equipment are increased.
  - Tolerance of positions and activities is increased.
- Impact on disabilities
  - Ability to assume or resume required self-care, home management, work (job/school/play), community, and leisure roles is improved.
- Risk reduction/prevention
  - Preoperative and postoperative complications are reduced.
  - Risk factors are reduced.
  - Risk of recurrence of condition is reduced.
  - Risk of secondary impairment is reduced.
  - Safety is improved.
  - Self-management of symptoms is improved.
- Impact on health, wellness, and fitness
  - Health status is improved.
  - Physical capacity is increased.
  - Physical function is improved.
- Impact on societal resources
  - Utilization of physical therapy services is optimized.
  - Utilization of physical therapy services results in efficient use of health care dollars.
- Patient/client satisfaction
  - Access, availability, and services provided are acceptable to patient/client.
  - Administrative management of practice is acceptable to patient/client.
  - Clinical proficiency of physical therapist is acceptable to patient/client.
  - Coordination of care is acceptable to patient/client.
  - Cost of health care services is decreased.
  - Intensity of care is decreased.
  - Interpersonal skills of physical therapist are acceptable to patient/client, family, and significant others.
  - Sense of well-being is improved.
  - Stressors are decreased.

Interventions Continued

Functional Training in Self-Care and Home Management (Including Activities of Daily Living [ADL] and Instrumental Activities of Daily Living [IADL])

Interventions

- Injury prevention or reduction
  - injury prevention education during self-care and home management
  - injury prevention or reduction with use of devices and equipment
  - safety awareness training during self-care and home management

Anticipated Goals and Expected Outcomes

- Impact on pathology/pathophysiology (disease, disorder, or condition)
  - Pain is decreased.
- Impact on impairments
  - Balance is improved.
  - Sensory awareness is increased.
  - Weight-bearing status is improved.
- Impact on functional limitations
  - Ability to perform physical actions, tasks, or activities related to self-care and home management is improved.
  - Level of supervision required for task performance is decreased.
  - Performance of and independence in ADL and IADL with or without devices and equipment are increased.
  - Tolerance of positions and activities is increased.
- Impact on disabilities
  - Ability to assume or resume required self-care and home management roles is improved.
- Risk reduction/prevention
  - Risk factors are reduced.
  - Risk of secondary impairments is reduced.
  - Safety is improved.
  - Self-management of symptoms is improved.
- Impact on health, wellness, and fitness
  - Health status is improved.
  - Physical function is improved.
- Impact on societal resources
  - Utilization of physical therapy services is optimized.
  - Utilization of physical therapy services results in efficient use of health care dollars.
- Patient/client satisfaction
  - Access, availability, and services provided are acceptable to patient/client.
  - Administrative management of practice is acceptable to patient/client.
  - Clinical proficiency of physical therapist is acceptable to patient/client.
  - Coordination of care is acceptable to patient/client.
  - Cost of health care services is decreased.
  - Intensity of care is decreased.
  - Interpersonal skills of physical therapist are acceptable to patient/client, family, and significant others.
  - Sense of well-being is improved.
  - Stressors are decreased.

Functional Training in Work (Job/School/Play), Community, and Leisure Integration or Reintegration (Including Instrumental Activities of Daily Living [IADL], Work Hardening, and Work Conditioning)

Interventions

- Injury prevention or reduction
  - injury prevention education during work (job/school/play), community, and leisure integration or reintegration
  - injury prevention or reduction with use of devices and equipment
  - safety awareness training during work (job/school/play), community, and leisure integration or reintegration

Anticipated Goals and Expected Outcomes

- Impact on pathology/pathophysiology (disease, disorder, or condition)
  - Pain is decreased.
- Impact on impairments
  - Balance is improved.
  - Sensory awareness is increased.
  - Weight-bearing status is improved.
- Impact on functional limitations
  - Ability to perform physical actions, tasks, or activities related to work (job/school/play), community, and leisure integration or reintegration is improved.
  - Level of supervision required for task performance is decreased.
  - Performance of and independence in IADL with or without devices and equipment are increased.
  - Tolerance of positions and activities is increased.
- Impact on disabilities
  - Ability to assume or resume required work (job/school/play), community, and leisure roles is improved.
- Risk reduction/prevention
  - Risk factors are reduced.
  - Risk of secondary impairment is reduced.
  - Safety is improved.
  - Self-management of symptoms is improved.
- Impact on health, wellness, and fitness
  - Health status is improved.
  - Physical function is improved.
- Impact on societal resources
  - Costs of work-related injury or disability are reduced.
  - Utilization of physical therapy services is optimized.
  - Utilization of physical therapy services results in efficient use of health care dollars.
- Patient/client satisfaction
  - Access, availability, and services provided are acceptable to patient/client.
  - Administrative management of practice is acceptable to patient/client.
  - Clinical proficiency of physical therapist is acceptable to patient/client.
  - Coordination of care is acceptable to patient/client.
  - Cost of health care services is decreased.
  - Intensity of care is decreased.
  - Interpersonal skills of physical therapist are acceptable to patient/client, family, and significant others.
  - Sense of well-being is improved.
  - Stressors are decreased.

Manual Therapy Techniques (Including Mobilization/Manipulation)

Interventions

- Manual lymphatic drainage
- Massage
  - therapeutic massage

Anticipated Goals and Expected Outcomes

- Impact on pathology/pathophysiology (disease, disorder, or condition)
  - Edema, lymphedema, or effusion is reduced.
  - Joint swelling, inflammation, or restriction is reduced.
  - Pain is decreased.
  - Soft tissue swelling, inflammation, or restriction is reduced.
- Impact on impairments
  - Integumentary integrity is improved.
  - Relaxation is increased.
  - Sensory awareness is increased.
- Impact on functional limitations
  - Ability to perform movement tasks is improved.
  - Ability to perform physical actions, tasks, or activities related to self-care, home management, work (job/school/play), community, and leisure is improved.
  - Tolerance of positions and activities is increased.
- Impact on disabilities
  - Ability to assume or resume required self-care, home management, work (job/school/play), community, and leisure roles is improved.
- Risk reduction/prevention
  - Risk factors are reduced.
  - Risk of recurrence of condition is reduced.
  - Risk of secondary impairment is reduced.
  - Self-management of symptoms is improved.
- Impact on health, wellness, and fitness
  - Physical function is improved.
- Impact on societal resources
  - Utilization of physical therapy services is optimized.
  - Utilization of physical therapy services results in efficient use of health care dollars.
- Patient/client satisfaction
  - Access, availability, and services provided are acceptable to patient/client.
  - Administrative management of practice is acceptable to patient/client.
  - Clinical proficiency of physical therapist is acceptable to patient/client.
  - Coordination of care is acceptable to patient/client.
  - Cost of health care services is decreased.
  - Intensity of care is decreased.
  - Interpersonal skills of physical therapist are acceptable to patient/client, family, and significant others.
  - Sense of well-being is improved.
  - Stressors are decreased.

Prescription, Application, and, as Appropriate, Fabrication of Devices and Equipment (Assistive, Adaptive, Orthotic, Protective, Supportive, and Prosthetic)

Interventions

- Adaptive devices
  - hospital beds
  - seating systems
- Assistive devices
  - canes
  - crutches
  - long-handled reachers
  - power devices
  - static and dynamic splints
  - walkers
  - wheelchairs
- Orthotic devices
  - braces
  - casts
  - shoe inserts
  - splints
- Prosthetic devices (lower-extremity and upper-extremity)
- Protective devices
  - braces
  - cushions
  - protective taping
- Supportive devices
  - compression garments
  - elastic wraps
  - supportive taping

Anticipated Goals and Expected Outcomes

- Impact on pathology/pathophysiology (disease, disorder, or condition)
  - Edema, lymphedema, or effusion is reduced.
  - Joint swelling, inflammation, or restriction is reduced.
  - Pain is decreased.
  - Soft tissue swelling, inflammation, or restriction is reduced.
- Impact on impairments
  - Balance is improved.
  - Energy expenditure per unit of work is decreased.
  - Gait, locomotion, and balance are improved.
  - Integumentary integrity is improved.
  - Joint stability is improved.
  - Optimal joint alignment is achieved.
  - Optimal loading on a body part is achieved.
  - Quality and quantity of movement between and across body segments are improved.
  - Weight-bearing status is improved.
- Impact on functional limitations
  - Ability to perform physical actions, tasks, or activities related to self-care, home management, work (job/school/play), community, and leisure is improved.
  - Level of supervision required for task performance is decreased.
  - Performance of and independence in activities of daily living (ADL) and instrumental activities of daily living (IADL) with or without devices and equipment are increased.
  - Tolerance of positions and activities is improved.
- Impact on disabilities
  - Ability to assume or resume required self-care, home management, work (job/school/play), community, and leisure roles is improved.
- Risk reduction/prevention
  - Pressure on body tissues is reduced.
  - Protection of body parts is increased.
  - Risk factors are reduced.
  - Risk of secondary impairment is reduced.
  - Safety is improved.
  - Self-management of symptoms is improved.
  - Stresses precipitating injury are decreased.
- Impact on health, wellness, and fitness
  - Health status is improved.
  - Physical function is improved.
- Impact on societal resources
  - Utilization of physical therapy services is optimized.
  - Utilization of physical therapy services results in efficient use of health care dollars.
- Patient/client satisfaction
  - Access, availability, and services provided are acceptable to patient/client.
  - Administrative management of practice is acceptable to patient/client.
  - Clinical proficiency of physical therapist is acceptable to patient/client.
  - Coordination of care is acceptable to patient/client.
  - Cost of health care services is decreased.
  - Intensity of care is decreased.
  - Interpersonal skills of physical therapist are acceptable to patient/client, family, and significant others.
  - Sense of well-being is improved.
  - Stressors are decreased.

Integumentary Repair and Protection Techniques

Interventions

- Debridement—nonselective
  - enzymatic debridement
  - wet dressings
  - wet-to-dry dressings
  - wet-to-moist dressings
- Debridement—selective
  - debridement with other agents (eg, autolysis)
  - enzymatic debridement
  - sharp debridement
- Dressings
  - hydrogels
  - vacuum-assisted closure
  - wound coverings
- Oxygen therapy
  - supplemental
  - topical
- Topical agents
  - cleansers
  - creams
  - moisturizers
  - ointments
  - sealants

Anticipated Goals and Expected Outcomes

- Impact on pathology/pathophysiology (disease, disorder, or condition)
  - Debridement of nonviable tissue is achieved.
  - Pain is decreased.
  - Soft tissue or wound healing is enhanced.
  - Tissue perfusion and oxygenation are enhanced.
  - Wound size is reduced.
- Impact on impairments
  - Integumentary integrity is improved.
  - Weight-bearing status is improved.
- Impact on functional limitations
  - Ability to perform physical actions, tasks, or activities related to self-care, home management, work (job/ school/ play), community, and leisure is improved.
  - Level of supervision required for task performance is decreased.
  - Performance of and independence in activities of daily living (ADL) and instrumental activities of daily living (IADL) with or without devices and equipment are increased.
  - Tolerance of positions and activities is increased.
- Impact on disabilities
  - Ability to assume or resume required self-care, home management, work (job/school/play), community, and leisure roles is improved.
- Risk reduction/prevention
  - Preoperative and postoperative complications are reduced.
  - Risk factors are reduced.
  - Risk of secondary impairment is reduced.
  - Self-management of symptoms is improved.
- Impact on health, wellness, and fitness
  - Health status is improved.
  - Physical function is improved.
- Impact on societal resources
  - Utilization of physical therapy services is optimized.
  - Utilization of physical therapy services results in efficient use of health care dollars.
- Patient/client satisfaction
  - Access, availability, and services provided are acceptable to patient/client.
  - Administrative management of practice is acceptable to patient/client.
  - Clinical proficiency of physical therapist is acceptable to patient/client.
  - Coordination of care is acceptable to patient/client.
  - Cost of health care services is decreased.
  - Intensity of care is decreased.
  - Interpersonal skills of physical therapist are acceptable to patient/client, family, and significant others.
  - Sense of well-being is improved.
  - Stressors are decreased.

Electrotherapeutic Modalities

Interventions

- Electrical stimulation
  - electrical muscle stimulation (EMS)
  - high voltage pulsed current (HVPC)
  - transcutaneous electrical nerve stimulation (TENS)

Anticipated Goals and Expected Outcomes

- Impact on pathology/pathophysiology (disease, disorder, or condition)
  - Edema, lymphedema, or effusion is reduced.
  - Joint swelling, inflammation, or restriction is reduced.
  - Nutrient delivery to tissue is increased.
  - Pain is decreased.
  - Soft tissue or wound healing is enhanced.
  - Soft tissue swelling, inflammation, or restriction is reduced.
  - Tissue perfusion and oxygenation are enhanced.
- Impact on impairments
  - Integumentary integrity is improved.
  - Sensory awareness is increased.
- Impact on functional limitations
  - Ability to perform physical actions, tasks, or activities related to self-care, home management, work (job/school/play), community, and leisure is improved.
  - Level of supervision required for task performance is decreased.
  - Performance of and independence in activities of daily living (ADL) and instrumental activities of daily living (IADL) with or without devices and equipment are increased.
  - Tolerance of positions and activities is increased.
- Impact on disabilities
  - Ability to assume or resume required self-care, home management, work (job/school/play), community, and leisure roles is improved.
- Risk reduction/prevention
  - Preoperative and postoperative complications are reduced.
  - Risk factors are reduced.
  - Risk of secondary impairment is reduced.
  - Self-management of symptoms is improved.
- Impact on health, wellness, and fitness
  - Physical function is improved.
- Impact on societal resources
  - Utilization of physical therapy services is optimized.
  - Utilization of physical therapy services results in efficient use of health care dollars.
- Patient/client satisfaction
  - Access, availability, and services provided are acceptable to patient/client.
  - Administrative management of practice is acceptable to patient/client.
  - Clinical proficiency of physical therapist is acceptable to patient/client.
  - Coordination of care is acceptable to patient/client.
  - Interpersonal skills of physical therapist are acceptable to patient/client, family, and significant others.
  - Sense of well-being is improved.
  - Stressors are decreased.

Physical Agents and Mechanical Modalities

Interventions

Physical agents may include:

- Hydrotherapy
  - pulsatile lavage
  - whirlpool tanks
- Light agents
  - laser
  - ultraviolet
- Sound agents
  - phonophoresis
  - ultrasound
- Thermotherapy
  - diathermy
  - dry heat
  - hot packs
  - paraffin baths

Mechanical modalities may include:

- Compression therapies
  - compression bandaging
  - compression therapies
  - taping
  - total contact casting
  - vasopneumatic compression devices

Anticipated Goals and Expected Outcomes

- Impact on pathology/pathophysiology (disease, disorder, or condition)
  - Debridement of nonviable tissue is achieved.
  - Edema, lymphedema, or effusion is reduced.
  - Joint swelling, inflammation, or restriction is reduced.
  - Nutrient delivery to tissue is increased.
  - Pain is decreased.
  - Soft tissue swelling, inflammation, or restriction is reduced.
  - Tissue perfusion and oxygenation are enhanced.
- Impact on impairments
  - Integumentary integrity is improved.
  - Range of motion is improved.
  - Weight-bearing status is improved.
- Impact on functional limitations
  - Ability to perform physical actions, tasks, or activities related to self-care, home management, work (job/school/play), community, and leisure is improved.
  - Performance of and independence in activities of daily living (ADL) and instrumental activities of daily living (IADL) with or without devices and equipment are increased.
  - Tolerance of positions and activities is increased.
- Impact on disabilities
  - Ability to assume or resume required self-care, home management, work (job/school/play), community, and leisure roles is improved.
- Risk reduction/prevention
  - Complications of soft tissue and circulatory disorders are decreased.
  - Risk of secondary impairment is reduced.
  - Self-management of symptoms is improved.
  - Stresses precipitating injury are decreased.
- Impact on health, wellness, and fitness
  - Physical function is improved.
- Impact on societal resources
  - Utilization of physical therapy services is optimized.
- Patient/client satisfaction
  - Access, availability, and services provided are acceptable to patient/client.
  - Administrative management of practice is acceptable to patient/client.
  - Clinical proficiency of physical therapist is acceptable to patient/client.
  - Coordination of care is acceptable to patient/client.
  - Interpersonal skills of physical therapist are acceptable to patient/client, family, and significant others.
  - Sense of well-being is improved.
  - Stressors are decreased.

Reexamination

Reexamination is the process of performing selected tests and measures after the initial examination to evaluate progress and to modify or redirect interventions. Reexamination may be indicated more than once during a single episode of care. It also may be performed over the course of a disease, disorder, or condition, which for some patients/clients may be over the life span. Indications for reexamination include new clinical findings or failure to respond to physical therapy interventions.

Global Outcomes for Patients/Clients in This Pattern

Throughout the entire episode of care, the physical therapist determines the anticipated goals and expected outcomes for each intervention. These anticipated goals and expected outcomes are delineated in shaded boxes that accompany the lists of interventions in each preferred practice pattern. As the patient/client reaches the termination of physical therapy services and the end of the episode of care, the physical therapist measures the global outcomes of the physical therapy services by characterizing or quantifying the impact of the physical therapy interventions in the following domains:

- Pathology/pathophysiology (disease, disorder, or condition)
- Impairments
- Functional limitations
- Disabilities
- Risk reduction/prevention
- Health, wellness, and fitness
- Societal resources
- Patient/client satisfaction

In some instances, a particular anticipated goal or expected outcome is thoroughly achieved through implementation of a single form of intervention. More commonly, however, the anticipated goals and expected outcomes are achieved as a result of the combined effects of several forms of interventions, leading to enhancement of both health status and health-related quality of life.

Criteria for Termination of Physical Therapy Services

Discharge is the process of ending physical therapy services that have been provided during a single episode of care. It occurs when the anticipated goals and expected outcomes have been achieved. Discharge does *not* occur with a *transfer* (defined as the time when a patient is moved from one site to another site within the same setting or across settings during a single episode of care). Although there may be facility-specific or payer-specific requirements for documentation regarding the conclusion of physical therapy services, *discharge occurs based on the physical therapist's analysis of the achievement of anticipated goals and expected outcomes.*

Discontinuation is the process of ending physical therapy services that have been provided during a single episode of care when (1) the patient/client, caregiver, or legal guardian declines to continue intervention; (2) the patient/client is unable to continue to progress toward outcomes because of medical or psychosocial complications or because financial/insurance resources have been expended; or (3) the physical therapist determines that the patient/client will no longer benefit from physical therapy. When physical therapy services are terminated prior to achievement of anticipated goals and expected outcomes, patient/client status and the rationale for termination are documented.

For patients/clients who require multiple episodes of care, periodic follow-up is needed over the life span to ensure safety and effective adaptation following changes in physical status, caregivers, environment, or task demands. In consultation with appropriate individuals, and in consideration of the outcomes, the physical therapist plans for discharge or discontinuation and provides for appropriate follow-up or referral.

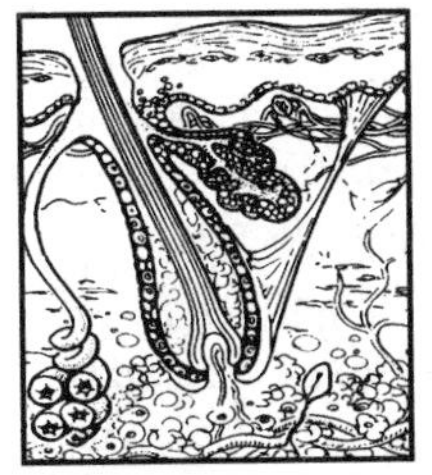

Impaired Integumentary Integrity Associated With Full-Thickness Skin Involvement and Scar Formation

This preferred practice pattern describes the generally accepted elements of patient/client management that physical therapists provide for patients/clients who are classified in this pattern. The pattern title reflects the diagnosis made by the physical therapist. APTA emphasizes that preferred practice patterns are the boundaries within which a physical therapist may select any of a number of clinical alternatives, based on consideration of a wide variety of factors, such as individual patient/client needs; the profession's code of ethics and standards of practice; and patient/client age, culture, gender roles, race, sex, sexual orientation, and socioeconomic status.

Patient/Client Diagnostic Classification

Patients/clients will be classified into this pattern—for impaired integumentary integrity associated with full-thickness skin involvement and scar formation—as a result of the physical therapist's evaluation of the examination data. The findings from the examination (history, systems review, and tests and measures) may indicate the presence or risk of pathology/ pathophysiology, impairments, functional limitations, or disabilities or the need for health, wellness, or fitness programs. The physical therapist integrates, synthesizes, and interprets the data to determine the diagnostic classification.

Inclusion

The following examples of examination findings may support the inclusion of patients/clients in this pattern:

Risk Factors or Consequences of Pathology/Pathophysiology (Disease, Disorder, or Condition)

- Abscess
- Amputation
- Burns
- Frostbite
- Hematoma
- Immature, hypertrophic, or keloid scar
- Lymphostatic ulcer
- Malnutrition
- Neoplasm
- Neuropathic ulcers (grade 2)
- Pressure ulcers (stage 3)
- Prior scar
- Surgical wounds
- Toxic epidermal necrolysis
- Vascular ulcers
  - Arterial
  - Diabetic
  - Venous

Impairments, Functional Limitations, or Disabilities

- Impairments associated with abnormal fluid distribution
- Impaired sensation
- Impaired skin
- Muscle weakness

Note:

Some risk factors or consequences of pathology/ pathophysiology— such as *infection* and *traumatic wounds*— may be severe and complex; *however, they do not necessarily exclude patients/clients from this pattern.* Severe and complex risk factors or consequences may require modification of the frequency of visits and duration of care. (See "Evaluation, Diagnosis, and Prognosis," page 642.)

Exclusion or Multiple-Pattern Classification

The following examples of examination findings may support exclusion from this pattern or classification into additional patterns. Depending on the level of severity or complexity of the examination findings, the physical therapist may determine that the patient/client would be more appropriately managed through (1) classification in an entirely different pattern or (2) classification in both this and another pattern.

Findings That May Require Classification in a Different Pattern

- Crushing injury
- Electricity related injury
- Lymphedema
- Recent amputation

Findings That May Require Classification in Additional Patterns

- Diabetic neuropathy

ICD-9-CM Codes

The listing below contains the current (as of press time) and most typical 3- and 4-digit ICD-9-CM codes related to this preferred practice pattern. Because patient/client diagnostic classification is based on impairments, functional limitations, and disabilities—not on codes—patients/clients may be classified into the pattern even though the codes listed with the pattern may not apply to those clients.

This listing is intended for general information only and should not be used for coding purposes. The codes should be confirmed by referring to the World Health Organization's *International Classification of Diseases, 9th Revision, Clinical Modification (ICD-9-CM 2001)*, Volumes 1 and 3 (Chicago, Ill: American Medical Association; 2000) or subsequent revisions or by referring to other ICD-9-CM coding manuals that contain exclusion notes and instructions regarding fifth-digit requirements.

017 Tuberculosis of other organs
- **017.0** Skin and subcutaneous cellular tissue

031 Diseases due to other mycobacteria
- **031.1** Cutaneous

036 Meningococcal infection
- **036.1** Meningococcal encephalitis

040 Other bacterial diseases
- **040.0** Gas gangrene

172 Malignant melanoma of skin
- **172.5** Trunk, except scrotum
- **172.6** Upper limb, including shoulder
- **172.7** Lower limb, including hip
- **172.8** Other specified sites of skin

173 Other malignant neoplasm of skin
- **173.5** Skin of trunk, except scrotum
- **173.6** Skin of upper limb, including shoulder
- **173.7** Skin of lower limb, including hip
- **173.8** Other specified sites of skin

176 Kaposi's sarcoma
- **176.0** Skin

216 Benign neoplasm of skin

232 Carcinoma in situ of skin

239 Neoplasms of unspecified nature

263 Other and unspecified protein-calorie malnutrition

269 Other nutritional deficiencies

443 Other peripheral vascular disease
- **443.1** Thromboangiitis obliterans [Buerger's disease]

454 Varicose veins of lower extremities
- **454.0** With ulcer
- **454.2** With ulcer and inflammation

459 Other disorders of circulatory system

680 Carbuncle and furuncle
- **680.2** Trunk
- **680.3** Upper arm and forearm
- **680.4** Hand
- **680.5** Buttock
- **680.6** Leg, except foot
- **680.7** Foot

681 Cellulitis and abscess of finger and toe
- **681.0** Finger
- **681.1** Toe

682 Other cellulitis and abscess
- **682.0** Face
- **682.2** Trunk
- **682.3** Upper arm and forearm
- **682.4** Hand, except fingers and thumb
- **682.5** Buttock
- **682.6** Leg, except foot
- **682.7** Foot, except toes

686 Other local infections of skin and subcutaneous tissue
- **686.0** Pyoderma
- **686.1** Pyogenic granuloma
- **686.8** Other specified local infections of skin and subcutaneous tissue

694 Bullous dermatoses

695 Erythematous conditions
- **695.1** Erythema multiforme
  Toxic epidermal nectolysis
- **695.4** Lupus erythematosus

701 Other hypertrophic and atrophic conditions of skin
- **701.0** Circumscribed scleroderma
- **701.4** Keloid scar
- **701.5** Other abnormal granulation tissue

707 Chronic ulcer of skin
- **707.1** Ulcer of lower limbs, except decubitus
- **707.8** Chronic ulcer of other specified sites

709 Other disorders of skin and subcutaneous tissue
- **709.2** Scar conditions and fibrosis of skin
- **709.3** Degenerative skin disorders

941 Burn of face, head, and neck
- **941.3** Full-thickness skin loss [third degree, not otherwise specified]

942 Burn of trunk
- **942.3** Full-thickness skin loss [third degree, not otherwise specified]

943 Burn of upper limb, except wrist and hand
- **943.3** Full-thickness skin loss [third degree, not otherwise specified]

944 Burn of wrist(s) and hand(s)
- **944.3** Full-thickness skin loss [third degree, not otherwise specified]

945 Burn of lower limb(s)
- **945.3** Full-thickness skin loss [third degree, not otherwise specified]

946 Burns of multiple specified sites
- **946.3** Full-thickness skin loss [third degree, not otherwise specified]

948 Burns classified according to extent of body surface involved

949 Burn, unspecified
- **949.3** Full-thickness skin loss [third degree, not otherwise specified]

991 Effects of reduced temperature
- **991.1** Frostbite of hand
- **991.2** Frostbite of foot
- **991.3** Frostbite of other and unspecified sites

997 Complications affecting specified body system, not elsewhere classified
- **997.6** Amputation stump complication

Examination

Examination is a comprehensive screening and specific testing process that leads to a diagnostic classification or, when appropriate, to a referral to another practitioner. Examination is required prior to the initial intervention and is performed for all patients/clients. Through the examination, the physical therapist may identify impairments, functional limitations, disabilities, changes in physical function or overall health status, and needs related to restoration of health and to prevention, wellness, and fitness. The physical therapist synthesizes the examination findings to establish the diagnosis and the prognosis (including the plan of care). The patient/client, family, significant others, and caregivers may provide information during the examination process.

Examination has three components: the patient/client history, the systems review, and tests and measures. The *history* is a systematic gathering of past and current information (often from the patient/client) related to why the patient/client is seeking the services of the physical therapist. The *systems review* is a brief or limited examination of (1) the anatomical and physiological status of the cardiovascular/pulmonary, integumentary, musculoskeletal, and neuromuscular systems and (2) the communication ability, affect, cognition, language, and learning style of the patient/client. *Tests and measures* are the means of gathering data about the patient/client.

The selection of examination procedures and the depth of the examination vary based on patient/client age; severity of the problem; stage of recovery (acute, subacute, chronic); phase of rehabilitation (early, intermediate, late, return to activity); home, work (job/school/play), or community situation; and other relevant factors. *For clinical indications in selecting tests and measures and for listings of tests and measures, tools used to gather data, and the types of data generated by tests and measures, refer to Chapter 2.*

Patient/Client History

The history may include:

General Demographics
- Age
- Sex
- Race/ethnicity
- Primary language
- Education

Social History
- Cultural beliefs and behaviors
- Family and caregiver resources
- Social interactions, social activities, and support systems

Employment/Work (Job/School/Play)
- Current and prior work (job/school/play), community, and leisure actions, tasks, or activities

Growth and Development
- Developmental history
- Hand dominance

Living Environment
- Devices and equipment (eg, assistive, adaptive, orthotic, protective, supportive, prosthetic)
- Living environment and community characteristics
- Projected discharge destinations

General Health Status (Self-Report, Family Report, Caregiver Report)
- General health perception
- Physical function (eg, mobility, sleep patterns, restricted bed days)
- Psychological function (eg, memory, reasoning ability, depression, anxiety)
- Role function (eg, community, leisure, social, work)
- Social function (eg, social activity, social interaction, social support)

Social/Health Habits (Past and Current)
- Behavioral health risks (eg, smoking, drug abuse)
- Level of physical fitness

Family History
- Familial health risks

Medical/Surgical History
- Cardiovascular
- Endocrine/metabolic
- Gastrointestinal
- Genitourinary
- Gynecological
- Integumentary
- Musculoskeletal
- Neuromuscular
- Obstetrical
- Prior hospitalizations, surgeries, and preexisting medical and other health-related conditions
- Psychological
- Pulmonary

Current Condition(s)/Chief Complaint(s)
- Concerns that led patient/client to seek the services of a physical therapist
- Concerns or needs of patient/client who requires the services of a physical therapist
- Current therapeutic interventions
- Mechanisms of injury or disease, including date of onset and course of events
- Onset and pattern of symptoms
- Patient/client, family, significant other, and caregiver expectations and goals for the therapeutic intervention
- Patient/client, family, significant other, and caregiver perceptions of patient's/client's emotional response to the current clinical situation
- Previous occurrence of chief complaint(s)
- Prior therapeutic interventions

Functional Status and Activity Level
- Current and prior functional status in self-care and home management activities, including activities of daily living (ADL) and instrumental activities of daily living (IADL)
- Current and prior functional status in work (job/school/play), community, and leisure actions, tasks, or activities

Medications
- Medications for current condition
- Medications previously taken for current condition
- Medications for other conditions

Other Clinical Tests
- Laboratory and diagnostic tests
- Review of available records (eg, medical, education, surgical)
- Review of other clinical findings (eg, nutrition and hydration)

Systems Review

The systems review may include:

Anatomical and Physiological Status

- Cardiovascular/Pulmonary
  - Blood pressure
  - Edema
  - Heart rate
  - Respiratory rate
- Integumentary
  - Pliability (texture)
  - Presence of scar formation
  - Skin color
  - Skin integrity
- Musculoskeletal
  - Gross range of motion
  - Gross strength
  - Gross symmetry
  - Height
  - Weight
- Neuromuscular
  - Gross coordinated movements (eg, balance, gait, locomotion, transfers, transitions)
  - Motor function (motor control, motor learning)

Communication, Affect, Cognition, Language, and Learning Style

- Ability to make needs known
- Consciousness
- Expected emotional/behavioral responses
- Learning preferences (eg, education needs, learning barriers)
- Orientation (person, place, time)

Tests and Measures

Tests and measures for this pattern may include those that characterize or quantify:

Anthropometric Characteristics

- Body composition (eg, body mass index, impedance measurement, skinfold thickness measurement)
- Body dimensions (eg, girth measurement, length measurement)
- Edema (eg, girth measurement, palpation, scales, volume measurement)

Circulation (Arterial, Venous, and Lymphatic)

- Cardiovascular signs, including heart rate, rhythm, and sounds; pressures and flow; and superficial vascular responses (eg, auscultation, girth measurement, observations, palpation, sphygmomanometry, thermography)
- Cardiovascular symptoms (eg, angina, claudication, and perceived exertion scales)

Cranial and Peripheral Nerve Integrity

- Motor distribution of the cranial nerves (eg, dynamometry, muscle tests, observations)
- Motor distribution of the peripheral nerves (eg, dynamometry, muscle tests, observations, thoracic outlet tests)
- Sensory distribution of the cranial nerves (eg, discrimination tests; tactile tests, including coarse and light touch, cold and heat, pain, pressure, and vibration)
- Sensory distribution of the peripheral nerves (eg, discrimination tests; tactile tests, including coarse and light touch, cold and heat, pain, pressure, and vibration; thoracic outlet tests)

Gait, Locomotion, and Balance

- Gait and locomotion during functional activities with or without the use of assistive, adaptive, orthotic, protective, supportive, or prosthetic devices or equipment (eg, ADL scales, gait indexes, IADL scales, mobility skill profiles, observations, videographic assessments)
- Gait and locomotion with or without the use of assistive, adaptive, orthotic, protective, supportive, or prosthetic devices or equipment (eg, dynamometry, electroneuromyography, footprint analyses, gait indexes, mobility skill profiles, observations, photographic assessments, technology-assisted assessments, videographic assessments, weight-bearing scales, wheelchair mobility tests)
- Safety during gait, locomotion, and balance (eg, confidence scales, diaries, fall scales, functional assessment profiles, logs, reports)

Integumentary Integrity

Associated skin

- Activities, positioning, and postures that produce or relieve trauma to the skin (eg, observations, pressure-sensing maps, scales)
- Assistive, adaptive, orthotic, protective, supportive, or prosthetic devices and equipment that may produce or relieve trauma to the skin (eg, observations, pressure-sensing maps, risk assessment scales)
- Skin characteristics, including blistering, continuity of skin color, dermatitis, hair growth, mobility, nail growth, sensation, temperature, texture, and turgor (eg, observations, palpation, photographic assessments, thermography)

Wound

- Activities, positioning, and postures that aggravate the wound or scar or that produce or relieve trauma (eg, observations, pressure-sensing maps)
- Burn (eg, body charts, planimetry)
- Signs of infection (eg, cultures, observations, palpation)
- Wound characteristics, including bleeding, contraction, depth, drainage, exposed anatomical structures, location, odor, pigment, shape, size, staging and progression, tunneling, and undermining (eg, digital and grid measurement, grading of sores and ulcers, observations, palpation, photographic assessments, wound tracing)
- Wound scar tissue characteristics, including banding, pliability, sensation, and texture (eg, observations, scar-rating scales)

Muscle Performance (Including Strength, Power, and Endurance)

- Muscle strength, power, and endurance during functional activities (eg, ADL scales, functional muscle tests, IADL scales, observations, videographic assessments)

Orthotic, Protective, and Supportive Devices

- Components, alignment, fit, and ability to care for orthotic, protective, and supportive devices and equipment (eg, interviews, logs, observations, pressure-sensing maps, reports)
- Orthotic, protective, and supportive devices and equipment use during functional activities (eg, ADL scales, functional scales, IADL scales, interviews, observations, profiles)
- Remediation of impairments, functional limitations, or disabilities with use of orthotic, protective, and supportive devices and equipment (eg, activity status indexes, ADL scales, aerobic capacity tests, functional performance inventories, health assessment questionnaires, IADL scales, pain scales, play scales, videographic assessments)
- Safety during use of orthotic, protective, and supportive devices and equipment (eg, diaries, fall scales, interviews, logs, observations, reports)

Pain

- Pain, soreness, and nociception (eg, angina scales, analog scales, discrimination tests, pain drawings and maps, provocation tests, verbal and pictorial descriptor tests)
- Pain in specific body parts (eg, pain indexes, pain questionnaires, structural provocation tests)

Prosthetic Requirements

- Components, alignment, fit, and ability to care for the prosthetic device (eg, interviews, logs, observations, pressure-sensing maps, reports)
- Safety during use of the prosthetic device (eg, diaries, fall scales, interviews, logs, observations, reports)

Range of Motion (ROM) (Including Muscle Length)

- Functional ROM (eg, observations, squat testing, toe touch tests)
- Joint active and passive movement (eg, goniometry, inclinometry, observations, photographic assessments, technology-assisted assessments, videographic assessments)
- Muscle length, soft tissue extensibility, and flexibility (eg, contracture tests, goniometry, inclinometry, ligamentous tests, linear measurement, multisegment flexibility tests, palpation)

Sensory Integrity

- Deep sensations (eg, kinesthesiometry, observations, photographic assessments, vibration tests)

Work (Job/School/Play), Community, and Leisure Integration or Reintegration (Including IADL)

- Safety in work (job/school/play), community, and leisure activities and environments (eg, diaries, fall scales, interviews, logs, observations, videographic assessments)

Evaluation, Diagnosis, and Prognosis (Including Plan of Care)

Physical therapists perform *evaluations* (make clinical judgments) based on the data gathered from the history, systems review, and tests and measures. In the evaluation process, physical therapists synthesize the examination data to establish the diagnosis and prognosis (including the plan of care). Factors that influence the complexity of the evaluation include the clinical findings, extent of loss of function, chronicity or severity of the problem, possibility of multisite or multisystem involvement, preexisting condition(s), potential discharge destination, social considerations, physical function, and overall health status.

A *diagnosis* is a label encompassing a cluster of signs and symptoms, syndromes, or categories. It is the result of the systematic diagnostic process, which includes integrating and evaluating the data from the examination. The diagnostic label indicates the primary dysfunction(s) toward which the therapist will direct interventions. The *prognosis* is the determination of the predicted optimal level of improvement in function and the amount of time needed to reach that level and may also include a prediction of levels of improvement that may be reached at various intervals during the course of therapy. During the prognostic process, the physical therapist develops the plan of care. The *plan of care* identifies specific interventions, proposed frequency and duration of the interventions, anticipated goals, expected outcomes, and discharge plans. The plan of care identifies realistic anticipated goals and expected outcomes, taking into consideration the expectations of the patient/client and appropriate others. These anticipated goals and expected outcomes should be measureable and time limited.

The frequency of visits and duration of the episode of care may vary from a short episode with a high intensity of intervention to a longer episode with a diminishing intensity of intervention. Frequency and duration may vary greatly among patients/clients based on a variety of factors that the physical therapist considers throughout the evaluation process, such as anatomical and physiological changes related to growth and development; caregiver consistency or expertise; chronicity or severity of the current condition; living environment; multisite or multisystem involvement; social support; potential discharge destinations; probability of prolonged impairment, functional limitation, or disability; and stability of the condition.

Prognosis

Over the course of 4 to 12 weeks, patient/client will demonstrate optimal wound integumentary integrity and the highest level of functioning in home, work (job/school/play), community, and leisure environments.

Over the course of 6 to 18 months, patient/client will demonstrate optimal scar maturity and the highest level of functioning in home, work (job/school/ play), community, and leisure environments.

During the episode of care, patient/client will achieve (1) the anticipated goals and expected outcomes of the interventions that are described in the plan of care and (2) the global outcomes for patients/ clients who are classified in this pattern.

Expected Range of Number of Visits Per Episode of Care

12 to 50

This range represents the lower and upper limits of the number of physical therapist visits required to achieve anticipated goals and expected outcomes. *It is anticipated that 80% of patients/clients who are classified into this pattern will achieve the anticipated goals and expected outcomes within 12 to 50 visits during a single continuous episode of care.* Frequency of visits and duration of the episode of care should be determined by the physical therapist to maximize effectiveness of care and efficiency of service delivery.

Factors That May Require New Episode of Care or That May Modify Frequency of Visits/ Duration of Episode

- Accessibility and availability of resources
- Adherence to the intervention program
- Age
- Anatomical and physiological changes related to growth and development
- Caregiver consistency or expertise
- Chronicity or severity of the current condition
- Cognitive status
- Comorbitities, complications, or secondary impairments
- Concurrent medical, surgical, and therapeutic interventions
- Decline in functional independence
- Level of impairment
- Level of physical function
- Living environment
- Multisite or multisystem involvement
- Nutritional status
- Overall health status
- Potential discharge destinations
- Premorbid conditions
- Probability of prolonged impairment, functional limitation, or disability
- Psychological and socioeconomic factors
- Psychomotor abilities
- Social support
- Stability of the condition

Intervention

Intervention is the purposeful interaction of the physical therapist with the patient/client and, when appropriate, with other individuals involved in patient/client care, using various physical therapy procedures and techniques to produce changes in the condition consistent with the diagnosis and prognosis. Decisions about interventions are contingent on the timely monitoring of patient/client response and the progress made toward achieving the anticipated goals and expected outcomes.

Communication, coordination, and documentation and patient/client-related instruction are provided for all patients/clients across all settings. Procedural interventions are selected or modified based on the examination data and the evaluation, the diagnosis and the prognosis, and the anticipated goals and expected outcomes for a particular patient/client. *For clinical considerations in selecting interventions, listings of interventions, and listings of anticipated goals and expected outcomes, refer to Chapter 3.*

Coordination, Communication, and Documentation

Coordination, communication, and documentation may include:

Interventions

- Addressing required functions
  - advance directives
  - individualized family service plans (IFSPs) or individualized education plans (IEPs)
  - informed consent
  - mandatory communication and reporting (eg, patient advocacy and abuse reporting)
- Admission and discharge planning
- Case management
- Collaboration and coordination with agencies, including:
  - equipment suppliers
  - home care agencies
  - payer groups
  - schools
  - transportation agencies
- Communication across settings, including:
  - case conferences
  - documentation
  - education plans
- Cost-effective resource utilization
- Data collection, analysis, and reporting
  - outcome data
  - peer review findings
  - record reviews
- Documentation across settings, following APTA's *Guidelines for Physical Therapy Documentation* (Appendix 5), including:
  - changes in impairments, functional limitations, and disabilities
  - changes in interventions
  - elements of patient/client management (examination, evaluation, diagnosis, prognosis, intervention)
  - outcomes of intervention
- Interdisciplinary teamwork
  - case conferences
  - patient care rounds
  - patient/client family meetings
- Referrals to other professionals or resources

Anticipated Goals and Expected Outcomes

- Accountability for services is increased.
- Admission data and discharge planning are completed.
- Advance directives, individualized family service plans (IFSPs) or individualized education plans (IEPs), informed consent, and mandatory communication and reporting (eg, patient advocacy and abuse reporting) are obtained or completed.
- Available resources are maximally utilized.
- Care is coordinated with patient/client, family, significant others, caregivers, and other professionals.
- Case is managed throughout the episode of care.
- Collaboration and coordination occurs with agencies, including equipment suppliers, home care agencies, payer groups, schools, and transportation agencies.
- Communication enhances risk reduction and prevention.
- Communication occurs across settings through case conferences, education plans, and documentation.
- Data are collected, analyzed, and reported, including outcome data, peer review findings, and record reviews.
- Decision making is enhanced regarding health, wellness, and fitness needs.
- Decision making is enhanced regarding patient/client health and the use of health care resources by patient/client, family, significant others, and caregivers.
- Documentation occurs throughout patient/client management and across settings and follows APTA's *Guidelines for Physical Therapy Documentation* (Appendix 5).
- Interdisciplinary collaboration occurs through case conferences, patient care rounds, and patient/client family meetings.
- Patient/client, family, significant other, and caregiver understanding of anticipated goals and expected outcomes is increased.
- Placement needs are determined.
- Referrals are made to other professionals or resources whenever necessary and appropriate.
- Resources are utilized in a cost-effective way.

Patient/Client-Related Instruction

Patient/client-related instruction may include:

Interventions

- Instruction, education and training of patients/clients and caregivers regarding:
  - current condition (pathology/pathophysiology [disease, disorder, or condition], impairments, functional limitations, or disabilities)
  - enhancement of performance
  - health, wellness, and fitness programs
  - plan of care
  - risk factors for pathology/pathophysiology (disease, disorder, or condition), impairments, functional limitations, or disabilities
  - transitions across settings
  - transitions to new roles

Anticipated Goals and Expected Outcomes

- Ability to perform physical actions, tasks, or activities is improved.
- Awareness and use of community resources are improved.
- Behaviors that foster healthy habits, wellness, and prevention are acquired.
- Decision making is enhanced regarding patient/client health and the use of health care resources by patient/client, family, significant others, and caregivers.
- Disability associated with acute or chronic illnesses is reduced.
- Functional independence in activities of daily living (ADL) and instrumental activities of daily living (IADL) is increased.
- Health status is improved.
- Intensity of care is decreased.
- Level of supervision required for task performance is decreased.
- Patient/client, family, significant other, and caregiver knowledge and awareness of the diagnosis, prognosis, interventions, and anticipated goals and expected outcomes are increased.
- Patient/client knowledge of personal and environmental factors associated with the condition is increased.
- Performance levels in self-care, home management, work (job/school/play), community, or leisure actions, tasks, or activities are improved.
- Physical function is improved.
- Risk of recurrence of condition is reduced.
- Risk of secondary impairment is reduced.
- Safety of patient/client, family, significant others, and caregivers is improved.
- Self-management of symptoms is improved.
- Utilization and cost of health care services are decreased.

Procedural Interventions

Procedural interventions for this pattern may include:

Therapeutic Exercise

Interventions

- Balance, coordination, and agility training
  - perceptual training
  - posture awareness training
  - sensory training or retraining
  - task-specific performance training
- Body mechanics and postural stabilization
  - posture awareness training
- Flexibility exercises
  - muscle lengthening
  - range of motion
  - stretching
- Gait and locomotion training
  - perceptual training
  - standardized, programmatic, complementary exercise approaches
- Strength, power, and endurance training for head, neck, limb, pelvic-floor, trunk, and ventilatory muscles
  - active assistive, active, and resistive exercises (including concentric, dynamic/isotonic, eccentric, isokinetic, isometric, and plyometric)
  - task-specific performance training

Anticipated Goals and Expected Outcomes

- Impact on pathology/pathophysiology (disease, disorder, or condition)
  - Joint swelling, inflammation, or restriction is reduced.
  - Nutrient delivery to tissue is increased.
  - Osteogenic effects of exercise are maximized.
  - Pain is decreased.
  - Physiological response to increased oxygen demand is improved.
  - Soft tissue swelling, inflammation, or restriction is reduced.
  - Tissue perfusion and oxygenation are enhanced.
- Impact on impairments
  - Balance is improved.
  - Endurance is increased.
  - Gait, locomotion, and balance are improved.
  - Integumentary integrity is improved.
  - Joint integrity and mobility are improved.
  - Muscle performance (strength, power, and endurance) is increased.
  - Postural control is improved.
  - Range of motion is improved.
  - Sensory awareness is increased.
  - Weight-bearing status is improved.
- Impact on functional limitations
  - Ability to perform physical actions, tasks, or activities related to self-care, home management, work (job/school/play), community, and leisure is improved.
  - Level of supervision required for task performance is decreased.
  - Performance of and independence in activities of daily living (ADL) and instrumental activities of daily living (IADL) with or without devices and equipment are increased.
  - Tolerance of positions and activities is increased.
- Impact on disabilities
  - Ability to assume or resume required self-care, home management, work (job/school/play), community, and leisure roles is improved.
- Risk reduction/prevention
  - Preoperative and postoperative complications are reduced.
  - Risk factors are reduced.
  - Risk of secondary impairment is reduced.
  - Safety is improved.
  - Self-management of symptoms is improved.
- Impact on health, wellness, and fitness
  - Fitness is improved.
  - Health status is improved.
  - Physical capacity is increased.
  - Physical function is improved.
- Impact on societal resources
  - Utilization of physical therapy services is optimized.
  - Utilization of physical therapy services results in efficient use of health care dollars.
- Patient/client satisfaction
  - Access, availability, and services provided are acceptable to patient/client.
  - Administrative management of practice is acceptable to patient/client.
  - Clinical proficiency of physical therapist is acceptable to patient/client.
  - Coordination of care is acceptable to patient/client.
  - Cost of health care services is decreased.
  - Intensity of care is decreased.
  - Interpersonal skills of physical therapist are acceptable to patient/client, family, and significant others.
  - Sense of well-being is improved.
  - Stressors are decreased.

Functional Training in Self-Care and Home Management (Including Activities of Daily Living [ADL] and Instrumental Activities of Daily Living [IADL])

Interventions

- ADL training
  - bathing
  - bed mobility and transfer training
  - developmental activities
  - dressing
  - eating
  - grooming
  - toileting
- IADL training
  - caring for dependents
  - home maintenance
  - household chores
  - shopping
  - structured play for infants and children
  - yard work
- Injury prevention or reduction
  - injury prevention education during self-care and home management
  - injury prevention or reduction with use of devices and equipment
  - safety awareness training during self-care and home management

Anticipated Goals and Expected Outcomes

- Impact on pathology/pathophysiology (disease, disorder, condition)
  - Pain is decreased.
  - Physiological response to increased oxygen demand is improved.
- Impact on impairments
  - Balance is improved.
  - Endurance is increased.
  - Sensory awareness is increased.
  - Weight-bearing status is improved.
- Impact on functional limitations
  - Ability to perform physical actions, tasks, or activities related to self-care and home management is improved.
  - Level of supervision required for task performance is decreased.
  - Performance of and independence in ADL and IADL with or without devices and equipment are increased.
  - Tolerance of positions and activities is increased.
- Impact on disabilities
  - Ability to assume or resume required self-care and home management roles is improved.
- Risk reduction/prevention
  - Risk factors are reduced.
  - Risk of secondary impairments is reduced.
  - Safety is improved.
  - Self-management of symptoms is improved.
- Impact on health, wellness, and fitness
  - Health status is improved.
  - Physical capacity is increased.
  - Physical function is improved.
- Impact on societal resources
  - Utilization of physical therapy services is optimized.
  - Utilization of physical therapy services results in efficient use of health care dollars.
- Patient/client satisfaction
  - Access, availability, and services provided are acceptable to patient/client.
  - Administrative management of practice is acceptable to patient/client.
  - Clinical proficiency of physical therapist is acceptable to patient/client.
  - Coordination of care is acceptable to patient/client.
  - Cost of health care services is decreased.
  - Intensity of care is decreased.
  - Interpersonal skills of physical therapist are acceptable to patient/client, family, and significant others.
  - Sense of well-being is improved.
  - Stressors are decreased.

Functional Training in Work (Job/School/Play), Community, and Leisure Integration or Reintegration (Including Instrumental Activities of Daily Living [IADL], Work Hardening, and Work Conditioning)

Interventions

- IADL training
  - community service training involving instruments
  - school and play activities training including tools and instruments
  - work training with tools
- Injury prevention or reduction
  - injury prevention education during work (job/school/play), community, and leisure integration or reintegration
  - injury prevention or reduction with use of devices and equipment
  - safety awareness training during during work (job/school/play), community, and leisure integration or reintegration

Anticipated Goals and Expected Outcomes

- Impact on pathology/pathophysiology (disease, disorder, or condition)
  - Pain is decreased.
  - Physiological response to increased oxygen demand is improved.
- Impact on impairments
  - Balance is improved.
  - Endurance is increased.
  - Muscle performance (strength, power, and endurance) is increased.
  - Sensory awareness is increased.
  - Weight-bearing status is improved.
- Impact on functional limitations
  - Ability to perform physical actions, tasks, or activities related to work (job/school/play), community, and leisure integration or reintegration is improved.
  - Level of supervision required for task performance is decreased.
  - Performance of and independence in IADL with or without devices and equipment are increased.
  - Tolerance of positions and activities is increased.
- Impact on disabilities
  - Ability to assume or resume required work (job/school/play), community, and leisure roles is improved.
- Risk reduction/prevention
  - Risk factors are reduced.
  - Risk of secondary impairment is reduced.
  - Safety is improved.
  - Self-management of symptoms is improved.
- Impact on health, wellness, and fitness
  - Fitness is improved.
  - Health status is improved.
  - Physical capacity is increased.
  - Physical function is improved.
- Impact on societal resources
  - Costs of work-related injury or disability are reduced.
  - Utilization of physical therapy services is optimized.
  - Utilization of physical therapy services results in efficient use of health care dollars.
- Patient/client satisfaction
  - Access, availability, and services provided are acceptable to patient/client.
  - Administrative management of practice is acceptable to patient/client.
  - Clinical proficiency of physical therapist is acceptable to patient/client.
  - Coordination of care is acceptable to patient/client.
  - Cost of health care services is decreased.
  - Intensity of care is decreased.
  - Interpersonal skills of physical therapist are acceptable to patient/client, family, and significant others.
  - Sense of well-being is improved.
  - Stressors are decreased.

Manual Therapy Techniques (Including Mobilization/Manipulation)

Interventions

- Manual lymphatic drainage
- Massage
  - connective tissue massage
  - therapeutic massage
- Mobilization/manipulation
  - soft tissue

Anticipated Goals and Expected Outcomes

- Impact on pathology/pathophysiology (disease, disorder, or condition)
  - Edema, lymphedema, or effusion is reduced.
  - Joint swelling, inflammation, or restriction is reduced.
  - Pain is decreased.
  - Soft tissue swelling, inflammation, or restriction is reduced.
- Impact on impairments
  - Integumentary integrity is improved.
  - Joint integrity and mobility are improved.
  - Range of motion is improved.
  - Relaxation is increased.
  - Sensory awareness is increased.
- Impact on functional limitations
  - Ability to perform movement tasks is improved.
  - Ability to perform physical actions, tasks, or activities related to self-care, home management, work (job/school/play), community, and leisure is improved.
  - Tolerance of positions and activities is increased.
- Impact on disabilities
  - Ability to assume or resume required self-care, home management, work (job/school/play), community, and leisure roles is improved.
- Risk reduction/prevention
  - Risk factors are reduced.
  - Risk of secondary impairment is reduced.
  - Self-management of symptoms is improved.
- Impact on health, wellness, and fitness
  - Physical capacity is increased.
  - Physical function is improved.
- Impact on societal resources
  - Utilization of physical therapy services is optimized.
  - Utilization of physical therapy services results in efficient use of health care dollars.
- Patient/client satisfaction
  - Access, availability, and services provided are acceptable to patient/client.
  - Administrative management of practice is acceptable to patient/client.
  - Clinical proficiency of physical therapist is acceptable to patient/client.
  - Coordination of care is acceptable to patient/client.
  - Cost of health care services is decreased.
  - Intensity of care is decreased.
  - Interpersonal skills of physical therapist are acceptable to patient/client, family, and significant others.
  - Sense of well-being is improved.
  - Stressors are decreased.

Procedural Interventions continued

Prescription, Application, and, as Appropriate, Fabrication of Devices and Equipment (Assistive, Adaptive, Orthotic, Protective, Supportive, and Prosthetic)

Interventions

- Adaptive devices
  - environmental controls
  - hospital beds
  - raised toilet seats
  - seating systems
- Assistive devices
  - canes
  - crutches
  - long-handled reachers
  - power devices
  - static and dynamic splints
  - walkers
  - wheelchairs
- Orthotic devices
  - braces
  - casts
  - shoe inserts
  - splints
- Prosthetic devices (lower-extremity and upper-extremity)
- Protective devices
  - braces
  - cushions
  - protective taping
- Supportive devices
  - compression garments
  - elastic wraps
  - neck collars
  - serial casts
  - slings
  - supplemental oxygen
  - supportive taping

Anticipated Goals and Expected Outcomes

- Impact on pathology/pathophysiology (disease, disorder, or condition)
  - Edema, lymphedema, or effusion is reduced.
  - Joint swelling, inflammation, or restriction is reduced.
  - Pain is decreased.
  - Physiological response to increased oxygen demand is improved.
  - Soft tissue swelling, inflammation, or restriction is reduced.
- Impact on impairments
  - Balance is improved.
  - Energy expenditure per unit of work is decreased.
  - Gait, locomotion, and balance are improved.
  - Integumentary integrity is improved.
  - Joint stability is improved.
  - Optimal joint alignment is achieved.
  - Optimal loading on a body part is achieved.
  - Quality and quantity of movement between and across body segments are improved.
  - Weight-bearing status is improved.
- Impact on functional limitations
  - Ability to perform physical actions, tasks, or activities related to self-care, home management, work (job/school/play), community, and leisure is improved.
  - Level of supervision required for task performance is decreased.
  - Performance of and independence in activities of daily living (ADL) and instrumental activities of daily living (IADL) with or without devices and equipment are increased.
  - Tolerance of positions and activities is improved.
- Impact on disabilities
  - Ability to assume or resume required self-care, home management, work (job/school/play), community, and leisure roles is improved.
- Risk reduction/prevention
  - Pressure on body tissues is reduced.
  - Protection of body parts is increased.
  - Risk factors are reduced.
  - Risk of secondary impairment is reduced.
  - Safety is improved.
  - Self-management of symptoms is improved.
- Impact on health, wellness, and fitness
  - Health status is improved.
  - Physical capacity is increased.
  - Physical function is improved.
- Impact on societal resources
  - Utilization of physical therapy services is optimized.
  - Utilization of physical therapy services results in efficient use of health care dollars.
- Patient/client satisfaction
  - Access, availability, and services provided are acceptable to patient/client.
  - Administrative management of practice is acceptable to patient/client.
  - Clinical proficiency of physical therapist is acceptable to patient/client.
  - Coordination of care is acceptable to patient/client.
  - Cost of health care services is decreased.
  - Intensity of care is decreased.
  - Interpersonal skills of physical therapist are acceptable to patient/client, family, and significant others.
  - Sense of well-being is improved.
  - Stressors are decreased.

Integumentary Repair and Protection Techniques

Interventions

- Debridement—nonselective
  - enzymatic debridement
  - wet dressings
  - wet-to-dry dressings
  - wet-to-moist dressings
- Debridement—selective
  - debridement with other agents (eg, autolysis)
  - enzymatic debridement
  - sharp debridement
- Dressings
  - hydrogels
  - vacuum-assisted closure
  - wound coverings
- Oxygen therapy
  - supplemental
  - topical
- Topical agents
  - cleansers
  - creams
  - moisturizers
  - ointments
  - sealants

Anticipated Goals and Expected Outcomes

- Impact on pathology/pathophysiology (disease, disorder, or condition)
  - Debridement of nonviable tissue is achieved.
  - Pain is decreased.
  - Soft tissue or wound healing is enhanced.
  - Tissue perfusion and oxygenation are enhanced.
  - Wound size is reduced.
- Impact on impairments
  - Integumentary integrity is improved.
  - Weight-bearing status is improved.
- Impact on functional limitations
  - Ability to perform physical actions, tasks, or activities related to self-care, home management, work (job/ school/ play), community and leisure is improved.
  - Level of supervision required for task performance is decreased.
  - Performance of and independence in activities of daily living (ADL) and instrumental activities of daily living (IADL) with or without devices and equipment are increased.
  - Tolerance of positions and activities is increased.
- Impact on disabilities
  - Ability to assume or resume required self-care, home management, work (job/school/play), community, and leisure roles is improved.
- Risk reduction/prevention
  - Preoperative and postoperative complications are reduced.
  - Risk factors are reduced.
  - Risk of secondary impairment is reduced.
  - Self-management of symptoms is improved.
- Impact on health, wellness, and fitness
  - Health status is improved.
  - Physical function is improved.
- Impact on societal resources
  - Utilization of physical therapy services is optimized.
  - Utilization of physical therapy services results in efficient use of health care dollars.
- Patient/client satisfaction
  - Access, availability, and services provided are acceptable to patient/client.
  - Administrative management of practice is acceptable to patient/client.
  - Clinical proficiency of physical therapist is acceptable to patient/client.
  - Coordination of care is acceptable to patient/client.
  - Cost of health care services is decreased.
  - Intensity of care is decreased.
  - Interpersonal skills of physical therapist are acceptable to patient/client, family, and significant others.
  - Sense of well-being is improved.
  - Stressors are decreased.

Electrotherapeutic Modalities

Interventions

- Electrical stimulation
  - electrical muscle stimulation (EMS)
  - high voltage pulsed current (HVPC)
  - transcutaneous electrical nerve stimulation (TENS)

Anticipated Goals and Expected Outcomes

- Impact on pathology/pathophysiology (disease, disorder, or condition)
  - Edema, lymphedema, or effusion is reduced.
  - Joint swelling, inflammation, or restriction is reduced.
  - Nutrient delivery to tissue is increased.
  - Pain is decreased.
  - Soft tissue or wound healing is enhanced.
  - Soft tissue swelling, inflammation, or restriction is reduced.
  - Tissue perfusion and oxygenation are enhanced.
- Impact on impairments
  - Integumentary integrity is improved.
  - Sensory awareness is increased.
- Impact on functional limitations
  - Ability to perform physical actions, tasks, or activities related to self-care, home management, work (job/school/play), community, and leisure is improved.
  - Level of supervision required for task performance is decreased.
  - Performance of and independence in activities of daily living (ADL) and instrumental activities of daily living (IADL) with or without devices and equipment are increased.
  - Tolerance of positions and activities is increased.
- Impact on disabilities
  - Ability to assume or resume required self-care, home management, work (job/school/play), community, and leisure roles is improved.
- Risk reduction/prevention
  - Complications of immobility are reduced.
  - Preoperative and postoperative complications are reduced.
  - Risk factors are reduced.
  - Risk of secondary impairment is reduced.
  - Self-management of symptoms is improved.
- Impact on health, wellness, and fitness
  - Physical capacity is increased.
  - Physical function is improved.
- Impact on societal resources
  - Utilization of physical therapy services is optimized.
  - Utilization of physical therapy services results in efficient use of health care dollars.
- Patient/client satisfaction
  - Access, availability, and services provided are acceptable to patient/client.
  - Administrative management of practice is acceptable to patient/client.
  - Clinical proficiency of physical therapist is acceptable to patient/client.
  - Coordination of care is acceptable to patient/client.
  - Interpersonal skills of physical therapist are acceptable to patient/client, family, and significant others.
  - Sense of well-being is improved.
  - Stressors are decreased.

Physical Agents and Mechanical Modalities

Interventions

Physical agents may include:

- Hydrotherapy
  - pulsatile lavage
  - whirlpool tanks
- Light agents
  - laser
  - ultraviolet
- Sound agents
  - phonophoresis
  - ultrasound
- Thermotherapy
  - diathermy
  - dry heat
  - hot packs
  - paraffin baths

Mechanical modalities may include:

- Compression therapies
  - compression bandaging
  - compression garments
  - taping
  - total contact casting
  - vasopneumatic compression devices
- Gravity-assisted compression devices
  - tilt table
- Mechanical motion devices
  - continuous passive motion (CPM)

Anticipated Goals and Expected Outcomes

- Impact on pathology/pathophysiology (disease, disorder, or condition)
  - Debridement of nonviable tissue is achieved.
  - Edema, lymphedema, or effusion is reduced.
  - Joint swelling, inflammation, or restriction is reduced.
  - Nutrient delivery to tissue is increased.
  - Pain is decreased.
  - Soft tissue swelling, inflammation, or restriction is reduced.
  - Tissue perfusion and oxygenation are enhanced.
- Impact on impairments
  - Integumentary integrity is improved.
  - Range of motion is improved.
  - Weight-bearing status is improved.
- Impact on functional limitations
  - Ability to perform physical actions, tasks, or activities related to self-care, home management, work (job/school/play), community, and leisure is improved.
  - Performance of and independence in activities of daily living (ADL) and instrumental activities of daily living (IADL) with or without devices and equipment are increased.
  - Tolerance of positions and activities is increased.
- Impact on disabilities
  - Ability to assume or resume required self-care, home management, work (job/school/play), community, and leisure roles is improved.
- Risk reduction/prevention
  - Complications of soft tissue and circulatory disorders are decreased.
  - Risk of secondary impairment is reduced.
  - Self-management of symptoms is improved.
  - Stresses precipitating injury are decreased.
- Impact on health, wellness, and fitness
  - Physical function is improved.
- Impact on societal resources
  - Utilization of physical therapy services is optimized.
- Patient/client satisfaction
  - Access, availability, and services provided are acceptable to patient/client.
  - Administrative management of practice is acceptable to patient/client.
  - Clinical proficiency of physical therapist is acceptable to patient/client.
  - Coordination of care is acceptable to patient/client.
  - Interpersonal skills of physical therapist are acceptable to patient/client, family, and significant others.
  - Sense of well-being is improved.
  - Stressors are decreased.

Reexamination

Reexamination is the process of performing selected tests and measures after the initial examination to evaluate progress and to modify or redirect interventions. Reexamination may be indicated more than once during a single episode of care. It also may be performed over the course of a disease, disorder, or condition, which for some patients/clients may be over the life span. Indications for reexamination include new clinical findings or failure to respond to physical therapy interventions.

Global Outcomes for Patients/Clients in This Pattern

Throughout the entire episode of care, the physical therapist determines the anticipated goals and expected outcomes for each intervention. These anticipated goals and expected outcomes are delineated in shaded boxes that accompany the lists of interventions in each preferred practice pattern. As the patient/client reaches the termination of physical therapy services and the end of the episode of care, the physical therapist measures the global outcomes of the physical therapy services by characterizing or quantifying the impact of the physical therapy interventions in the following domains:

- Pathology/pathophysiology (disease, disorder, or condition)
- Impairments
- Functional limitations
- Disabilities
- Risk reduction/prevention
- Health, wellness, and fitness
- Societal resources
- Patient/client satisfaction

In some instances, a particular anticipated goal or expected outcome is thoroughly achieved through implementation of a single form of intervention. More commonly, however, the anticipated goals and expected outcomes are achieved as a result of the combined effects of several forms of interventions, leading to enhancement of both health status and health-related quality of life.

Criteria for Termination of Physical Therapy Services

Discharge is the process of ending physical therapy services that have been provided during a single episode of care. It occurs when the anticipated goals and expected outcomes have been achieved. Discharge does *not* occur with a *transfer* (defined as the time when a patient is moved from one site to another site within the same setting or across settings during a single episode of care). Although there may be facility-specific or payer-specific requirements for documentation regarding the conclusion of physical therapy services, *discharge occurs based on the physical therapist's analysis of the achievement of anticipated goals and expected outcomes.*

Discontinuation is the process of ending physical therapy services that have been provided during a single episode of care when (1) the patient/client, caregiver, or legal guardian declines to continue intervention; (2) the patient/client is unable to continue to progress toward outcomes because of medical or psychosocial complications or because financial/insurance resources have been expended; or (3) the physical therapist determines that the patient/client will no longer benefit from physical therapy. When physical therapy services are terminated prior to achievement of anticipated goals and expected outcomes, patient/client status and the rationale for termination are documented.

For patients/clients who require multiple episodes of care, periodic follow-up is needed over the life span to ensure safety and effective adaptation following changes in physical status, caregivers, environment, or task demands. In consultation with appropriate individuals, and in consideration of the outcomes, the physical therapist plans for discharge or discontinuation and provides for appropriate follow-up or referral.

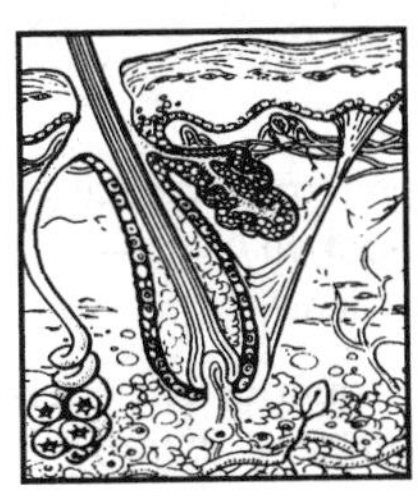

Impaired Integumentary Integrity Associated With Skin Involvement Extending Into Fascia, Muscle, or Bone and Scar Formation

This preferred practice pattern describes the generally accepted elements of patient/client management that physical therapists provide for patients/clients who are classified in this pattern. The pattern title reflects the diagnosis made by the physical therapist. APTA emphasizes that preferred practice patterns are the boundaries within which a physical therapist may select any of a number of clinical alternatives, based on consideration of a wide variety of factors, such as individual patient/client needs; the profession's code of ethics and standards of practice; and patient/client age, culture, gender roles, race, sex, sexual orientation, and socioeconomic status.

Patient/Client Diagnostic Classification

Patients/clients will be classified into this pattern—for impaired integumentary integrity associated with skin involvement extending into fascia, muscle, or bone and scar formation—as a result of the physical therapist's evaluation of the examination data. The findings from the examination (history, systems review, and tests and measures) may indicate the presence or risk of pathology/pathophysiology, impairments, functional limitations, or disabilities or the need for health, wellness, or fitness programs. The physical therapist integrates, synthesizes, and interprets the data to determine the diagnostic classification.

Inclusion

The following examples of examination findings may support the inclusion of patients/clients in this pattern:

Risk Factors or Consequences of Pathology/Pathophysiology (Disease, Disorder, or Condition)

- Abscess
- Burns
- Chronic surgical wound
- Electrical burns
- Frostbite
- Hematoma
- Kaposi's sarcoma
- Lymphostatic ulcer
- Necrotizing fasciitis
- Neoplasm
- Neuropathic ulcers (grades 3, 4, 5)
- Pressure ulcers (stage 4)
- Recent amputation
- Subcutaneous arterial ulcer
- Surgical wounds
- Vascular ulcers
  - Diabetic
  - Venous

Impairments, Functional Limitations, or Disabilities

- Impaired joint integrity
- Impaired sensation
- Impaired skin
- Impairments associated with abnormal fluid distribution
- Muscle weakness
- Decreased range of motion

Note:

Some risk factors or consequences of pathology/pathophysiology—such as *paralysis*—may be severe and complex; *however, they do not necessarily exclude patients/clients from this pattern.* Severe and complex risk factors or consequences may require modification of the frequency of visits and duration of care. (See "Evaluation, Diagnosis, and Prognosis," page 662.)

Exclusion or Multiple-Pattern Classification

The following examples of examination findings may support exclusion from this pattern or classification into additional patterns. Depending on the level of severity or complexity of the examination findings, the physical therapist may determine that the patient/client would be more appropriately managed through (1) classification in an entirely different pattern or (2) classification in both this and another pattern.

Findings That May Require Classification in a Different Pattern

- Impairments associated with lymphedema

Findings That May Require Classification in Additional Patterns

- Fracture
- Impairments associated with diabetes

ICD-9-CM Codes

The listing below contains the current (as of press time) and most typical 3- and 4-digit ICD-9-CM codes related to this preferred practice pattern. Because patient/client diagnostic classification is based on impairments, functional limitations, and disabilities—not on codes—patients/clients may be classified into the pattern even though the codes listed with the pattern may not apply to those clients.

This listing is intended for general information only and should not be used for coding purposes. The codes should be confirmed by referring to the World Health Organization's *International Classification of Diseases, 9th Revision, Clinical Modification (ICD-9-CM 2001)*, Volumes 1 and 3 (Chicago, Ill: American Medical Association; 2000) or subsequent revisions or by referring to other ICD-9-CM coding manuals that contain exclusion notes and instructions regarding fifth-digit requirements.

017 Tuberculosis of other organs
- **017.0** Skin and subcutaneous cellular tissue

036 Meningococcal infection
- **036.2** Meningococcemia

171 Malignant neoplasm of connective and other soft tissue
- **171.2** Upper limb, including shoulder
- **171.3** Lower limb, including hip
- **171.5** Abdomen
- **171.6** Pelvis
- **171.8** Other specified sites of connective and other soft tissue

172 Malignant melanoma of skin
- **172.5** Trunk, except scrotum
- **172.6** Upper limb, including shoulder
- **172.7** Lower limb, including hip
- **172.8** Other specified sites of skin

173 Other malignant neoplasm of skin
- **173.5** Skin of trunk, except scrotum
- **173.6** Skin of upper limb, including shoulder
- **173.7** Skin of lower limb, including hip
- **173.8** Other specified sites of skin

176 Kaposi's sarcoma
- **176.0** Skin
- **176.1** Soft tissue

215 Other benign neoplasm of connective and other soft tissue
- **215.2** Upper limb, including shoulder
- **215.3** Lower limb, including hip
- **215.6** Pelvis

239 Neoplasms of unspecified nature
- **239.2** Bone, soft tissue, and skin

263 Other and unspecified protein-calorie malnutrition

269 Other nutritional deficiencies

440 Atherosclerosis
- **440.2** Of native arteries of the extremities
  - **440.24** Atherosclerosis of the extremities with gangrene

443 Other peripheral vascular disease
- **443.1** Thromboangiitis obliterans [Buerger's disease]

454 Varicose veins of lower extremities
- **454.0** With ulcer
- **454.2** With ulcer and inflammation

459 Other disorders of circulatory system

674 Other and unspecified complications of the puerperium, not elsewhere classified
- **674.1** Disruption of cesarean wound

680 Carbuncle and furuncle
- **680.2** Trunk
- **680.3** Upper arm and forearm
- **680.4** Hand
- **680.5** Buttock
- **680.6** Leg, except foot
- **680.7** Foot

681 Cellulitis and abscess of finger and toe
- **681.0** Finger

686 Other local infections of skin and subcutaneous tissue
- **686.8** Other specified local infections of skin and subcutaneous tissue

707 Chronic ulcer of skin
- **707.0** Decubitus ulcer
- **707.1** Ulcer of lower limbs, except decubitus
- **707.8** Chronic ulcer of other specified sites

710 Diffuse diseases of connective tissue
- **710.0** Systemic lupus erythematosus
- **710.1** Systemic sclerosis
- **710.3** Dermatomyositis

728 Disorders of muscle, ligament, and fascia
- **728.8** Other disorders of muscle, ligament, and fascia
  - **728.86** Necrotizing fasciitis

880 Open wound of shoulder and upper arm

881 Open wound of elbow, forearm, and wrist

882 Open wound of hand except finger(s) alone

883 Open wound of finger(s)

884 Multiple and unspecified open wound of upper limb

885 Traumatic amputation of thumb (complete) (partial)

886 Traumatic amputation of other finger(s) (complete) (partial)

887 Traumatic amputation of arm and hand (complete) (partial)

890 Open wound of hip and thigh

891 Open wound of knee, leg [except thigh], and ankle

892 Open wound of foot except toe(s) alone

893 Open wound of toe(s)

894 Multiple and unspecified open wound of lower limb

895 Traumatic amputation of toe(s) (complete) (partial)

896 Traumatic amputation of foot (complete) (partial)

897 Traumatic amputation of leg(s) (complete) (partial)

927 Crushing injury of upper limb

928 Crushing injury of lower limb

929 Crushing injury of multiple and unspecified sites

941 Burn of face, head, and neck

- **941.4** Deep necrosis of underlying tissues [deep third degree] without mention of loss of a body part
- **941.5** Deep necrosis of underlying tissues [deep third degree] with loss of a body part

942 Burn of trunk

- **942.4** Deep necrosis of underlying tissues [deep third degree] without mention of loss of a body part
- **942.5** Deep necrosis of underlying tissues [deep third degree] with loss of a body part

943 Burn of upper limb, except wrist and hand

- **943.4** Deep necrosis of underlying tissues [deep third degree] without mention of loss of a body part
- **943.5** Deep necrosis of underlying tissues [deep third degree] with loss of a body part

944 Burn of wrist(s) and hand(s)

- **944.4** Deep necrosis of underlying tissues [deep third degree] without mention of loss of a body part
- **944.5** Deep necrosis of underlying tissues [deep third degree] with loss of a body part

946 Burns of multiple specified sites

- **946.4** Deep necrosis of underlying tissues [deep third degree] without mention of loss of a body part
- **946.5** Deep necrosis of underlying tissues [deep third degree] with loss of a body part

948 Burns classified according to extent of body surface involved

991 Effects of reduced temperature

- **991.1** Frostbite of hand
- **991.2** Frostbite of foot
- **991.3** Frostbite of other and unspecified sites
- **991.4** Immersion foot
- **991.5** Chilblains

997 Complications affecting specified body system, not elsewhere classified

- **997.6** Amputation stump complication

998 Other complications of procedures, not elsewhere classified

- **998.3** Disruption of operation wound

Examination

Examination is a comprehensive screening and specific testing process that leads to a diagnostic classification or, when appropriate, to a referral to another practitioner. Examination is required prior to the initial intervention and is performed for all patients/clients. Through the examination, the physical therapist may identify impairments, functional limitations, disabilities, changes in physical function or overall health status, and needs related to restoration of health and to prevention, wellness, and fitness. The physical therapist synthesizes the examination findings to establish the diagnosis and the prognosis (including the plan of care). The patient/client, family, significant others, and caregivers may provide information during the examination process.

Examination has three components: the patient/client history, the systems review, and tests and measures. The *history* is a systematic gathering of past and current information (often from the patient/client) related to why the patient/client is seeking the services of the physical therapist. The *systems review* is a brief or limited examination of (1) the anatomical and physiological status of the cardiovascular/pulmonary, integumentary, musculoskeletal, and neuromuscular systems and (2) the communication ability, affect, cognition, language, and learning style of the patient/client. *Tests and measures* are the means of gathering data about the patient/client.

The selection of examination procedures and the depth of the examination vary based on patient/client age; severity of the problem; stage of recovery (acute, subacute, chronic); phase of rehabilitation (early, intermediate, late, return to activity); home, work (job/school/play), or community situation; and other relevant factors. *For clinical indications in selecting tests and measures and for listings of tests and measures, tools used to gather data, and the types of data generated by tests and measures, refer to Chapter 2.*

Patient/Client History

The history may include:

General Demographics
- Age
- Sex
- Race/ethnicity
- Primary language
- Education

Social History
- Cultural beliefs and behaviors
- Family and caregiver resources
- Social interactions, social activities, and support systems

Employment/Work (Job/School/Play)
- Current and prior work (job/school/play), community, and leisure actions, tasks, or activities

Growth and Development
- Developmental history
- Hand dominance

Living Environment
- Devices and equipment (eg, assistive, adaptive, orthotic, protective, supportive, prosthetic)
- Living environment and community characteristics
- Projected discharge destinations

General Health Status (Self-Report, Family Report, Caregiver Report)
- General health perception
- Physical function (eg, mobility, sleep patterns, restricted bed days)
- Psychological function (eg, memory, reasoning ability, depression, anxiety)
- Role function (eg, community, leisure, social, work)
- Social function (eg, social activity, social interaction, social support)

Social/Health Habits (Past and Current)
- Behavioral health risks (eg, smoking, drug abuse)
- Level of physical fitness

Family History
- Familial health risks

Medical/Surgical History
- Cardiovascular
- Endocrine/metabolic
- Gastrointestinal
- Genitourinary
- Gynecological
- Integumentary
- Musculoskeletal
- Neuromuscular
- Obstetrical
- Prior hospitalizations, surgeries, and preexisting medical and other health-related conditions
- Psychological
- Pulmonary

Current Condition(s)/Chief Complaint(s)
- Concerns that led patient/client to seek the services of a physical therapist
- Concerns or needs of patient/client who requires the services of a physical therapist
- Current therapeutic interventions
- Mechanisms of injury or disease, including date of onset and course of events
- Onset and pattern of symptoms
- Patient/client, family, significant other, and caregiver expectations and goals for the therapeutic intervention
- Patient/client, family, significant other, and caregiver perceptions of patient's/client's emotional response to the current clinical situation
- Previous occurrence of chief complaint(s)
- Prior therapeutic interventions

Functional Status and Activity Level
- Current and prior functional status in self-care and home management activities, including activities of daily living (ADL) and instrumental activities of daily living (IADL)
- Current and prior functional status in work (job/school/play), community, and leisure actions, tasks, or activities

Medications
- Medications for current condition
- Medications previously taken for current condition
- Medications for other conditions

Other Clinical Tests
- Laboratory and diagnostic tests
- Review of available records (eg, medical, education, surgical)
- Review of other clinical findings (eg, nutrition and hydration)

Systems Review

The systems review may include:

Anatomical and Physiological Status

- Cardiovascular/Pulmonary
  - Blood pressure
  - Edema
  - Heart rate
  - Respiratory rate
- Integumentary
  - Pliability (texture)
  - Presence of scar formation
  - Skin color
  - Skin integrity
- Musculoskeletal
  - Gross range of motion
  - Gross strength
  - Gross symmetry
  - Height
  - Weight
- Neuromuscular
  - Gross coordinated movements (eg, balance, gait, locomotion, transfers, transitions)
  - Motor function (motor control, motor learning)

Communication, Affect, Cognition, Language, and Learning Style

- Ability to make needs known
- Consciousness
- Expected emotional/behavioral responses
- Learning preferences (eg, education needs, learning barriers)
- Orientation (person, place, time)

Tests and Measures

Tests and measures for this pattern may include those that characterize or quantify:

Anthropometric Characteristics

- Body composition (eg, body mass index, impedance measurement, skinfold thickness measurement)
- Body dimensions (eg, girth measurement, length measurement)
- Edema (eg, girth measurement, palpation, scales, volume measurement)

Arousal, Attention, and Cognition

- Arousal and attention (eg, adaptability tests, arousal and awareness scales, indexes, profiles, questionnaires)
- Motivation (eg, adaptive behavior scales)
- Recall, including memory and retention (eg, assessment scales, interviews, questionnaires)

Circulation (Arterial, Venous, and Lymphatic)

- Cardiovascular signs, including heart rate, rhythm, and sounds; pressures and flow; and superficial vascular responses (eg, auscultation, electrocardiography, girth measurement, observations, palpation, sphygmomanometry, thermography)
- Cardiovascular symptoms (eg, angina, claudication, and perceived exertion scales)
- Physiological responses to position change, including autonomic responses, central and peripheral pressures, heart rate and rhythm, respiratory rate and rhythm, ventilatory pattern (eg, auscultation, electrocardiography, observations, palpation, sphygmomanometry)

Cranial and Peripheral Nerve Integrity

- Motor distribution of the cranial nerves (eg, dynamometry, muscle tests, observations)
- Motor distribution of the peripheral nerves (eg, dynamometry, muscle tests, observations, thoracic outlet tests)
- Sensory distribution of the cranial nerves (eg, discrimination tests; tactile tests, including coarse and light touch, cold and heat, pain, pressure, and vibration)
- Sensory distribution of the peripheral nerves (eg, discrimination tests; tactile tests, including coarse and light touch, cold and heat, pain, pressure, and vibration; thoracic outlet tests)

Gait, Locomotion, and Balance

- Gait and locomotion during functional activities with or without the use of assistive, adaptive, orthotic, protective, supportive, or prosthetic devices or equipment (eg, ADL scales, gait indexes, IADL scales, mobility skill profiles, observations, videographic assessments)
- Gait and locomotion with or without the use of assistive, adaptive, orthotic, protective, supportive, or prosthetic devices or equipment (eg, dynamometry, electroneuromyography, footprint analyses, gait indexes, mobility skill profiles, observations, photographic assessments, technology-assisted assessments, videographic assessments, weight-bearing scales, wheelchair mobility tests)
- Safety during gait, locomotion, and balance (eg, confidence scales, diaries, fall scales, functional assessment profiles, logs, reports)

Integumentary Integrity

Associated skin

- Activities, positioning, and postures that produce or relieve trauma to the skin (eg, observations, pressure-sensing maps, scales)
- Assistive, adaptive, orthotic, protective, supportive, or prosthetic devices and equipment that may produce or relieve trauma to the skin (eg, observations, pressure-sensing maps, risk assessment scales)
- Skin characteristics, including blistering, continuity of skin color, dermatitis, hair growth, mobility, nail growth, sensation, temperature, texture, and turgor (eg, observations, palpation, photographic assessments, thermography)

Wound

- Activities, positioning, and postures that aggravate the wound or scar or that produce or relieve trauma (eg, observations, pressure-sensing maps)
- Burn (eg, body charting, planimetry)
- Signs of infection (eg, cultures, observations, palpation)
- Wound characteristics, including bleeding, contraction, depth, drainage, exposed anatomical structures, location, odor, pigment, shape, size, staging and progression, tunneling, and undermining (eg, digital and grid measurement, grading of sores and ulcers, observations, palpation, photographic assessments, wound tracing)
- Wound scar tissue characteristics, including banding, pliability, sensation, and texture (eg, observations, scar-rating scales)

Muscle Performance (Including Strength, Power, and Endurance)

- Muscle strength, power, and endurance during functional activities (eg, ADL scales, functional muscle tests, IADL scales, observations, videographic assessments)

Orthotic, Protective, and Supportive Devices

- Components, alignment, fit, and ability to care for orthotic, protective, and supportive devices and equipment (eg, interviews, logs, observations, pressure-sensing maps, reports)
- Orthotic, protective, and supportive devices and equipment use during functional activities (eg, ADL scales, functional scales, IADL scales, interviews, observations, profiles)
- Remediation of impairments, functional limitations, or disabilities with use of orthotic, protective, and supportive devices and equipment (eg, activity status indexes, ADL scales, aerobic capacity tests, functional performance inventories, health assessment questionnaires, IADL scales, pain scales, play scales, videographic assessments)
- Safety during use of orthotic, protective, and supportive devices and equipment (eg, diaries, fall scales, interviews, logs, observations, reports)

Pain

- Pain, soreness, and nociception (eg, analog scales, discrimination tests, pain drawings and maps, provocation tests, verbal and pictorial descriptor tests)
- Pain in specific body parts (eg, pain indexes, pain questionnaires, structural provocation tests)

Posture

- Postural alignment and position (static and dynamic), including symmetry and deviation from midline (eg, grid measurements, observations, photographic assessments, technology-assisted assessments, videographic assessments)
- Specific body parts (eg, angle assessment, forward-bending test, goniometry, observations, palpation, positional tests)

Prosthetic Requirements

- Components, alignment, fit, and ability to care for the prosthetic device (eg, interviews, logs, observations, pressure-sensing maps, reports)
- Safety during use of the prosthetic device (eg, diaries, fall scales, interviews, logs, observations, reports)

Range of Motion (ROM) (Including Muscle Length)

- Functional ROM (eg, observations, squat testing, toe touch tests)
- Joint active and passive movement (eg, goniometry, inclinometry, observations, photographic assessments, technology-assisted assessments, videographic assessments)
- Muscle length, soft tissue extensibility, and flexibility (eg, contracture tests, goniometry, inclinometry, ligamentous tests, linear measurement, multisegment flexibility tests, palpation)

Self-Care and Home Management (Including ADL and IADL)

- Safety in self-care and home management activities and environments (eg, diaries, fall scales, interviews, logs, observations, reports, videographic assessments)

Sensory Integrity

- Combined/cortical sensations (eg, stereognosis tests, tactile discrimination tests)
- Deep sensations (eg, kinesthesiometry, observations, photographic assessments, vibration tests)

Work (Job/School/Play), Community, and Leisure Integration or Reintegration (Including IADL)

- Safety in work (job/school/play), community, and leisure activities and environments (eg, diaries, fall scales, interviews, logs, observations, videographic assessments)

Evaluation, Diagnosis, and Prognosis (Including Plan of Care)

Physical therapists perform *evaluations* (make clinical judgments) based on the data gathered from the history, systems review, and tests and measures. In the evaluation process, physical therapists synthesize the examination data to establish the diagnosis and prognosis (including the plan of care). Factors that influence the complexity of the evaluation include the clinical findings, extent of loss of function, chronicity or severity of the problem, possibility of multisite or multisystem involvement, preexisting condition(s), potential discharge destination, social considerations, physical function, and overall health status.

A *diagnosis* is a label encompassing a cluster of signs and symptoms, syndromes, or categories. It is the result of the systematic diagnostic process, which includes integrating and evaluating the data from the examination. The diagnostic label indicates the primary dysfunction(s) toward which the therapist will direct interventions. The *prognosis* is the determination of the predicted optimal level of improvement in function and the amount of time needed to reach that level and may also include a prediction of levels of improvement that may be reached at various intervals during the course of therapy. During the prognostic process, the physical therapist develops the plan of care. The *plan of care* identifies specific interventions, proposed frequency and duration of the interventions, anticipated goals, expected outcomes, and discharge plans. The plan of care identifies realistic anticipated goals and expected outcomes, taking into consideration the expectations of the patient/client and appropriate others. These anticipated goals and expected outcomes should be measureable and time limited.

The frequency of visits and duration of the episode of care may vary from a short episode with a high intensity of intervention to a longer episode with a diminishing intensity of intervention. Frequency and duration may vary greatly among patients/clients based on a variety of factors that the physical therapist considers throughout the evaluation process, such as anatomical and physiological changes related to growth and development; caregiver consistency or expertise; chronicity or severity of the current condition; living environment; multisite or multisystem involvement; social support; potential discharge destinations; probability of prolonged impairment, functional limitation, or disability; and stability of the condition.

Prognosis	Expected Range of Number of Visits Per Episode of Care
Over the course of 4 to 16 weeks, patient/client will demonstrate optimal wound integumentary integrity and the highest level of functioning in home, work (job/school/play), community, and leisure environments.	**12 to 90**
Over the course of 6 to 24 months, patient/client will demonstrate mature scar and the highest level of functioning in home, work (job/school/play), community, and leisure environments.	**12 to 90**
During the episode of care, patient/client will achieve (1) the anticipated goals and expected outcomes of the interventions that are described in the plan of care and (2) the global outcomes for patients/clients who are classified in this pattern.	These ranges represent the lower and upper limits of the number of physical therapist visits required to achieve the anticipated goals and expected outcomes. *It is anticipated that 80% of patients/clients who are classified into this pattern will achieve the anticipated goals and expected outcomes within these ranges during a single continuous episode of care.* Frequency of visits and duration of the episode of care should be determined by the physical therapist to maximize effectiveness of care and efficiency of service delivery.

Factors That May Require New Episode of Care or That May Modify Frequency of Visits/Duration of Episode

- Accessibility and availability of resources
- Adherence to the intervention program
- Age
- Anatomical and physiological changes related to growth and development
- Caregiver consistency or expertise
- Chronicity or severity of the current condition
- Cognitive status
- Comorbitities, complications, or secondary impairments
- Concurrent medical, surgical, and therapeutic interventions
- Decline in functional independence
- Level of impairment
- Level of physical function
- Living environment
- Multisite or multisystem involvement
- Nutritional status
- Overall health status
- Potential discharge destinations
- Premorbid conditions
- Probability of prolonged impairment, functional limitation, or disability
- Psychological and socioeconomic factors
- Psychomotor abilities
- Social support
- Stability of the condition

Intervention

Intervention is the purposeful interaction of the physical therapist with the patient/client and, when appropriate, with other individuals involved in patient/client care, using various physical therapy procedures and techniques to produce changes in the condition consistent with the diagnosis and prognosis. Decisions about interventions are contingent on the timely monitoring of patient/client response and the progress made toward achieving the anticipated goals and expected outcomes.

Communication, coordination, and documentation and patient/client-related instruction are provided for all patients/clients across all settings. Procedural interventions are selected or modified based on the examination data and the evaluation, the diagnosis and the prognosis, and the anticipated goals and expected outcomes for a particular patient/client. *For clinical considerations in selecting interventions, listings of interventions, and listings of anticipated goals and expected outcomes, refer to Chapter 3.*

Coordination, Communication, and Documentation

Coordination, communication, and documentation may include:

Interventions

- Addressing required functions
  - advance directives
  - individualized family service plans (IFSPs) or individualized education plans (IEPs)
  - informed consent
  - mandatory communication and reporting (eg, patient advocacy and abuse reporting)
- Admission and discharge planning
- Case management
- Collaboration and coordination with agencies, including:
  - equipment suppliers
  - home care agencies
  - payer groups
  - schools
  - transportation agencies
- Communication across settings, including:
  - case conferences
  - documentation
  - education plans
- Cost-effective resource utilization
- Data collection, analysis, and reporting
  - outcome data
  - peer review findings
  - record reviews
- Documentation across settings, following APTA's *Guidelines for Physical Therapy Documentation* (Appendix 5), including:
  - changes in impairments, functional limitations, and disabilities
  - changes in interventions
  - elements of patient/client management (examination, evaluation, diagnosis, prognosis, intervention)
  - outcomes of intervention
- Interdisciplinary teamwork
  - case conferences
  - patient care rounds
  - patient/client family meetings
- Referrals to other professionals or resources

Anticipated Goals and Expected Outcomes

- Accountability for services is increased.
- Admission data and discharge planning are completed.
- Advance directives, individualized family service plans (IFSPs) or individualized education plans (IEPs), informed consent, and mandatory communication and reporting (eg, patient advocacy and abuse reporting) are obtained or completed.
- Available resources are maximally utilized.
- Care is coordinated with patient/client, family, significant others, caregivers, and other professionals.
- Case is managed throughout the episode of care.
- Collaboration and coordination occurs with agencies, including equipment suppliers, home care agencies, payer groups, schools, and transportation agencies.
- Communication enhances risk reduction and prevention.
- Communication occurs across settings through case conferences, education plans, and documentation.
- Data are collected, analyzed, and reported, including outcome data, peer review findings, and record reviews.
- Decision making is enhanced regarding health, wellness, and fitness needs.
- Decision making is enhanced regarding patient/client health and the use of health care resources by patient/client, family, significant others, and caregivers.
- Documentation occurs throughout patient/client management and across settings and follows APTA's *Guidelines for Physical Therapy Documentation* (Appendix 5).
- Interdisciplinary collaboration occurs through case conferences, patient care rounds, and patient/client family meetings.
- Patient/client, family, significant other, and caregiver understanding of anticipated goals and expected outcomes is increased.
- Placement needs are determined.
- Referrals are made to other professionals or resources whenever necessary and appropriate.
- Resources are utilized in a cost-effective way.

Patient/Client-Related Instruction

Patient/client-related instruction may include:

Interventions

- Instruction, education, and training of patients/clients and caregivers regarding:
  - current condition (pathology/pathophysiology [disease, disorder, or condition], impairments, functional limitations, or disabilities)
  - enhancement of performance
  - health, wellness, and fitness programs
  - plan of care
  - risk factors for pathology/pathophysiology (disease, disorder, or condition), impairments, functional limitations, or disabilities
  - transitions across settings
  - transitions to new roles

Anticipated Goals and Expected Outcomes

- Ability to perform physical actions, tasks, or activities is improved.
- Awareness and use of community resources are improved.
- Behaviors that foster healthy habits, wellness, and prevention are acquired.
- Decision making is enhanced regarding patient/client health and the use of health care resources by patient/client, family, significant others, and caregivers.
- Disability associated with acute or chronic illnesses is reduced.
- Functional independence in activities of daily living (ADL) and instrumental activities of daily living (IADL) is increased.
- Health status is improved.
- Intensity of care is decreased.
- Level of supervision required for task performance is decreased.
- Patient/client, family, significant other, and caregiver knowledge and awareness of the diagnosis, prognosis, interventions, and anticipated goals and expected outcomes are increased.
- Patient/client knowledge of personal and environmental factors associated with the condition is increased.
- Performance levels in self-care, home management, work (job/school/play), community, or leisure actions, tasks, or activities are improved.
- Physical function is improved.
- Risk of recurrence of condition is reduced.
- Risk of secondary impairment is reduced.
- Safety of patient/client, family, significant others, and caregivers is improved.
- Self-management of symptoms is improved.
- Utilization and cost of health care services are decreased.

Procedural Interventions

Procedural interventions for this pattern may include:

Therapeutic Exercise

Interventions

- Balance, coordination, and agility training
  - perceptual training
  - posture awareness training
  - sensory training or retraining
  - task-specific performance training
- Body mechanics and postural stabilization
  - postural stabilization activities
  - posture awareness training
- Flexibility exercises
  - muscle lengthening
  - range of motion
  - stretching
- Gait and locomotion training
  - perceptual training
  - standardized, programmatic, complementary exercise approaches
- Strength, power, and endurance training for head, neck, limb, pelvic-floor, trunk, and ventilatory muscles
  - active assistive, active, and resistive exercises (including concentric, dynamic/isotonic, eccentric, isokinetic, isometric, and plyometric)
  - task-specific performance training

Anticipated Goals and Expected Outcomes

- Impact on pathology/pathophysiology (disease, disorder, or condition)
  - Joint swelling, inflammation, or restriction is reduced.
  - Nutrient delivery to tissue is increased.
  - Osteogenic effects of exercise are maximized.
  - Pain is decreased.
  - Physiological response to increased oxygen demand is improved.
  - Soft tissue swelling, inflammation, or restriction is reduced.
  - Tissue perfusion and oxygenation are enhanced.
- Impact on impairments
  - Balance is improved.
  - Endurance is increased.
  - Gait, locomotion, and balance are improved.
  - Integumentary integrity is improved.
  - Joint integrity and mobility are improved.
  - Muscle performance (strength, power, and endurance) is increased.
  - Postural control is improved.
  - Range of motion is improved.
  - Sensory awareness is increased.
  - Weight-bearing status is improved.
- Impact on functional limitations
  - Ability to perform physical actions, tasks, or activities related to self-care, home management, work (job/school/play), community, and leisure is increased.
  - Level of supervision required for task performance is decreased.
  - Performance of and independence in activities of daily living (ADL) and instrumental activities of daily living (IADL) with or without devices and equipment are increased.
  - Tolerance of positions and activities is increased.
- Impact on disabilities
  - Ability to assume or resume required self-care, home management, work (job/school/play), community, and leisure roles is improved.
- Risk reduction/prevention
  - Preoperative and postoperative complications are reduced.
  - Risk factors are reduced.
  - Risk of recurrence of condition is reduced.
  - Risk of secondary impairment is reduced.
  - Safety is improved.
  - Self-management of symptoms is improved.
- Impact on health, wellness, and fitness
  - Fitness is improved.
  - Health status is improved.
  - Physical capacity is increased.
  - Physical function is improved.
- Impact on societal resources
  - Utilization of physical therapy services is optimized.
  - Utilization of physical therapy services results in efficient use of health care dollars.
- Patient/client satisfaction
  - Access, availability, and services provided are acceptable to patient/client.
  - Administrative management of practice is acceptable to patient/client.
  - Clinical proficiency of physical therapist is acceptable to patient/client.
  - Coordination of care is acceptable to patient/client.
  - Cost of health care services is decreased.
  - Intensity of care is decreased.
  - Interpersonal skills of physical therapist are acceptable to patient/client, family, and significant others.
  - Sense of well-being is improved.
  - Stressors are decreased.

Functional Training in Self-Care and Home Management (Including Activities of Daily Living [ADL] and Instrumental Activities of Daily Living [IADL])

Interventions

- ADL training
  - bathing
  - bed mobility and transfer training
  - developmental activities
  - dressing
  - eating
  - grooming
  - toileting
- IADL training
  - caring for dependents
  - home maintenance
  - household chores
  - shopping
  - structured play for infants and children
  - yard work
- Injury prevention or reduction
  - injury prevention education during self-care and home management
  - injury prevention or reduction with use of devices and equipment
  - safety awareness training during self-care and home management

Anticipated Goals and Expected Outcomes

- Impact on pathology/pathophysiology (disease, disorder, or condition)
  - Pain is decreased.
  - Physiological response to increased oxygen demand is improved.
- Impact on impairments
  - Balance is improved.
  - Endurance is increased.
  - Energy expenditure per unit of work is decreased.
  - Motor function (motor control and motor learning) is improved.
  - Muscle performance (strength, power, and endurance) is increased.
  - Postural control is improved.
  - Sensory awareness is increased.
  - Weight-bearing status is improved.
  - Work of breathing is decreased.
- Impact on functional limitations
  - Ability to perform physical actions, tasks, or activities related to self-care and home management is improved.
  - Level of supervision required for task performance is decreased.
  - Performance of and independence in ADL and IADL) with or without devices and equipment are increased.
  - Tolerance of positions and activities is increased.
- Impact on disabilities
  - Ability to assume or resume required self-care and home management roles is improved.
- Risk reduction/prevention
  - Risk factors are reduced.
  - Risk of secondary impairments is reduced.
  - Safety is improved.
  - Self-management of symptoms is improved.
- Impact on health, wellness, and fitness
  - Health status is improved.
  - Physical capacity is increased.
  - Physical function is improved.
- Impact on societal resources
  - Utilization of physical therapy services is optimized.
  - Utilization of physical therapy services results in efficient use of health care dollars.
- Patient/client satisfaction
  - Access, availability, and services provided are acceptable to patient/client.
  - Administrative management of practice is acceptable to patient/client.
  - Clinical proficiency of physical therapist is acceptable to patient/client.
  - Coordination of care is acceptable to patient/client.
  - Cost of health care services is decreased.
  - Intensity of care is decreased.
  - Interpersonal skills of physical therapist are acceptable to patient/client, family, and significant others.
  - Sense of well-being is improved.
  - Stressors are decreased.

Functional Training in Work (Job/School/Play), Community, and Leisure Integration or Reintegration (Including Instrumental Activities of Daily Living [IADL], Work Hardening, and Work Conditioning)

Interventions

- IADL training
  - community service training involving instruments
  - school and play activities training including tools and instruments
  - work training with tools
- Injury prevention or reduction
  - injury prevention education during work (job/school/play), community, and leisure integration or reintegration
  - injury prevention or reduction with use of devices and equipment
  - safety awareness training during during work (job/school/play), community, and leisure integration or reintegration

Anticipated Goals and Expected Outcomes

- Impact on pathology/pathophysiology (disease, disorder, or condition)
  - Pain is decreased.
  - Physiological response to increased oxygen demand is improved.
- Impact on impairments
  - Balance is improved.
  - Endurance is increased.
  - Muscle performance (strength, power, and endurance) is increased.
  - Sensory awareness is increased.
  - Weight-bearing status is improved.
- Impact on functional limitations
  - Ability to perform physical actions, tasks, or activities related to work (job/school/play), community, and leisure integration or reintegration is improved.
  - Level of supervision required for task performance is decreased.
  - Performance of and independence in IADL with or without devices and equipment are increased.
  - Tolerance of positions and activities is increased.
- Impact on disabilities
  - Ability to assume or resume required work (job/school/play), community, and leisure roles is improved.
- Risk reduction/prevention
  - Risk factors are reduced.
  - Risk of secondary impairment is reduced.
  - Safety is improved.
- Impact on health, wellness, and fitness
  - Fitness is improved.
  - Health status is improved.
  - Physical capacity is increased.
  - Physical function is improved.
- Impact on societal resources
  - Costs of work-related injury or disability are reduced.
  - Utilization of physical therapy services is optimized.
  - Utilization of physical therapy services results in efficient use of health care dollars.
- Patient/client satisfaction
  - Access, availability, and services provided are acceptable to patient/client.
  - Administrative management of practice is acceptable to patient/client.
  - Clinical proficiency of physical therapist is acceptable to patient/client.
  - Coordination of care is acceptable to patient/client.
  - Cost of health care services is decreased.
  - Intensity of care is decreased.
  - Interpersonal skills of physical therapist are acceptable to patient/client, family, and significant others.
  - Sense of well-being is improved.
  - Stressors are decreased.

Manual Therapy Techniques (Including Mobilization/Manipulation)

Interventions

- Manual lymphatic drainage
- Massage
  - connective tissue massage
  - therapeutic massage
- Mobilization/manipulation
  - soft tissue

Anticipated Goals and Expected Outcomes

- Impact on pathology/pathophysiology (disease, disorder, or condition)
  - Edema, lymphedema, or effusion is reduced.
  - Joint swelling, inflammation, or restriction is reduced.
  - Pain is decreased.
  - Soft tissue swelling, inflammation, or restriction is reduced.
- Impact on impairments
  - Integumentary integrity is improved.
  - Joint integrity and mobility are improved.
  - Range of motion is improved.
  - Relaxation is increased.
  - Sensory awareness is increased.
- Impact on functional limitations
  - Ability to perform movement tasks is improved.
  - Ability to perform physical actions, tasks, or activities related to self-care, home management, work (job/school/play), community, and leisure is improved.
  - Tolerance of positions and activities is increased.
- Impact on disabilities
  - Ability to assume or resume required self-care, home management, work (job/school/play), community, and leisure roles is improved.
- Risk reduction/prevention
  - Risk factors are reduced.
  - Risk of secondary impairment is reduced.
  - Self-management of symptoms is improved.
- Impact on health, wellness, and fitness
  - Physical capacity is increased.
  - Physical function is improved.
- Impact on societal resources
  - Utilization of physical therapy services is optimized.
  - Utilization of physical therapy services results in efficient use of health care dollars.
- Patient/client satisfaction
  - Access, availability, and services provided are acceptable to patient/client.
  - Administrative management of practice is acceptable to patient/client.
  - Clinical proficiency of physical therapist is acceptable to patient/client.
  - Coordination of care is acceptable to patient/client.
  - Cost of health care services is decreased.
  - Intensity of care is decreased.
  - Interpersonal skills of physical therapist are acceptable to patient/client, family, and significant others.
  - Sense of well-being is improved.
  - Stressors are decreased.

Prescription, Application, and, as Appropriate, Fabrication of Devices and Equipment (Assistive, Adaptive, Orthotic, Protective, Supportive, and Prosthetic)

Interventions

- Adaptive devices
  - environmental controls
  - hospital beds
  - raised toilet seats
  - seating systems
- Assistive devices
  - canes
  - crutches
  - long-handled reachers
  - power devices
  - static and dynamic splints
  - walkers
  - wheelchairs
- Orthotic devices
  - braces
  - casts
  - shoe inserts
  - splints
- Prosthetic devices (lower-extremity and upper-extremity)
- Protective devices
  - braces
  - cushions
  - protective taping
- Supportive devices
  - compression garments
  - elastic wraps
  - neck collars
  - serial casts
  - slings
  - supportive taping

Anticipated Goals and Expected Outcomes

- Impact on pathology/pathophysiology (disease, disorder, or condition)
  - Edema, lymphedema, or effusion is reduced.
  - Joint swelling, inflammation, or restriction is reduced.
  - Pain is decreased.
  - Physiological response to increased oxygen demand is improved.
  - Soft tissue swelling, inflammation, or restriction is reduced.
- Impact on impairments
  - Balance is improved.
  - Energy expenditure per unit of work is decreased.
  - Gait, locomotion, and balance are improved.
  - Integumentary integrity is improved.
  - Joint stability is improved.
  - Optimal joint alignment is achieved.
  - Optimal loading on a body part is achieved.
  - Quality and quantity of movement between and across body segments are improved.
  - Weight-bearing status is improved.
- Impact on functional limitations
  - Ability to perform physical actions, tasks, or activities related to self-care, home management, work (job/school/play), community, and leisure is improved.
  - Level of supervision required for task performance is decreased.
  - Performance of and independence in activities of daily living (ADL) and instrumental activities of daily living (IADL) with or without devices and equipment are increased.
  - Tolerance of positions and activities is improved.
- Impact on disabilities
  - Ability to assume or resume required self-care, home management, work (job/school/play), community, and leisure roles is improved.
- Risk reduction/prevention
  - Pressure on body tissues is reduced.
  - Protection of body parts is increased.
  - Risk factors are reduced.
  - Risk of secondary impairment is reduced.
  - Safety is improved.
  - Self-management of symptoms is improved.
- Impact on health, wellness, and fitness
  - Health status is improved.
  - Physical capacity is increased.
  - Physical function is improved.
- Impact on societal resources
  - Utilization of physical therapy services is optimized.
  - Utilization of physical therapy services results in efficient use of health care dollars.
- Patient/client satisfaction
  - Access, availability, and services provided are acceptable to patient/client.
  - Administrative management of practice is acceptable to patient/client.
  - Clinical proficiency of physical therapist is acceptable to patient/client.
  - Coordination of care is acceptable to patient/client.
  - Cost of health care services is decreased.
  - Intensity of care is decreased.
  - Interpersonal skills of physical therapist are acceptable to patient/client, family, and significant others.
  - Sense of well-being is improved.
  - Stressors are decreased.

Integumentary Repair and Protection Techniques

Interventions

- Debridement—nonselective
  - wet-to-dry dressings
- Debridement—selective
  - debridement with other agents (eg, autolysis)
  - enzymatic debridement
  - sharp debridement
- Dressings
  - hydrogels
  - vacuum-assisted closure
  - wound coverings
- Oxygen therapy
  - supplemental
  - topical
- Topical agents
  - cleansers
  - creams
  - moisturizers
  - ointments
  - sealants

Anticipated Goals and Expected Outcomes

- Impact on pathology/pathophysiology (disease, disorder, or condition)
  - Debridement of nonviable tissue is achieved.
  - Pain is decreased.
  - Soft tissue or wound healing is enhanced.
  - Tissue perfusion and oxygenation are enhanced.
  - Wound size is reduced.
- Impact on impairments
  - Integumentary integrity is improved.
  - Weight-bearing status is improved.
- Impact on functional limitations
  - Ability to perform physical actions, tasks, or activities related to self-care, home management, work (job/ school/ play), community, and leisure is improved.
  - Level of supervision required for task performance is decreased.
  - Performance of and independence in activities of daily living (ADL) and instrumental activities of daily living (IADL) with or without devices and equipment are increased.
  - Tolerance of positions and activities is increased.
- Impact on disabilities
  - Ability to assume or resume required self-care, home management, work (job/school/play), community, and leisure roles is improved.
- Risk reduction/prevention
  - Preoperative and postoperative complications are reduced.
  - Risk factors are reduced.
  - Risk of secondary impairment is reduced.
  - Self-management of symptoms is improved.
- Impact on health, wellness, and fitness
  - Health status is improved.
  - Physical function is improved.
- Impact on societal resources
  - Utilization of physical therapy services is optimized.
  - Utilization of physical therapy services results in efficient use of health care dollars.
- Patient/client satisfaction
  - Access, availability, and services provided are acceptable to patient/client.
  - Administrative management of practice is acceptable to patient/client.
  - Clinical proficiency of physical therapist is acceptable to patient/client.
  - Coordination of care is acceptable to patient/client.
  - Cost of health care services is decreased.
  - Intensity of care is decreased.
  - Interpersonal skills of physical therapist are acceptable to patient/client, family, and significant others.
  - Sense of well-being is improved.
  - Stressors are decreased.

Electrotherapeutic Modalities

Interventions

- Electrical stimulation
    - electrical muscle stimulation (EMS)
    - high voltage pulsed current (HVPC)
    - transcutaneous electrical nerve stimulation (TENS)

Anticipated Goals and Expected Outcomes

- Impact on pathology/pathophysiology (disease, disorder, or condition)
    - Edema, lymphedema, or effusion is reduced.
    - Joint swelling, inflammation, or restriction is reduced.
    - Nutrient delivery to tissue is increased.
    - Pain is decreased.
    - Soft tissue or wound healing is enhanced.
    - Soft tissue swelling, inflammation, or restriction is reduced.
    - Tissue perfusion and oxygenation are enhanced.
- Impact on impairments
    - Integumentary integrity is improved.
    - Sensory awareness is increased.
- Impact on functional limitations
    - Ability to perform physical actions, tasks, or activities related to self-care, home management, work (job/school/play), community, and leisure is improved.
    - Level of supervision required for task performance is decreased.
    - Performance of and independence in activities of daily living (ADL) and instrumental activities of daily living (IADL) with or without devices and equipment are increased.
    - Tolerance of positions and activities is increased.
- Impact on disabilities
    - Ability to assume or resume required self-care, home management, work (job/school/play), community, and leisure roles is improved.
- Risk reduction/prevention
    - Complications of immobility are reduced.
    - Preoperative and postoperative complications are reduced.
    - Risk factors are reduced.
    - Risk of secondary impairment is reduced.
    - Self-management of symptoms is improved.
- Impact on health, wellness, and fitness
    - Physical capacity is increased.
    - Physical function is improved.
- Impact on societal resources
    - Utilization of physical therapy services is optimized.
    - Utilization of physical therapy services results in efficient use of health care dollars.
- Patient/client satisfaction
    - Access, availability, and services provided are acceptable to patient/client.
    - Administrative management of practice is acceptable to patient/client.
    - Clinical proficiency of physical therapist is acceptable to patient/client.
    - Coordination of care is acceptable to patient/client.
    - Interpersonal skills of physical therapist are acceptable to patient/client, family, and significant others.
    - Sense of well-being is improved.
    - Stressors are decreased.

Physical Agents and Mechanical Modalities

Interventions

Physical agents may include:

- Hydrotherapy
  - pulsatile lavage
  - whirlpool tanks
- Light agents
  - laser
  - ultraviolet
- Sound agents
  - phonophoresis
  - ultrasound
- Thermotherapy
  - diathermy
  - dry heat
  - hot packs
  - paraffin baths

Mechanical modalities may include:

- Compression therapies
  - compression bandaging
  - compression garments
  - taping
  - total contact casting
  - vasopneumatic compression devices
- Gravity-assisted compression devices
  - tilt table
- Mechanical motion devices
  - continuous passive motion (CPM)

Anticipated Goals and Expected Outcomes

- Impact on pathology/pathophysiology (disease, disorder, or condition)
  - Debridement of nonviable tissue is achieved.
  - Edema, lymphedema, or effusion is reduced.
  - Joint swelling, inflammation, or restriction is reduced.
  - Nutrient delivery to tissue is increased.
  - Pain is decreased.
  - Soft tissue swelling, inflammation, or restriction is reduced.
  - Tissue perfusion and oxygenation are enhanced.
- Impact on impairments
  - Integumentary integrity is improved.
  - Range of motion is improved.
  - Weight-bearing status is improved.
- Impact on functional limitations
  - Ability to perform physical actions, tasks, or activities related to self-care, home management, work (job/school/play), community, and leisure is improved.
  - Performance of and independence in activities of daily living (ADL) and instrumental activities of daily living (IADL) with or without devices and equipment are increased.
  - Tolerance of positions and activities is increased.
- Impact on disabilities
  - Ability to assume or resume required self-care, home management, work (job/school/play), community, and leisure roles is improved.
- Risk reduction/prevention
  - Complications of soft tissue and circulatory disorders are decreased.
  - Risk of secondary impairment is reduced.
  - Self-management of symptoms is improved.
  - Stresses precipitating injury are decreased.
- Impact on health, wellness, and fitness
  - Physical function is improved.
- Impact on societal resources
  - Utilization of physical therapy services is optimized.
- Patient/client satisfaction
  - Access, availability, and services provided are acceptable to patient/client.
  - Administrative management of practice is acceptable to patient/client.
  - Clinical proficiency of physical therapist is acceptable to patient/client.
  - Coordination of care is acceptable to patient/client.
  - Interpersonal skills of physical therapist are acceptable to patient/client, family, and significant others.
  - Sense of well-being is improved.
  - Stressors are decreased.

Reexamination

Reexamination is the process of performing selected tests and measures after the initial examination to evaluate progress and to modify or redirect interventions. Reexamination may be indicated more than once during a single episode of care. It also may be performed over the course of a disease, disorder, or condition, which for some patients/clients may be over the life span. Indications for reexamination include new clinical findings or failure to respond to physical therapy interventions.

Global Outcomes for Patients/Clients in This Pattern

Throughout the entire episode of care, the physical therapist determines the anticipated goals and expected outcomes for each intervention. These anticipated goals and expected outcomes are delineated in shaded boxes that accompany the lists of interventions in each preferred practice pattern. As the patient/client reaches the termination of physical therapy services and the end of the episode of care, the physical therapist measures the global outcomes of the physical therapy services by characterizing or quantifying the impact of the physical therapy interventions in the following domains:

- Pathology/pathophysiology (disease, disorder, or condition)
- Impairments
- Functional limitations
- Disabilities
- Risk reduction/prevention
- Health, wellness, and fitness
- Societal resources
- Patient/client satisfaction

In some instances, a particular anticipated goal or expected outcome is thoroughly achieved through implementation of a single form of intervention. More commonly, however, the anticipated goals and expected outcomes are achieved as a result of the combined effects of several forms of interventions, leading to enhancement of both health status and health-related quality of life.

Criteria for Termination of Physical Therapy Services

Discharge is the process of ending physical therapy services that have been provided during a single episode of care. It occurs when the anticipated goals and expected outcomes have been achieved. Discharge does *not* occur with a *transfer* (defined as the time when a patient is moved from one site to another site within the same setting or across settings during a single episode of care). Although there may be facility-specific or payer-specific requirements for documentation regarding the conclusion of physical therapy services, *discharge occurs based on the physical therapist's analysis of the achievement of anticipated goals and expected outcomes.*

Discontinuation is the process of ending physical therapy services that have been provided during a single episode of care when (1) the patient/client, caregiver, or legal guardian declines to continue intervention; (2) the patient/client is unable to continue to progress toward outcomes because of medical or psychosocial complications or because financial/insurance resources have been expended; or (3) the physical therapist determines that the patient/client will no longer benefit from physical therapy. When physical therapy services are terminated prior to achievement of anticipated goals and expected outcomes, patient/client status and the rationale for termination are documented.

For patients/clients who require multiple episodes of care, periodic follow-up is needed over the life span to ensure safety and effective adaptation following changes in physical status, caregivers, environment, or task demands. In consultation with appropriate individuals, and in consideration of the outcomes, the physical therapist plans for discharge or discontinuation and provides for appropriate follow-up or referral.

APPENDIXES:

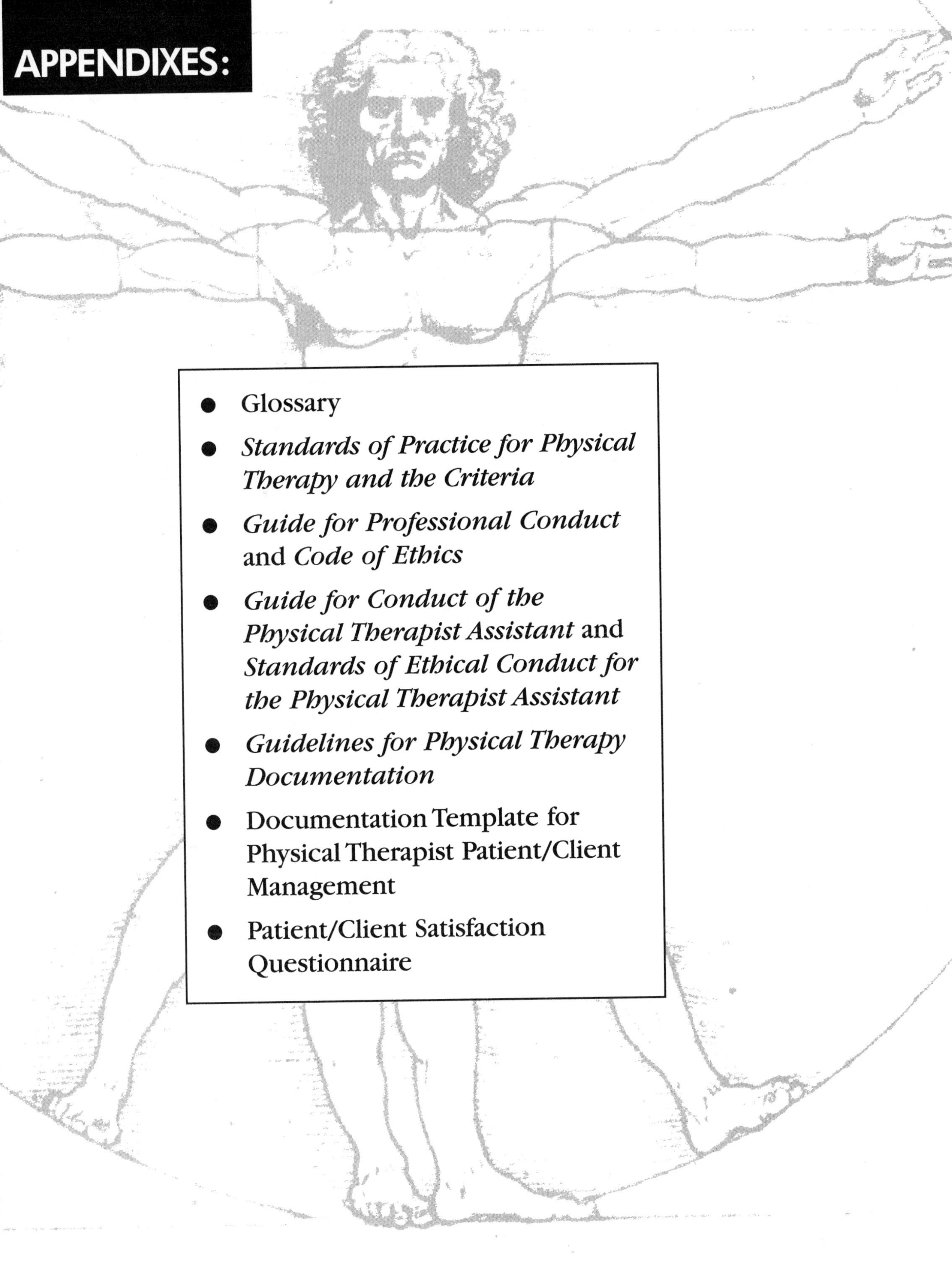

- Glossary
- *Standards of Practice for Physical Therapy and the Criteria*
- *Guide for Professional Conduct* and *Code of Ethics*
- *Guide for Conduct of the Physical Therapist Assistant* and *Standards of Ethical Conduct for the Physical Therapist Assistant*
- *Guidelines for Physical Therapy Documentation*
- Documentation Template for Physical Therapist Patient/Client Management
- Patient/Client Satisfaction Questionnaire

Glossary

A

Activities of daily living (ADL) The self-care, communication, and mobility skills (eg, bathing, bed mobility, dressing, eating, grooming, toileting, and transfers) required for independence in everyday living.

Adaptive devices A variety of implements or equipment used to aid patients/clients in performing actions, tasks, activities, or movements. Adaptive devices include environmental controls, raised toilet seats, and seating systems.

Aerobic conditioning The performance of therapeutic exercise and activities to increase endurance.

Aerobic capacity/endurance The ability to perform work or participate in activities over time using the body's oxygen uptake, delivery, and energy release mechanisms.

Airway clearance techniques A group of therapeutic activities intended to manage or prevent the consequences of impaired mucociliary transport or the inability to protect the airway (eg, impaired cough).

Anthropometric characteristics Those traits that describe body dimensions, such as height, weight, girth, and body fat composition.

Anticipated goals See Goals.

Arousal A state of responsiveness to stimulation or action or of physiological readiness for activity.

Arthrokinematic The accessory or joint play movements of a joint that cannot be performed voluntarily and that are defined by the structure and shape of the joint surfaces, without regard to the forces producing motion or resulting from motion.

Assessment The measurement or quantification of a variable or the placement of a value on something. Assessment should not be confused with examination or evaluation.

Assistive devices A variety of implements or equipment used to aid patients/clients in performing actions, activities, movements or tasks. Assistive devices include canes, crutches, long-handled reachers, power devices, static and dynamic splints, walkers, and wheelchairs.

Associated skin Skin that is not disrupted, including skin either contiguous to a wound or skin at risk of injury or breakdown.

Attention Selective awareness of the environment or selective responsiveness to stimuli.

Auscultation The act of listening to internal body sounds (eg, heart, lungs).

Autogenic drainage Airway clearance through the patient's/client's own efforts (eg, coughing).

B

Back school A structured educational program about back problems, usually offered to a group of patients/clients.

Balance The ability to maintain the body in equilibrium with gravity both statically (ie, while stationary) and dynamically (ie, while moving).

Barriers See Environmental, home, and work (job/school/play) barriers.

Biofeedback A training technique that enables an individual to gain some element of voluntary control over muscular or autonomic nervous system functions using a device that produces auditory or visual stimuli.

Body mechanics The interrelationships of the muscles and joints as they maintain or adjust posture in response to forces placed on or generated by the body.

C

Cardiovascular pump Structures responsible for maintaining cardiac output, including the cardiac muscle, valves, arterial smooth muscle, and venous smooth muscle.

Cardiovascular pump dysfunction Abnormalities of the cardiac muscles, valves, conduction, or circulation that interrupt or interfere with cardiac output or circulation.

Caregivers Individuals who are responsible for the patient's/client's care, including home health aides, day-care providers, teachers, or educational aides.

Cicatrix Scar; the fibrous tissue replacing the normal tissues destroyed by injury or disease.

Circulation The movement of blood through organs and tissues to deliver oxygen and to remove carbon dioxide and the passive movement (drainage) of lymph through channels, organs, and tissues for removal of cellular byproducts and inflammatory wastes.

Clients Individuals who engage the services of a physical therapist and who can benefit from the physical therapist's consultation, interventions, professional advice, health promotion, fitness, wellness, or prevention services. Clients also are businesses, school systems, and others to whom physical therapists provide services.

Cognition The act or process of knowing, including both awareness and judgment.

Communication The exchange of information.

Community integration or reintegration The process of assuming or resuming roles and functions in the community, such as gaining access to transportation (eg, driving a car, boarding a bus, negotiating a neighborhood), to community businesses and services (eg, banks, shops, parks), and to public facilities (eg, attending theaters, town hall meetings, parks, places of worship).

Complementary exercise approaches A broad range of nonconventional exercise systems used in combination with conventional therapeutic exercise to enhance control of the body and sense of well-being.

Compression therapy Treatment using devices or techniques that decrease the density of a part of the body through the application of pressure.

Conditioning Improvement of physical and mental capacity with a program of exercises or a course of training.

Consultation The rendering of professional or expert opinion or advice by a physical therapist. The consulting physical therapist applies highly specialized knowledge and skills to identify problems, recommend solutions, or produce a specified outcome or product in a given amount of time on behalf of a patient/client.

Continuous passive motion (CPM) The use of a device that allows a joint (eg, the knee) to be exercised without the involvement of the patient/client, often in the early postoperative period.

Contrast bath The immersion of an extremity in alternating hot and cold water.

Coordination The working together of all parties involved with the patient/client.

Cosmesis A concern in rehabilitation, especially regarding surgical operations or burns, for the appearance of the patient/client.

Cranial nerve integrity The intactness of the twelve pairs of nerves connected with the brain, including their somatic, visceral, and afferent and efferent components.

Cryotherapy Therapeutic application of cold (eg, ice).

D

Debridement *Non-selective debridement* is the removal of nonspecific areas of devitalized tissue with prior tissue preparation. Non-selective debridement may include the use of enzymatic debridement, wet dressings, wet-to-dry dressings, and wet-to-moist dressings. *Selective debridement* is the removal of specific areas of devitalized tissue without prior tissue preparation. Selective debridement may include use of autolytic or enzymatic agents or sharp instruments. *Selective sharp debridement*, which often occurs at the line of demarcation between viable and non-viable tissue, is the use of sharp instruments for tissue removal.

Deconditioning The physiologic changes in systemic function following prolonged periods of rest or inactivity.

Deficit A lack or deficiency. *Developmental deficit:* The difference between the expected level of peformance and the actual (lower) level of performance in an aspect of development (eg, motor, communication, social).

Developmental delay The failure to reach expected age-specific performance in one or more areas of development (eg, motor, sensory-perceptual).

Diagnosis Diagnosis is both a process and a label. The diagnostic process includes integrating and evaluating the data that are obtained during the examination to describe the patient/client condition in terms that will guide the prognosis, the plan of care, and intervention strategies. Physical therapists use diagnostic labels that identify the impact of a condition on function at the level of the system (especially the movement system) and at the level of the whole person.

Disability The inability to perform or a limitation in the performance of actions, tasks, and activities usually expected in specific social roles that are customary for the individual or expected for the person's status or role in a specific sociocultural context and physical environment. In the Guide, the categories of required roles are self-care, home management, work (job/school/play), and community/leisure.

Discharge The process of ending physical therapy services that have been provided during a single episode of care, when the anticipated goals and expected outcomes have been achieved. Discharge does *not* occur with a transfer (that is, when the patient is moved from one site to another site within the same setting or across setting during a single episode of care).

Discontinuation The process of ending physical therapy services that have been provided during a single episode of care when: (1) the patient/client, caregiver, or legal guardian declines to continue intervention, (2) the patient/client is unable to continue to progress toward anticipated goals and expected outcomes because of medical or psychosocial complications or because financial/insurance resources have been expended, or (3) the physical therapist determines that the patient/client will no longer benefit from physical therapy.

Disease A pathological condition or abnormal entity with a characteristic group of signs and symptoms affecting the body and with known or unknown etiology.

Disorder Derangement or abnormality of function (anatomic or physiologic); pathology.

Documentation Any entry into the patient/client record—such as consultation reports, initial examination reports, progress notes, flow sheets, checklists, reexamination reports, or summations of care—that identifies the care or service provided.

Dynamometry Measurement of the degree of muscle power.

Dysfunction Disturbance, impairment, or abnormality of function of an organ.

E

Electrical potential The amount of electrical energy residing in specific tissues.

Electrical stimulation An intervention using electricity to produce a therapeutic effect.

Electrophysiologic testing The process of examining and recording the electrical responses of the body.

Electromyography (EMG) The examining and recording of the electrical activity of a muscle.

Electrotherapeutic modalities A broad group of agents that use electricity and are intended to assist functional training; assist muscle force generation and contraction; decrease unwanted muscular activity; increase the rate of healing of open wounds and soft tissue; maintain strength after injury or surgery; modulate or decrease pain; or reduce or eliminate soft tissue swelling, inflammation, or restriction.

Endurance See Aerobic capacity; see Muscle endurance.

Environmental, home, and work (job/school/play) barriers The physical impediments that keep patients/clients from functioning optimally in their surroundings, including safety hazards (eg, throw rugs, slippery surfaces), access problems (eg, narrow doors, thresholds, high steps, absence of power doors or elevators), and home or office design barriers (eg, excessive distances to negotiate, multistory environments, sinks, bathrooms, counters, placement of controls or switches).

Episode of physical therapy care All physical therapy services that are (1) provided by a physical therapist, (2) provided in an unbroken sequence, and (3) related to the physical therapy interventions for a given condition or problem or related to a request from the patient/client, family, or other health care provider. A defined number or identified range of number of visits will be established for an episode of care. The episode of care may include transfers between sites within or across settings or reclassification of the patient/client from one preferred practice pattern to another.

Episode of physical therapy maintenance A series of occasional clinical, educational, and administrative services related to maintenance of current function. Programs for maintenance of function are a vital part of the practice of physical therapy. No defined number or range of number of visits is established for this type of episode.

Episode of physical therapy prevention A series of occasional clinical, educational, and administrative services related to prevention, to the promotion of health, wellness, and fitness, and to the preservation of optimal function. Prevention services and programs that promote health, wellness, and fitness are a vital part of the practice of physical therapy. No defined number or range of number of visits is established for this type of episode.

Ergonomics The relationship among the worker; the work that is done; the actions, tasks, or activities inherent in that work (job/school/play); and the environment in which the work (job/school/play) is performed. Ergonomics uses scientific and engineering principles to improve safety, efficiency, and quality of movement involved in work (job/school/play).

Evaluation A dynamic process in which the physical therapist makes clinical judgments based on data gathered during the examination.

Examination A comprehensive screening and specific testing process leading to diagnostic classification or, as appropriate, to a referral to another practitioner. The examination has three components: the patient/client history, the systems review, and tests and measures.

Expected outcomes The intended results of patient/client management, which indicate the changes in impairments, functional limitations, and disabilities and the changes in health, wellness, and fitness needs that are expected as the result of implementing the plan of care. The expected outcomes in the plan should be measurable and time limited.

F

Fitness A dynamic physical state—comprising cardiovascular/pulmonary endurance; muscle strength, power, endurance, and flexibility; relaxation; and body composition—that allows optimal and efficient performance of daily and leisure activities.

Flexibility The pliability of a portion of the body that is determined by joint integrity, soft tissue extensibility, and muscle length.

Force plate An embedded plate used to measure the force that a person exerts when walking.

Function Those activities identified by an individual as essential to support physical, social, and psychological well-being and to create a personal sense of meaningful living.

Functional assessment The measurement or quantification of those activities identified by an individual as essential to support physical, social, and psychological well-being and to create a personal sense of meaningful living.

Functional limitation The restriction of the ability to perform, at the level of the whole person, a physical action, task, or activity in an efficient, typically expected, or competent manner.

Functional muscle testing Performance-based muscle assessment in particular positions simulating functional tasks and activities and usually under specific test conditions.

Functional training The education and training of patients/clients in activities of daily living (ADL) and instrumental activities of daily living (IADL) that are intended to improve the ability to perform physical actions, tasks, or activities in an efficient, typically expected, or competent manner.

G

Gait The manner in which a person walks, characterized by rhythm, cadence, step, stride, and speed.

Goniometry Measurement of the angle of a joint or a series of joints.

Goals The intended results of patient/client management. Goals indicate changes in impairment, functional limitations, and disabilities and changes in health, wellness, and fitness needs that are expected as a result of implementing the plan of care. Goals should be measurable and time limited. (If required, goals may be expressed as short-term and long-term goals.)

H

Health status The state or status of the conditions that comprise good health.

History A systematic gathering of data—from both the past and the present—related to why the patient/client is seeking the services of the physical therapist. The data that are obtained (eg, through interview, through review of the patient/client record, or from other sources) include demographic information, social history, employment and work (job/school/play), growth and development, living environments, general health status, social and health habits (past and current), family history, medical/surgical history, current conditions or chief complaints, functional status and activity level, medications, and other clinical tests. While taking the history, the physical therapist also identifies health restoration and prevention needs and coexisting health problems that may have implications for intervention.

Home management The ability to perform the more complex instrumental activities of daily living (IADL), such as, structured play (for infants and children), maintaining a home, shopping, performing heavy household chores, caring for dependents, and performing yard work.

Hydrotherapy An intervention using water to produce a therapeutic effect.

I

Impairment A loss or abnormality of anatomical, physiological, mental, or psychological structure or function. *Secondary impairment:* Impairment that originates from other, preexisting impairments.

Instruction See Patient/client-related instruction.

Instrumental activities of daily living (IADL) The more complex skills—such as caring for dependents, maintaining a home, performing household chores and yardwork, shopping, and structured play (for infants and children)—that are important components of maintaining independent living.

Integumentary integrity The intactness of the skin, including the ability of the skin to serve as a barrier to environmental threats (eg, bacteria, parasites).

Integumentary repair and protection techniques The application of therapeutic procedures and modalities that are intended to enhance wound perfusion, manage scar, promote an optimal wound environment, remove excess exudate from a wound complex, and eliminate nonviable tissue from a wound bed.

Intervention The purposeful interaction of the physical therapist with the patient/client and, when appropriate, with other individuals involved in patient/client care, using various physical therapy procedures and techniques to produce changes in the condition.

Iontophoresis The introduction of ions into tissues by means of electric current to produce a therapeutic effect.

J

Joint integrity The intactness of the structure and shape of the joint, including its osteokinematic and arthrokinematic characteristics.

Joint mobility The capacity of the joint to be moved passively, taking into account the structure and shape of the joint surface in addition to characteristics of the tissue surrounding the joint.

K

Kinesthesia The awareness of movement.

L

Leisure integration or reintegration The process of assuming or resuming roles and functions of avocational and enjoyable pastimes, such as recreational activities (eg, playing a sport) and age-appropriate hobbies (eg, collecting antiques, gardening, or making crafts).

Locomotion The ability to move from one place to another.

M

Maintenance See Episode of physical therapy maintenance.

Manual therapy techniques Skilled hand movements intended to improve tissue extensibility; increase range of motion; induce relaxation; mobilize or manipulate soft tissue and joints; modulate pain; and reduce soft tissue swelling, inflammation, or restriction.

Mechanical modalities A group of devices that use forces such as approximation, compression, and distraction and that are intended to improve circulation, increase range of motion, modulate pain, or stabilize an area that requires temporary support.

Mobilization/manipulation A manual therapy technique comprising a continuum of skilled passive movements to the joints and/or related soft tissues that are applied at varying speeds and amplitudes, including a small-amplitude/high-velocity therapeutic movement.

Modality A broad group of agents that may include thermal, acoustic, radiant, mechanical, or electrical energy to produce physiologic changes in tissues for therapeutic purposes.

Motor control The ability of the central nervous system to control or direct the neuromotor system in purposeful movement and postural adjustment by selective allocation of muscle tension across appropriate joint segments.

Motor deficit A lack or deficiency of normal motor function (motor control and motor function) that may be the result of pathology or other disorder. Weaknesses, paralysis, abnormal movement patterns, abnormal timing, coordination, clumsiness, involuntary movements, or abnormal postures may be manifestations of impaired motor function (motor control and motor learning).

Motor function (motor control and motor learning) The ability to learn or demonstrate the skillful and efficient assumption, maintenance, modification, and control of voluntary postures and movement patterns.

Motor learning A set of processes associated with practice or experience leading to relatively permanent changes in the capability for producing skilled action.

Muscle endurance The ability to sustain forces repeatedly or to generate forces over a period of time.

Muscle length The maximum extensibility of a muscle-tendon unit.

Muscle performance The capacity of a muscle or a group of muscles to generate forces.

Muscle power The work produced per unit of time or the product of strength and speed.

Muscle strength The muscle force exerted by a muscle or a group of muscles to overcome a resistance under a specific set of circumstances.

Muscle tension State of partial muscle contraction that is characterized by persistent, involuntary contraction of muscle fibers or of a muscle or muscles and that is usually associated with pain and excessive irritability.

Muscle tone The velocity-dependent resistance to stretch that muscle exhibits.

N

Neuromotor development The acquisition and evolution of movement skills throughout the life span.

O

Orthotic devices A variety of implements and equipment used to support or protect weak or ineffective joints or muscles and serve to enhance performance. Orthotic devices include braces, casts, shoe inserts, and splints.

Osteokinematics Gross angular motions of the shafts of bones in sagittal, frontal, and transverse planes.

Outcome See Expected outcomes.

Oxygen saturation The amount of oxygen combined with hemoglobin as measured in arterial blood.

P

Pain A disturbed sensation that causes suffering or distress.

Pallesthesia The ability to sense mechanical vibration.

Palpation Examination using the hands (eg, palpation of muscle spasm, palpation of the thoracic cage).

Paraffin bath A superficial thermal modality using paraffin wax and mineral oil to produce a therapeutic effect.

Patient/client-related instruction The process of informing, educating, or training patients/clients, families, significant others, and caregivers with the intent to promote and optimize physical therapy services.

Patients Individuals who are the recipients of physical therapy examination, evaluation, diagnosis, prognosis, and intervention and who have a disease, disorder, condition, impairment, functional limitation, or disability.

Pathology/pathophysiology (disease, disorder, condition) An abnormality characterized by a particular cluster of signs and symptoms and recognized by either the patient/client or practitioner as "abnormal." It is primarily identified at the cellular level.

Percussion (diagnostic) A procedure in which the clinician taps a body part manually or with an instrument to estimate its density or its resonance.

Percussion A procedure utilized with pulmonary postural drainage to lossen secretions from the bronchial walls. The therapist uses slightly cupped hands to percuss the chest wall.

Performance-based assessment The measurement and quantification of a variable during completion of a task or activity.

Peripheral nerve integrity The intactness of the spinal nerves, including their afferent and efferent components.

Phototherapy An intervention using the application of light to produce a therapeutic effect.

Physical agents A broad group of procedures using various forms of energy that are applied to tissues in a systematic manner and that are intended to increase connective tissue extensibility; increase the healing rate of open wounds and soft tissue; modulate pain; reduce or eliminate soft tissue swelling, inflammation, or restriction associated with musculoskeletal injury or circulatory dysfunction; remodel scar tissue; or treat skin conditions. These agents may include athermal, cryotherapy, hydrotherapy, light, sound, and thermotherapy agents.

Physical capacity The ability of the body or body parts to process and execute physical tasks.

Physical function Fundamental component of health status describing the state of those sensory and motor skills necessary for usual daily activities, including work and recreation.

Physical performance Whole body effort intended to accomplish an action, task, or activity.

Physical therapist/physiotherapist A person who is a graduate of an accredited physical therapist education program and is licensed to practice physical therapy. The terms "physical therapist" and "physiotherapist" are synonymous.

Physical therapist assistant A technically educated health care provider who assists the physical therapist in the provision of selected physical therapy interventions. The physical therapist assistant is the only individual who provides selected physical therapy interventions under the direction and supervision of the physical therapist. The physical therapist assistant is a graduate of a physical therapist assistant associate degree program accredited by the Commission on Accreditation in Physical Therapy (CAPTE).

Physical therapy/physiotherapy Physical therapy is examination, evaluation, diagnosis, prognosis, and intervention provided by physical therapists/physiotherapists. Physical therapy includes diagnosis and management of movement dysfunction and enhancement of physical and functional abilities; restoration, maintenance, and promotion of optimal physical function, optimal fitness and wellness, and optimal quality of life as it relates to movement and health; and prevention of the onset, symptoms, and progression of impairments, functional limitations, and disabilities that may result from diseases, disorders, conditions, or injuries. The terms "physical therapy" and "physiotherapy" are synonymous.

Plan of care Statements that specify the anticipated goals and the expected outcomes, predicted level of optimal improvement, specific interventions to be used, and proposed duration and frequency of the interventions that are required to reach the goals and outcomes. The plan of care includes the anticipated discharge plans.

Postural drainage See Pulmonary postural drainage.

Posture The alignment and positioning of the body in relation to gravity, center of mass, and base of support.

Power See Muscle power.

Prevention Activities that are directed toward (1)achieving and restoring optimal functional capacity, (2) minimizing impairments, functional limitations, and disabilities, (3) maintaining health (thereby preventing further deterioration or future illness), (4) creating appropriate environmental adaptations to enhance independent function. *Primary prevention:* Prevention of disease in a susceptible or potentially susceptible population through specific measures such as general health promotion efforts. *Secondary prevention:* Efforts to decrease the duration of illness, severity of diseases, and sequelae through early diagnosis and prompt intervention. *Tertiary prevention:* Efforts to limit the degree of disability and promote rehabilitation and restoration of function in patients/clients with chronic and irreversible diseases. Also see Episode of physical therapy prevention.

Primary care The provision of integrated, accessible health care services by clinicians who are accountable for addressing a large majority of personal health care needs, developing a sustained partnership with patients and practicing within the context of family and community. [*Defining Primary Care:An Interim Report*. Washington, DC: Institute of Medicine, National Academy Press; 1995]

Prognosis The determination of the predicted optimal level of improvement in function and the amount of time needed to reach that level.

Proprioception The reception of stimuli from within the body (eg, from muscles and tendons) and includes position sense (the awareness of joint position) and kinesthesia (the awareness of movement).

Prosthesis An artificial device used to replace a missing part of the body.

Prosthetic requirements The biomechanical elements necessitated by the loss of a body part.

Protective devices A variety of devices and equipment used to support or protect weak or ineffective joints or muscles and serve to enhance performance. Protective devices include braces, cushions, helmets, and protective taping.

Pulmonary postural drainage Placing the body in a position that uses gravity to drain fluid from segments of the lungs.

R

Range of motion (ROM) The arc through which movement occurs at a joint or a series of joints.

Reconditioning Restoration to good physical and mental condition.

Reexamination The process of performing selected tests and measures after the inital examination to evaluate progress and to modify or redirect interventions.

Referral A recommendation that a patient/client seek service from another health care provider or resource.

Reflex A stereotypic, involuntary reaction to any of a variety of sensory stimuli.

Reflex integrity The intactness of the neural path involved in a reflex.

Respiration/gas exchange The exchange of oxygen and carbon dioxide across a membrane either in the lungs or at the cellular level.

S

Scar Disposition of connective tissue as a result of the healing process.

Screening Determining the need for further examination or consultation by a physical therapist or for referral to another health professional. *Cognitive screening:* Brief assessment of the patient's/client's thinking process (eg, ability to process commands).

Self-care management The ability to perform activities of daily living (ADL), such as bed mobility, transfers, dressing, grooming, bathing, eating, and toileting.

Sensory Having to do with sensations or the senses, including peripheral sensory processing (eg, sensitivity to touch) and cortical sensory processing (eg, two-point and sharp/dull discrimination).

Sensory integration The ability to integrate information that is derived from the environment and that relates to movement.

Sensory integrity The intactness of cortical sensory processing, including proprioception, pallesthesia, stereognosis, and topognosis.

Serial casting A process in which the patient is recasted over a period of time, typically to achieve increased range of motion of a particular body part.

Signs Objective evidence of physical abnormality.

Splinting Support of a body segment through application of an external device. *Static:* Customized and prefabricated splints, inhibitory casts, and spinal and other braces that are designed to maintain joints in a desired position. *Dynamic:* Customized and prefabricated supports that allow for or control motion while providing support.

Stereognosis The ability to perceive, recognize, and name familiar objects.

Strength See Muscle strength.

Strengthening The process of making stronger. *Active:* A form of strength-building exercise in which the patient/client actively contracts the muscle(s) through the range of motion of active movement. Movement may begin with gravity eliminated and progress to movement against gravity. *Assistive:* A form of strength-building exercise in which the physical therapist assists the patient/client through the available range of motion. *Resistive:* Any form of active exercise in which a dynamic or static muscular contraction is resisted by an outside force. The external force may be applied manually or mechanically.

Supportive devices A variety of devices and equipment used to support or protect weak or ineffective joints or muscles and serve to enhance performance. Supportive devices include compression garments, corsets, elastic wraps, neck collars, serial casts, slings, supplemental oxygen, and supportive taping.

Symptoms Subjective evidence of physical abnormality.

T

Tests and measures Specific standardized methods and techniques used to gather data about the patient/client after the history and systems review have been performed.

Therapeutic exercise The systematic performance or execution of planned physical movements, postures, or activities intended to enable the patient/client to (1) remediate or prevent impairments, (2) enhance function, (3) reduce risk, (4) optimize overall health, and (5) enhance fitness and well-being.

Thermistor An electrical resistor that uses a semiconductor whose resistance varies sharply in a known manner with the ambient temperature; used in determining temperature.

Thermotherapy An intervention using heat to cause vasodilation to produce a therapeutic effect.

Topognosis The ability to localize exactly a cutaneous sensation.

Traction The therapeutic use of manual or mechanical tension created by a pulling force to produce a combination of distraction and gliding to relieve pain and increase tissue flexibility.

Transcutaneous electrical nerve stimulation (TENS) An intervention using electrical energy to stimulate cutaneous and peripheral nerves via electrodes on the skin's surface.

Transfer The process of relocating a body from one object or surface to another (eg, getting into or out of bed, moving from a wheelchair to a chair).

Travel training Instruction provided to develop an awareness of the environment and to learn skills necessary to move effectively and safely from place to place within that environment.

Treatment The sum of all interventions provided by the physical therapist to a patient/client during an episode of care.

U

Ultrasound A diagnostic or therapeutic technique using high-frequency sound waves to produce heat. *Pulsed ultrasound:* The application of therapeutic ultrasound using predetermined interrupted frequencies.

Ultraviolet A form of radiant energy using light rays with wavelengths beyond the violet end of the visible spectrum.

V

Vasopneumatic compression device A device to decrease edema by using compressive forces that are applied to the body part.

Ventilation The movement of a volume of gas into and out of the lungs.

Ventilatory pump Thoracic skeleton and skeletal muscles and their innervation responsible for ventilation. The muscles include the diaphragm; the intercostal, scalene, and sternocleidomastoid muscles; the accessory muscles of ventilation; and the abdominal, triangular, and quadratus lumborum muscles.

Ventilatory pump dysfunction Abnormalities of the thoracic skeleton, respiratory muscles, airways, or lungs that interrupt or interfere with the work of breathing or ventilation.

Vestibular Describing the sense of balance located in the inner ear.

Visit All physical therapy services provided in a 24-hour period. *Range of number of visits:* All visits within a single episode of care. The range may be adjusted based on factors that may require a new episode of care or that may modify frequency of visits and duration of episode.

Visual analog scale A tool used in a pain examination that allows the patient/client to indicate degree of pain by pointing to a visual representation of pain intensity.

Volume measurement The amount of fluid that has been displaced from a container (of any size) following the introduction of part or all of the body.

W

Wellness Concepts that embrace positive health behaviors that promote a state of physical and mental balance and fitness.

Work conditioning An intensive, work-related, goal-oriented conditioning program designed specifically to restore systemic neuromusculoskeletal functions (eg, strength, endurance, movement, flexibility, motor control) and cardiopulmonary functions. The objective of the work conditioning program is to restore physical capacity and function to enable the patient/client to return to work.

Work hardening A highly structured, goal-oriented, individualized treatment program designed to return the client to work. Work hardening programs, which are often interdisciplinary in nature, use real or simulated work activities designed to restore physical, behavioral, and vocational functions. Work hardening addresses issues of productivity, safety, physical tolerances, and worker behaviors.

Work (job/school/play) integration or reintegration The process of assuming or resuming roles and functions at work (job/school/play), such as gaining access to work (job/school /play) environments and workstations, negotiating school environments, and participating in age-appropriate play activities or work hardening or work conditioning programs.

Wound An area of disrupted or discontinuous skin or tissue.

Wound care Procedures used to achieve a clean wound bed, promote a moist environment or facilitate autolytic debridement, or absorb excessive exudation from a wound complex. Also see Integumentary repair and protection techniques.

Standards of Practice for Physical Therapy and the Criteria

The *Standards of Practice for Physical Therapy* are promulgated by APTA's House of Delegates; Criteria for the Standards are promulgated by APTA's Board of Directors. Criteria are italicized beneath the Standards to which they apply. To view the most recent version of the *Standards of Practice for Physical Therapy and the Criteria*, visit the APTA Web site at www.apta.org. OR: To obtain a copy of the most recent version of the *Standards of Practice for Physical Therapy and the Criteria*, contact APTA at 800/399-2782, ext. 3395.

The physical therapy profession is committed to providing an optimum level of service delivery and to striving for excellence in practice. The House of Delegates of the American Physical Therapy Association, as the formal body that represents the profession, attests to this commitment by adopting and promoting the following *Standards of Practice for Physical Therapy*. These Standards are the profession's statement of conditions and performances that are essential for provision of high-quality physical therapy. The Standards provide a foundation for assessment of physical therapy practice.

I. LEGAL/ETHICAL CONSIDERATIONS

A. Legal Considerations

The physical therapist complies with all the legal requirements of jurisdictions regulating the practice of physical therapy.

The physical therapist assistant complies with all the legal requirements of jurisdictions regulating the work of the assistant.

B. Ethical Considerations

The physical therapist practices according to the *Code of Ethics* of the American Physical Therapy Association.

The physical therapist assistant complies with the *Standards of Ethical Conduct for the Physical Therapist Assistant* of the American Physical Therapy Association.

II. ADMINISTRATION OF THE PHYSICAL THERAPY SERVICE

A. Statement of Mission, Purposes, and Goals

The physical therapy service has a statement of mission, purposes, and goals that reflects the needs and interests of the patients/clients served, the physical therapy personnel affiliated with the service, and the community.

The statement of mission, purposes, and goals:

- *Defines the scope and limitations of the physical therapy service.*
- *Identifies the goals and objectives of the service.*
- *Is reviewed annually.*

B. Organizational Plan

The physical therapy service has a written organizational plan.

The organizational plan:

- *Describes relationships among components within the physical therapy service and, where the service is part of a larger organization, between the service and other components of that organization.*
- *Ensures that the service is directed by a physical therapist.*
- *Defines supervisory structures within the service.*
- *Reflects current personnel functions.*

C. Policies and Procedures

The physical therapy service has written policies and procedures that reflect the operation of the service and that are consistent with the mission, purposes, and goals of the service.

The written policies and procedures:

- *Are reviewed regularly and revised as necessary.*
- *Meet the requirements of federal and state law and external agencies.*
- *Apply to, but are not limited to:*
  - *Clinical education*
  - *Clinical research*
  - *Interdisciplinary collaboration*
  - *Criteria for access to care*
  - *Criteria for initiation and continuation of care*
  - *Criteria for referral to other appropriate health care providers*
  - *Criteria for termination of care*
  - *Equipment maintenance*
  - *Environmental safety*
  - *Fiscal management*
  - *Infection control*
  - *Job/position descriptions*
  - *Competency assessment*
  - *Medical emergencies*
  - *Care of patients/clients, including guidelines*
  - *Rights of patients/clients*
  - *Personnel-related policies*
  - *Improvement of quality of care and performance of services*
  - *Documentation*
  - *Staff orientation*

D. Administration

A physical therapist is responsible for the direction of the physical therapy service.

The director of the physical therapy service:

- *Ensures compliance with local, state, and federal requirements.*
- *Ensures compliance with current APTA documents, including* Standards of Practice for Physical Therapy and the Criteria, Code of Ethics, Guide for Professional Conduct, Standards of Ethical Conduct for the Physical Therapist Assistant, *and* Guide for Conduct of the Physical Therapist Assistant.

- *Ensures that services are consistent with the mission, purposes, and goals of the physical therapy service.*
- *Ensures that services are provided in accordance with established policies and procedures.*
- *Reviews and updates policies and procedures.*
- *Provides training that ensures continued competence of physical therapist assistants and support personnel who are involved in the provision on physical therapist-directed support services.*
- *Provides for continuous in-service training on safety issues and for periodic safety inspection of equipment by qualified individuals.*

E. Fiscal Management

The director of the physical therapy service, in consultation with physical therapy staff and appropriate administrative personnel, participates in planning for, and allocation of, resources. Fiscal planning and management of the service are based on sound accounting principles.

The fiscal management plan:

- *Includes a budget that provides for optimal use of resources.*
- *Ensures accurate recording and reporting of financial information.*
- *Ensures compliance with legal requirements.*
- *Allows for cost-effective utilization of resources.*
- *Uses a fee schedule that is consistent with the cost of physical therapy services and that is within customary norms of fairness and reasonableness.*

F. Improvement of Quality of Care and Performance

The physical therapy service has a written plan for continuous improvement of quality of care and performance of services.

The improvement plan:

- *Provides evidence of ongoing review and evaluation of the physical therapy service.*
- *Provides a mechanism for documenting improvement in quality of care and performance.*
- *Is consistent with requirements of external agencies, as applicable.*

G. Staffing

The physical therapy personnel affiliated with the physical therapy service have demonstrated competence and are sufficient to achieve the mission, purposes, and goals of the service.

The physical therapy service:

- *Meets all legal requirements regarding licensure and certification of appropriate personnel.*
- *Ensures that the level of expertise within the service is appropriate to the needs of the patients/clients served.*
- *Provides for appropriate ratios of personnel to patients/clients.*
- *Provides for appropriate rations of support personnel to professional personnel.*

H. Staff Development

The physical therapy service has a written plan that provides for appropriate and ongoing staff development.

The staff development plan:

- *Includes self-assessment, individual goal setting, and organizational needs in directing continuing education and learning activities.*
- *Includes strategies for lifelong learning and professional career development.*

I. Physical Setting

The physical setting is designed to provide a safe and accessible environment that facilitates fulfillment of the mission, purposes, and goals of the physical therapy service. The equipment is safe and sufficient to achieve the purposes and goals of physical therapy.

The physical setting:

- *Meets all applicable legal requirements for health and safety.*
- *Meets space needs appropriate for the number and type of patients/clients served.*
- *Meets all applicable legal requirements for health and safety.*
- *Is inspected routinely.*

J. Collaboration

The physical therapy service collaborates with all appropriate disciplines.

The collaboration:

- *Uses an interdisciplinary team approach to the care of patients/clients.*
- *Provides interdisciplinary instruction of patients and clients and families.*
- *Ensures interdisciplinary professional development and continuing education.*

III. PROVISION OF SERVICES

A. Informed Consent

The physical therapist has sole responsibility for providing information to the patient/client and for obtaining informed consent in accordance with jurisdictional law before initiating intervention.

The information provided to patients/clients:

- *Clearly describes the proposed intervention.*
- *Delineates material (decisional) risks associated with the proposed intervention.*
- *Identifies expected benefits of the proposed intervention.*
- *Compares the benefits and risks possible both with and without the proposed intervention*
- *Explains reasonable alternatives to the proposed intervention.*

Informed consent:

- *Requires consent of a competent adult.*
- *Requires consent of a parent/legal guardian as the surrogate decision maker when the adult patient is not competent or when the patient/client is a minor.*
- *Requires the patient/client or legal guardian to acknowledge understanding of the intervention and to give consent before intervention is initiated.*

B. Initial Examination/Evaluation/Diagnosis/ Prognosis

The physical therapist performs an initial examination and evaluates to establish a diagnosis and prognosis prior to intervention.

The physical therapist examination:

- *Identifies the physical therapy needs of the patient/client.*
- *Incorporates appropriate tests and measures to facilitate outcome measurement.*
- *Produces data that are sufficient to allow evaluation, diagnosis, prognosis, and the establishment of a plan of care.*
- *May result in recommendations for additional services to meet the needs of the patient/client.*

C. Plan of Care

The physical therapist establishes a plan of care for the patient/client based on the examination, evaluation, diagnosis, prognosis, anticipated goals, and expected outcomes of the planned interventions for identified impairments, functional limitations, and disabilities.

The physical therapist involves the patient/client and appropriate others in the planning, implementation, and assessment of the intervention program.

The physical therapist, in consultation with appropriate disciplines, plans for discharge of the patient/client, taking into consideration achievement of anticipated goals and expected outcomes, and provides for appropriate follow-up or referral.

The plan of care:

- *Identifies realistic long-term and short-term goals and expected outcomes, taking into consideration the expectations of the patient/client and appropriate others.*
- *Describes the proposed intervention, including frequency and duration.*

D. Intervention

The physical therapist provides, or directs and supervises, the physical therapy intervention consistent with the results of the examination, evaluation, diagnosis, prognosis, and the plan of care.

The intervention:

- *Is provided under the ongoing the direct care of or under the direction and supervision of the physical therapist.*
- *Is provided in such a way that responsibilities are commensurate with the qualifications and the legal limitations of the physical therapist assistant and of the support personnel who may be involved in the provision of physical therapist-directed support services.*
- *Is altered in accordance with changes in response or status.*
- *Is provided at a level that is consistent with current physical therapy practice.*
- *Is interdisciplinary when necessary to meet the needs of the patient/client.*

E. Reexamination

The physical therapist reexamines the patient/client as necessary during an episode of care to evaluate progress or change in patient's/client's status and modifies the plan of care accordingly or discontinues physical therapy services.

The physical therapist reexamination:

- *Identifies ongoing patient/client needs.*
- *May result in recommendations for additional services, discharge, or discontinuation of physical therapy services.*

F. Discharge/Discontinuation of Intervention

The physical therapist discharges the patient/client from physical therapy services when the anticipated goals or expected outcomes for the patient/client have been achieved.

The physical therapist discontinues intervention when the patient/client is unable to continue to progress toward goals or when the physical therapist determines that the patient/client will no longer benefit from physical therapy.

Discharge:

- *Occurs at the end of an episode of care and is the end of physical therapy services that have been provided during that episode.*

Discontinuation:

- *Also occurs when the patient/client, caregiver, or legal guardian declines to continue intervention.*

G. Communication/Coordination/Documentation

The physical therapist communicates, coordinates, and documents all aspects of patient/client management, including the results of the initial examination and evaluation, diagnosis, prognosis, plan of care, interventions, response to interventions, changes in patient/client status relative to the interventions, reexamination, and discharge/discontinuation of intervention.

Physical therapist documentation:

- *Is dated and appropriately authenticated by the physical therapist who performed the examination and established the plan of care.*
- *Is dated and appropriately aauthenticated by the physical therapist who performed the intervention or, when allowable by law or regulations, by the physical therapist assistant who performed specific components of the intervention as selected by the supervising physical therapist.*
- *Is dated and appropriately aauthenticated by the physical therapist who performed the reexamination, and includes modifications to the plan of care.*
- *Is dated and appropriately aauthenticated by the physical therapist who performed the discharge, and includes the status of the patient/client and the goals and outcomes achieved.*
- *Includes, when a patient/client is discharged prior to achievement of goals and outcomes, the status of the patient/client and the rationale for discontinuation.*

IV. EDUCATION

The physical therapist is responsible for individual professional development. The physical therapist assistant is responsible for individual career development.

The physical therapist participates in the education of physical therapist students, physical therapist assistant students, and students in other health professions.

The physical therapist educates and provides consultation to consumers and the general public regarding the purposes and benefits of physical therapy.

The physical therapist educates and provides consultation to consumers and the general public regarding the roles of the physical therapist and the physical therapist assistant.

The physical therapist:

- *Educates and provides consultation to consumers and the general public regarding the roles of the physical therapist, the physical therapist assistant, and other support personnel.*

V. RESEARCH

The physical therapist applies research findings to practice and encourages, participates in, and promotes activities that establish the outcomes of patient/client management provided by the physical therapist.

The physical therapist supports collaborative research.

VI. COMMUNITY RESPONSIBILITY

The physical therapist demonstrates community responsibility by participating in community and community agency activities, educating the public, formulating public policy, or providing pro bono physical therapy services.

The physical therapist:

- *Participates in community and community agency activities.*
- *Educates the public, including prevention education and health promotion.*
- *Helps formulate public policy.*
- *Provides pro bono physical therapy services.*

Adopted by the House of Delegates, APTA, June 1980
Amended June 2002, June 2000, June 1999, June 1996, June 1991, June 1985

Guide for Professional Conduct

Purpose

This *Guide for Professional Conduct* (Guide) is intended to serve physical therapists in interpreting the *Code of Ethics* (Code) of the American Physical Therapy Association (Association) in matters of professional conduct. The Guide provides guidelines by which physical therapists may determine the propriety of their conduct. It is also intended to guide the professional development of physical therapist students. The Code and the Guide apply to all physical therapists. These guidelines are subject to changes as the dynamics of the profession change and as new patterns of health care delivery are developed and accepted by the professional community and the public. This Guide is subject to monitoring and timely revision by the Ethics and Judicial Committee of the Association.

Interpreting Ethical Principles

The interpretations expressed in this Guide reflect the opinions, decisions, and advice of the Ethics and Judicial Committee. These interpretations are intended to assist an physical therapist in applying general ethical principals to specific situations. They should not be considered inclusive of all situations that could evolve.

PRINCIPLE 1

A physical therapist shall respect the rights and dignity of all individuals and shall provide compassionate care.

1.1 Attitudes of a Physical Therapist

A. A physical therapist shall recognize individual and cultural differences and shall respect and be responsive to those differences.

B. A physical therapist shall be guided by concern for the physical, psychological, and socioeconomic welfare of patients/clients.

C. A physical therapist shall not harass, abuse, or discriminate against others.

D. A physical therapist shall be aware of the patient's health-related needs and act in a manner that facilitates meeting those needs.

PRINCIPLE 2

A physical therapist shall act in a trustworthy manner towards patients/clients, and in all other aspects of physical therapy practice.

2.1 Patient/Physical Therapist Relationship

A. To act in a trustworthy manner the physical therapist shall act in the patient's/client's best interest. Working in the patient's/client's best interest requires knowledge of the patient's/client's needs from the patient's/client's perspective. Patients/clients often come to the physical therapist in a vulnerable state and normally will rely on the physical therapist's advice, which they perceive to be based on superior knowledge, skill, and experience. The trustworthy physical therapist acts to ameliorate the patient's/client's vulnerability, not to exploit it.

B. A physical therapist shall not exploit any aspect of the physical therapist/patient relationship.

C. A physical therapist shall not engage in any sexual relationship or activity, whether consensual or nonconsensual, with any patient while a physical therapist/patient relationship exists.

D. The physical therapist shall create an environment that encourages an open dialogue with the patient/client.

Code of Ethics

Preamble

This *Code of Ethics* of the American Physical Therapy Association sets forth principles for the ethical practice of physical therapy. All physical therapists are responsible for maintaining and promoting ethical practice. To this end, the physical therapist shall act in the best interest of the patient/client. This *Code of Ethics* shall be binding on all physical therapists.

Principle 1

A physical therapist shall respect the rights and dignity of all individuals and shall provide compassionate care.

Principle 2

A physical therapist shall act in a trustworthy manner towards patients/clients, and in all other aspects of physical therapy practice.

Principle 3

A physical therapist shall comply with laws and regulations governing physical therapy and shall strive to effect changes that benefit patients/clients.

Principle 4

A physical therapist shall exercise sound professional judgment.

Principle 5

A physical therapist shall achieve and maintain professional competence.

Principle 6

A physical therapist shall maintain and promote high standards for physical therapy practice, education, and research.

Principle 7

A physical therapist shall seek only such remuneration as is deserved and reasonable for physical therapy services.

Principle 8

A physical therapist shall provide and make available accurate and relevant information to patients/clients about their care and to the public about physical therapy services.

Principle 9

A physical therapist shall protect the public and the profession from unethical, incompetent, and illegal acts.

Principle 10

A physical therapist shall endeavor to address the health needs of society.

Principle 11

A physical therapist shall respect the rights, knowledge, and skills of colleagues and other health care professionals.

Adopted by the House of Delegates, APTA, June 1973
Amended June 2002, June 2000, June 1991, June 1987, June 1981, June 1978, June 1977

E. In the event the physical therapist or patient terminates the physical therapist/patient relationship while the patient continues to need physical therapy services, the physical therapist should take steps to transfer the care of the patient to another provider.

2.2 Truthfulness

A physical therapist shall not make statements that he/she knows or should know are false, deceptive, fraudulent, or unfair. See Section 8.2.D.

2.3 Confidential Information

A. Information relating to the physical therapist/patient relationship is confidential and may not be communicated to a third party not involved in that patient's care without the prior consent of the patient, subject to applicable law.

B. Information derived from peer review shall be held confidential by the reviewer unless the physical therapist who was reviewed consents to the release of the information.

C. A physical therapist may disclose information to appropriate authorities when it is necessary to protect the welfare of an individual or the community or when required by law. Such disclosure shall be in accordance with applicable law.

2.4 Patient Autonomy and Consent

A. A physical therapist shall not restrict patients' freedom to select their provider of physical therapy.

B. A physical therapist shall communicate to the patient/client the findings of his/her examination, evaluation, diagnosis, and prognosis.

C. A physical therapist shall collaborate with the patient/client to establish the goals of treatment and the plan of care.

D. A physical therapist shall use sound professional judgment in informing the patient/client of any substantial risks of the recommended examination and intervention.

E. A physical therapist shall respect the patient's/client's right to make decisions regarding the recommended plan of care, including consent, modification, or refusal.

PRINCIPLE 3

A physical therapist shall comply with laws and regulations governing physical therapy and shall strive to effect changes that benefit patients/clients.

3.1 Professional Practice

A physical therapist shall provide examination, evaluation, diagnosis, prognosis, and intervention. A physical therapist shall not engage in any unlawful activity that substantially relates to the qualifications, functions, or duties of a physical therapist.

3.2 Just Laws and Regulations

A physical therapist shall advocate the adoption of laws, regulations, and policies by providers, employers, third party payers, legislatures, and regulatory agencies to provide and improve access to necessary health care services for all individuals.

3.3 Unjust Laws and Regulations

A physical therapist shall endeavor to change unjust laws, regulations, and policies that govern the practice of physical therapy. See Section 10.2.

PRINCIPLE 4

A physical therapist shall exercise sound professional judgment.

4.1 Professional Responsibility

A. A physical therapist shall make professional judgments that are in the patient/client's best interests.

B. Regardless of practice setting, a physical therapist has primary responsibility for the physical therapy care of a patient and shall make independent judgments regarding that care consistent with accepted professional standards. See Section 2.4.

C. A physical therapist shall not provide physical therapy services to a patient/client while his/her ability to do so safely is impaired.

D. A physical therapist shall exercise sound professional judgment based upon his/her knowledge, skill, education, training, and experience.

E. Upon accepting a patient/client for physical therapy services, a physical therapist shall be responsible for: the examination, evaluation, and diagnosis of that individual; the prognosis and intervention; reexamination and modification of the plan of care; and the maintenance of adequate records, including progress reports. A physical therapist shall establish the plan of care and shall provide and/or supervise and direct the appropriate interventions. See Section 2.4.

F. If the diagnostic process reveals findings that are outside the scope of the physical therapist's knowledge, experience, or expertise, the physical therapist shall so inform the patient/client and refer to an appropriate practitioner.

G. When the patient has been referred from another practitioner, the physical therapist shall communicate the findings of the examination and evaluation, the diagnosis, the proposed intervention, and reexamination findings (as indicated) to the referring practitioner.

H. A physical therapist shall determine when a patient/client will no longer benefit from physical therapy services.

4.2 Direction and Supervision

A. The supervising physical therapist has primary responsibility for the physical therapy care rendered to a patient/client.

B. A physical therapist shall not delegate to a less qualified person any activity that requires the unique skill, knowledge, and judgment of the physical therapist.

C. A physical therapist shall have regular and ongoing communications with the physical therapist assistant to whom he/she has delegated specific interventions.

4.3 Practice Arrangements

A. Participation in a business, partnership, corporation, or other entity does not exempt physical therapists, whether employers, partners, or stockholders, either individually or collectively, from the obligation to promote, maintain and comply with the ethical principles of the Association.

B. A physical therapist shall advise his/her employer(s) of any employer practice that causes a physical therapist to be in conflict with the ethical principles of the Association. A physical therapist shall seek to eliminate aspects of his/her employment that are in conflict with the ethical principles of the Association.

4.4 Gifts and Other Considerations

A physical therapist shall not accept or offer gifts or other considerations that affect or give an appearance of affecting his/her professional judgment.

PRINCIPLE 5

A physical therapist shall achieve and maintain professional competence.

5.1 Scope of Competence

A physical therapist shall practice within the scope of his/her competence and commensurate with his/her level of education, training, and experience.

5.2 Self-Assessment

A physical therapist shall engage in self-assessment, which is a lifelong professional responsibility for maintaining competence.

5.3 Professional Development

A physical therapist shall participate in educational activities that enhance his/her basic knowledge and skills.

PRINCIPLE 6

A physical therapist shall maintain and promote high standards for physical therapy practice, education, and research.

6.1 Professional Standards

A physical therapist shall know the accepted professional standards when engaging in physical therapy practice, education and/or research. A physical therapist shall continuously engage in assessment activities to determine compliance with these standards. If a physical therapist is not in compliance with these standards, he/she shall engage in activities designed to reach compliance with the standards. When a physical therapist is in compliance with these standards, he/she shall engage in activities designed to maintain such compliance.

6.2 Practice

A. A physical therapist shall achieve and maintain professional competence. See Section 5.

B. A physical therapist shall demonstrate his/her commitment to quality improvement by engaging in peer and utilization review and other self-assessment activities.

6.3 Professional Education

A. A physical therapist shall support high-quality education in academic and clinical settings.

B. A physical therapist participating in the educational process is responsible to the students, the academic institutions, and the clinical settings for promoting ethical conduct. A physical therapist shall model ethical behavior and provide the student with information about the *Code of Ethics*, opportunities to discuss ethical conflicts, and procedures for reporting unresolved ethical conflicts. See Section 9.

6.4 Continuing Education

A. A physical therapist providing continuing education must be competent in the content area.

B. When a physical therapist provides continuing education, he/she shall ensure that course content, objectives, faculty credentials, and responsibilities of the instructional staff are accurately stated in the promotional and instructional course materials.

C. A physical therapist shall evaluate the efficacy and effectiveness of information and techniques presented in continuing education programs before integrating them into his or her practice.

6.5 Research

A. A physical therapist shall support research activities that contribute knowledge for improved patient care.

B. A physical therapist shall critically evaluate published studies related to physical therapy practice, research, and education before integrating them into his or her practice.

C. A physical therapist shall report to appropriate authorities any acts in the conduct or presentation of research that appear unethical or illegal. See Section 9.

PRINCIPLE 7

A physical therapist shall seek only such remuneration as is deserved and reasonable for physical therapy services.

7.1 Business and Employment Practices

A. A physical therapist's business/employment practices shall be consistent with the ethical principles of the Association.

B. A physical therapist shall never place her/his own financial interest above the welfare of individuals under his/her care.

C. A physical therapist shall recognize that third-party payer contracts may limit, in one form or another, the provision of physical therapy services. Third-party limitations do not absolve the physical therapist from making sound professional judgments that are in the patient's best interest. A physical therapist shall avoid underutilization of physical therapy services.

D. When a physical therapist's judgment is that a patient will receive negligible benefit from physical therapy services, the physical therapist shall not provide or continue to provide such services if the primary reason for doing so is to further the financial self-interest of the physical therapist or his/her employer. A physical therapist shall avoid overutilization of physical therapy services.

E. Fees for physical therapy services should be reasonable for the service performed, considering the setting in which it is provided, practice costs in the geographic area, judgment of other organizations, and other relevant factors.

F. A physical therapist shall not directly or indirectly request, receive, or participate in the dividing, transferring, assigning, or rebating of an unearned fee.

G. A physical therapist shall not profit by means of a credit or other valuable consideration, such as an unearned commission, discount, or gratuity, in connection with the furnishing of physical therapy services.

H. Unless laws impose restrictions to the contrary, physical therapists who provide physical therapy services within a business entity may pool fees and monies received. Physical therapists may divide or apportion these fees and monies in accordance with the business agreement.

I. A physical therapist may enter into agreements with organizations to provide physical therapy services if such agreements do not violate the ethical principles of the Association or applicable laws.

7.2 Endorsement of Products or Services

A. A physical therapist shall not exert influence on individuals under his/her care or their families to use products or services based on the direct or indirect financial interest of the physical therapist in such products or services. Realizing that these individuals will normally rely on the physical therapist's advice, their best interest must always be maintained, as must their right of free choice relating to the use of any product or service. Although it cannot be considered unethical for physical therapists to own or have a financial interest in the production, sale, or distribution of products/services, they must act in accordance with law and make full disclosure of their interest whenever individuals under their care use such products/services.

B. A physical therapist may receive remuneration for endorsement or advertisement of products or services to the public, physical therapists, or other health professionals provided he/she discloses any financial interest in the production, sale, or distribution of said products or services.

C. When endorsing or advertising products or services, a physical therapist shall use sound professional judgment and shall not give the appearance of Association endorsement unless the Association has formally endorsed the products or services.

7.3 Disclosure

A physical therapist shall disclose to the patient if the referring practitioner derives compensation from the provision of physical therapy.

PRINCIPLE 8

A physical therapist shall provide and make available accurate and relevant information to patients/clients about their care and to the public about physical therapy services.

8.1 Accurate and Relevant Information to the Patient

A. A physical therapist shall provide the patient/client information about his/her condition and plan of care. See Section 2.4.

B. Upon the request of the patient, the physical therapist shall provide, or make available, the medical record to the patient or a patient-designated third party.

C. A physical therapist shall inform patients of any known financial limitations that may affect their care.

D. A physical therapist shall inform the patient when, in his/her judgment, the patient will receive negligible benefit from further care. See Section 7.1.C.

8.2 Accurate and Relevant Information to the Public

A. A physical therapist shall inform the public about the societal benefits of the profession and who is qualified to provide physical therapy services.

B. Information given to the public shall emphasize that individual problems cannot be treated without individualized examination and plans/programs of care.

C. A physical therapist may advertise his/her services to the public.

D. A physical therapist shall not use, or participate in the use of, any form of communication containing a false, plagiarized, fraudulent, deceptive, unfair, or sensational statement or claim.

E. A physical therapist who places a paid advertisement shall identify it as such unless it is apparent from the context that it is a paid advertisement.

PRINCIPLE 9

A physical therapist shall protect the public and the profession from unethical, incompetent, and illegal acts.

9.1 Consumer Protection

A. A physical therapist shall provide care that is within the scope of practice as defined by the state practice act.

B. A physical therapist shall not engage in any conduct that is unethical, incompetent, or illegal.

C. A physical therapist shall report any conduct that appears to be unethical, incompetent, or illegal.

D. A physical therapist may not participate in any arrangements in which patients are exploited due to the referring sources' enhancing their personal incomes as a result of referring for, prescribing, or recommending physical therapy. See Section 5.

PRINCIPLE 10

A physical therapist shall endeavor to address the health needs of society.

10.1 Pro Bono Service

A physical therapist shall render pro bono publico (reduced or no fee) services to patients lacking the ability to pay for services, as each physical therapist's practice permits.

10.2 Community Health

A physical therapist shall endeavor to support activities that benefit the health status of the community. See Section 3.

PRINCIPLE 11

A physical therapist shall respect the rights, knowledge, and skills of colleagues and other health care professionals.

11.1 Consultation

A physical therapist shall seek consultation whenever the welfare of the patient will be safeguarded or advanced by consulting those who have special skills, knowledge, and experience.

11.2 Patient/Provider Relationships

A physical therapist shall not undermine the relationship(s) between his/her patient and other healthcare professionals.

11.3 Disparagement

Physical therapists shall not disparage colleagues and other health care professionals. See Section 9 and Section 2.4.A.

Issued by Ethics and Judicial Committee, APTA, October 1981
Last Amended, January 2002

Guide for Conduct of the Physical Therapist Assistant

Purpose

This *Guide for Conduct of the Physical Therapist Assistant* (Guide) is intended to serve physical therapist assistants in interpreting the *Standards of Ethical Conduct for the Physical Therapist Assistant* (Standards) of the American Physical Therapy Association (APTA). The Guide provides guidelines by which physical therapist assistants may determine the propriety of their conduct. It is also intended to guide the development of physical therapist assistant students. The Standards and Guide apply to all physical therapist assistants. These guidelines are subject to change as the dynamics of the profession change and as new patterns of health care delivery are developed and accepted by the professional community and the public. This Guide is subject to monitoring and timely revision by the Ethics and Judicial Committee of the Association.

Interpreting Standards

The interpretations expressed in this Guide reflect the opinions, decisions, and advice of the Ethics and Judicial Committee. These interpretations are intended to guide a physical therapist assistant in applying general ethical principles to specific situations. They should not be considered inclusive of all situations that could evolve.

STANDARD 1

A physical therapist assistant shall respect the rights and dignity of all individuals and shall provide compassionate care.

1.1 Attitude of a Physical Therapist Assistant

A. A physical therapist assistant shall demonstrate sensitivity to individual and cultural differences.

B. A physical therapist assistant shall be guided at all times by concern for the physical and psychological welfare of patients/clients.

C. A physical therapist assistant shall not harass, abuse, or discriminate against others.

STANDARD 2

A physical therapist assistant shall act in a trustworthy manner towards patients/clients.

2.1 Trustworthiness

A. To act in a trustworthy manner a physical therapist assistant shall act in the patient's/client's best interest. Working in the patient's/client's best interest requires sensitivity to the patient's/client's vulnerability and an effective working relationship between the physical therapist and the physical therapist assistant.

B. A physical therapist assistant shall act to ameliorate the patient's/client's vulnerability, not to exploit it.

C. A physical therapist assistant shall clearly identify himself/herself as a physical therapist assistant to patients/clients.

D. A physical therapist assistant shall conduct himself/herself in a manner that supports the physical therapist/patient relationship.

E. A physical therapist assistant shall not engage in any sexual relationship or activity, whether consensual or nonconsensual, with any patient/client entrusted to his/her care.

F. A physical therapist assistant shall not invite, accept, or offer gifts or other considerations that affect or give an appearance of affecting his/her provision of physical therapy interventions.

Standards of Ethical Conduct for the Physical Therapist Assistant

Preamble

This document of the American Physical Therapy Association sets forth standards for the ethical conduct of the physical therapist assistant. All physical therapist assistants are responsible for maintaining high standards of conduct while assisting physical therapists. The physical therapist assistant shall act in the best interest of the patient/client. These standards of conduct shall be binding on all physical therapist assistants.

STANDARD 1

A physical therapist assistant shall respect the rights and dignity of all individuals and shall provide compassionate care.

STANDARD 2

A physical therapist assistant shall act in a trustworthy manner toward patients/clients.

STANDARD 3

A physical therapist assistant shall provide selected physical therapy interventions only under the supervision and direction of a physical therapist.

STANDARD 4

A physical therapist assistant shall comply with laws and regulations governing physical therapy.

STANDARD 5

A physical therapist assistant shall achieve and maintain competence in the provision of selected physical therapy interventions.

STANDARD 6

A physical therapist assistant shall make judgments that are commensurate with his or her educational and legal qualifications as a physical therapist assistant.

STANDARD 7

A physical therapist assistant shall protect the public and the profession from unethical, incompetent, and illegal acts.

Adopted by the House of Delegates, APTA, June 1982
Amended June 2000, June 1991

2.2 Exploitation of Patients

A physical therapist assistant shall not participate in any arrangements in which patients/clients are exploited. Such arrangements include situations where referring sources enhance their personal incomes as a result of referring for, delegating, prescribing, or recommending physical therapy services.

2.3 Truthfulness

A. A physical therapist assistant shall not make statements that he/she knows or should know are false, deceptive, fraudulent, or unfair.

B. Although it cannot be considered unethical for a physical therapist assistant to own or have a financial interest in the production, sale, or distribution of products/services, he/she must act in accordance with law and make full disclosure of his/her interest to patients/clients.

2.4 Confidential Information

A. Information relating to the patient/client is confidential and may not be communicated to a third party not involved in that patient's/client's care without the prior consent of the patient/client, subject to applicable law.

B. A physical therapist assistant shall refer all requests for release of confidential information to the supervising physical therapist.

STANDARD 3

A physical therapist assistant shall provide selected physical therapy interventions only under the supervision and direction of a physical therapist.

3.1 Supervisory Relationship

A. A physical therapist assistant shall provide services only under the supervision and direction of a physical therapist.

B. A physical therapist assistant shall provide only those physical therapy interventions that have been selected by the physical therapist.

C. A physical therapist assistant shall not carry out any selected physical therapy interventions that are outside his/her education, training, experience, or skill and shall notify the physical therapist.

D. A physical therapist assistant may adjust specific interventions within the plan of care established by the physical therapist in response to changes in the patient's/client's status.

E. A physical therapist assistant shall not perform examinations or evaluations, interpret data, determine diagnosis or prognosis, or establish or alter a plan of care.

F. Consistent with the physical therapist assistant's education, training, knowledge, and experience, he/she may respond to the patient's/client's inquiries regarding interventions that are within the established plan of care.

G. A physical therapist assistant shall have regular and ongoing communication with the physical therapist regarding the patient's/client's status.

STANDARD 4

A physical therapist assistant shall comply with laws and regulations governing physical therapy.

4.1 Supervision

A physical therapist assistant shall know and comply with applicable law. Regardless of the content of any law, a physical therapist assistant shall provide services only under the supervision and direction of a physical therapist.

4.2 Representation

A physical therapist assistant shall not hold himself/herself out as a physical therapist.

STANDARD 5

A physical therapist assistant shall achieve and maintain competence in the provision of selected physical therapy interventions.

5.1 Competence

A physical therapist assistant shall provide interventions consistent with his/her level of education, training, experience, and skill.

5.2 Self-assessment

A physical therapist assistant shall engage in self-assessment in order to maintain competence.

5.3 Development

A physical therapist assistant shall participate in educational activities that enhance his/her basic knowledge and skills.

STANDARD 6

A physical therapist assistant shall make judgments that are commensurate with his/her educational and legal qualifications as a physical therapist assistant.

6.1 Patient Safety

A. A physical therapist assistant shall discontinue immediately any components of interventions that, in his/her judgment, appear to be harmful to the patient/client and shall discuss his/her concerns with the physical therapist.

B. A physical therapist assistant shall not carry out any selected physical therapy interventions that are outside his/her education, training, experience, or skill and shall notify the physical therapist.

C. A physical therapist assistant shall not perform interventions while his/her ability to do so safely is impaired.

6.2 Patient Status Judgments

A physical therapist assistant participates in patient/client status judgments by reporting changes to the physical therapist and requesting patient/client reexamination or revision of the plan of care. See Section 3.1.

6.3 Gifts and Other Considerations

A physical therapist assistant shall not invite, accept, or offer gifts or other considerations that affect or give the appearance of affecting his/her provision of physical therapy interventions or that exploit the patient/client in any way. See Section 2.1.B.

STANDARD 7

A physical therapist assistant shall protect the public and the profession from unethical, incompetent, and illegal acts.

7.1 Consumer Protection

A physical therapist assistant shall report any conduct that appears to be unethical or illegal.

7.2 Organizational Employment

A. A physical therapist assistant shall inform his/her employer(s) and/or appropriate physical therapist of any employer practice that causes him or her to be in conflict with the *Standards of Ethical Conduct for the Physical Therapist Assistant.*

B. A physical therapist assistant shall not engage in any activity that puts him or her in conflict with the Standards, regardless of directives from a physical therapist or employer.

Issued by Ethics and Judicial Committee, APTA, October 1981
Last Amended July 2001

Guidelines for Physical Therapy Documentation

Preamble

The American Physical Therapy Association (APTA) is committed to meeting the physical therapy needs of society, to meeting the needs and interests of its members, and to developing and improving the art and science of physical therapy, including practice, education, and research. To help meet these responsibilities, the APTA Board of Directors has approved the following guidelines for physical therapy documentation. It is recognized that these guidelines do not reflect all of the unique documentation requirements associated with the many specialty areas within the physical therapy profession. Applicable for both handwritten and electronic documentation systems, these guidelines are intended to be used as a foundation for the development of more specific documentation guidelines in specialty areas, while at the same time providing guidance for the physical therapy profession across all practice settings.

It is the position of APTA that physical therapist examination, evaluation, diagnosis, and prognosis shall be documented, dated, and authenticated by the physical therapist who performs the service. Intervention provided by the physical therapist or physical therapist assistant, under the direction and supervision of a physical therapist, is documented, dated, and authenticated by the physical therapist or, when permissible by law, the physical therapist assistant.

Other notations or flow charts are considered a component of the documented record but do not meet the requirements of documentation in, or of, themselves (*Position on Authority for Physical Therapy Documentation*, HOD 06-00-20-05).

Operational Definitions

Guidelines: APTA defines "guidelines" as approved, non-binding statements of advice.

Documentation: Any entry into the client record, such as consultation report, initial examination report, progress note, flow sheet/checklist that identifies the care/service provided, re-examination, or summation of care.

Authentication: The process used to verify that an entry is complete, accurate, and final. Indications of authentication can include original written signatures and computer "signatures" on secured electronic record systems only.

I. General Guidelines

A. All documentation must comply with the applicable jurisdictional/regulatory requirements.
   1. All handwritten entries shall be made in ink and will include original signatures. Electronic entries are made with appropriate security and confidentiality provisions.
   2. Charting errors should be corrected by drawing a single line through the error and initialing and dating the chart or through the appropriate mechanism for electronic documentation that clearly indicates that a change was made without deletion of the original record.
   3. Identification.
      - 3.1 Include patient's/client's full name and identification number, if applicable, on all official documents.
      - 3.2 All entries must be dated and authenticated with the provider's full name and appropriate designation (ie, PT or PTA).
      - 3.3 Documentation by graduates or others pending receipt of an unrestricted license shall be authenticated by a licensed physical therapist.
      - 3.4 Documentation by students (SPT/SPTA) in physical therapist or physical therapist assistant programs must be additionally authenticated by the physical therapist or, when permissible by law, documentation by physical therapist assistant students may be authenticated by a physical therapist assistant.
   4. Documentation should include the referral mechanism by which physical therapy services are initiated. Examples include:
      - Ex 4.1 Self-referral/direct access.
      - Ex 4.2 Request for consultation from a practitioner.

II. Initial Patient/Client Management

A. Documentation is required at the onset of each episode of physical therapy care and shall include the elements of examination, evaluation, diagnosis, and prognosis.

B. Documentation of the initial episode of physical therapy care shall include the elements of examination, a comprehensive screening and specific testing process leading to diagnostic classification, or, as appropriate, to a referral to another practitioner. The examination has three components: the patient/client history, the systems review, and tests and measures:
   1. Documentation of appropriate history:
      - 1.1 General demographics
      - 1.2 Social history
      - 1.3 Employment/work (job/school/play)
      - 1.4 Growth and development
      - 1.5 Living environment
      - 1.6 General health status (self-report, family report, caregiver report)
      - 1.7 Social/health habits (past and current)
      - 1.8 Family history
      - 1.9 Medical/surgical history
      - 1.10 Current condition(s)/Chief complaint(s)
      - 1.11 Functional status and activity level
      - 1.12 Medications
      - 1.13 Other clinical tests
   2. Documentation of systems review
      - 2.1 Documentation of physiologic and anatomical status to include the following systems:
        - *2.1.1 Cardiovascular/pulmonary*
          - 2.1.1.1 Blood pressure
          - 2.1.1.2 Edema
          - 2.1.1.3 Heart rate
          - 2.1.1.4 Respiratory rate
        - *2.1.2 Integumentary*
          - 2.1.2.1 Presence of scar formation
          - 2.1.2.2 Skin color
          - 2.1.2.3 Skin integrity
        - *2.1.3 Musculoskeletal*
          - 2.1.3.1 Gross range of motion
          - 2.1.3.2 Gross strength
          - 2.1.3.3 Gross symmetry
          - 2.1.3.4 Height
          - 2.1.3.5 Weight

2.1.4 Neuromuscular

2.1.4.1 Gross coordinated movement (eg, balance, locomotion, transfers, and transitions)

2.2 A review of communication, affect, cognition, language, and learning style.

2.2.1 Ability to make needs known

2.2.2 Consciousness

2.2.3 Orientation (person, place, time)

2.2.4 Expected emotional/behavioral responses

2.2.5 Learning preferences

3. Documentation of selection and administration of appropriate tests and measures to determine patient/client status in a number of areas and documentation of findings. The following is a list of the areas to be addressed in the documented examination and evaluation, including illustrative tests and measures for each area:

3.1 Aerobic Capacity/Endurance

Examples of examination findings include:

Ex 3.1.1 Aerobic capacity during functional activities

Ex 3.1.2 Aerobic capacity during standardized exercise test protocols

Ex 3.1.3 Cardiovascular signs and symptoms in response to increased oxygen demand with exercise or activity

Ex 3.1.4 Pulmonary signs and symptoms in response to increased oxygen demand with exercise or activity

3.2 Anthropometric Characteristics

Examples of examination findings include:

Ex 3.2.1 Body composition

Ex 3.2.2 Body dimensions

Ex 3.2.3 Edema

3.3 Arousal, Attention, and Cognition

Examples of examination findings include:

Ex 3.3.1 Arousal and attention

Ex 3.3.2 Cognition

Ex 3.3.3 Communication

Ex 3.3.4 Consciousness

Ex 3.3.5 Motivation

Ex 3.3.6 Orientation to time, person, place, and situation

Ex 3.3.7 Recall

3.4 Assistive and Adaptive Devices

Examples of examination findings include:

Ex 3.4.1 Assistive or adaptive devices and equipment use during functional activities

Ex 3.4.2 Components, alignment, fit, and ability to care for the assistive or adaptive devices and equipment

Ex 3.4.3 Remediation of impairments, functional limitations, or disabilities with use of assistive or adaptive devices and equipment

Ex. 3.4.4 Safety during use of assistive or adaptive devices and equipment

3.5 Circulation (Arterial, Venous, Lymphatic)

Examples of examination findings include:

Ex 3.5.1 Cardiovascular signs

Ex 3.5.2 Cardiovascular symptoms

Ex 3.5.3 Physiological responses to position change

3.6 Cranial and Peripheral Nerve Integrity

Examples of examination findings include:

Ex 3.6.1 Electrophysiological integrity

Ex 3.6.2 Motor distribution of the cranial nerves

Ex 3.6.3 Motor distribution of the peripheral nerves

Ex 3.6.4 Response to neural provocation

Ex 3.6.5 Response to stimuli, including auditory, gustatory, olfactory, pharyngeal, vestibular, and visual

Ex 3.6.6 Sensory distribution of the cranial nerves

Ex 3.6.7 Sensory distribution of the peripheral nerves

3.7 Environmental, Home, and Work (Job/School/Play) Barriers

Examples of examination findings include:

Ex 3.7.1 Current and potential barriers

Ex 3.7.2 Physical space and environment

3.8 Ergonomics and Body Mechanics

Examples of examination findings for ergonomics include:

Ex 3.8.1 Dexterity and coordination during work

Ex 3.8.2 Functional capacity and performance during work actions, tasks, or activities

Ex 3.8.3 Safety in work environments

Ex 3.8.4 Specific work conditions or activities

Ex 3.8.5 Tools, devices, equipment, and workstations related to work actions, tasks, or activities

Examples of examination findings for body mechanics include:

Ex 3.8.6 Body mechanics during self-care, home management, work, community, or leisure actions, tasks, or activities

3.9 Gait, Locomotion, and Balance

Examples of examination findings include:

Ex 3.9.1 Balance during functional activities with or without the use of assistive, adaptive, orthotic, protection, supportive, or prosthetic devices or equipment

Ex 3.9.2 Balance (dynamic and static) with or without the use of assistive, adaptive, orthotic, protective, supportive, or prosthetic devices or equipment

Ex 3.9.3 Gait and locomotion during functional activities with or without the use of assis tive, adaptive, orthotic, protective, supportive, or prosthetic devices or equipment

Ex 3.9.4 Gait and locomotion with or without the use of assistive, adaptive, orthotic, protective, supportive, or prosthetic devices or equipment

Ex 3.9.5 Safety during gait, locomotion, and balance

3.10 Integumentary Integrity

Examples of examination findings include:

Ex 3.10.1 Associated skin:

Ex 3.10.1.1 Activities, positioning, and postures that produce or relieve trauma to the skin

Ex 3.10.1.2 Assisitve, adaptive, orthotic, protective, supportive, or prosthetic devices and equipment that may produce or relieve trauma to the skin

Ex 3.10.1.3 Skin characteristics

Ex 3.10.2 Wound:

Ex 3.10.2.1 Activities, positioning, and postures that aggravate the wound or scar or that produce or relieve trauma

Ex 3.10.2.2 Burn

Ex 3.10.2.3 Signs of infection
Ex 3.10.2.4 Wound characteristics
Ex 3.10.2.5 Wound scar tissue characteristics

3.11 Joint Integrity and Mobility
Examples of examination findings include:
Ex 3.11.1 Joint integrity and mobility
Ex 3.11.2 Joint play movements
Ex 3.11.3 Specific body parts

3.12 Motor Function
Examples of examination findings include:
Ex 3.12.1 Dexterity, coordination, and agility
Ex 3.12.2 Electrophysiological integrity
Ex 3.12.3 Hand function
Ex 3.12.4 Initiation, modification, and control of movement patterns and voluntary postures

3.13 Muscle Performance
Examples of examination findings include:
Ex 3.13.1 Electrophysiological integrity
Ex 3.13.2 Muscle strength, power, and endurance
Ex 3.13.3 Muscle strength, power, and endurance during functional activities
Ex 3.13.4 Muscle tension

3.14 Neuromotor Development and Sensory Integration
Examples of examination findings include:
Ex 3.14.1 Acquisition and evolution of motor skills
Ex 3.14.2 Oral motor function, phonation, and speech production
Ex 3.14.3 Sensorimotor integration

3.15 Orthotic, Protective, and Supportive Devices
Examples of examination findings include:
Ex 3.15.1 Components, alignment, fit, and ability to care for the orthotic, protective, and supportive devices and equipment
Ex 3.15.2 Orthotic, protective, and supportive devices and equipment use during functional activities
Ex 3.15.3 Remediation of impairments, functional limitations, or disabilities with use of orthotic, protective, and supportive devices and equipment
Ex 3.15.4 Safety during use of orthotic, protective, and supportive devices and equipment

3.16 Pain
Examples of examination findings include:
Ex 3.16.1 Pain, soreness, and nociception
Ex 3.16.2 Pain in specific body parts

3.17 Posture
Examples of examination findings include:
Ex 3.17.1 Postural alignment and position (dynamic)
Ex 3.17.2 Postural alignment and position (static)
Ex 3.17.3 Specific body parts

3.18 Prosthetic Requirements
Examples of examination findings include:
Ex 3.18.1 Components, alignment, fit, and ability to care for prosthetic device
Ex 3.18.2 Prosthetic device use during functional activities
Ex 3.18.3 Remediation of impairments, functional limitations, or disabilities with use of the prosthetic device
Ex 3.18.4 Residual limb or adjacent segment
Ex 3.18.5 Safety during use of the prosthetic device

3.19 Range of Motion (Including Muscle Length)
Examples of examination findings include:
Ex 3.19.1 Functional ROM
Ex 3.19.2 Joint active and passive movement
Ex 3.19.3 Muscle length, soft tissue extensibility, and flexibility

3.20 Reflex Integrity
Examples of examination findings include:
Ex 3.20.1 Deep reflexes
Ex 3.20.2 Electrophysiological integrity
Ex 3.20.3 Postural reflexes and reactions, including righting, equilibrium, and protective reactions
Ex 3.20.4 Primitive reflexes and reactions
Ex 3.20.5 Resistance to passive stretch
Ex 3.20.6 Superficial reflexes and reactions

3.21 Self-Care and Home Management
Examples of examination findings include:
Ex 3.21.1 Ability to gain access to home environments
Ex 3.21.2 Ability to perform self-care and home managment activities with or without assistive, adaptive, orthotic, protective, supportive, or prosthetic devices and equipment
Ex 3.21.3 Safety in self-care and home management activities and environments

3.22 Sensory Integrity
Examples of examination findings include:
Ex 3.22.1 Combined/cortical sensations
Ex 3.22.2 Deep sensations
Ex 3.22.3 Electrophysiological integrity

3.23 Ventilation and Respiration
Examples of examination findings include:
Ex 3.23.1 Pulmonary signs of respiration/gas exchange
Ex 3.23.2 Pulmonary signs of ventilatory function
Ex 3.23.3 Pulmonary symptoms

3.24 Work (Job/School/Play), Community, and Leisure Integration or Reintegration
Examples of examination findings include:
Ex 3.24.1 Ability to assume or resume work (job/school/play), community, and leisure activities with or without assistive, adaptive, orthotic, protective, supportive, or prosthetic devices and equipment
Ex 3.24.2 Ability to gain access to work (job/school/play), community, and leisure environments
Ex 3.24.3 Safety in work (job/school/play), community, and leisure activities and environments

C. Documentation of evaluation (a dynamic process in which the physical therapist makes clinical judgements based on data gathered during the examination).

D. Documentation of diagnosis, a label that identifies the impact of a condition on function at the level of the system, especially the movement system, and at the level of the whole person in terms that can guide the prognosis, the plan of care, and intervention strategies.

E. Documentation of prognosis (determination of the level of optimal improvement that might be attained through intervention and the amount of time required to reach that level. Documentation shall include goals, outcomes, and plan of care).
1. Patient/client (and family members and significant others, if appropriate) is involved in establishing goals and outcomes.
2. All goals and outcomes are stated in measurable terms.

3. Goals and outcomes are related to impairments, functional limitations, and disabilities and the changes in health, wellness, and fitness needs identified in the examination.
4. The plan of care:
   4.1 Is based on the examination, evaluation, diagnosis, and prognosis.
   4.2. Identifies goals and outcomes of all proposed interventions.
   4.3 Describes the proposed interventions taking into consideration the expectations of the patient/client and others as appropriate.
   4.4. Includes frequency and duration of all proposed interventions to achieve the anticipated goals and expected outcomes.
   4.5 Involves appropriate coordination and communication of care with other professionals/services.
   4.6 Includes plan for discharge.

F. Authentication by and appropriate designation of the physical therapist.

III. Documentation of the Continuation of Care

A. Documentation of intervention or services provided and current patient/client status.
1. Documentation is required for every visit/encounter.
   1.1 Authentication and appropriate designation of the physical therapist or the physical therapist assistant providing the service under the direction and supervision of a physical therapist.
2. Documentation of each visit/encounter shall include the following elements:
   2.1 Patient/client self-report (as appropriate).
   2.2 Identification of specific interventions provided, including frequency, intensity, and duration as appropriate.
   Examples include:
   2.2.1 Knee extension, 3 sets, 10 repetitions, 10-lb weight.
   2.2.2 Transfer training bed to chair with sliding board.
   2.3 Equipment provided.
   2.4 Changes in patient/client status as they relate to the plan of care.
   2.5 Adverse reaction to interventions, if any.
   2.6 Factors that modify frequency or intensity of intervention and progression toward anticipated goals, including patient/client adherence to patient/client-related instructions.
   2.7 Communication/consultation with providers/patient/client/family/significant other.

B. Documentation of re-examination
1. Documentation of re-examination is provided as appropriate to evaluate progress and to modify or redirect intervention.
2. Documentation of re-examination shall include the following elements:
   2.1 Documentation of selected components of examination to update patient's/client's status.
   2.2 Interpretation of findings and, when indicated, revision of goals and outcomes.
   2.3 When indicated, revision of plan of care as directly correlated with goals and outcomes as documented.
   2.4 Authentication by and appropriate designation of the physical therapist.

IV. Documentation of Summation of Episode of Care

A. Documentation is required following conclusion of the current episode in the physical therapy intervention sequence.

B. Documentation of the summation of the episode of care shall include the following elements:
1. Criteria for termination of services:
   Examples of discharge include:
   Ex 1.1 Anticipated goals and expected outcomes have been achieved.
   Examples of discontinuation include:
   Ex 1.2 Patient/client, caregiver, or legal guardian declines to continue intervention.
   Ex 1.3 Patient/client is unable to continue to progress toward anticipated goals due to medical or psychosocial complications or because financial/insurance resources have been expended.
   Ex 1.4 Physical therapist determines that the patient/client will no longer benefit from physical therapy.
2. Current physical/functional status.
3. Degree of goals and outcomes achieved and reasons for goals and outcomes not being achieved.
4. Discharge or discontinuation plan that includes written and verbal communication related to the patient's/client's continuing care.
   Examples include:
   Ex 4.1 Home program.
   Ex 4.2 Referrals for additional services.
   Ex 4.3 Recommendations for follow-up physical therapy care.
   Ex 4.4 Family and caregiver training.
   Ex 4.5 Equipment provided.
5. Authentication by and appropriate designation of the physical therapist.

Additional References:

1 *Direction and Supervision of the Physical Therapist Assistant* (HOD 06-00-16-27).

2 *Comprehensive Accreditation Manual for Hospitals.* Oakbrook Terrace, Ill: Joint Commission on the Accreditation of Healthcare Organizations; 1996.

3 *Glossary of Terms Related to Information Security.* Schaumburg, Ill: Computer-based Patient Record Institute; 1996.

4 *Guidelines for Establishing Information Security Policies at Organizations Using Computer-based Patient Records.* Schaumburg, Ill: Computer-based Patient Record Institute; 1995.

5 *Current Procedural Terminology.* Chicago, Ill: American Medical Association (AMA); 2000.

6 *Coding and Payment Guide for the Physical Therapist.* Washington, DC: St Anthony's Publishing; 2000.

7 Healthcare Finance Administration (HCFA): Minimal Data Set (MDS) Regulations, HCFA/AMA Documentation Guidelines, Home Health Regulations. Available at: www.hcfa.gov.

8 State Practice Acts. Available at: www.fsbpt.org.

Adopted by the Board of Directors, APTA, March 1993
Amended February 2002, November 2001, March 2000, November 1998, March 1997, March 1995, November 1994, June 1993, March 1993

APTA documents are revised on a regular basis. For the most recent revisions, contact www.apta.org or APTA's Service Center at 800/399-2782, ext. 3395.

Documentation Template

As a framework for organizing the patient/client management that physical therapists provide—and as the source of standardized terminology for communicating what physical therapists do—the *Guide to Physical Therapist Practice* provides a logical structure for documentation.

The template includes an inpatient history form, which would be completed by the physical therapist; an outpatient history form, which would be completed by the patient/client; and the forms that apply to both inpatient and outpatient settings: systems review, tests and measures, evaluation, diagnosis, prognosis, anticipated goals, expected outcomes, interventions, and discharge plan.

DOCUMENTATION TEMPLATE FOR PHYSICAL THERAPIST PATIENT/CLIENT MANAGEMENT
Inpatient Form, Page 1

Today's Date: ____________
Patient ID#: ____________

IDENTIFICATION INFORMATION

1 **Name:**

a Last ____________

b First ____________ c MI ____ d Jr/Sr ____

2 **Admission Date:** Month ☐☐ Day ☐☐ Year ☐☐☐☐

3 **Date of Birth:** Month ☐☐ Day ☐☐ Year ☐☐☐☐

4 **Sex:** a ☐ Male b ☐ Female

5 **Dominant Hand:** a ☐ Right b ☐ Left c ☐ Unknown

6 **Race**
- a ☐ American Indian or Alaska Native
- b ☐ Asian
- c ☐ Black or African American
- d ☐ Hispanic or Latino
- e ☐ Native Hawaiian or Other Pacific Islander
- f ☐ White

7 **Ethnicity**
- a ☐ Hispanic or Latino
- b ☐ Not Hispanic or Latino

8 **Language**
- a ☐ English understood
- b ☐ Interpreter needed
- c ☐ Primary language: ____________

9 **Education**
- a Highest grade completed (Circle one): 1 2 3 4 5 6 7 8 9 10 11 12
- b ☐ Some college/technical school
- c ☐ College graduate
- d ☐ Graduate school/advanced degree

10 **Has patient completed an advance directive?** a ☐ Yes b ☐ No

11 **Referred by:** ____________

12 **Reasons for referral to physical therapy:** ____________

SOCIAL HISTORY

13 **Cultural/Religious**
Any customs or religious beliefs or wishes that might affect care?
____

14 **Lives(d) With**

	(1)–Admission	(2)–Expected at Discharge
a Alone	☐	☐
b Spouse only	☐	☐
c Spouse and other(s)	☐	☐
d Child (not spouse)	☐	☐
e Other relative(s) (not spouse or children)	☐	☐
f Group setting	☐	☐
g Personal care attendant	☐	☐
h Unknown	☐	☐
i Other ____________		

15 **Available Social Supports (family/friends)**
0=No 1=Possibly yes 2=Definitely

	Now	Willing/Able Postdischarge
a Emotional support	☐	☐
b Intermittent physical support with ADLs or IADLs—less than daily	☐ ☐	☐ ☐
c Intermittent physical support with ADLs or IADLs—daily	☐	☐
d Full-time physical support (as needed) with ADLs or IADLs	☐	☐
e All or most of necessary transportation	☐	☐

16 **Caregiver Status** Presence of family member/friend willing and able to assist patient/client? a ☐ Yes b ☐ No

17 **EMPLOYMENT/WORK (Job/School/Play)**
- a ☐ Working full-time outside of home
- b ☐ Working part-time outside of home
- c ☐ Working full-time from home
- d ☐ Working part-time from home
- e ☐ Homemaker
- f ☐ Student
- g ☐ Retired
- h ☐ Unemployed
- i Occupation: ____________

LIVING ENVIRONMENT

18 **Devices and Equipment (eg, cane, glasses, hearing aids, walker)**
____
____
____
____
____
____

19 **Type of Residence**

	(1)–Admission	(2)–Expected at Discharge
a Private home	☐	☐
b Private apartment	☐	☐
c Rented room	☐	☐
d Board and care/assisted living/group home	☐	☐
e Homeless (with or without shelter)	☐	☐
f Long-term care facility (nursing home)	☐	☐
g Hospice	☐	☐
h Unknown	☐	☐
i Other ____________		

20 **Environment**

a Stairs, no railing	☐	☐
b Stairs, railing	☐	☐
c Ramps	☐	☐
d Elevator	☐	☐
e Uneven terrain	☐	☐
f Other obstacles: ____________		

21 **Past Use of Community Services 0=No 1=Unknown 2=Yes**

a Day services/programs	☐	f Mental health services	☐
b Home health services	☐	g Respiratory therapy	☐
c Homemaking services	☐	h Therapies—PT, OT, SLP	☐
d Hospice	☐	i Other (eg, volunteer) ____________	☐
e Meals on Wheels	☐		

22 **GENERAL HEALTH STATUS**
- a Patient/client rates health as:
  ☐ Excellent ☐ Good ☐ Fair ☐ Poor
- b Major life changes during past year? (1) ☐ Yes (2) ☐ No

23 SOCIAL/HEALTH HABITS (Past and Current)

a Alcohol

(1) How many days per week does patient/client drink beer, wine, or other alcoholic beverages, on average? ______

(2) If one beer, one glass of wine, or one cocktail equals one drink, how many drinks does patient/client have on an average day? _____

b Smoking

(1) Currently smokes tobacco?

(a) ☐ Yes

1. ☐ Cigarettes: # of packs per day _____

2. ☐ Cigars/pipes: # per day ____

(b) ☐ No

(2) Smoked in past? (a) ☐ Yes Year quit: ☐☐☐☐

(b) ☐ No

c Exercise

(1) Exercises beyond normal daily activities and chores?

(a) ☐ Yes

Describe the exercise: ________________________

1. On average, how many days per week does patient/client exercise or do physical activity? _____

2. For how many minutes, on an average day? __

(b) ☐ No

24 FAMILY HISTORY

Condition:	Relationship to Patient/Client:	Age at Onset (if known):
a Heart disease	______	______
b Hypertension	______	______
c Stroke	______	______
d Diabetes	______	______
e Cancer	______	______
f Other: ______	______	______
______	______	______

25 PATIENT/CLIENT MEDICAL/SURGICAL HISTORY: ____

____

____

____

____

____

26 FUNCTIONAL STATUS/ACTIVITY LEVEL (Check all that apply):

a ☐ Difficulty with locomotion/movement:

(1) ☐ Bed mobility

(2) ☐ Transfers

(3) ☐ Gait (walking)

(a) ☐ On level

(b) ☐ On stairs

(c) ☐ On ramps

(d) ☐ On uneven terrain

b ☐ Difficulty with self-care (such as bathing, dressing, eating, toileting)

c ☐ Difficulty with home management (such as household chores, shopping, driving/transportation)

d ☐ Difficulty with community and work activities/integration

(1) ☐ Work/school

(2) ☐ Recreation or play activity

27 MEDICATIONS (List): ________________________

____

____

____

____

____

____

____

____

____

28 OTHER CLINICAL TESTS (List):

	Month	Year	Findings
______	☐☐	☐☐☐☐	______
______	☐☐	☐☐☐☐	______
______	☐☐	☐☐☐☐	______
______	☐☐	☐☐☐☐	______

DOCUMENTATION TEMPLATE FOR PHYSICAL THERAPIST PATIENT/CLIENT MANAGEMENT

Outpatient Form 1, Page 1

Today's Date: ____________
Patient ID#: ____________

1 **Name:**

a Last

b First c MI d Jr/Sr

2 **Street Address:** ____________

City State Zip

3 **Date of Birth:** Month Day Year ☐☐ ☐☐ ☐☐☐☐

4 **Sex:** a ☐ Male b ☐ Female

5 **Are you:** a ☐ Right-handed b ☐ Left-handed

6 **Type of Insurance:** a ☐ Insurer ____________
b ☐ Workers' Comp c ☐ Medicare d ☐ Self-pay e ☐ Other

7 **Race:**
a ☐ American Indian or Alaska Native
b ☐ Asian
c ☐ Black or African American
d ☐ Hispanic or Latino
e ☐ Native Hawaiian or Other Pacific Islander
f ☐ White

8 **Ethnicity:**
a ☐ Hispanic or Latino
b ☐ Not Hispanic or Latino

9 **Language:**
a ☐ English understood
b ☐ Interpreter needed
c ☐ Language you speak most often: ____________

10 **Education:**
a Highest grade completed (Circle one): 1 2 3 4 5 6 7 8 9 10 11 12
b ☐ Some college / technical school
c ☐ College graduate
d ☐ Graduate school / advanced degree

SOCIAL HISTORY

11 **Cultural/Religious:** Any customs or religious beliefs or wishes that might affect care?
____

12 **With whom do you live:**
a ☐ Alone
b ☐ Spouse only
c ☐ Spouse and other(s)
d ☐ Child (not spouse)
e ☐ Other relative(s) (not spouse or children)
f ☐ Group setting
g ☐ Personal care attendant
h ☐ Other:

13 **Have you completed an advance directive?** a ☐ Yes b ☐ No

14 **Who referred you to the physical therapist?**
____

15 **Employment/Work (Job/School/Play)**
a ☐ Working full-time outside of home
b ☐ Working part-time outside of home
c ☐ Working full-time from home
d ☐ Working part-time from home
e ☐ Homemaker f ☐ Student g ☐ Retired h ☐ Unemployed
i Occupation: ____________

LIVING ENVIRONMENT

16 **Does your home have:**
a ☐ Stairs, no railing
b ☐ Stairs, railing
c ☐ Ramps
d ☐ Elevator
e ☐ Uneven terrain
f ☐ Assistive devices (eg, bathroom): ____________
g ☐ Any obstacles: ____________

17 **Do you use:**
a ☐ Cane
b ☐ Walker or rollator
c ☐ Manual wheelchair
d ☐ Motorized wheelchair
e ☐ Glasses, hearing aids
f ☐ Other: ____________

18 **Where do you live:**
a ☐ Private home
b ☐ Private apartment
c ☐ Rented room
d ☐ Board and care / assisted living / group home
e ☐ Homeless (with or without shelter)
f ☐ Long-term care facility (nursing home)
g ☐ Hospice
h ☐ Other: ____________

19 **GENERAL HEALTH STATUS**
a Please rate your health:
(1) ☐ Excellent (2) ☐ Good (3) ☐ Fair (4) ☐ Poor
b Have you had any major life changes during past year? (eg, new baby, job change, death of a family member) (1) ☐ Yes (2) ☐ No

20 **SOCIAL/HEALTH HABITS**
a Smoking
(1) Currently smoke tobacco? (a) ☐ Yes 1. ☐ Cigarettes: # of packs per day __
2. ☐ Cigars/Pipes: # per day __
(b) ☐ No
(2) Smoked in past? (a) ☐ Yes Year quit: ☐☐☐☐ (b) ☐ No

b Alcohol
(1) How many days per week do you drink beer, wine, or other alcoholic beverages, on average? ___
(2) If one beer, one glass of wine, or one cocktail equals one drink, how many drinks do you have on an average day? ___

c Exercise
Do you exercise beyond normal daily activities and chores?
(a) ☐ Yes Describe the exercise: ____________
1. On average, how many days per week do you exercise or do physical activity? ______
2. For how many minutes, on an average day? ____
(b) ☐ No

21 **FAMILY HISTORY** (Indicate whether mother, father, brother/sister, aunt/uncle, or grandmother/grandfather, and age of onset if known)
a Heart disease: ____________
b Hypertension: ____________
c Stroke: ____________
d Diabetes: ____________
e Cancer: ____________
f Psychological: ____________
g Arthritis: ____________
h Osteoporosis: ____________
i Other: ____________

22 MEDICAL/SURGICAL HISTORY

a Please check if you have ever had:

(1) ☐ Arthritis
(2) ☐ Broken bones/fractures
(3) ☐ Osteoporosis
(4) ☐ Blood disorders
(5) ☐ Circulation/vascular problems
(6) ☐ Heart problems
(7) ☐ High blood pressure
(8) ☐ Lung problems
(9) ☐ Stroke
(10) ☐ Diabetes/high blood sugar
(11) ☐ Low blood sugar/hypoglycemia
(12) ☐ Head injury
(13) ☐ Multiple sclerosis
(14) ☐ Muscular dystrophy
(15) ☐ Parkinson disease
(16) ☐ Seizures/epilepsy
(17) ☐ Allergies
(18) ☐ Developmental or growth problems
(19) ☐ Thyroid problems
(20) ☐ Cancer
(21) ☐ Infectious disease (eg, tuberculosis, hepatitis)
(22) ☐ Kidney problems
(23) ☐ Repeated infections
(24) ☐ Ulcers/stomach problems
(25) ☐ Skin diseases
(26) ☐ Depression
(27) ☐ Other:_______________

b Within the past year, have you had any of the following symptoms? (Check all that apply)

(1) ☐ Chest pain
(2) ☐ Heart palpitations
(3) ☐ Cough
(4) ☐ Hoarseness
(5) ☐ Shortness of breath
(6) ☐ Dizziness or blackouts
(7) ☐ Coordination problems
(8) ☐ Weakness in arms or legs
(9) ☐ Loss of balance
(10) ☐ Difficulty walking
(11) ☐ Joint pain or swelling
(12) ☐ Pain at night
(13) ☐ Difficulty sleeping
(14) ☐ Loss of appetite
(15) ☐ Nausea/vomiting
(16) ☐ Difficulty swallowing
(17) ☐ Bowel problems
(18) ☐ Weight loss/gain
(19) ☐ Urinary problems
(20) ☐ Fever/chills/sweats
(21) ☐ Headaches
(22) ☐ Hearing problems
(23) ☐ Vision problems
(24) ☐ Other:_______________

c Have you ever had surgery? (1) ☐ Yes (2) ☐ No
If yes, please describe, and include dates:

	Month	Year
_______________	☐☐	☐☐☐☐
_______________	☐☐	☐☐☐☐
_______________	☐☐	☐☐☐☐

For men only: d Have you been diagnosed with prostate disease?
(1) ☐ Yes (2) ☐ No

For women only:
Have you been diagnosed with:

e Pelvic inflammatory disease?
(1) ☐ Yes (2) ☐ No

f Endometriosis?
(1) ☐ Yes (2) ☐ No

g Trouble with your period?
(1) ☐ Yes (2) ☐ No

h Complicated pregnancies or deliveries?
(1) ☐ Yes (2) ☐ No

i Pregnant, or think you might be pregnant?
(1) ☐ Yes (2) ☐ No

j Other gynecological or obstetrical difficulties?
(1) ☐ Yes (2) ☐ No
If yes, please describe:
____

23 CURRENT CONDITION(S)/CHIEF COMPLAINT(S)

a Describe the problem(s) for which you seek physical therapy:
____
____

b When did the problem(s) begin (date)? Month ☐☐ Year ☐☐☐☐

c What happened?_______________
____

d Have you ever had the problem(s) before?

(1) ☐ Yes

(a) What did you do for the problem(s)? _______________
____

(b) Did the problem(s) get better?
1. ☐ Yes 2. ☐ No

(c) About how long did the problem(s) last? _______________

(2) ☐ No

23 Current Condition(s)/Chief Complaint(s) (continued)

e How are you taking care of the problem(s) now? _______________
____

f What makes the problem(s) better? _______________
____

g What makes the problem(s) worse? _______________
____
____

h What are your goals for physical therapy? _______________
____

i Are you seeing anyone else for the problem(s)? (Check all that apply)

(1) ☐ Acupuncturist
(2) ☐ Cardiologist
(3) ☐ Chiropractor
(4) ☐ Dentist
(5) ☐ Family practitioner
(6) ☐ Internist
(7) ☐ Massage therapist
(8) ☐ Neurologist
(9) ☐ Obstetrician/gynecologist
(10) ☐ Occupational therapist
(11) ☐ Orthopedist
(12) ☐ Osteopath
(13) ☐ Pediatrician
(14) ☐ Podiatrist
(15) ☐ Primary care physician
(16) ☐ Rheumatologist
Other: _______________

24 FUNCTIONAL STATUS/ACTIVITY LEVEL (Check all that apply)

a ☐ Difficulty with locomotion/movement:
(1) ☐ Bed mobility
(2) ☐ Transfers (such as moving from bed to chair, from bed to commode)
(3) ☐ Gait (walking)
(a) ☐ On level
(b) ☐ On stairs
(c) ☐ On ramps
(d) ☐ On uneven terrain

b ☐ Difficulty with self-care (such as bathing, dressing, eating, toileting)

c ☐ Difficulty with home management (such as household chores, shopping, driving/transportation, care of dependents)

d ☐ Difficulty with community and work activities/integration
(1) ☐ Work/school
(2) ☐ Recreation or play activity

25 MEDICATIONS

a Do you take any prescription medications? (1) ☐ Yes (2) ☐ No
If yes, please list: _______________
____

b Do you take any nonprescription medications? (Check all that apply)

(1) ☐ Advil/Aleve
(2) ☐ Antacids
(3) ☐ Ibuprofen/Naproxen
(4) ☐ Antihistamines
(5) ☐ Aspirin
(6) ☐ Decongestants
(7) ☐ Herbal supplements
(8) ☐ Tylenol
(9) ☐ Other: _______________
____
____

c Have you taken any medications previously for the condition for which you are seeing the physical therapist?
(1) ☐ Yes (2) ☐ No If yes, please list:
____

26 OTHER CLINICAL TESTS

Within the past year, have you had any of the following tests? (Check all that apply)

a ☐ Angiogram
b ☐ Arthroscopy
c ☐ Biopsy
d ☐ Blood tests
e ☐ Bone scan
f ☐ Bronchoscopy
g ☐ CT scan
h ☐ Doppler ultrasound
i ☐ Echocardiogram
j ☐ EEG (electroencephalogram)
k ☐ EKG (electrocardiogram)
l ☐ EMG (electromyogram)
m ☐ Mammogram
n ☐ MRI
o ☐ Myelogram
p ☐ NCV (nerve conduction velocity)
q ☐ Pap smear
r ☐ Pulmonary function test
s ☐ Spinal tap
t ☐ Stool tests
u ☐ Stress test (eg, treadmill, bicycle)
v ☐ Urine tests
w ☐ X-rays
x ☐ Other:_______________

DOCUMENTATION TEMPLATE FOR PHYSICAL THERAPIST PATIENT/CLIENT MANAGEMENT

Systems Review

	Not Impaired	Impaired
CARDIOVASCULAR/PULMONARY SYSTEM	☐	☐

Blood pressure: ____________________

Edema: ____________________

Heart rate: ____________________

Respiratory rate: ____________________

	Not Impaired	Impaired
INTEGUMENTARY SYSTEM	☐	☐

Integrity

Pliability (texture): ____________________

Presence of scar formation: ____________________

Skin color: ____________________

Skin integrity: ____________________

MUSCULOSKELETAL SYSTEM	Not Impaired	Impaired
Gross Range of Motion	☐	☐
Gross Strength	☐	☐
Gross Symmetry	☐	☐

Standing: ____________________

Sitting: ____________________

Activity specific: ____________________

Other: ____________________

Height ____________________

Weight ____________________

NEUROMUSCULAR SYSTEM

Gross Coordinated Movements	Not Impaired	Impaired
Balance	☐	☐
Gait	☐	☐
Locomotion	☐	☐
Transfers	☐	☐
Transitions	☐	☐
Motor function (motor control, motor learning)	☐	☐

COMMUNICATION, AFFECT, COGNITION, LEARNING STYLE

	Not Impaired	Impaired
Communication (eg, age-appropriate)	☐	☐
Orientation x 3 (person/place/time)	☐	☐
Emotional/behavioral responses	☐	☐

Learning barriers:

- ☐ None
- ☐ Vision
- ☐ Hearing
- ☐ Unable to read
- ☐ Unable to understand what is read
- ☐ Language/needs interpreter
- ☐ Other: ____________________

Education needs:

- ☐ Disease process
- ☐ Safety
- ☐ Use of devices/equipment
- ☐ Activities of daily living
- ☐ Exercise program
- ☐ Other: ____________________

How does patient/client best learn? ☐ Pictures ☐ Reading ☐ Listening ☐ Demonstration ☐ Other: ____________________

DOCUMENTATION TEMPLATE FOR PHYSICAL THERAPIST PATIENT/CLIENT MANAGEMENT

Tests and Measures

KEY TO TESTS AND MEASURES:

1 Aerobic Capacity/Endurance
2 Anthropometric Characteristics
3 Arousal, Attention, and Cognition
4 Assistive and Adaptive Devices
5 Circulation (Arterial, Venous, Lymphatic)
6 Cranial and Peripheral Nerve Integrity
7 Environmental, Home, and Work (Job/School/Play) Barriers
8 Ergonomics and Body Mechanics
9 Gait, Locomotion, and Balance
10 Integumentary Integrity
11 Joint Integrity and Mobility
12 Motor Function (Motor Control and Motor Learning)
13 Muscle Performance (Including Strength, Power, and Endurance)
14 Neuromotor Development and Sensory Integration
15 Orthotic, Protective, and Supportive Devices
16 Pain
17 Posture
18 Prosthetic Requirements
19 Range of Motion (Including Muscle Length)
20 Reflex Integrity
21 Self-Care and Home Management (Including Activities of Daily Living and Instrumental Activities of Daily Living)
22 Sensory Integrity
23 Ventilation and Respiration/Gas Exchange
24 Work (Job/School/Play), Community, and Leisure Integration or Reintegration (Including Instrumental Activities of Daily Living)

NOTES:

DOCUMENTATION TEMPLATE FOR PHYSICAL THERAPIST PATIENT/CLIENT MANAGEMENT

Evaluation

PREFERRED PHYSICAL THERAPIST PRACTICE PATTERNS℠

DIAGNOSIS:

Musculoskeletal Patterns

- ☐ A: Primary Prevention/Risk Reduction for Skeletal Demineralization
- ☐ B: Impaired Posture
- ☐ C: Impaired Muscle Performance
- ☐ D: Impaired Joint Mobility, Motor Function, Muscle Performance, and Range of Motion Associated With Connective Tissue Dysfunction
- ☐ E: Impaired Joint Mobility, Motor Function, Muscle Performance, and Range of Motion Associated With Localized Inflammation
- ☐ F: Impaired Joint Mobility, Motor Function, Muscle Performance, Range of Motion, and Reflex Integrity Associated With Spinal Disorders
- ☐ G: Impaired Joint Mobility, Muscle Performance, and Range of Motion Associated With Fracture
- ☐ H: Impaired Joint Mobility, Motor Function, Muscle Performance, and Range of Motion Associated With Joint Arthroplasty
- ☐ I: Impaired Joint Mobility, Motor Function, Muscle Performance, and Range of Motion Associated With Bony or Soft Tissue Surgery
- ☐ J: Impaired Motor Function, Muscle Performance, Range of Motion, Gait, Locomotion, and Balance Associated With Amputation

Neuromuscular Patterns

- ☐ A: Primary Prevention/Risk Reduction for Loss of Balance and Falling
- ☐ B: Impaired Neuromotor Development
- ☐ C: Impaired Motor Function and Sensory Integrity Associated With Nonprogressive Disorders of the Central Nervous System—Congenital Origin or Acquired in Infancy or Childhood
- ☐ D: Impaired Motor Function and Sensory Integrity Associated With Nonprogressive Disorders of the Central Nervous System—Acquired in Adolescence or Adulthood
- ☐ E: Impaired Motor Function and Sensory Integrity Associated With Progressive Disorders of the Central Nervous System
- ☐ F: Impaired Peripheral Nerve Integrity and Muscle Performance Associated With Peripheral Nerve Injury
- ☐ G: Impaired Motor Function and Sensory Integrity Associated With Acute or Chronic Polyneuropathies
- ☐ H: Impaired Motor Function, Peripheral Nerve Integrity, and Sensory Integrity Associated With Nonprogressive Disorders of the Spinal Cord
- ☐ I: Impaired Arousal, Range of Motion, and Motor Control Associated With Coma, Near Coma, or Vegetative State

Cardiovascular/Pulmonary Patterns

- ☐ A: Primary Prevention/Risk Reduction for Cardiovascular/Pulmonary Disorders
- ☐ B: Impaired Aerobic Capacity/Endurance Associated With Deconditioning
- ☐ C: Impaired Ventilation, Respiration/Gas Exchange, and Aerobic Capacity/Endurance Associated With Airway Clearance Dysfunction
- ☐ D: Impaired Aerobic Capacity/Endurance Associated With Cardiovascular Pump Dysfunction or Failure
- ☐ E: Impaired Ventilation and Respiration/Gas Exchange Associated With Ventilatory Pump Dysfunction or Failure
- ☐ F: Impaired Ventilation and Respiration/Gas Exchange Associated With Respiratory Failure
- ☐ G: Impaired Ventilation, Respiration/Gas Exchange, and Aerobic Capacity/Endurance Associated With Respiratory Failure in the Neonate
- ☐ H: Impaired Circulation and Anthropometric Dimensions Associated With Lymphatic System Disorders

Integumentary Patterns

- ☐ A: Primary Prevention/Risk Reduction for Integumentary Disorders
- ☐ B: Impaired Integumentary Integrity Associated With Superficial Skin Involvement
- ☐ C: Impaired Integumentary Integrity Associated With Partial-Thickness Skin Involvement and Scar Formation
- ☐ D: Impaired Integumentary Integrity Associated With Full-Thickness Skin Involvement and Scar Formation
- ☐ E: Impaired Integumentary Integrity Associated With Skin Involvement Extending Into Fascia, Muscle, or Bone and Scar Formation

PROGNOSIS: ____

____

____

____

____

____

____

____

____

____

____

DOCUMENTATION TEMPLATE FOR PHYSICAL THERAPIST PATIENT/CLIENT MANAGEMENT

Plan of Care

Anticipated Goals: ______________________________

____

____

____

____

Expected Outcomes: ______________________________

____

____

____

Interventions: ______________________________

____

____

____

____

Frequency of Visits/Duration of Episode of Care:

____

____

____

Education (including safety, exercise, and disease information): ______________________________

____

____

Who was educated? ☐ Patient/client ☐ Family (name and relationship): ______________________________

How did patient/family demonstrate learning:

- ☐ Patient/client verbalized understanding
- ☐ Family/significant other verbalized understanding
- ☐ Patient/client demonstrated correctly
- ☐ Demonstration was unsuccessful (describe): ______________________________

____

____

Discharge Plan: ______________________________

____

____

____

____

____

____

____

____

____

Patient/Client Satisfaction

Physical therapists recognize the importance of patient/client satisfaction and value patient/client feedback. Health care providers, in general, must rely on sources of information that include the perspective of the patient/client in the definition of quality of care.

In 2000, the American Physical Therapy Association published an instrument to measure satisfaction following physical therapy intervention.[1] Other instruments, specific to physical therapist practice, have been published or are under development.[2]

References

1 Goldstein MS, Elliott SD, Guccione AA. The development of an instrument to measure satisfaction with physical therapy. *Phys Ther.* 2000;80:853-863.

2 Roush SE, Sonstroem RJ. Development of the Physical Therapy Outpatient Satisfaction Survey (PTOPS). *Phys Ther*. 1999;79:159-170.

APTA's Physical Therapy Patient Satisfaction Questionnaire[a]

Dear Patient/Client,

You recently received physical therapy services at our facility. Because we strive to deliver the best possible physical therapy services, we are interested in learning from patients/clients how we might improve or enhance our services. Please take a few minutes to complete and return this questionnaire.

Please place an X in the appropriate box to indicate your rating, or answer the descriptive questions on the appropriate line. Any additional comments you wish to make are welcome; write in the "Comments" section at the end of the questionnaire, or attach additional pages if you require more space. Please return the questionnaire to us at your earliest convenience.

Thank you very much for your feedback!

Descriptive Questions

1. Your age: _____ Years
2. Your sex: ☐ Male ☐ Female
3. How did you learn about this facility? (*Check all that apply.*)
   - ☐ Physician
   - ☐ Friend
   - ☐ Telephone book
   - ☐ Insurance company recommendation
   - ☐ Former patient
   - ☐ Other, please indicate ______________________________
4. Was this your first experience with physical therapy? ☐ Yes ☐ No
5. Was this your first experience with this facility? ☐ Yes ☐ No
6. Please check the location of the problem for which you received physical therapy. (*Check all that apply.*)
   - ☐ Neck
   - ☐ Lower back
   - ☐ Shoulder
   - ☐ Elbow
   - ☐ Hip
   - ☐ Foot
   - ☐ Hand
   - ☐ Knee
   - ☐ Other, please indicate ______________________________

Please rate your degree of satisfaction with each of the following statements. *(1=strongly disagree, 2=disagree, 3=neither agree nor disagree, 4=agree, 5=strongly agree. Please check 9 if you have no opinion on the subject.)*

	1	2	3	4	5	9
7. My privacy was respected during my physical therapy care.	☐	☐	☐	☐	☐	☐
8. My physical therapist was courteous.	☐	☐	☐	☐	☐	☐
9. All other staff members were courteous.	☐	☐	☐	☐	☐	☐
10. The clinic scheduled appointments at convenient times.	☐	☐	☐	☐	☐	☐
11. I was satisfied with the treatment provided by my physical therapist.	☐	☐	☐	☐	☐	☐
12. My first visit for physical therapy was scheduled quickly.	☐	☐	☐	☐	☐	☐
13. It was easy to schedule visits after my first appointment.	☐	☐	☐	☐	☐	☐
14. I was seen promptly when I arrived for treatment.	☐	☐	☐	☐	☐	☐
15. The location of the facility was convenient for me.	☐	☐	☐	☐	☐	☐
16. My bills were accurate.	☐	☐	☐	☐	☐	☐
17. I was satisfied with the services provided by my physical therapist assistant(s).	☐	☐	☐	☐	☐	☐
18. Parking was available for me.	☐	☐	☐	☐	☐	☐
19. My physical therapist understood my problem or condition.	☐	☐	☐	☐	☐	☐
20. The instructions my physical therapist gave me were helpful.	☐	☐	☐	☐	☐	☐
21. I was satisfied with the overall quality of my physical therapy care.	☐	☐	☐	☐	☐	☐
22. I would recommend this facility to family or friends.	☐	☐	☐	☐	☐	☐
23. I would return to this facility if I required physical therapy care in the future.	☐	☐	☐	☐	☐	☐
24. The cost of the physical therapy treatment received was reasonable.	☐	☐	☐	☐	☐	☐
25. If I had to, I would pay for these physical therapy services myself.	☐	☐	☐	☐	☐	☐
27. Overall, I was satisfied with my experience with physical therapy.	☐	☐	☐	☐	☐	☐

Comments:

____

____

____

____

[a] Adapted with permission of the American Physical Therapy Association from Goldstein MS, Elliott SD, Guccione AA. The development of an instrument to measure satisfaction with physical therapy. *Phys Ther*. 2000;80:853–863.

Numerical Index to ICD-9-CM Codes

100

200

300

400

442 Other aneurysm . . . 4J, 5D, 5I
  442.3 Of artery of lower extremity . . . 4J
  442.8 Of other specified artery . . . 5D, 5I
443 Other peripheral vascular disease . . . 4C, 4J, 6B, 6D, 7A, 7D, 7E
  443.0 Raynaud's syndrome . . . 7A
  443.1 Thromboangiitis obliterans [Buerger's disease] . . . 7A, 7D, 7E
  443.9 Peripheral vascular disease, unspecified . . . 6B, 7A
444 Arterial embolism and thrombosis . . . 5D, 5I, 6D
  444.9 Of unspecified artery . . . 5D, 5I
447 Other disorders of arteries and arterioles . . . 5D, 5I
  447.1 Stricture of artery . . . 5D, 5I
454 Varicose veins of lower extremities . . . 7A, 7B, 7C, 7D, 7E
454 With ulcer . . . 7C, 7D, 7E
  454.1 With inflammation . . . 7B
  454.2 With ulcer and inflammation . . . 7C, 7D, 7E
457 Noninfectious disorders of lymphatic channels . . . 6H, 7A
  457.0 Postmastectomy lymphedema syndrome . . . 6H, 7A
  457.1 Other lymphedema . . . 6H, 7A
  457.8 Other noninfectious disorders of lymphatic channels . . . 6H
  457.9 Unspecified noninfectious disorder of lymphatic channels . . . 6H
459 Other disorders of circulatory system . . . 4J, 7A
  459.1 Postphlebitic syndrome . . . 7A
  459.8 Other specified disorders of circulatory system . . . 4J, 7A
  459.81 Venous (peripheral) insufficiency, unspecified . . . 7A
  459.9 Unspecified circulatory system disorder . . . 7A
480 Viral pneumonia . . . 6F
481 Pneumococcal pneumonia [Streptococcus pneumoniae pneumonia] . . . 6F
482 Other bacterial pneumonia . . . 6B, 6C, 6F
  482.2 Pneumonia due to Hemophilus influenzae . . . 6B, 6C
  482.9 Bacterial pneumonia unspecified . . . 6B, 6C
483 Pneumonia due to other specified organism . . . 6F
484 Pneumonia in infectious diseases classified elsewhere . . 6F
485 Bronchopneumonia, organism unspecified . . . 6F
486 Pneumonia, organism unspecified . . . 6F
491 Chronic bronchitis . . . 6B, 6C, 6F
  491.8 Other chronic bronchitis . . . 6C
  491.9 Unspecified chronic bronchitis . . . 6B, 6C
492 Emphysema . . . 6B, 6C, 6E, 6F
  492.8 Other emphysema . . . 6B, 6C, 6E, 6F
493 Asthma . . . 6B, 6C, 6E, 6F
494 Bronchiectasis . . . 6B, 6C, 6F
495 Extrinsic allergic alveolitis . . . 6F
  495.7 Ventilation pneumonitis . . . 6F
496 Chronic airway obstruction, not elsewhere classified . . . 6B, 6C, 6F

500

500 Coal workers' pneumoconiosis . . . 6C
501 Asbestosis . . . 6C
502 Pneumoconiosis due to other silica or silicates . . . 6C
503 Pneumoconiosis due to other inorganic dust . . . 6C
504 Pneumonopathy due to inhalation of other dust . . . 6C
505 Pneumoconiosis, unspecified . . . 6C, 6E
507 Pneumonitis due to solids and liquids . . . 6C, 6F
  507.0 Due to inhalation of food or vomitus . . . 6C, 6F
508 Respiratory conditions due to other and unspecified external agents . . . 6B, 6C, 6G
  508.9 Respiratory conditions due to unspecified external agent . . . 6B, 6C, 6G
510 Empyema . . . 6C
511 Pleurisy . . . 6C, 6F
  511.8 Other specified forms of effusion, except tuberculous . . . 6F
512 Pneumothorax . . . 6F
  512.8 Other spontaneous pneumothorax . . . 6F
513 Abscess of lung and mediastinum . . . 6B, 6C, 6F
  513.0 Abscess of lung . . . 6B, 6C
514 Pulmonary congestion and hypostasis . . . 6B, 6C, 6F, 6G
515 Postinflammatory pulmonary fibrosis . . . 6C, 6E
516 Other alveolar and parietoalveolar pneumonopathy . . . 6B, 6C, 6F, 6G
  516.9 Unspecified alveolar and parietoalveolar pneumonopathy . . . 6b, 6C, 6F, 6G
517 Lung involvement in conditions classified elsewhere . . . 6B, 6F
  517.8 Lung involvement in other diseases classified elsewhere . . . 6B
518 Other diseases of lung . . . 6B, 6C, 6E, 6F, 6G
  518.0 Pulmonary collapse . . . 6B, 6C, 6F, 6G
  518.5 Pulmonary insufficiency following trauma and surgery . . . 6F
  518.8 Other diseases of lung . . . 6B, 6C, 6F, 6G
    518.81 Acute respiratory failure . . . 6F
    518.82 Other pulmonary insufficiency, not elsewhere classified . . . 6F
    518.89 Other diseases of lung, not elsewhere classified . . . 6C, 6G
519 Other diseases of respiratory system . . . 6B, 6E, 6F
  519.4 Disorders of diaphragm . . . 6B, 6E, 6F
524 Dentofacial anomalies, including malocclusion . . . 4B, 4D, 4E, 4H
  524.6 Temporomandibular joint disorders . . . 4B, 4D, 4E, 4H
553 Other hernia of abdominal cavity without mention of obstruction or gangrene . . . 6G
  553.3 Diaphragmatic hernia . . . 6G
564 Functional digestive disorders, not elsewhere classified . . . 4C
  564.0 Constipation . . . 4C
568 Other disorders of peritoneum . . . 4B
  568.0 Peritoneal adhesions (postoperative) (postinfection) . . . 4B
569 Other disorders of intestine . . . 4C
  569.4 Other specified disorders of rectum and anus . . . 4C
    569.42 Anal or rectal pain . . . 4C
581 Nephrotic syndrome . . . 4C, 7A
  581.9 Nephrotic syndrome with unspecified pathological lesion in kidney . . . 7A
582 Chronic glomerulonephritis . . . 4C
583 Nephritis and nephropathy, not specified as acute or chronic . . . 4C

716 Other and unspecified arthropathies . . . 4D, 4E, 4F, 4H, 4I, 7A
- **716.5** Unspecified polyarthropathy or polyarthritis . . . 4D
- **716.6** Unspecified monoarthritis . . . 4E, 7A
- **716.8** Other specified arthropathy . . . 4H, 4I
- **716.9** Arthropathy, unspecified . . . 4D, 4E, 4F

717 Internal derangement of knee . . . 4E, 4H, 4I
- **717.7** Chondromalacia of patella . . . 4E
- **717.8** Other internal derangement of knee . . . 4I
- **717.9** Unspecified internal derangement of knee . . . 4H, 4I

718 Other derangement of joint . . . 4B, 4D, 4E, 4F, 4H, 4I
- **718.0** Articular cartilage disorder . . . 4I
- **718.2** Pathological dislocation . . . 4I
- **718.3** Recurrent dislocation of joint . . . 4F, 4I
- **718.4** Contracture of joint . . . 4I
- **718.5** Ankylosis of joint . . . 4I
- **718.8** Other joint derangement, not elsewhere classified . . . 4B, 4E
- **718.9** Unspecified derangement of joint . . . 4F, 4H, 4I

719 Other and unspecified disorders of joint . . . 4A, 4B, 4C, 4D, 4E, 4F, 4G, 4H, 4I, 7A
- **719.0** Effusion of joint . . . 4E
- **719.2** Villonodular synovitis . . . 4E
- **719.4** Pain in joint . . . 4D, 7A
- **719.5** Stiffness of joint, not elsewhere classified . . . 4A, 4B, 4G, 4H, 4I
- **719.7** Difficulty in walking . . . 4A, 4B, 4C, 4H, 4I
- **719.8** Other specified disorders of joint . . . 4A, 4D, 4F, 4G, 4H, 4I

720 Ankylosing spondylitis and other inflammatory spondylopathies . . . 4E, 4F
- **720.2** Sacroiliitis, not elsewhere classified . . . 4E

721 Spondylosis and allied disorders . . . 4F, 4I, 5H
- **721.1** Cervical spondylosis with myelopathy . . . 4F, 5H
- **721.4** Thoracic or lumbar spondylosis with myelopathy . . . 4F, 5H
- **721.9** Spondylosis of unspecified site . . . 5H
  - 721.91 With myelopathy . . . 5H

722 Intervertebral disk disorders . . . 4B, 4E, 4F, 4I, 5H
- **722.1** Displacement of thoracic or lumbar intervertebral disk without myelopathy . . . 5H
- **722.4** Degeneration of cervical intervertebral disk . 4B, 4F
- **722.5** Degeneration of thoracic or lumbar intervertebral disk . . . 4B, 4F
- **722.6** Degeneration of intervertebral disk, site unspecified . . . 4F, 4B
- **722.7** Intervertebral disk disorder with myelopathy . . . 4F, 4I, 5H
- **722.8** Postlaminectomy syndrome . . . 4F

723 Other disorders of cervical region . . . 4B, 4F, 4I
- **723.0** Spinal stenosis in cervical region . . . 4F
- **723.1** Cervicalgia . . . 4B, 4F
- **723.5** Torticollis, unspecified . . . 4B

724 Other and unspecified disorders of back . . . 4B, 4D, 4E, 4F, 4I
- **724.0** Spinal stenosis, other than cervical . . . 4E, 4F, 4I
- **724.1** Pain in thoracic spine . . . 4B
- **724.2** Lumbago . . . 4B, 4E, 4F
- **724.3** Sciatica . . . 4I, 4F
- **724.6** Disorders of sacrum . . . 4B, 4D
- **724.9** Other unspecified back disorders . . . 4B, 4D, 4F

725 Polymyalgia rheumatica . . . 4B

726 Peripheral enthesopathies and allied syndromes . . . 4D, 4E, 4I
- **726.0** Adhesive capsulitis of shoulder . . . 4D, 4E, 4I
- **726.1** Rotator cuff syndrome of shoulder and allied disorders . . . 4D, 4E, 4I
  - **726.10** Disorders of bursae and tendons in shoulder region, unspecified . . . 4E
- **726.2** Other affections of shoulder region, not elsewhere classified . . . 4D, 4E, 4I
- **726.3** Enthesopathy of elbow region . . . 4E
  - **726.31** Medial epicondylitis . . . 4E
  - **726.32** Lateral epicondylitis . . . 4E
- **726.5** Enthesopathy of hip region . . . 4E
- **726.6** Enthesopathy of knee . . . 4E
  - **726.60** Enthesopathy of knee, unspecified . . . 4E
- **726.9** Enthesopathy of unspecified site . . . 4E
- **726.9** Unspecified enthesopathy . . . 4D, 4E, 4I

727 Other disorders of synovium, tendon, and bursa . . . 4D, 4E, 4F, 4I
- **727.0** Synovitis and tenosynovitis . . . 4D, 4E, 4F, 4I
  - **727.04** Radial styloid tenosynovitis . . . 4E
- **727.1** Bunion . . . 4I
- **727.3** Other bursitis . . . 4E
- **727.4** Ganglion and cyst of synovium, tendon, and bursa . . . 4I
- **727.6** Rupture of tendon, nontraumatic . . . 4D, 4E, 4I
  - **727.61** Complete rupture of rotator cuff . . . 4E
- **727.8** Other disorders of synovium, tendon, and bursa 4D
- **727.9** Unspecified disorder of synovium, tendon, and bursa . . . 4E

728 Disorders of muscle, ligament, and fascia . . . 4A, 4B, 4C, 4D, 4E, 4F, 4G, 4I, 5B, 7A, 7E
- **728.1** Muscular calcification and ossification . . . 4G
- **728.2** Muscular wasting and disuse atrophy, not elsewhere classified . . . 4A, 4B, 4C, 4F
- **728.3** Other specific muscle disorders . . . 4A
- **728.3** Other specific muscle disorders . . . 5B
- **728.4** Laxity of ligament . . . 4D
- **728.6** Contracture of palmar fascia . . . 4D, 4I
- **728.7** Other fibromatoses . . . 4D, 4E
  - **728.71** Plantar fascial fibromatosis . . . 4E
- **728.8** Other disorders of muscle, ligament, and fascia . . . 4D, 4F, 4B, 4C
- **728.8** Other disorders of muscle, ligament, and fascia . . . 7E
  - **728.85** Spasm of muscle . . . 4B, 4C, 4F
  - **728.86** Necrotizing fasciitis . . . 7E
- **728.9** Unspecified disorder of muscle, ligament, and fascia . . . 4C, 4E, 4F, 7A

800

900

914 Superficial injury of hand(s), except finger(s) alone 7C
- 914.0 Abrasion or friction burn without mention of infection 7C
- 914.1 Abrasion or friction burn, infected 7C
- 914.2 Blister without mention of infection 7C
- 914.3 Blister, infected 7C

915 Superficial injury of finger(s) .7C
- 915.0 Abrasion or friction burn without mention of infection 7C
- 915.1 Abrasion or friction burn, infected 7C
- 915.2 Blister without mention of infection 7C
- 915.3 Blister, infected 7C

916 Superficial injury of hip, thigh, leg, and ankle 7C
- 916.0 Abrasion or friction burn without mention of infection 7C
- 916.1 Abrasion or friction burn, infected 7C
- 916.2 Blister without mention of infection 7C
- 916.3 Blister, infected 7C

917 Superficial injury of foot and toe(s) 7C
- 917.0 Abrasion or friction burn without mention of infection 7C
- 917.1 Abrasion or friction burn, infected 7C
- 917.2 Blister without mention of infection 7C
- 917.3 Blister, infected 7C

920 Contusion of face, scalp, and neck except eye(s) 7B

922 Breast 7B

922 Contusion of trunk 4F, 7B
- 922.1 Chest wall 7B
- 922.2 Abdominal wall 7B
- 922.3 Back 4F, 7B
- 922.8 Multiple sites of trunk 7B

923 Contusion of upper limb 4E, 7B
- 923.0 Shoulder and upper arm 7B
- 923.1 Elbow and forearm 7B
- 923.2 Wrist and hand(s), except finger(s) alone 7B
- 923.3 Finger 7B
- 923.8 Multiple sites of upper limb 7B

924 Contusion of lower limb and of other and unspecified sites 4E, 7B
- 924.0 Hip and thigh 7B
- 924.1 Knee and lower leg 7B
- 924.2 Ankle and foot, excluding toe(s) 7B
- 924.3 Toe 7B
- 924.4 Multiple sites of lower limb 7B

927 Crushing injury of upper limb 4E, 4J, 7E

928 Crushing injury of lower limb 4E, 4J, 7E

929 Crushing injury of multiple and unspecified sites 4J, 7E

941 Burn of face, head, and neck 4D, 6C, 6E, 7D, 7E
- 941.0 Unspecified degree 4D
- 941.1 Erythema [first degree] 4D
- 941.2 Blisters, epidermal loss [second degree] 4D
- 941.3 Full-thickness skin loss [third degree, not otherwise specified] 4D, 7D
- 941.4 Deep necrosis of underlying tissues [deep third degree] without mention of loss of a body part .4D, 7E
- 941.5 Deep necrosis of underlying tissues [deep third degree] with loss of a body part 4D, 7E

942 Burn of trunk 4D, 6C, 6E, 7B, 7C, 7D, 7E
- 942.0 Unspecified degree 4D
- 942.1 Erythema [first degree] 4D, 7B
- 942.2 Blisters, epidermal loss [second degree] . . .4D, 7C
- 942.3 Full-thickness skin loss [third degree, not otherwise specified] 4D, 7D
- 942.4 Deep necrosis of underlying tissues [deep third degree] without mention of loss of a body part 4D, 7E
- 942.5 Deep necrosis of underlying tissues [deep third degree] with loss of a body part 4D, 7E

943 Burn of upper limb, except wrist and hand4D, 7B, 7C, 7D, 7E
- 943.0 Unspecified degree 4D
- 943.1 Erythema [first degree] 4D, 7B
- 943.2 Blisters, epidermal loss [second degree] . . .4D, 7C
- 943.3 Full-thickness skin loss [third degree, not otherwise specified] 4D, 7D
- 943.4 Deep necrosis of underlying tissues [deep third degree] without mention of loss of a body part 4D, 7E
- 943.5 Deep necrosis of underlying tissues [deep third degree] with loss of a body part 4D, 7E

944 Burn of wrist(s) and hand(s) 4D, 7B, 7C, 7D, 7E
- 944.0 Unspecified degree 4D
- 944.1 Erythema [first degree] 4D, 7B
- 944.2 Blisters, epidermal loss [second degree] . . .4D, 7C
- 944.3 Full-thickness skin loss [third degree, not otherwise specified] 4D, 7D
- 944.4 Deep necrosis of underlying tissues [deep third degree] without mention of loss of a body part 4D, 7E
- 944.5 Deep necrosis of underlying tissues [deep third degree] with loss of a body part 4D, 7E

945 Burn of lower limb(s) 4D, 7B, 7C, 7D
- 945.0 Unspecified degree 4D
- 945.1 Erythema [first degree] 4D, 7B
- 945.2 Blisters, epidermal loss [second degree] . . .4D, 7C
- 945.3 Full-thickness skin loss [third degree, not otherwise specified] 4D, 7D

946 Burns of multiple specified sites 4D, 6E, 7B, 7C, 7D, 7E
- 946.0 Unspecified degree 4D
- 946.1 Erythema [first degree] 4D, 7B
- 946.2 Blisters, epidermal loss [second degree] . . .4D, 7C
- 946.3 Full-thickness skin loss [third degree, not otherwise specified] 4D, 7D
- 946.4 Deep necrosis of underlying tissues [deep third degree] without mention of loss of a body part .7E
- 946.5 Deep necrosis of underlying tissues [deep third degree] with loss of a body part 4D, 7E

947 Burn of internal organs 6C, 6E
- 947.0 Mouth and pharynx 4D
- 947.1 Larynx, trachea, and lung 4D, 6C
- 947.2 Esophagus 4D
- 947.3 Gastrointestinal tract .4D
- 947.4 Vagina and uterus 4D
- 947.8 Other unspecified parts 4D
- 947.9 Unspecified site 4D, 6C

948 Burns classified according to extent of body surface involved 4D, 6E, 7B, 7C, 7D, 7E

949 Burn, unspecified 4D, 6E, 7B, 7C, 7D

Supplemental Classification of Factors Influencing Health Status and Contact With Health Services

Alphabetical Index to ICD-9-CM Codes

A

B

C

D

E

F

G

H

I

J

K

L

M

N

O

P

Q

R

S

T

U

V

W

Notes:

Notes:

Notes:

Notes:

Notes: